Review of Medical Dosimetry

William Amestoy

Review of Medical Dosimetry

A Study Guide

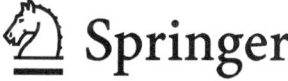

William Amestoy
University of Miami Sylvester Cancer Center
Miami
Florida
USA

ISBN 978-3-319-13625-7   ISBN 978-3-319-13626-4 (eBook)
DOI 10.1007/978-3-319-13626-4
Springer Cham Heidelberg New York Dordrecht London

Library of Congress Control Number: 2015933636

© Springer International Publishing Switzerland 2015
This work is subject to copyright. All rights are reserved by the Publisher, whether the whole or part of the material is concerned, specifically the rights of translation, reprinting, reuse of illustrations, recitation, broadcasting, reproduction on microfilms or in any other physical way, and transmission or information storage and retrieval, electronic adaptation, computer software, or by similar or dissimilar methodology now known or hereafter developed. Exempted from this legal reservation are brief excerpts in connection with reviews or scholarly analysis or material supplied specifically for the purpose of being entered and executed on a computer system, for exclusive use by the purchaser of the work. Duplication of this publication or parts thereof is permitted only under the provisions of the Copyright Law of the Publisher's location, in its current version, and permission for use must always be obtained from Springer. Permissions for use may be obtained through RightsLink at the Copyright Clearance Center. Violations are liable to prosecution under the respective Copyright Law.
The use of general descriptive names, registered names, trademarks, service marks, etc. in this publication does not imply, even in the absence of a specific statement, that such names are exempt from the relevant protective laws and regulations and therefore free for general use.
While the advice and information in this book are believed to be true and accurate at the date of publication, neither the authors nor the editors nor the publisher can accept any legal responsibility for any errors or omissions that may be made. The publisher makes no warranty, express or implied, with respect to the material contained herein.

Printed on acid-free paper

Springer is part of Springer Science+Business Media (www.springer.com)

With Love to:
My wife, Vivian Amestoy,
And our twin,
Brandon Amestoy and Brianna Amestoy
(3 years old)

Preface

The field of radiation oncology has significantly changed in recent decades, mainly due to the implementation of new medical instruments, and hence the corresponding new treatment strategies. The field of radiotherapy has been a technology-driven field and in recent years this trend has continued with the use of VMAT, protons and different imaging and motion tracking devices. The field of medical physics ensures that all of these new technologies are implemented safely and used to their fullest potential to deliver the most accurate and effective treatments to patients. As medical physics has evolved, so has medical dosimetry. From the very primitive treatment planning, which was based on x-ray films and hand-calculations, medical dosimetry has transformed to include modern treatment planning based on tomographic images (CT, MRI and PET) and computer optimizations.

To make sure that the individuals who practice in radiation oncology have the appropriate knowledge and skills to safely and effectively treat patients, groups like the American Board of Radiology (ABR) and the American Association of Medical Dosimetrists (AAMD) have developed tests to ensure this level of competence. To prepare for these tests a huge amount of preparation is required and it can be difficult to know where to begin when preparing to take one of these exams. With this in mind, this study guide was written mainly for candidates who will take Medical Dosimetrist Certification Board (MDCB) exam but is also beneficial to medical physicists who will take the ABR written exams (part I and part II) and for radiation oncology residents who must pass a physics exam as well.

The knowledge and skills for medical dosimetrists, medical physicists and radiation oncologists is very similar in terms of the required physics knowledge, except that medical physicists have much more in-depth and extensive training. Considering this difference, the questions are catalogued into three levels: 1, 2 and 3. Questions at level 1 are very essential, questions at level 2 are clinical related and slightly more in depth and questions at level 3 are advanced questions, mainly for ABR candidates. However, MDCB candidates and radiation oncology residents are encouraged to challenge those topics for advanced studies. Each quiz is labeled to which level it belongs.

This study guide was not written to be the only document that is going to be studied before the exam, it was developed to guide the candidate to see what type of material is important to understand and also to test how much knowledge the candidate currently possesses. There are a plethora of resources available that delve deeply into all of these topics, and that is one of the difficulties in studying for these board examinations as it is hard to figure out what topics are important. To effectively accomplish this goal, not only were questions written, but explanations of the answer to each question were included to clarify some of the important *concepts* that are critical to passing the examinations. Again, the goal of this study guide is not to repeat what can be found in a textbook, but to provide a framework that the candidate can use. When a topic is reached where the candidate feels that needs further explanation, other resources can be used. The final section of the book includes three practice tests with the same amount of questions given by the MDCB to work on the applicant speed as well as score. Each examination contains 155 multiple choice questions and the time allowed for completion is 3 h and 50 min.

Remember, this study guide is not intended to replace textbooks or duplicate a specific test, and the questions and answers have been prepared by the author and chief editor. This guide provides a solid framework to address important concepts covered in radiation oncology physics board exams.

Acknowledgements

I dedicate this book to my family; my wife Vivian and our twins Brandon and Brianna (3 years old). My adorable twins helped me by sitting next to me and drawing while daddy was working.

I am grateful to my chief editor, Dr. Matthew Studenski, the other reviewers, contributors, test examiners and institutions who contributed to this guide. I also want to thank Dr. Kelin Wang, Maria Irene Monterroso, Karen Brown and Alex Iglesias who helped me prepare and organize the chapters and put a lot of effort in reviewing this book. They all worked as hard as I did to make this workbook possible for you. Thanks are also due to our families, who endured our hard work in the planning of this workbook and some of the faculty and residents at University of Miami and Innovative Cancer Center who provided great encouragement towards the completion of this project. I am very appreciative to everyone who helped me in this journey and hope it becomes a great tool for all of you.

As per MDCB history, the current pass rate is around 57 % (past 5 years). Let's bring that pass rate up.

William Amestoy, RTT (R) (T), CMD

Contents

1 Radiation Physics 1
   1.1   Atomic and Nuclear Structure (Questions) 1
   1.2   Radioactivity (Questions) 10
   1.3   Production of X-Ray (Questions) 18
   1.4   Interaction of Radiation with Matter (Questions) 26
   1.5   Treatment Machine Characteristics (Questions) 35
   1.6   Radiation Units (Questions) 48
   1.7   Atomic and Nuclear Structure (Answers) 60
   1.8   Radioactivity (Answers) 68
   1.9   Production of X-Ray (Answers) 76
   1.10 Interaction of Radiation with Matter (Answer) 84
   1.11 Treatment Machine Characteristics (Answers) 89
   1.12 Radiation Units (Answers) 100

2 Dose Calculation Methods 109
   2.1   Dose Calculation (Questions) 110
   2.2   Applied Mathematics (Questions) 133
   2.3   External Beam Calculations (Questions) 144
   2.4   Effects of Beam-Modifying Devices (Questions) 145
   2.5   Irregular Field Calculations (Questions) 148
   2.6   Special Calculations (Questions) 155
   2.7   Manual Corrections for Tissue Inhomogeneities (Questions) .. 162
   2.8   Dose Calculation (Answers) 164
   2.9   Applied Mathematics (Answers) 180
   2.10 External Beam Calculations (Answers) 199
   2.11 Effects of Beam-Modifying Devices (Answers) 200
   2.12 Irregular Field Calculations (Answers) 204
   2.13 Special Calculations (Answers) 212
   2.14 Manual Corrections for Tissue Inhomogeneity (Answers) 219

3 Treatment Planning and Treatment Planning System (TPS) 221
   3.1   Isodose Curve Parameters and Isodose
         Distributions (Questions) 222
   3.2   Electron Beam Dose Distributions (Questions) 236

3.3	IMRT and VMAT (Questions)	246
3.4	Special Procedures and SRS (Questions)	251
3.5	Nuclear Medicine Therapy (Questions)	266
3.6	Isodose Curve Parameters and Isodose Distributions (Answers)	268
3.7	Electron Beam Dose Distributions (Answers)	281
3.8	IMRT and VMAT (Answers)	288
3.9	Special Procedures and SRS (Answers)	291
3.10	Nuclear Medicine Therapy (Answers)	301

4 Patient Immobilization ... 305

4.1	Patient Positioning and Treatment Devices (Questions)	306
4.2	Image-Guided Radiotherapy (Questions)	308
4.3	Margins Accounting for Positioning (Questions)	312
4.4	Patient Positioning and Treatment Devices (Answers)	314
4.5	Image-Guided Radiotherapy (Answers)	316
4.6	Margins Accounted for Positioning (Answers)	318

5 Brachytherapy ... 321

5.1	General Concepts on Brachytherapy (Questions)	322
5.2	Radioactive Source Characteristics (Questions)	326
5.3	Implant Methods (Questions)	335
5.4	Temporary Implant Procedures (Questions)	340
5.5	Permanent Implant Procedures (Questions)	348
5.6	Dose Delivery (Questions)	351
5.7	Brachytherapy Dose Calculations (Questions)	354
5.8	ICRU and AAPM TG Reports on Brachytherapy (Questions)	364
5.9	General Concepts on Brachytherapy (Answers)	368
5.10	Radioactive Source Characteristics (Answers)	370
5.11	Implant Methods (Answers)	377
5.12	Temporary Implant Procedures (Answers)	380
5.13	Permanent Implant Procedures (Answers)	384
5.14	Dose Delivery (Answers)	386
5.15	Brachytherapy Dose Calculations (Answers)	388
5.16	ICRU and AAPM TG Reports on Brachytherapy (Answers)	403

6 Radiobiology ... 407

6.1	Cellular Biology (Questions)	408
6.2	Cell Death Due to Irradiation (Questions)	410
6.3	Normal Tissue Complication (NTC) (Questions)	412
6.4	Cell Survival Curves and Models (Questions)	422
6.5	BED and Fractionations (Questions)	425
6.6	Oxygen Enhancement and Hyperthermia Treatments (Questions)	427
6.7	Summary (Questions)	430
6.8	Cellular Biology (Answers)	432

6.9	Cell Death Due to Irradiations (Answers)	433
6.10	Normal Tissue Complication (NTC) (Answers)	435
6.11	Cell Survival Curves and Models (Answers)	442
6.12	BED and Fractionations (Answers)	444
6.13	Oxygen Enhancement and Hyperthermia Treatments (Answers)	446
6.14	Summary (Answers)	447

7 Radiation Safety ... 449

7.1	Maximum Permissible Dose Equivalent (Questions)	450
7.2	Time, Distance, and Shielding (Questions)	457
7.3	Brachytherapy Source Handling and Storage (Questions)	459
7.4	Dose Survey and Exposure Monitoring (Questions)	469
7.5	Nuclear Medicine Procedures (Questions)	474
7.6	Structural Shielding Design (Questions)	476
7.7	Radioactive Material Shipping (Questions)	481
7.8	Summary (Questions)	483
7.9	Maximum Permissible Dose Equivalent (Answers)	488
7.10	Time, Distance, and Shielding (Answers)	493
7.11	Brachytherapy Source Handling and Storage (Answers)	494
7.12	Dose Survey and Exposure Monitoring (Answers)	500
7.13	Nuclear Medicine Procedures (Answers)	504
7.14	Structural Shielding Design (Answers)	506
7.15	Radioactive Material Shipping (Answers)	509
7.16	Summary (Answers)	510

8 Quality Assurance ... 513

8.1	QA Guidance and Protocols (Questions)	513
8.2	Requirements and Tolerance for QA Procedures (Questions)	516
8.3	QA for Treatment Planning System (Questions)	525
8.4	Equipment or Devices for Measurement (Questions)	527
8.5	QA Procedures (Questions)	532
8.6	QA Guidance and Protocols (Answers)	534
8.7	Requirements and Tolerance for QA Procedures (Answers)	535
8.8	QA for Treatment Planning System (Answers)	541
8.9	Equipment or Devices for Measurement (Answers)	542
8.10	QA Procedures (Answers)	545

9 Fundamentals of Computer Technologies ... 549

9.1	Basic Computer Terminology (Questions)	549
9.2	Internet and Telecommunication (Questions)	553
9.3	Medical Images (Questions)	554
9.4	Basic Computer Terminology (Answers)	556
9.5	Internet and Telecommunication (Answers)	558
9.6	Medical Images (Answers)	559

10	**Professional Responsibilities**..	561
	10.1 Working as Professionals at Health System (Questions).......	561
	10.2 Professional Medical Dosimetrists (Questions)..............	570
	10.3 Working as Professionals at Health System (Answers)........	574
	10.4 Professional Medical Dosimetrists (Answers)...............	581
11	**Radiation Oncology**..	585
	11.1 The Brain (Questions)..	585
	11.2 The Head and Neck Region (Questions)......................	591
	11.3 The Thorax (Questions).......................................	607
	11.4 The Abdomen (Questions).....................................	619
	11.5 The Pelvis (Questions)..	622
	11.6 The Spinal Canal (Questions).................................	631
	11.7 Children (Questions)..	633
	11.8 Benign Diseases (Questions)..................................	642
	11.9 The Skin (Questions)..	643
	11.10 Soft Tissue Sarcomas (Questions)............................	645
	11.11 Extras (Questions)..	646
	11.12 The Brain (Answers)..	647
	11.13 The Head and Neck Region (Answers)........................	650
	11.14 The Thorax (Answers)...	658
	11.15 The Abdomen (Answers).......................................	666
	11.16 The Pelvis (Answers)..	668
	11.17 The Spinal Canal (Answers)...................................	672
	11.18 Children (Answers)..	673
	11.19 Benign Diseases (Answers)....................................	678
	11.20 The Skin (Answers)..	679
	11.21 Soft Tissue Sarcomas (Answers)..............................	680
	11.22 Extras (Answers)..	681
12	**Anatomy**..	683
	12.1 Brain (Questions)...	683
	12.2 Head and Neck (Questions)..................................	685
	12.3 Thorax (Questions)...	687
	12.4 Abdomen (Questions)..	690
	12.5 Pelvis (Questions)...	693
	12.6 Brain (Answers)...	697
	12.7 Head and Neck (Answers).....................................	700
	12.8 Thorax (Answers)...	704
	12.9 Abdomen (Answers)..	709
	12.10 Pelvis (Answers)...	715
13	**Imaging Modalities**...	723
	13.1 Imaging Modalities (Questions)...............................	723
	13.2 Ultrasound (Questions).......................................	733
	13.3 Nuclear Medicine (Questions).................................	737

	13.4	Positron Emission Tomography (PET) (Questions)	739
	13.5	Imaging Modalities (Answers)	742
	13.6	Ultrasound (Answers)	749
	13.7	Nuclear Medicine (Answers)	752
	13.8	Positron Emission Tomography (PET) (Answers)	754

14 Practice Test 757
    14.1 Practice Test I: Questions 757
    14.2 Practice Test II: Questions 785
    14.3 Practice Test III: Questions 813
    14.4 Practice Test IA: Answers 842
    14.5 Practice Test IIA: Answers 850
    14.6 Practice Test IIIA: Answers 858

References 867

Contributors

Matthew Studenski, PhD, DABR Assistant Professor of Medical Physics, University of Miami Sylvester Cancer Center; Department of Radiation Oncology Physics

Reviewers:
Kelin Wang, PhD, DABR Assistant Professor of Medical Physics, University of Miami Sylvester Cancer Center; Department of Radiation Oncology Physics

Maria Irene Monterroso, MS, DABR University of Miami Sylvester Cancer Center; Department of Radiation Oncology Physics

Karen Brown, B.A. ARRT, R.T. (T) University of Miami Sylvester Cancer Center; Department of Radiation Oncology

Contributors:
Joseph Both, PhD, DABR Assistant Professor of Medical Physics, University of Miami Sylvester Cancer Center; Department of Radiation Oncology Physics

Kyle Padgett, PhD, DABR Assistant Professor of Medical Physics, University of Miami Sylvester Cancer Center; Department of Radiation Oncology Physics

Alejandro Iglesias, CMD Chief Dosimetrist and Director of Innovative Cancer Center

Test examiners:
Bret Adams, MD PhD Radiation Oncology Resident, University of Miami Sylvester Cancer Center

Hao Sha, PhD Student of Medical Physics, University of Miami

Pablo Pereira ARRT, R.T. (T) Medical dosimetrist, Innovative Cancer Center

Institutions:
University of Miami, Sylvester Cancer Center
Innovative Cancer Center

180.1

Radiation Physics

Contents

1.1	Atomic and Nuclear Structure (Questions)	1
1.2	Radioactivity (Questions)	10
1.3	Production of X-Ray (Questions)	18
1.4	Interaction of Radiation with Matter (Questions)	26
1.5	Treatment Machine Characteristics (Questions)	35
1.6	Radiation Units (Questions)	48
1.7	Atomic and Nuclear Structure (Answers)	60
1.8	Radioactivity (Answers)	68
1.9	Production of X-Ray (Answers)	76
1.10	Interaction of Radiation with Matter (Answer)	84
1.11	Treatment Machine Characteristics (Answers)	89
1.12	Radiation Units (Answers)	100

1.1 Atomic and Nuclear Structure (Questions)

Quiz-1 (Level 1)

1. One atomic mass unit is equal to:
   A. 1.66×10^{-27} kg
   B. 1.862 MeV
   C. 1.602×10^{-19} J
   D. 0.511 MeV/c²

2. What is the conversion factor from amu to MeV/c2?
   A. 939
   B. 0.511
   C. 938
   D. 931

© Springer International Publishing Switzerland 2015
W. Amestoy, *Review of Medical Dosimetry: A Study Guide*,
DOI 10.1007/978-3-319-13626-4_1

3. What is the number of charge of a proton?
A. +1
B. −1
C. 0
D. 0.511

4. The nucleus of an atom is composed of
A. I, II, and III only
B. I and III only
C. II and III only
D. IV only
E. All are correct
I. Electrons
II. Protons
III. Neutrons
IV. Positron

5. What is the force that binds electrons to the atom?
A. Strong force
B. Electromagnetic force
C. Gravitational force
D. Weak force

6. The energy needed to remove an electron from the shell is called:
A. The balance electrons
B. The binding energy
C. Transitions
D. Energy levels

7. Electron binding energy increases:
A. I, II, and III only
B. I and III only
C. II and III and IV only
D. IV only
E. All are correct
I. As the electron orbits get farther from the nucleus
II. In the K shell compared with N shell
III. And is proportional to Z2
IV. With increasing charge of the nucleus

8. The chemical properties of an atom are determined by:
A. Valence electrons
B. Shielding electrons
C. Effective nuclear charge
D. Nuclear diameter

1.1 Atomic and Nuclear Structure (Questions)

9. The maximum number of electrons that can occupy a specific energy level is determined using the formula:
A. E^{kl}photon $= E_k - E_l$
B. $E = mc^2$
C. $2n^2$
D. $T_{1/2} = \text{Ln}2/\lambda$

10. What is the maximum number of electrons that can hold in L shell?
A. 12
B. 2
C. 18
D. 8

11. The atoms are designated by atomic symbols; the symbol "A" represents:
A. I, II, and III only
B. I and III only
C. III and IV only
D. IV only
E. All are correct
I. Atomic number
II. Number of electrons
III. Mass number
IV. Number of protons and neutrons

12. In a neutral atom, the number of electrons is equals to:
A. Atomic number
B. Number of photons
C. Symbol "A"
D. Number of nucleons

13. The number of neutrons in an atom is equal to:
A. A only
B. $A + Z$
C. Z only
D. $A - Z$

14. In chronological order, identify the number of electron, number of protons, number of neutrons, its mass number, atomic number, and number of nucleons in the following element [gold ($^{197}_{79}$Au)]:
A. 79, 79, 118, 197, 79, and 197
B. 118, 79, 197, 118, 79, and 197
C. 79, 79, 197, 118, 79, and 118
D. 197, 79, 118, 197, 79, and 118

15. The rest mass of an electron (MeV/c²) is equal to:
A. 938
B. 0.511
C. 939
D. No rest mass

16. A transition is said to have taken placed on an atom when:
A. An electron is removed from an atom
B. All electrons are in the lowest allowable energy levels
C. An electron moves from its original shell to another
D. Electrons are attracted by the nucleus

17. What is the maximum number of electrons allowed in M shell?
A. 2
B. 18
C. 12
D. 32

18. An atom which is ionized and loses an electron is called a/an:
A. Negative ion
B. Electrically neutral
C. Positive ion
D. Characteristic radiation

19. Atoms who have nuclei with the same number of protons but different number of neutrons are called:
A. Isomers
B. Isobars
C. Isotones
D. Isotopes

20. Which of the following is an isotone?
A. $^{131m}_{54}Xe - ^{131}_{54}Xe$
B. $^{76}_{32}Ce - ^{76}_{34}Se$
C. $^{12}_{6}C, ^{14}_{6}C$
D. $^{37}_{17}C, ^{39}_{19}P$

Quiz-2 (Level 2)

1. What is the maximum number of electrons the 2p subshell can hold?
A. 2
B. 6
C. 8
D. 18

1.1 Atomic and Nuclear Structure (Questions)

2–9. Match the following elements with its corresponding classification (answers may be used more than once):
A. Isotopes
B. Isotones
C. Isobars
D. Isomers
2. Same number of protons, but different number of neutrons
3. Same number of neutrons, but different number of protons
4. Same number of nucleons, but different number of protons
5. Same number of protons and neutrons, but different nuclear energy state
6. Same Z number, but different A number
7. Different A number, different Z number, but same number of neutrons
8. Same A number, but different Z number
9. Same A and Z, but different nuclear energy state

10. A breakup of an unstable nucleus into two more stable nuclei of comparable mass with the release of large amount of energy in the form of heat and radiation is called:
A. Fusion
B. Fission
C. Internal conversion
D. Gamma emission

11. The relationship between wavelength, frequency, and velocity for photons is given by the formula:
A. $E = h\nu$
B. $E = hc/\lambda$
C. $c = \nu \lambda$
D. $A = -\lambda N$

12. The most stable atoms are:
A. Atoms with even number of protons, odd number of neutrons
B. Atoms with odd number of protons, even number of neutrons
C. Atoms with even number of protons, even number of neutrons
D. Atoms with odd number of protons, odd number of neutrons

13. Avogadro's number (N_A) refers to:
A. The ratio of the number of constituent particles in a sample to the amount of substance
B. The smaller quantity of an element
C. The amount of energy required to remove an electron from an atom
D. The number of electrons per unit cubic distance

14. The accepted value of Avogadro's number (N_A) is:
A. 3×10^8
B. 1.602×10^{-19}
C. 1.66×10^{-27}
D. 6.0228×10^{23}

15. Avogadro's number (N_A) can be used to calculate:
A. I, II, and III only
B. I and III only
C. III and IV only
D. IV only
E. All are correct
I. Number of atoms per gram
II. Number of grams per atom
III. Number of electrons per gram
IV. Amount of energy

16. Calculate the number of atoms/g of Cobalt if its atomic weight (A_w) is 58.93 g/mol:
A. 3.549×10^{25}
B. 1.0220×10^{22}
C. 1.220×10^{23}
D. 9.7845×10^{23}

17. Which of the following formulas is used to calculate grams/atom of a material?
A. N_A / A_w
B. $N_A \times A_w$
C. A_w / N_A
D. $N_A \times Z / A_w$

18. According to the atomic mass unit, the mass of a neutron is:
A. No mass
B. 1.00727 amu
C. 0.000548 amu
D. 1.00866 amu

19. The mass defect is defined as:
A. A defect in the number of protons in the nucleus
B. Every gram atomic weight of a substance contains the same number of atoms
C. The different in mass between an atom and the sum of the masses of its constituent particles
D. The propagation of energy through space or a material medium

1.1 Atomic and Nuclear Structure (Questions)   7

20. Which of the following is/are properties of an electron?
A. I, II, and III only
B. I and III only
C. III and IV only
D. IV only
E. All are correct
I. It can undergo collision interactions.
II. It is a fundamental particle.
III. It possesses mass, charge, and spin.
IV. It has a magnetic field.

21. The smallest component of an element having the chemical properties of the element is:
A. Element
B. Atom
C. Nucleus
D. Quarks

22. The structure or model of an atom was discovered by:
A. Wilhelm Roentgen
B. Niels Bohr
C. Henri Becquerel
D. Pierre Curie

23. Which of the following is/are characteristics of ions?
A. I, II, and III only
B. I and III only
C. III and IV only
D. IV only
E. All are correct
I. They are charged atoms.
II. The number of electrons is different than the number of protons.
III. Ions are named cation if the number of electrons is less than the number of protons.
IV. Ions are named anion if the number of electrons exceeds the number of protons.

24. Which of the following bond occurs between two nonmetallic atoms?
A. Ionic bond
B. Van der Waals bond
C. Covalent bond
D. Metallic bond

25. Which of the following is true about ^{137}Cs and ^{137m}Ba?
A. I, II, and III only
B. I and III only
C. III and IV only
D. II only
E. All are correct
I. They belong to the same element.
II. They possess the same mass number.
III. They are considered isotopes.
IV. They possess the same atomic number.

Quiz-3 (Level 3)

1. Suppose the rest mass of electron is m_0 and the speed is $v=0.6c$; its kinetic energy is:
A. $m_0v^2/2$
B. Smaller than $m_0v^2/2$
C. Larger than $m_0v^2/2$
D. 0.511 MeV/c^2

2. A meson is composed of
A. A quark and an antiquark of the same flavor
B. A quark and an antiquark of different flavor
C. 2 quarks or 2 antiquarks of different flavor
D. 2 quarks or 2 antiquarks of same flavor

3. Neutrinos or antineutrinos are generated in standard beta decays. The energy spectrum of beta particles is consecutive, suggesting neutrinos or antineutrinos may carry rather large energy. However, in dosimetry there is never a dose calculation related to neutrinos; the reason is
A. It is too hard to calculate because neutrinos have different energy
B. The dose related to neutrinos is negligible thus it is never counted
C. Neutrinos never interact with tissue by Compton scattering or any other interactions
D. Actually we should calculate the dose, but unfortunately little research has been done

4. A radiation oncology clinic plans to use a muon beam ($v=0.999c$) pipe from a high-energy (GeV) synchrotron located 1 km away. The lifetime for muons is about 2 μs. This plan sounds impossible, right?
A. Right. At the speed of light, it takes muons about 3 μs to travel through the 1 km pipe so all muons will decay to electrons and antineutrino before treatment. Therefore, this plan is impossible

1.1 Atomic and Nuclear Structure (Questions)

B. Still possible. Because after 3 μs, which is 1.5 lifetime, only some muons decay. This can be calculated by simple math. The plan is still possible since the remaining muons can be used.

C. Right. A muon decays into an electron and an antineutrino with random directions; thus, the beam quality is too bad to be used, even though some muons remain from decay.

D. The lifetime for muons at 0.999c is much longer than 2 μs, so there is no decay and nothing to be worried about. The plan is possible.

5. Does a neutron have an antiparticle?
A. The term antiparticle means identical mass but opposite charge, like an electron and a positron. A neutron has no charge; thus a neutron does not have an antiparticle.
B. Yes, a neutron has an antiparticle, which is an antineutron, a different particle from a neutron.
C. Yes, however, a neutron's antiparticle is exactly itself.
D. A neutron is not an elementary particle; thus, the concept of an antiparticle does not apply to a neutron.

6. How many kind(s) of neutrino(s) exist in nature?
A. 6
B. 3
C. 1
D. 2

7. Electric force and magnetic force are actually the same type of interaction, so-called electromagnetic interaction. Which physicist unified those two interactions?
A. Einstein, with the theory of special relativity
B. Maxwell, with Maxwell equation group
C. Hertz, with the discovery of electromagnetic wave
D. Faraday, with his discovery of electromagnetic induction

8. There are four types of fields discovered in nature. Physicists tried to unify them by symmetry.
A. I and II
B. I, II, and III
C. II only
D. II and III
I. Photons change energies by blue shift or red shift when they travel in gravitational field; thus gravity is unified to electromagnetic field.
II. The weak field and the electromagnetic field are the same under electroweak interaction theory.
III. The Grand Unified Theory actually cannot unify gravitational field.

9. The fuel in a nuclear plant and the material to make a atomic bomb are similar; thus,
A. They can be mutually exchanged.
B. Fuel in a nuclear plant can be used to produce an atomic bomb, but not vice versa.
C. Material to make an atomic bomb can be used in a nuclear plant, but not vice versa.
D. They cannot be exchanged because of the different abundance of atoms to produce fission.

10. Electromagnetic interaction occurs by exchanging photons; nucleons interact to each other by exchanging:
A. Quarks
B. Mesons
C. Colors
D. W± or neutral vector bosons

11. In the standard model, a quark may have the following interactions:
A. Strong, electromagnetic, and weak
B. Strong and electromagnetic
C. Strong and weak
D. Strong only

1.2 Radioactivity (Questions)

Quiz-1 (Level 1)

1. Radioactivity was first discovered by
A. Wilhelm Roentgen
B. Marie Curie
C. Henri Becquerel
D. Pierre Curie

2. Radioactivity is defined as
A. An emission of radiation from unstable nuclei of element in the form of particles, electromagnetic radiation, or both
B. Radiation in which a particle carries energy is capable of removing electrons from an atom, thus producing free radicals
C. The rate of energy loss per unit path length
D. The rate of decay of a radioactive material

3. Which of the following is true?
A. I, II, and III only
B. II and IV only

1.2 Radioactivity (Questions)

C. I and II only
D. All are true
I. The activity per unit mass of a radionuclide is termed the half-life.
II. The number of atoms disintegrating per unit time is proportional to the number of radioactive atoms.
III. The time required for either the activity or the number of radioactive atoms to decay to half the initial value is termed specific activity.
IV. The average life or the mean life is the average lifetime for the decay of radioactive atoms.

4-13. Match the formula with its corresponding name (answer may be more than one).
A. Decay constant
B. Activity
C. Half-life
D. Mean life
E. Number of atoms with time
F. Specific activity
G. Number of atoms per gram
4. $\tau = 1.44\, T_{1/2}$
5. $N = N_0 e^{-\lambda t}$
6. $A = -\lambda N$
7. $T_{1/2} = 0.693/\lambda$
8. $\tau = 1/\lambda$
9. $T_{1/2} = \ln 2/\lambda$
10. $A = A_0 e^{-\lambda t}/A_n = A_0 \exp(-0.693 \times t/T_{1/2})$
11. $SA = \lambda\, (N_A/A_W)$
12. Number of atoms/g $= N_A/A_W$
13. $\lambda = 0.693/T_{1/2}$

14. Transient equilibrium is achieved when:
A. Half-life of daughter is much longer than half-life of parent
B. Half-life of parent is much longer than half-life of daughter
C. The parent and daughter decay at their own respective half-lives
D. Half-life of parent is not much longer than half-life of daughter

Quiz-2 (Level 2)

1. Match the following graphs with its radioactive equilibrium types:
A. Secular equilibrium
B. Transient equilibrium
C. No equilibrium

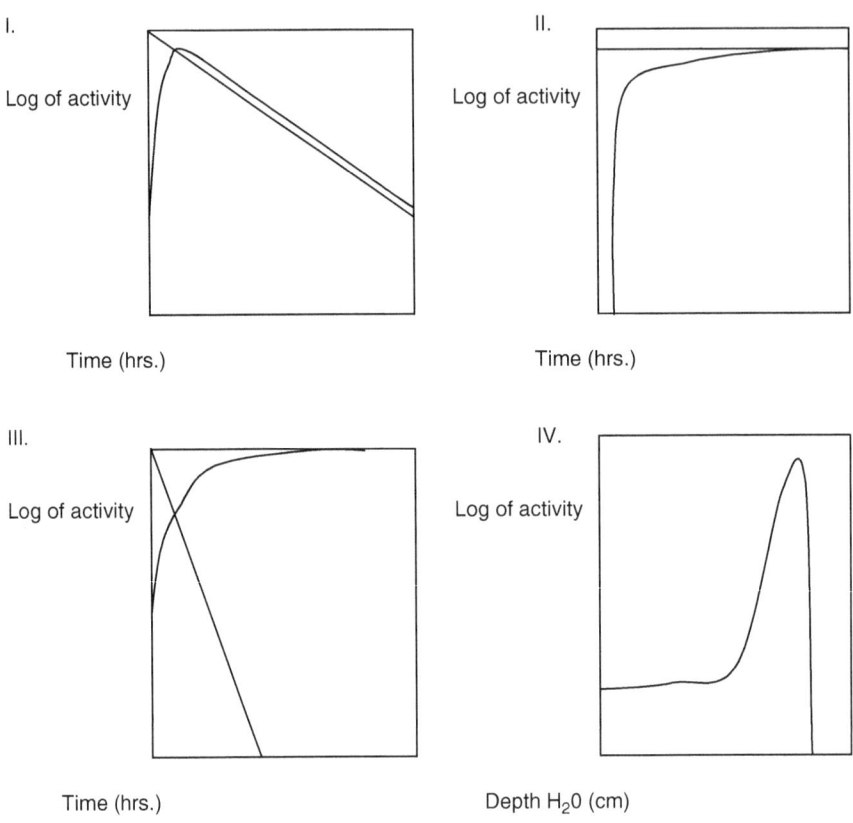

Fig. 1.2.1

2. Which of the following are modes of radioactive decay?
A. I only
B. II and III only
C. I, II, and III only
D. II and IV only
E. All answers are correct
I. Alpha particle decay
II. Beta particle decay
III. Electron capture
IV. Internal conversion

3. Match the following term with its corresponding symbol:
A. Alpha particle
B. Beta particle
C. Negatron
D. Positron
E. Gamma ray

1.2 Radioactivity (Questions)

I. γ
II. β⁻
III. β
IV. α
V. β⁺

4. Which of the following is a general reaction for α-particle decay process?

A. $^A_Z X \rightarrow \,^A_{Z+1}Y + \,^0_{-1}\beta + v' + Q$

B. $^A_Z X \rightarrow \,^A_{Z-1}Y + \,^0_{-1}\beta + v + Q$

C. $^A_Z X \rightarrow \,^{A-4}_{Z-2}Y + \,^4_2 He + Q$

D. $^A_Z X + \,^0_{-1}e \rightarrow \,^A_{Z-1}Y + v + Q$

5. Match the following reaction with its corresponding characteristics:

A. Internal conversion
B. Electron capture
C. Beta plus (positron) emission (β⁺)
D. Alpha particle (α)
E. Beta minus (negatron) emission (β⁻)

I. $Z \geq 82$, same nuclear structure of an $^4_2 He$, atomic number (Z) decrease by 2, atomic mass (A) decrease by 4, particle composed of two protons and two neutrons

II. Excessive number of neutrons; high neutron to proton (n/p) ratio; reduced n/p ratio by converting a neutron into a proton, negatron, and antineutrino; atomic number (Z) increases by 1, but atomic mass (A) remains the same

III. Deficit of neutrons, low neutron to proton (n/p) ratio, increase n/p ratio by converting a proton into a neutron and a positron; atomic number (Z) decreases by 1 but atomic mass (A) remains the same; consists of a continuous energy distribution

IV. Deficit of neutrons, low neutron to proton (n/p) ratio, increase n/p ratio by capturing one of the orbital electrons by the nucleus transforming a proton into a neutron; often called K capture; give rise to characteristic X-ray with emission of Auger electrons

V. Excess nuclear energy from the nucleus is passed on to one orbital electrons, which is then ejected from the atom and creates a vacancy which gives rise to characteristic X-ray with emission of Auger electrons; no change in atomic number

6. What is the decay constant of Ir-192 if its half-life is known to be 74.2 days?

I. 3.8915×10^{-5}/h
II. 0.000038915/h
III. 9.3396×10^{-3}/day
IV. 0.0093396/day

A. I and III only
B. II and IV only
C. I, II, and III only
D. All are correct

7. The decay constant of Co-60 is higher than the decay constant of Cs-137.
A. True
B. False

8. After 6 half-lives, the initial activity of a radionuclide is decreased to:
A. I only
B. I and IV only
C. II and III only
D. All are correct
I. $6^{.5}$
II. 0.0156
III. 0.5^6
IV. 2.4494

9. How many half-lives are needed for a radionuclide having an activity of 200 mCi to decay to 3.125 mCi?
A. $6\ T_{1/2}$
B. $4\ T_{1/2}$
C. $3\ T_{1/2}$
D. $7\ T_{1/2}$

10. The initial activity of Au-198 is 15 mCi; what is the activity in 20 days if its half-value layer is 2.5?
A. 0.2556 mCi
B. 0.09036 mCi
C. 2.8931 mCi
D. 2.490 mCi

11. The physicist in your department needs to use I-125 with an activity of 17.8095 mCi on November 10 for an implant, but he/she needs to place the order 10 days before (November 1). What is the activity of I-125 at the time of shipping (November 1)?
A. 20 mCi
B. 0.0116 mCi
C. 59.6 mCi
D. 25 mCi

12. When will the activity of 10 mCi of Rn-222 ($T_{1/2}=3.83$ days and decay constant $\lambda=1.8094\times 10^{-1}$/day) equal the activity of 5 mCi of Au-198 ($T_{1/2}=2.7$ days and a decay constant $\lambda=2.567\times 10^{-1}$ per day)
A. 915 days
B. 9.15 years
C. 9.15 days
D. 91.5 days

1.2 Radioactivity (Questions)

13. What is the mean life of Co-60 in years if its photon energy is 1.25 MeV?
A. 1.80
B. 7.57
C. 3.64
D. 5.62

14. The (α, n) reaction is:
A. A proton being captured by the nucleus with the emission of a γ-ray
B. A bombardment of a nucleus by an α-particle with the subsequent emission of a neutron
C. A bombardment of a nucleus by a proton with the subsequent emission of an α-particle
D. A bombardment of a nucleus by a proton with the subsequent emission of deuteron

15. Which of the following statements are true?
A. I only
B. I and III only
C. I and IV only
D. All are correct
I. λ_b is the fraction of the isotope removed biologically per unit time.
II. λ_{eff} is the fraction eliminated per unit time by biological and physiological process.
III. λ_p is the fraction that decays physically per unit time.
IV. $1/\lambda_{eff} = 1/\lambda_p + 1/\lambda_b$ is the formula used to find the fraction removal per unit time.

16. Which of the following statement(s) is true?
A. Physical half-life is longer than biological half-life.
B. Biological half-life is longer than physical half-life.
C. Effective half-life is shorter than the physical and biological half-life.
D. Effective half-life is longer than the physical and biological half-life.

17. Calculate the effective half-life of a radionuclide if the physical half-life is 7 h and the biological half-life is 14 h.
A. 15 h
B. 3.26 h
C. 16 h
D. 4.66 h

18. Which of the followings formulas are used to calculate effective half-life?
I. $1/\lambda_{eff} = 1/\lambda_p + 1/\lambda_b$
II. $T_a = 1.44 \times T_{1/2}$
III. $T_{eff} = T_p \times T_b / T_p + T_b$
IV. $A_0 = A_n e^{-\lambda \tau}$

A. I only
B. I and III only
C. II and IV only
D. All are correct

19. After how long will Ir-192 decay to 99.5 % of its original activity?
A. 5.37 days
B. 0.537 days
C. 53.7 h
D. 1 day

20. Which of the following is/are true about decay constant?
A. I only
B. II and III only
C. I, II, and III only
D. II and IV only
E. The process is considered a statistical event
I. The number of atoms disintegrating per unit time is proportional to the number of radioactive atoms.
II. The decay constant symbol is λ.
III. It is inversely proportional to half-life ($T_{1/2}$).
IV. It is the time required for the number of radioactive atoms to decay to half the initial value.

21. Which of the following decay processes is due to a deficit of neutrons?
A. Internal conversion
B. Electron capture
C. Alpha particles
D. β-

22. Which of the following decay processes is due to excess nuclear energy from the nucleus?
A. Internal conversion
B. Electron capture
C. Alpha particles
D. Beta minus

23. Which of the following decay processes gives rise to emission of Auger electrons?
A. I only
B. II and III only
C. I, II, and III only
D. II and IV only
E. All are correct

I. Beta plus decay
II. Internal conversion
III. Electron capture
IV. Beta minus decay

24. Which of the following particles is composed of two protons and two neutrons?
A. Hydrogen's nucleus
B. ^{3}He nucleus
C. Alpha particle
D. β- particle

25. Radioactivity or rate of decay can be affected by:
A. I only
B. II and III only
C. I, II, and III only
D. II and IV only
E. All are correct
I. Atomic nucleus composition
II. Pressure
III. Temperature
IV. Distance

26. The process by which an atomic nucleus of unstable atom becomes more stable by emitting particles and/or electromagnetic radiation is called:
A. Half-life
B. Transmutation
C. Radioactive decay
D. Electron equilibrium

27. Which of the following is considered beta decay?
A. I only
B. II and III only
C. I, II, and III only
D. II and IV only
E. All answers are correct
I. Helium emission
II. Positron emission
III. Electron capture
IV. Gamma emission

28. Which of the following particles is emitted on a beta plus (β$^+$) decay process?
A. Internal conversion
B. An electron
C. A positron
D. An alpha particle
E. A negatron

1.3 Production of X-Ray (Questions)

Quiz-1 (Level 2)

1. Which of the following scientist discovered X-Ray?
A. Henri Becquerel, 1896
B. Marie and Pierre Curie, 1898
C. Wilhelm Roentgen, 1895
D. Albert Einstein, 1915–1916

2. The X-ray tube consists of:
I. A cathode
II. An anode
III. A glass envelope
IV. A tissue compensator
A. I, II, and III only
B. I and III only
C. II and IV only
D. IV only
E. All are correct

3. Which of the following statements is false?
A. The anode is made of a tungsten target.
B. The cathode is a tungsten filament.
C. Electrons are accelerated toward the cathode.
D. X-ray emerges through a thin glass beryllium window.

4. The term thermionic emission refers to:
A. The ratio of output energy emitted as X-rays to the input energy deposit by electrons
B. The emission of electrons by the highly heated tungsten filament
C. The region, at the edge of a radiation beam, over which the dose rate changes rapidly as a function of distance from the beam axis
D. A neutral atom acquiring a positive or a negative charge

5. Which of the following statements about anode target are correct?
A. I, II, and III only
B. I and III only
C. II and IV only
D. IV only
E. All are correct
I. The anode target is made of tungsten.
II. The anode material atomic number (Z) is 74.
III. The target material must consist of a high atomic number and high melting point.
IV. The target material must consist of a high atomic number and low melting point.

1.3 Production of X-Ray (Questions)

6. The efficiency of X-ray production depends on what factor(s) of an anode:
A. Mass number (A)
B. The binding energy
C. Atomic number (Z)
D. Number of nucleons

7. To dissipate the heat from the target
A. The tungsten target is angled
B. An added filtration outside the tube is used
C. A cathode focusing cup is used
D. A rotating anode is used as well as oil outside the glass envelope.

8. From the following diagram, match all of the following parts of the X-ray tube.
A. Anode
B. Cathode
C. Focusing cup
D. Filament
E. Glass window
F. X-rays
G. Electron cloud
H. Tungsten target
I. Glass envelope

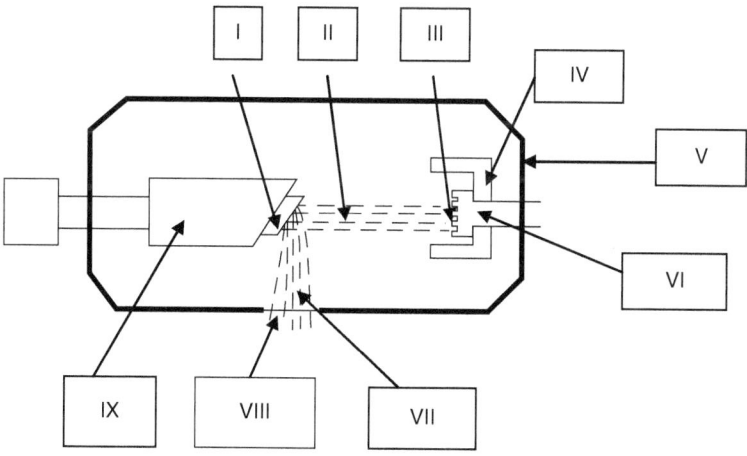

Fig. 1.3.1

9. Match all the X-ray tube parts with its corresponding function.
A. Anode
B. Cathode
C. Focusing cup
D. Filament
E. Glass window
F. X-rays
G. Electron cloud
H. Tungsten target
I. Glass envelope
J. Focal spot
I. It is made of molybdenum; negative electrode; directs the electrons toward the anode so that they strike the target in a well-defined area.
II. The anode and the cathode are inside; maintains a vacuum.
III. Allow the X-rays to escape from the vacuum tube.
IV. It is negative electrode; consists of a wire filament, a circuit to provide current, and a negatively charged focusing cup.
V. It is made of tungsten, located inside the focusing cup, when heated it emits electrons.
VI. It is a positive electrode; it is made of a tungsten target on a cylindrical copper base.
VII. It is positively charged and made of tungsten; electrons are slowed down through a process called Bremsstrahlung; X-rays are produced.
VIII. They are produced on the filament and travel from cathode to anode.
IX. Are produced in the target and travel outside through the glass window.
X. Area of the target where electrons collide and photons are emitted; it could be small or large.

10. What focal spot is used in therapy machines?
A. Small focal spot
B. Triangular focal spot
C. Stationary focal spot
D. Large focal spot

11. What is the target angle in a therapy machine?
A. 6–17°
B. 15–30°
C. 0.1–2 mm
D. 5–7 mm

12. Calculate the apparent focal spot if the size of the focal spot (A) is 2.5 mm and the target angle is 20°.
A. 5 mm
B. 8.5 cm

1.3 Production of X-Ray (Questions)

C. 0.85 mm
D. 3 mm

13. The function of the low-voltage circuit on an X-ray generator is?
A. Supply heating current to the filament.
B. Provide the accelerating potential for the electrons.
C. Control the tube current.
D. Provide a stepwise adjustment in voltage.

14. Match the following with its corresponding characteristics.
A. Self-rectified circuit
B. Half-wave rectification
C. Full-wave rectification
D. Step-up transformer
E. Step-down transformer
I. $N_1 > N_2$, where N_1 is the number of turns on the primary transformer and N_2 is the number of turns on the secondary transformer.
II. The current flows during both half-cycles.
III. $N_2 > N_1$, where N_2 is the number of turns on the secondary transformer and N_1 is the number of turns on the primary transformer.
IV. The tube current as well as the X-ray will be generated only during the half-cycle when the anode is positive.
V. The current will flow as usual during the cycle when the anode is positive related to the cathode.

15. What are the two mechanisms by which X-rays are produced?
A. Coherent scattering and photoelectric effect
B. Bremsstrahlung and characteristic
C. Compton effect and pair production
D. Annihilation radiation and photo disintegration

16. Which of the following statements are/is true about Bremsstrahlung X-ray radiation?
A. I, II, and III only
B. I and III only
C. II and IV only
D. IV only
E. All are correct
I. Photons are produced during a sudden deflection and acceleration of the electron when passing near the nucleus.
II. Results in either partial or complete loss of electron energy.
III. The resulting photon may have any energy up to the initial energy of the electron but not higher.
IV. The direction of emission of the photons depends on the energy of the incident electrons.

17. Which type of target is used by megavoltage X-rays tube accelerators?
A. Flattening filter
B. Transmission-type targets
C. Reflection targets
D. Filtration

18. The probability of Bremsstrahlung X-ray production fluctuates with:
A. The 1st power of the atomic number
B. Atomic mass² (A^2) of the target material
C. Atomic number² (Z^2) of the target material
D. Voltage applied to the tube

19. Which of the following is the result of removing an orbital electron in the K, L, or M shell by a direct hit of an incoming electron?
A. Photoelectric effect
B. Characteristic X-rays
C. Bremsstrahlung X-rays
D. Compton effect

20. Which of the following statement(s) is/are true about characteristic X-ray radiation?
A. I, II, and III only
B. I and III only
C. II and IV only
D. IV only
E. All are correct
I. It is a product of a direct interaction of an incoming electron with an orbital electron.
II. The orbital electron will move away from the collision with initial kinetic energy (E_0) minus the energy needed to eject the orbital electron (ΔE), $E_0 - \Delta E$.
III. A photon is produced when an outer orbital electron fills the vacancy created by the ejected orbital electron.
IV. Characteristic X-rays are created at discrete energies.

21. What is the energy of a photon emitted from the transition of an electron descending from the L shell with a binding energy of 1.100 KeV to the K shell with a binding energy of 8.980 KeV?
A. 8.163 keV
B. 7.880 keV
C. 10.08 keV
D. 9.878 keV

22. Match the following schematic illustration with its corresponding name.
A. Bremsstrahlung process
B. Characteristic radiation
C. Coherent scattering
D. Pair production

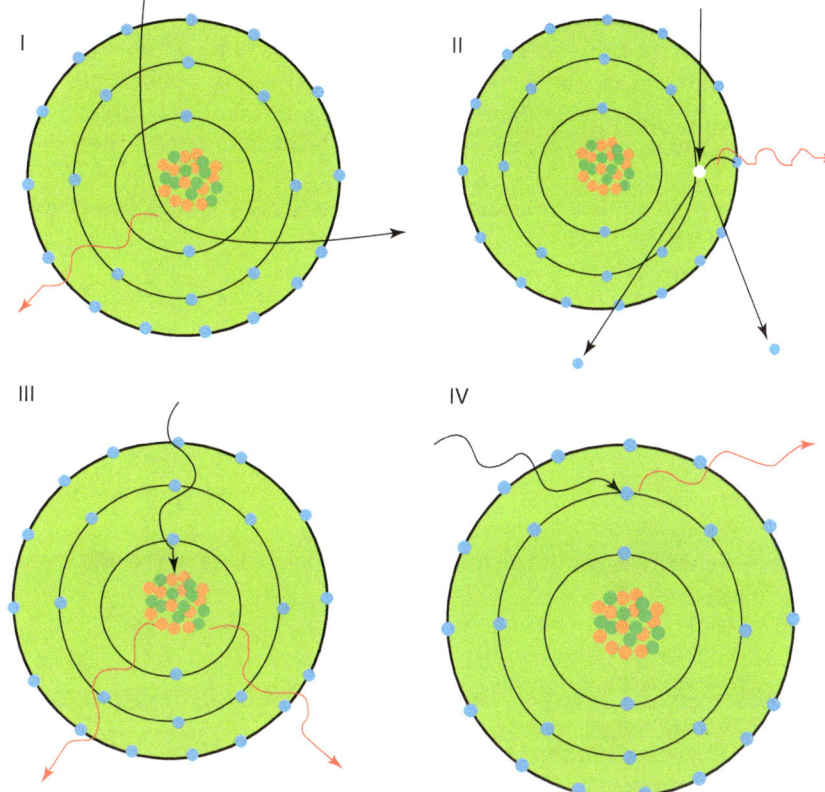

Fig. 1.3.2

23. The two types of filtration on an X-ray machine are:
A. Added and flattening filter
B. Added and magnetron
C. Inherent and added
D. Inherent and HVL

24. Inherent filtration refers to:
A. The absorption of the photons through a filter placed externally to the tube
B. The absorption of the photons through the target, glass walls of the tube, or a thin beryllium window
C. The placement of a flattening filter in the beam path
D. Shielding against leakage radiation

25. As filtration increases the X-ray beam has:
A. Higher average energy and lower penetrating power
B. Lower average energy and greater penetrating power
C. Higher average energy and greater penetrating power
D. Lower average energy and lower penetrating power

26. If additional penetration power of the beam is needed:
A. Added filtration and/or decreased voltage across the tube can be used.
B. Added filtration and/or increased voltage across the tube can be used.
C. Inherent filtration and/or decreased kVp across the tube can be used.
D. Inherent filtration and/or increased mAs can be used.

27. Which of the following factors can affect the X-ray emission spectrum?
A. I, II, and III only
B. I and III only
C. II and IV only
D. IV only
E. All are correct
I. kVp only
II. Distance and kVp only
III. kVp and mAs only
IV. Filtration and kVp only

28. The formula to approximate the mean or average energy of the photon is:
A. $E = h\nu$
B. $E_{avg} = 1/5\ E_{max}$
C. $E_{avg} = 0.5/E_{max}$
D. $E_{avg} = 1/3\ E_{max}$

29. What is the maximum and mean energy of a Bremsstrahlung photon spectrum that was generated using 110 kVp?
A. Max of 110 kV and mean of 3.66 kV
B. Max of 110 kV and mean of 36.66 kV
C. Max of 55 kV and mean of 0.003 kV
D. Max of 110 V and mean of 36.66 V

30. What is exposure?
A. The transmission of radiation through the edges of the collimator blocks
B. Used to bent the electron beam 90° or 270° from its original direction
C. Measure of ionization produce per unit mass on air
D. The energy absorbed in a material per unit mass

31. Which of the following materials is used to insulate an X-ray tube?
A. Water
B. Oil
C. Gas
D. Lead

32. Which of the following parts of the X-ray tube contains the filament and focusing cup?
A. The anode
B. The cathode
C. The transformer
D. The rectifier

1.3 Production of X-Ray (Questions)   25

33. Which of the formulas is used to determine the heat unit of an X-ray machine?
A. mA×kVp
B. mA×kVp/time
C. mA×kVp×time
D. kVp×time/mA

34. Which of the following determine the wavelength or energy of an X-ray?
A. Kilovoltage potential (kVp)
B. Milliamperage (mA)
C. Distance
D. Time

35. Which of the following is/are properties of X-rays?
A. I, II, and III only
B. I and III only
C. II and IV only
D. IV only
E. All are correct
I. X-rays are unaffected by gravity.
II. X-rays are unaffected by electric fields.
III. X-rays are unaffected by magnetic fields.
IV. X-rays cannot be focused.

36. How are X-rays produced?
A. By radioactive decay
B. By interaction of electrons with matter
C. By bombarding a proton into a nucleus
D. By interaction of a neutron with matter

37. An elastic collision is said to be
A. When momentum and kinetic energy are conserved
B. When momentum is conserved but kinetic energy is not conserved
C. When momentum and kinetic energy are not conserved
D. When momentum is not conserved but kinetic energy is conserved

38. The direction in which the X-ray beam is emitted from the target depends on:
A. I, II, and III only
B. I and III only
C. II and IV only
D. IV only
E. All are correct
I. The target design
II. The number of electrons striking the target
III. The energy of the incoming electrons
IV. The target focal spot size

39. Which of the following must be present in order for X-ray production to occur?
A. I, II, and III only
B. I and III only
C. II and IV only
D. IV only
E. All are correct
I. High-speed electrons
II. A large potential difference
III. A vacuum tube
IV. A means of electrons deceleration

40. The function(s) of the X-ray anode is/are:
A. I, II, and III only
B. I and III only
C. II and IV only
D. IV only
E. All are correct
I. Converts electronic energy into x-radiation
II. Serves as the target surface for the high-voltage electrons
III. Serves as the primary thermal conductor
IV. Serves as electron source

41. The function(s) of the X-ray housing is/are:
A. I, II, and III only
B. I and III only
C. II and IV only
D. IV only
E. All are correct
I. Absorbs scatter and leakage radiation
II. Dissipates most of the heat created within the tube
III. Isolates the high voltages
IV. Provides electrical insulation

1.4 Interaction of Radiation with Matter (Questions)

Quiz-1 (Level 2)

1. The process by which a neutral atom acquires a positive or a negative charge is known as:
A. Excitation
B. Ionization
C. LET
D. Bragg peak

1.4 Interaction of Radiation with Matter (Questions)

2. Which of the following particles is/are directly ionizing?
A. I, II, and III only
B. I and III only
C. II and IV only
D. IV only
E. All are correct
I. Electrons
II. Proton
III. Alpha particles
IV. Neutrons

3. Photons interact with the atoms of a material to produce high-speed electrons by which major processes?
A. I, II, and III only
B. I and III only
C. II and IV only
D. IV only
E. All are correct
I. Photoelectric effect
II. Compton effect
III. Pair production
IV. Characteristic X-ray production

4. The thickness of an absorber required to attenuate the intensity of the beam to half its original value is the:
A. Energy absorption coefficient
B. Energy transfer coefficient
C. Attenuation coefficient
D. Half-value layer (HVL)

5. Which of the following statement(s) is/are true?
A. I, II, and III only
B. I and III only
C. II and IV only
D. IV only
E. All are correct
I. For a heterogeneous beam, the first HVL is less than the subsequent HVLs.
II. As the filter thickness increases, the average energy of the transmitted beam increases.
III. As the filter thickness increases, the beam becomes increasingly harder.
IV. By increasing filtration of heterogeneous beam, penetration power or half-value layer of the beam increases.

6. Which of the following is the formula of HVL?
A. HVL=0.693/μ
B. HVL=0.693×μ
C. HVL=0.693/$T_{1/2}$
D. HVL=0.693/λ

7. Which of the following factors affect the amount of photon attenuation by a material?
A. I, II, and III only
B. I and III only
C. II and IV only
D. IV only
E. All are correct
I. Thickness or nature of the material in question
II. The energy of the photon
III. Linear attenuation coefficient (μ) of the material
IV. Density of the material in question

8. The main type(s) of interaction involving attenuation of a photon beam by an absorbing material is/are:
A. I, II, and III only
B. I and III only
C. II and IV only
D. IV only
E. All are correct
I. Coherent scattering and pair production
II. Bremsstrahlung and characteristic X-ray
III. Compton and photoelectric effect
IV. Half-value layer

9. In Coherent scattering:
A. The new photons have the same energy as the incoming photons, but are scattered in different directions.
B. The new photons have the more energy than the incoming photons, but are scattered in different directions.
C. The new photons have the same energy as the incoming photons, and are scattered in the same direction.
D. The new photons have the less energy as the incoming photons, but are scattered in different directions.

10. The probability of coherent scattering is increased by:
A. I, II, and III only
B. I and III only
C. II and IV only
D. IV only
E. All are correct

I. Low atomic number materials
II. High atomic number materials
III. High-energy photons
IV. Low-energy photons

11. The following are characteristics of the photoelectric effect:
A. I, II, and III only
B. I and III only
C. II and IV only
D. IV only
E. All are correct
I. An incoming photon is totally absorbed by an inner shell electron.
II. An atom is ionized when an electron is ejected from an orbital leaving a vacancy.
III. An electron from outer shell fills a vacancy in an inner shell producing a characteristic X-ray.
IV. The characteristic photon can be ejecting another electron called an Auger electron.

12. The main interaction responsible for diagnostic imaging is:
A. Coherent scattering
B. Compton effect
C. Photoelectric effect
D. Pair production

13. The probability of a photoelectric interaction depends on:
A. Atomic number (Z) and energy of the photon (E); the higher the Z of the material, the more likely the interaction, but the higher the energy of the photon, the less likely the interaction.
B. Atomic number (Z) and energy of the photon (E); the lower the Z of the material, the more likely the interaction, but the higher the energy of the photon, the less likely the interaction.
C. Atomic number (Z) and energy of the photon (E); the higher the Z of the material, the more likely the interaction, and the lower the energy of the photon, the less likely the interaction.
D. Atomic number (Z) and energy of the photon (E); the lower the Z of the material, the more likely the interaction, and the lower the energy of the photon, the less likely the interaction.

14. In which of the following types of interactions does a photon interact with an atomic electron as if it were a free electron?
A. Coherent scatter
B. Photoelectric effect
C. Compton effect
D. Pair production

15. Compton interaction depends on:
A. I, II, and III only
B. I and III only
C. II and IV only
D. IV only
E. All are correct
I. Atomic number (Z) of the material
II. Number of electrons per gram
III. Atomic mass (A) of the material
IV. Energy of the incident photon

16. Which of the following materials will attenuate more of an incoming photon beam in Compton interactions?
A. Bone
B. Soft tissue
C. Hydrogen
D. Water

17. For pair production to take place, the threshold energy of the incident photon must be:
A. Equal to 0.51 MeV
B. Greater than 1.02 MeV
C. Greater than 2.04 MeV
D. Less than 1.02 MeV

18. Which of the following statement(s) is/are true about pair production?
A. I, II, and III only
B. I and III only
C. II and IV only
D. IV only
E. All are correct
I. Incident photon energy must be greater than 1.02 MeV.
II. Photons interact with atom.
III. Photons give up all their energy in the process.
IV. An electron and a positron are created.

19. If a photon undergoes a Compton scattering event with an orbital electron by direct hit:
A. No energy is transferred to the electron.
B. The electron will receive maximum energy and the scattered photon will leave with the minimum energy.
C. A photon with energy of 0.511 MeV will be created.
D. This interaction is only possible with incoming photons of energy up to 50 keV.

20. Which of the following statement(s) is/are true?
A. I, II, and III only
B. I and III only

1.4 Interaction of Radiation with Matter (Questions)

C. II and IV only
D. IV only
E. All are correct
I. Coherent scattering probability increases with high atomic number (Z) materials and with photons of low energy.
II. Photoelectric effect probability increases with high atomic number (Z^3) materials and with lower-energy photons (E^{-3}).
III. Compton scattering probability also increases with decreasing energy (E^{-1}), and it depends on the number of electrons per gram of material and is independent of Z.
IV. Pair production probability increases with increasing atomic number (Z) and higher-energy photons greater or equal to 1.02 MeV.

21. Charged particles interact with matter by:
A. Compton interaction
B. Pair production interaction
C. Photoelectric effect interaction
D. Ionization and excitation

22. The rate of kinetic energy loss per unit path length of charged particle is
A. Mass stopping power
B. Stopping power
C. LET
D. Activity

23. Stopping power caused by ionization interaction for charge particles is:
A. Inversely proportional to the square of the particle charge and proportional to the square of its velocity.
B. Proportional to the square of the particle charge and inversely proportional to the square of its velocity.
C. Independent of the particle charge and its velocity.
D. As the particle slows down, its rate of energy loss decreases and so does the ionization to the medium.

24. The most efficient absorber material for neutron beams is
A. I, II, and III only
B. I and III only
C. II and IV only
D. IV only
E. All are correct
I. Paraffin wax
II. Polyethylene
III. Hydrogenous materials
IV. Lead

25. The dose absorbed by fat exposed to a neutron is
A. Lower than that of a muscle
B. Higher than that of a muscle
C. Same as the muscle
D. Lower than that of a bone

26. Match the energy range with its corresponding photon interaction:
A. Coherent scattering
B. Photoelectric effect
C. Compton effect
D. Pair production
I. 150 keV to over 50 MeV
II. Greater than 1.02 MeV
III. 1–50 keV
IV. Few electron volts to over 1 MeV in high atomic numbers elements

27. The reason that electrons do not deposit dose with a Bragg peak is due to:
A. Their relatively small mass
B. Their relatively large mass
C. Their negative charge
D. Their speed

28. What is an electron ejected from its orbit that receives sufficient energy to produce an ionization track of its own called?
A. I, II, and III only
B. I and III only
C. II and IV only
D. IV only
E. All are correct
I. Secondary electron
II. δ-ray
III. Delta ray
IV. Alpha ray

29. Which of the following is/are indirectly ionizing?
A. I, II, and III only
B. I and III only
C. II and IV only
D. IV only
E. All are correct
I. X-rays
II. γ-rays
III. Gamma rays
IV. Neutrons

1.4 Interaction of Radiation with Matter (Questions)

30. Match the diagram with its corresponding interaction.
A. Pair production
B. Photoelectric effect
C. Coherent scattering
D. Compton effect process

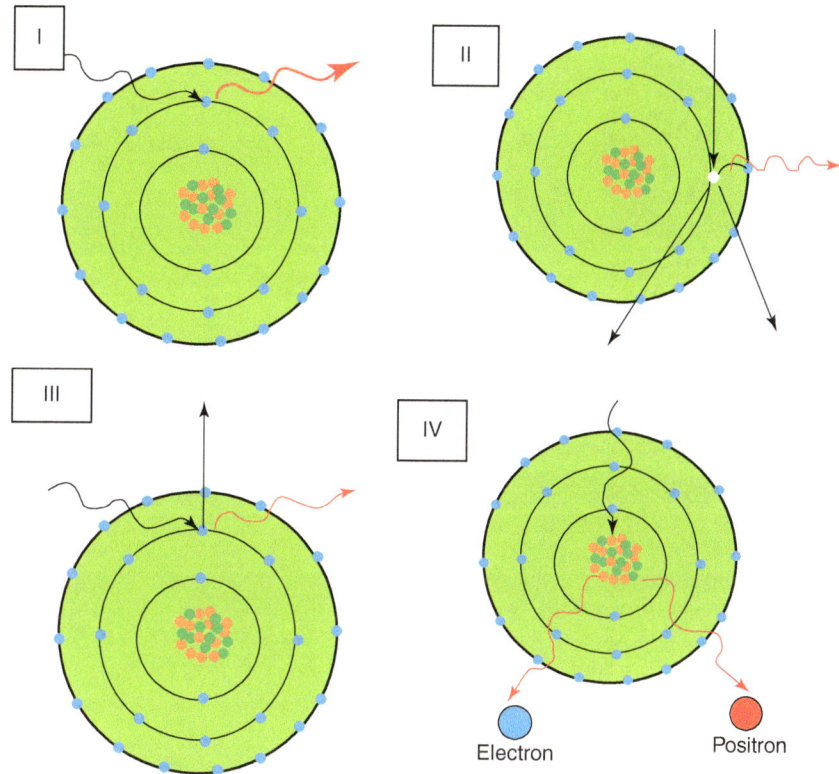

Fig. 1.4.1

31. Select the correct answer of the electromagnetic spectrum from the longest to the shorter wavelength:
A. Radio wave, infrared, ultraviolet wave, X-rays, and gamma rays
B. Ultraviolet wave, radio wave, infrared, X-rays, and gamma rays
C. Infrared, radio wave, ultraviolet wave, gamma rays, and X-rays
D. Radio wave, ultraviolet wave, infrared, gamma rays, and X-rays

32. Which of the following ionizing radiations have the highest energy?
A. Characteristic or diagnostic X-rays
B. Infrared light
C. γ-rays
D. Ultraviolet light

33. The higher the frequency:
A. The shorter the wavelength and the higher the energy
B. The longer the wavelength and the lower the energy
C. The shorter the wavelength and the lower the frequency
D. The longer the wavelength and the higher the energy

34. Which of the following interactions of photons with matter do not produce scattered photons?
A. I, II, and III only
B. I and III only
C. II and IV only
D. IV only
E. All are correct
I. Coherent scattering
II. Photoelectric effect
III. Compton effect
IV. Pair production

35. Coherent Scattering can be also called
A. I, II, and III only
B. I and III only
C. II and IV only
D. IV only
E. All are correct
I. Classical scattering
II. Photoelectric effect scattering
III. Rayleigh scattering
IV. Pair production scattering

36. Which of the following is/are properties of X-rays?
A. I, II, and III only
B. I and III only
C. II and IV only
D. IV only
E. All are correct
I. X-rays travel at the speed of light (3×10^8 m/s).
II. X-rays have a wide range of wavelengths.
III. X-rays propagate in straight lines in free space.
IV. X-rays can damage and kill living cells.

37. As the wavelength of an X-ray decreases:
A. Frequency increases and energy decreases.
B. Frequency decreases and energy increases.
C. Frequency increases and energy increases.
D. Frequency decreases and energy decreases.

38. Increasing the kVp in an X-ray generator will:
A. I, II, and III only
B. I and III only
C. II and IV only
D. IV only
E. All are correct
I. Increase the intensity of an X-ray beam
II. Decrease image noise
III. Increase the number of Compton interactions
IV. Maintain the same image contrast

1.5 Treatment Machine Characteristics (Questions)

Quiz-1 (Level 2)

1. Match the following therapy machines with its corresponding energy range.
A. Grenz-ray therapy
B. Contact therapy
C. Superficial therapy
D. Orthovoltage therapy
E. Supervoltage therapy
F. Megavoltage therapy
G. Van de Graaff generator
I. Greater than 1 MV
II. 40–50 kV
III. 50–150 kV
IV. Less than 20 kV
V. 500–1,000 kV
VI. 150–500 kV
VII. Typically at 2 MV

2. Which of the following therapy machines use 15–20 cm SSD (source to surface distance)?
A. Orthovoltage therapy
B. Superficial therapy
C. Contact therapy
D. Megavoltage therapy

3. Which of the following kilovoltage units can be used to treat a patient with a tumor at a depth of 3 cm?
A. Superficial therapy
B. Contact therapy
C. Grenz-ray therapy
D. Orthovoltage therapy

4. The greatest limitation in using orthovoltage or deep therapy is:
A. Skin sparing
B. Skin surface dose
C. Cone size
D. Size and cost of the machine

5. Match the following megavoltage therapy machines with its corresponding energy range.
A. Microtron therapy
B. Cyclotron therapy
C. Van de Graaff generator
D. Linear accelerator
E. Teletherapy C0-60
I. 15–50 MeV
II. 1.25 MeV
III. 2–10 MeV
IV. 4–40 MeV
V. 4–25 MeV

6. High-energy electron produced in a linear accelerator can be used to
A. I, II, and III only
B. I and III only
C. II and IV only
D. IV only
E. All are correct
I. Treat superficial tumors without the use of X-ray target and flattening filter
II. Treat superficial tumors when the X-ray target and flattening filter are inserted in the beam path
III. Treat deep-seated tumors when the X-ray target and flattening filter are inserted in the beam path
IV. Treat deep-seated tumors without the use of X-ray target and flattening filter

7. Match the major components and auxiliary systems of a linear accelerator with its corresponding letter.
I. Electron gun
II. Waveguide system
III. Modulator
IV. Accelerator tube
V. Treatment head (straight beam)
VI. Power supply
VII. Magnetron or klystron
VIII. Treatment head (bent beam)

1.5 Treatment Machine Characteristics (Questions)

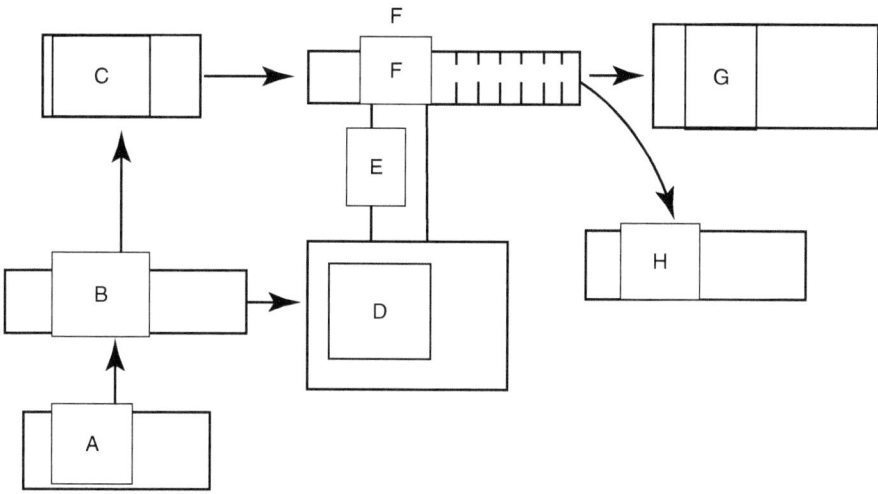

Fig. 1.5.1

8. Match the following linear accelerator components with its function.
A. Power supply
B. Modulator
C. Electron gun
D. Magnetron or klystron
E. Waveguide system
F. Accelerator tube
G. Treatment head
I. Provides a source of electrons.
II. Microwaves generated from the magnetron or klystron are sent into the accelerator structure throughout this component.
III. Generate control pulse to the electron gun and the magnetron or klystron.
IV. Electrons are accelerated to high energies in this component by the interaction with microwave radiation.
V. Provide direct current power to the modulator.
VI. Generate and/or amplify microwaves to accelerate the electrons through the waveguide.
VII. Contains an X-ray target, scattering foil, flattening filter, ion chamber, fixed and movable collimator, and light localizer system.

9. Treatment parameters (gantry, collimator, field size, dose per fraction, total dose) to be used for a patient's treatment are controlled by:
A. Ionization chamber
B. Calorimetry (calorimetry is a basic method of determining absorbed dose in a medium)
C. Beam handling section (after electrons have been accelerated, they are redirected by beam handling section which include the bending magnet, target, scattering foil, or flattening filter)
D. Record and verify section (the record and verify section controls treatment parameters)

10. Which of the following statements about magnetron and klystron are true?
A. Both devices produce microwaves.
B. Only a magnetron can be used in high-energy (>10 MV) linacs.
C. The magnetron produces microwaves, and the klystron is a microwave amplifier.
D. A magnetron is more expensive and has a longer life span than a klystron.

11. The two types of accelerator structure found in a linac machine are?
A. Traveling and standing waves
B. Traveling and horizontal waves
C. Standing wave and ion pump
D. Ion pump and electron gun

12. Match the major components treatment head of a linear accelerator with its corresponding letter.
A. Flattening filter
B. Ion chamber
C. Scattering foil
D. X-ray target
E. Primary collimator
F. Electron applicator
G. Secondary collimator
H. Bending magnet

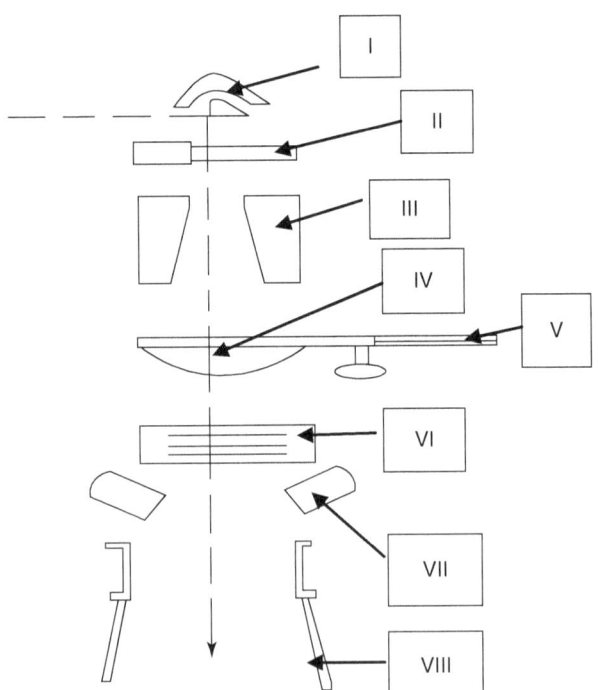

Fig. 1.5.2

1.5 Treatment Machine Characteristics (Questions)

13. What are the angles that electrons can be bent before striking the target?
A. I, II, and III only
B. I and III only
C. II and IV only
D. IV only
E. All are correct
I. Chromatic 90° bending magnet
II. Chromatic 180° bending magnet
III. Achromatic 270° bending magnet
IV. Achromatic 180° bending magnet

14. Match the following parts of the treatment head with its corresponding function:
A. Bending magnet
B. Monitor chamber
C. X-ray target
D. Flattening filter
E. Fixed primary collimator
F. Electron cone
G. Movable X-ray collimator
H. Light localizing system
I. Scattering foil
I. Consists of two pairs of lead or tungsten blocks (jaws) which provide a rectangular opening
II. Spreads the narrow electron beam and causes a fairly uniform electron distribution across the beam
III. Reduces the intensity of the forward peaked dose in the center of the field to produce dose uniformity across the radiation field at a specified depth
IV. Monitors the dose rate, integrates dose, and monitors beam flatness and symmetry
V. Produces a photon beam through the Bremsstrahlung process
VI. Bends the electron beam usually 90° or 270° from its original direction
VII. Used in electron mode to collimate electron beams since they scatter readily in air
VIII. Defines the X-ray beam
IX. Is congruent with the radiation field and is used in the alignment of the radiation beam and the treatment field marked on the patient's skin surface

15. Which of the following parts are moved aside when the linear accelerator is in the electron mode?
A. X-ray target and scattering foil
B. Flattening filter and X-ray target
C. Flattening filter and electron cone
D. Ion chamber and flattening filter

16. Which of the following parts are moved in front of the electron beam when the linear accelerator is in the electron mode?
A. Scattering foil
B. Flattening filter
C. X-ray target
D. Ion chamber

17. Ion chambers are made of:
A. High-Z materials
B. Low-Z materials
C. Tungsten
D. Lead

18. Which is the correct path of the beam when a linac accelerator is in the X-ray mode?
A. Bending magnet, X-ray target, primary collimator, scattering foils, monitor chamber, secondary collimator, and electron applicator
B. Bending magnet, X-ray target, primary collimator, flattening filter, monitor chamber, and secondary collimator
C. Bending magnet, primary collimator, scattering foils, monitor chamber, secondary collimator, electron applicator, and cutout
D. X-ray target, primary collimator, scattering foils, monitor chamber, secondary collimator, and electron applicator

19. The maximum field size projected at a standard distance of 100 cm focal spot to target by the secondary collimator is typically:
A. 50×50 cm
B. 80×80 cm
C. 40×40 cm
D. 10×10 cm

20. The point of intersection of the collimator axis and the axis of rotation of the gantry is known as:
A. Secondary collimator
B. SSD
C. Wiggler point
D. Isocenter

21. The main disadvantages of a betatron are:
A. Low dose rates and small field sizes
B. Easy energy selection and simplicity
C. Time error and wide penumbra
D. Low dose rates and penumbra

1.5 Treatment Machine Characteristics (Questions)

22. A microtron is:
A. A device that accelerates electrons in a circular orbit using a magnetic field with an accelerating tube shaped like a hollow doughnut
B. An electron accelerator that combines the principles of both the linear accelerator and the cyclotron
C. A charged particle accelerator, mainly used for nuclear physics research
D. A device that uses radioisotope sources to treat at extended distances

23. The most appropriate radionuclide for external beam radiotherapy is
A. Radium-226
B. Cesium-137
C. Cobalt-60
D. Iridium-192

24. Cobalt-60 is produced by:
A. Bombarding deuterons or protons against beryllium target in a deuterium tritium (D-T) generator, cyclotron, or linear accelerator
B. Irradiating stable ^{59}Co with neutrons in a nuclear reactor
C. A cyclotron or linear accelerator
D. Irradiating stable ^{61}Co with protons in a nuclear reactor

25. Which of the following statement(s) is/are true?
A. I, II, and III only
B. I and III only
C. II and IV only
D. IV only
E. All are correct
I. Co-60 $T_{1/2}$ is 30 years.
II. Co-60 photon energy is 5.26 MeV.
III. The exposure rate constant Γ (R-cm^2/mCi-h) of Co-60 is 8.25.
IV. Co-60 decays to ^{60}Ni with emission of electrons of 0.32 MeV and two photons of energy 1.17 and 1.33 MeV.

26. Which of the following is/are the advantage(s) of ^{60}Co over ^{226}Ra and ^{137}Cs?
A. I, II, and III only
B. I and III only
C. II and IV only
D. IV only
E. All are correct
I. Higher specific activity (curies per gram)
II. Greater radiation output per curie
III. Higher average photon energy
IV. Less expensive and has reduced self-absorption

27. The geometric penumbra associated with ^{60}Co is due to:
A. Machine characteristics
B. Finite size of the source
C. Field size
D. Edge of the collimator

28. The output of a ^{60}Co teletherapy source decreases by about:
A. 0.1 % monthly
B. 1.0 % monthly
C. 1.0 % each year
D. 10 % each month

29. Mechanisms to move the Co-60 source from the off to on position include:
A. I, II, and III only
B. I and III only
C. II and IV only
D. IV only
E. All are correct
I. Source mounted on a rotating wheel
II. Source mounted in a drawer plus its ability to slide horizontally
III. Mercury flows into the space immediately below the source to shut off the beam
IV. Source fixed in front of the aperture where heavy metal jaws shutter can be opened

30. The penumbra of a Cobalt-60 teletherapy beam is:
A. Smaller than that of a linear accelerator
B. Bigger than that of a linear accelerator
C. Same as that of a linear accelerator
D. Smaller on the on position and bigger on the off position than that of the linear accelerator

31. Transmission penumbra can be minimized if:
A. The inner surface of the blocks is made parallel to the central axis of the beam.
B. Larger collimator openings are used.
C. The inner surface of the blocks are shaped so that they remain parallel to the edge of the beam.
D. The outer surface of the blocks is made perpendicular to the central axis of the beam.

32. Match the correct graphic with its corresponding name.
A. Electron depth dose curve illustrating the R_p and R_{50}
B. Transmission penumbra
C. Geometry of two adjacent beams to calculate gap
D. Geometric penumbra

1.5 Treatment Machine Characteristics (Questions)

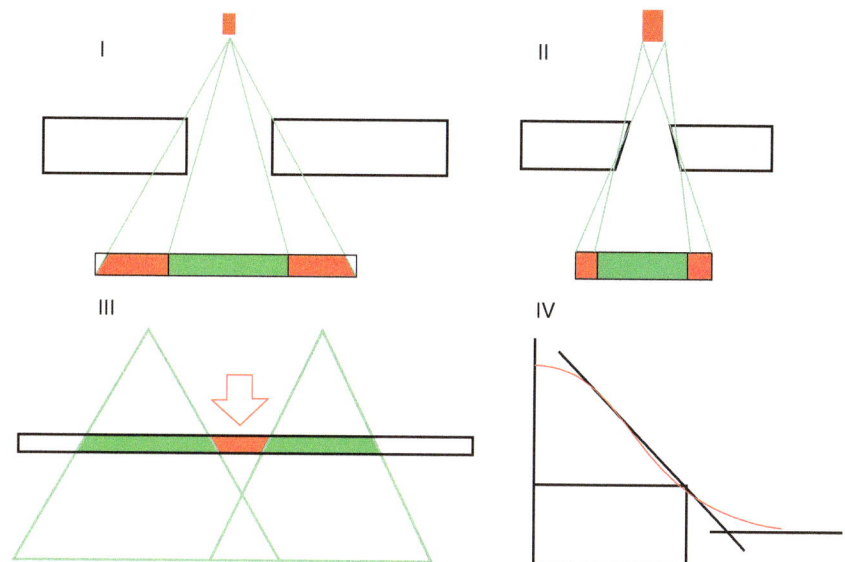

Fig. 1.5.3

33. Which of the following formulas is used to calculate geometric penumbra? (Geometric penumbra is equal to X.)
A. $X = a \times b / 2(a+b)$
B. $X = (\mu_{tissue} - \mu_{water}/\mu_{water})\ 1{,}000$
C. $X = s\ (SSD + d - SDD)/SDD$
D. $X = 0.5\ L_1 \times d/SSD_1 + 0.5\ L_2 \times d/SSD_2$

34. Which of the following statements about penumbra is false?
A. I, II, and III only
B. I and III only
C. II and IV only
D. IV only
E. None
I. As source diameter increases, penumbra increases.
II. As depth increases, penumbra increases.
III. As source diameter decreases, penumbra decreases.
IV. As source to diaphragm distance increases, penumbra decreases.

35. Geometric penumbra is independent of:
A. Source to diaphragm distance
B. Source diameter
C. Field size
D. Source to surface distance

36. The lateral distance between two specified isodose curves at a specified depth or the distance between the 80 % and the 20 % intensities of the beam profile is the definition of:
A. Physical penumbra
B. Transmission penumbra
C. Geometric penumbra
D. Trimmer bars

37. What is the penumbra size if the source measures 1.5 cm in diameter, the SSD is set at 90 cm, the depth is 10 cm, the SDD is 20 cm, and source to patient exit distance is 130 cm?
A. I, II, and III only
B. I and III only
C. II and IV only
D. IV only
E. All are correct
I. 4 cm to the right side and 2 cm to the left side
II. 6 cm to the right side and 6 cm to the left side
III. 3 cm to the right side and 3 cm to the left side
IV. 12 cm adding right and left side

38. The major disadvantages of high-energy protons over electrons or photons in radiotherapy are:
A. I, II, and III only
B. I and III only
C. II and IV only
D. IV only
E. All are correct
I. High cost of the machine
II. Low dose rates
III. Beam contamination
IV. Sharp penumbra

39. The major advantage of proton therapy is:
A. Distal dose falloff (Bragg peak)
B. Very sharp penumbra region
C. Range modulation
D. High-energy radiation therapy

40. Which of the following is/are true about orthovoltage X-ray units?
A. I, II, and III only
B. I and III only
C. II and IV only
D. IV only
E. All are correct

1.5 Treatment Machine Characteristics (Questions)

I. The SSD is usually set at 50 cm.
II. Their potential energy ranges from 150 to 500 kV.
III. The maximum dose usually occurs close to the skin surface.
IV. They are used to treat lesions *no* deeper than 2–3 cm.

41. Which of the following task group (TG) numbers is used on proton therapy machine QA?
A. Task group No.185
B. Task group No.224
C. Task group No.202
D. Task group No.140

Quiz-2 (Level 3)

1. What is the purpose of using a klystron?
A. I and II
B. III and IV
C. I, III, and IV
D. All
I. To increase the amplitude of accelerating voltage
II. To increase the total number of electrons in waveguide
III. To make electrons in waveguide into bunches, thus to pulse the X-ray
IV. To increase the energy of electrons in waveguide

2. After commissioning a new linear accelerator, what should the medical physicist do with the commission data?
A. I and III
B. II and III
C. III only
D. I and II
I. Input the commissioned data into the TPS and use this for dose calculation in planning.
II. Input the commissioned data into TPS and tweak the machine file in TPS before planning.
III. Keep a record as the baseline for annual and monthly QAs.

3. Most of energy of electrons in the accelerating waveguide will convert into heat instead of X-ray photons; thus a low duty factor is needed for heat dissipation. The duty factor is about:
A. 1 %
B. 3 %
C. 0.1 %
D. 0.5 %

4. To keep a low duty factor, what instrument is used?
A. Thyratron
B. Klystron
C. Phase shifter or automatic frequency control (AFC)
D. Triode gun

5. A standing wave (SW) accelerator has a shorter accelerating waveguide than a traveling wave (TW) accelerator. This is because:
A. In a SW accelerator, coupling cavities can be shifted off the central axis.
B. An SW is more energetic in accelerating electrons.
C. A TW accelerator has higher energy; thus it takes longer to accelerate electrons.
D. An SW has higher amplitude in accelerating voltage.

6. In a typical dual-energy traveling wave (TW) accelerator, to switch energy from 15 to 6 MV X-rays, what action is needed?
A. Beam loading.
B. Decrease beam current.
C. Reduce current in klystron.
D. Use a non-contact energy switch.

7. In a typical dual-energy stationed wave (SW) accelerator, to switch energy from 15 to 6 MV X-rays, what action is needed?
A. Beam loading.
B. Decrease beam current.
C. Reduce current in klystron.
D. Use non-contact energy switch in one-side coupling cavity.

8. What is the difference between automatic frequency control (AFC) and phase shifter?
A. No difference. Both are feedback circuit to adjust frequency.
B. AFC is for initial adjustment and phase shifter is for fine adjustment.
C. AFC is for fine adjustment and phase shifter is for an initial adjustment.
D. AFC and phase shifter are used together for SW accelerator.

9. What is the difference between triode gun and diode electron gun?
A. I and III
B. II and IV
C. I and IV
D. II and III
I. Triode gun has an extra control grid to control beam current.
II. Diode gun lacks a control grid for beam current control.
III. Diode gun cannot be used in SW accelerator.
IV. Diode gun cannot be used in TW accelerator.

1.5 Treatment Machine Characteristics (Questions)

10. What is major action to change the energies for electron mode in a traveling wave (SW) accelerator?
A. I and II
B. II and III
C. I and III
D. All
I. Change the wave amplitude.
II. Change the frequency phase.
III. Beam loading.

11. A thyratron is a high-speed switch for high-voltage control. What is its working frequency?
A. 300 Hz
B. 3,000 Hz
C. 30,000 Hz
D. 3 MHz

12. To keep a low duty factor by a thyratron, what is the actual pulse duration for accelerating in each 4 ms cycle?
A. 40 µs
B. 4 µs
C. 0.4 ms
D. 0.4 µs

13. What is the function of the circulator in the microwave transmission waveguide?
A. To block the microwave reflected from klystron to accelerating waveguide
B. To allow one-way passing of microwaves from klystron to accelerating waveguide
C. To isolate the N_2 (or Freon) in the transmission waveguide from the vacuum of accelerating waveguide
D. To avoid sparks (or arcing) inside the transmission waveguide

14. Once the beam of standing wave (SW) linear accelerator is pulsed on, the X-ray or electrons will come out after 1 µs; this is because:
A. It takes time for electrons to travel from electron gun through the waveguide.
B. It takes time for electrons to penetrate the target.
C. It takes time for the bending magnet to be ready.
D. It takes time to reach its maximum amplitude.

15. A thyratron is filled with hydrogen gas. What is the correct pressure and what is the gas for?
A. 0.5 psi, used as conductor
B. 0.5 Torr, used as conductor
C. 0.5 psi, used as insulator
D. 0.5 Torr, used as insulator

1.6 Radiation Units (Questions)

Quiz-1 (Level 2)

1. Which of the following is an International System of Units (SI unit) of mass?
   A. Seconds (s)
   B. Ampere (A)
   C. Kilograms (kg)
   D. Meter (m)

2. Which of the following statements is/are true?
   A. I, II, and III only
   B. I and III only
   C. II and IV only
   D. IV only
   E. All are correct
   I. The SI unit of force is Newton (N).
   II. The SI unit of frequency is Joule (J).
   III. The SI unit of power of work is a watt (W).
   IV. The SI unit of energy is hertz (Hz).

3. Which of the following formula is incorrect?
   A. Velocity (v) = distance (d)/time (t)
   B. Acceleration (a) = velocity (v)/time (t)
   C. Force (F) = mass (m) × acceleration (a)
   D. Power (P) = energy (E) × time (t)

4. Match the following electrical units with its corresponding SI unit.
   A. Electrical resistance (R)
   B. Charge (Q)
   C. Capacitance (C)
   D. Electric potential (V)
   I. Coulomb (C)
   II. Volt (V)
   III. Farad (F)
   IV. Ohm (Ω)

5. Match the following electrical units with its corresponding formula.
   A. Electrical resistance (R)
   B. Charge (Q)
   C. Capacitance (C)
   D. Electric potential (V)
   I. Current (I) × time (t)
   II. Energy (E)/charge (Q)
   III. Charge (Q)/electric potential (V)
   IV. Voltage (V)/current (I)

1.6 Radiation Units (Questions)

6. Match the radiation units with their corresponding SI unit; answer can be more than one.
A. Activity
B. Absorbed dose
C. Exposure (X)
D. KERMA (kinetic energy released per unit mass)
I. Gray (Gy)
II. C kg^{-1}
III. Becquerel (Bq)
IV. Sievert (Sv)

7. The definition of absorbed dose is
A. Energy loss by electrons per unit path length of a material
B. Energy absorbed from all ionizing radiations per unit mass of a material
C. Charge liberated by ionization radiation per unit mass air
D. Rate of decay of a radioactive material per unit time

8. What are some advantages of using absorbed dose rather than exposure?
A. I, II, and III only
B. I and III only
C. II and IV only
D. IV only
E. All are correct
I. Gy is applicable to all ionizing radiation.
II. Gy is applicable even in areas where electronic equilibrium does not exist.
III. Gy is directly related to radiation effects or measure of the biological effects produced by ionizing radiation.
IV. Gy is applicable to X-rays and gamma rays only.

9. The SI unit for absorbed dose is the Gray (Gy). The non-SI unit is the rad. One Gray is equal to what?
A. I, II, and III only
B. I and III only
C. II and IV only
D. IV only
E. All are correct
I. 1 Gy = 1 J of absorbed energy/1 kg of material
II. 1 Gy = 1 J/kg
III. 1 Gy = 100 rad
IV. 1 cGy = 1 rad

10. Ionization in AIR is measured in:
A. Absorbed dose
B. Roentgen
C. Specific activity
D. RBE

11. The unit, SI unit, and non-SI unit of KERMA are?
A. J/kg, Gy, and rad
B. J/kg, Gy, and C kg
C. Gy, Bq, and rad
D. J/kg, R, and C kg

12. KERMA is defined as?
A. I, II, and III only
B. I and III only
C. II and IV only
D. IV only
E. All are correct
I. Amount of kinetic energy transferred from photons to charged particles per unit mass
II. The sum of the initial kinetic energies of all the charged ionizing particles liberated by uncharged particles in a mass
III. Amount of kinetic energy transferred to electrons in a unit mass
IV. Quantity of radiation for all types of ionizing radiation

13. Ring dosimeters:
A. I, II, and III only
B. I and III only
C. II and IV only
D. IV only
E. All are correct
I. Should be worn when there is a possibility of significant exposure to the hand
II. Should be worn on the hand that is favored
III. Should be usually worn on the index finger, which receives the greatest exposure
IV. Should be worn under gloves to protect it from contamination

14. Which of the following statements are true?
A. I, II, and III only
B. I and III only
C. II and IV only
D. IV only
E. All are correct
I. Film badges will be issued to users of 10 mCi or more of gamma- or alpha-emitting radionuclides.
II. Film badges will be issued to users of 20 mCi or more of gamma- or beta-emitting radionuclides.

1.6 Radiation Units (Questions)

III. Ring badges will be issued to users of 0.5 mCi or more of gamma- or alpha-emitting radionuclides.
IV. Ring badges will be issued to users of 5 mCi or more of gamma- or beta-emitting radionuclides.

15. The quality of the radiation received by a personal film holder is determined by:
A. Film used inside the film badge
B. Filters used inside the film badge
C. Temperature used to develop the film
D. Pressure used after film badge is exposed

16. The f-factor is:
A. I, II, and III only
B. I and III only
C. II and IV only
D. IV only
E. All are correct
I. The roentgen-to-rad conversion factor
II. Relates dose in air to dose in tissue
III. A conversion of exposure to absorbed dose
IV. The rad-to-roentgen conversion factor

17. What is the dose delivered to bone if the exposure to the bone is 30 R and the f-factor is 6.17 R?
A. 0.21 cGy
B. 36.17 cGy
C. 185.1 cGy
D. 4.86 cGy

18. f-factor's constant for air is?
A. 0.693
B. 0.876 cGy/R (rad/R)
C. 876 cGy/R (rad/R)
D. 0.511 MeV

19. Disadvantages of radiographic film include?
A. I, II, and III only
B. I and III only
C. II and IV only
D. IV only
E. All are correct
I. Energy dependence
II. Physical, chemical, or thermal processing required
III. Environmental sensitivity
IV. Artifacts caused by air pockets adjacent to the film

20. Film can be used for:
A. I, II, and III only
B. I and III only
C. II and IV only
D. IV only
E. All are correct
I. Personal dosimetry
II. Detection of radiation leaks
III. Imaging and QA
IV. Detect betas, gamma rays, and neutrons

21. Radiation absorbed dose when measured on a film is related to:
A. The film base
B. The degree of blackening of the film
C. Emulsion
D. Silver bromide

22. The optical density of the film is measured by
A. Densitometer
B. Extrapolation chamber
C. Electrometer
D. TLD

23. Advantages of radiochromic films include
A. I, II, and III only
B. I and III only
C. II and IV only
D. IV only
E. All are correct
I. Tissue equivalence
II. High spatial resolution
III. Low spectral sensitivity variation or energy dependence
IV. No need for chemical processing

24. The most frequently used TLD material for clinical dosimetry is
A. Lithium borate ($Li_2B_4O_7$)
B. Calcium fluoride (CaF_2)
C. Calcium sulfate (C_aS_{o4}: Mn)
D. Lithium fluoride (LiF)

25. The optical density, OD, is defined as:
A. $\log (I_0 \times I_t)$
B. $\log (I_0/I_t)$
C. $\log (I_0 - I_t)$
D. $\log (I_0 + I_t)$

1.6 Radiation Units (Questions)

26. Film dosimetry is useful for
A. I, II, and III only
B. I and III only
C. II and IV only
D. IV only
E. All are correct
I. Patient-specific QA
II. Verifying light-field coincidence
III. Confirming field flatness and symmetry
IV. Obtaining quick qualitative patterns of a radiation distribution

27. A radiochromic film's response depends on
A. Humidity
B. Pressure
C. Temperature
D. Chemical processing

28. Which of the following statements are true about radiochromic films?
A. I, II, and III only
B. I and III only
C. II and IV only
D. IV only
E. All are correct
I. No physical, chemical, or thermal processing
II. Insensitive to visible light (although it should be stored in a dark envelope)
III. Sensitive to ultraviolet light and temperature
IV. Almost tissue equivalent

29. Where should body badges be worn?
A. Between the waist and the knees
B. Between the neck and the waist
C. On the neck all the time
D. On the finger

30. A control badge is usually shipped with a group of badges but is not worn by anyone. What is the purpose of the control badge?
A. I, II, and III only
B. I and III only
C. II and IV only
D. IV only
E. All are correct
I. To determine the background radiation exposure to the shipment of film badges
II. To count all the film badges when arrive to the lab
III. To serve to evaluate any exposures to the shipment during transit
IV. To estimate the number of film badges shipped from the lab

31. LET stands for:
A. Linear energy transfer
B. Lateral equivalent tumor
C. Linear electron therapy
D. Linear excitation tissue

32. Match the radiation measurement instruments with its corresponding measurement.
I. Absolute dosimetry
II. Relative dosimetry
A. Ion chamber
B. Film
C. Calorimetry dosimeter
D. TLD
E. Diodes

33. The most commonly used radiochromic films for dosimetry are:
A. I, II, and III only
B. I and III only
C. II and IV only
D. IV only
E. All are correct
I. GafChromic HD-810
II. TLD-700
III. Double-layer GafChromic MD-55-2
IV. DM-1260

34. A radiochromic film consists of:
A. I, II, and III only
B. I and III only
C. II and IV only
D. IV only
E. All are correct
I. Cellulose acetate or polyester resin coated with an emulsion containing small crystals of silver bromide (radiographic films)
II. Ultrathin colorless, radiosensitive leuco dye bonded onto a 100-μm-thick mylar base
III. Metallic silver (during development of radiographic films, the affected crystals are reduced to metallic silver)
IV. Thin layers of radiosensitive dye sandwiched between two pieces of polyester base

35. In the megavoltage range of photon energies, films have been used to measure isodose curves with acceptable accuracy of:
A. ±7 %
B. ±10 %

1.6 Radiation Units (Questions)

C. ±5 %
D. ±3 %

36. Thermoluminescence refers to:
A. I, II, and III only
B. I and III only
C. II and IV only
D. IV only
E. All are correct
I. Energy recovered as visible light when crystalline materials are heated
II. Release of electrons when crystalline materials are heated
III. Release of visible photons by thermal emission
IV. Energy recovered as protons by thermal emission

37. TLDs (or OSLDs) can be used for:
A. I, II, and III only
B. I and III only
C. II and IV only
D. IV only
E. All are correct
I. Direct insertion into tissues or body cavities
II. Measuring dose distribution in the buildup region
III. Measuring dose around brachytherapy sources
IV. Personal dose monitoring

38. A photomultiplier tube (PMT) is used to:
A. Measure the emitted light which converts light into an electrical current
B. Change resistance with temperature
C. Measure the change in molar amount of Fe^{2+}
D. Measure the radiation absorbed by a crystal

39. What is the optical density on a film if the amount of light collected without film is 100 and the amount of light transmitted through the film is 0.1 %?
A. 2 OD
B. 3 OD
C. 4 OD
D. 5 OD

40. The H-D curve or sensitometric curve plot in film dosimetry is:
A. The effective energy as a function of half-value layer
B. The total mass attenuation coefficient $(\mu/\rho)_{total}$ versus energy for different materials
C. Net optical density as a function of radiation exposure or dose from a dosimetry film
D. The relative dose rate as inverse square law function of distance from a point source

41. Which of the following is the most recent recommended protocol by the AAPM for calibration parameters of megavoltage beams?
A. TG-21 protocol
B. TG-51 protocol
C. TRS-398 protocol
D. TRS-277 protocol

42. The major changes from TG-21 to TG-51 are
A. I, II, and III only
B. I and III only
C. II and IV only
D. IV only
E. All are correct
I. The TG-51 protocol is based on absorbed-dose-to-water calibration factor instead of exposure or air KERMA calibration of the ion camber.
II. The TG-51 protocol does not need to calculate any theoretical dosimetry factors.
III. The TG-51 protocol does not need large tables of stopping-power ratios and mass-energy absorptions coefficients.
IV. The TG-51 protocol is more simply from the user's point of view.

43. According to the TG-51 protocol, which of the following is calibrated in water at R_{50}?
A. Photon beams
B. Electron beams
C. Neutron beams
D. Proton beams

44. Some disadvantages of diodes detectors include
A. I, II, and III only
B. I and III only
C. II and IV only
D. IV only
E. All are correct
I. Temperature dependence
II. Damage to diode occurs at each use due to radiation
III. Energy dependence in photon beams
IV. Directional dependence

45. Uses of silicon diodes include
A. I, II, and III only
B. I and III only
C. II and IV only
D. IV only
E. All are correct

1.6 Radiation Units (Questions)

I. Relative measurements in electron beams
II. Quick measurement for output constancy checks
III. In vivo patient dose monitoring
IV. Absolute dose measurements

46. Which of the following is the most sensitive instrument?
A. Thimble ionization chamber
B. Extrapolation chamber
C. Parallel-plate chamber
D. Silicon diodes

47. Which method of determining absorbed dose in the medium is used in a calorimetry instrument?
A. Chemical
B. Heat
C. Temperature
D. Pressure

48. According to the TG-51 protocol, which of the following is calibrated with an ionization chamber in water at a depth of 10 cm?
A. Electron beams
B. Photon beams
C. Proton beams
D. Neutron beams

49. Which of the following is the unit of absorbed radiation dose?
A. Becquerel (Bq)
B. Curie (Ci)
C. Gray (Gy)
D. Roentgen (R)

50. Which of the following radiation monitors can give instantaneous reading if needed?
A. I, II, and III only
B. I and III only
C. II and IV only
D. IV only
E. All are correct
I. Pocket dosimeter
II. Thermoluminescence dosimetry (TLD)
III. Silicon diode
IV. Film badge (radiographic film)

51. Energy absorbed per unit distance of ionizing particles passing through a material is known as?
A. Stopping power (S)
B. Linear energy transfer (LET)
C. Attenuation coefficient (μ)
D. Absorption

52. The time necessary for a radioactive material to decay to 50 % of its original activity is the definition of?
A. Half-life
B. Decay
C. Excitation
D. Half-value layer (HVL)

53. Which of the following is the most common type of personnel radiation monitoring device?
A. Pocket dosimeter
B. Thermoluminescence dosimetry (TLD)
C. Silicon diode
D. Film badge

54. Disadvantages of film badges include:
A. I, II, and III only
B. I and III only
C. II and IV only
D. IV only
E. All are correct
I. Very expensive.
II. One needs to wait until the results are reported.
III. Exposure cannot be reverified.
IV. Energy dependence.

55. Which kind of detector is used inside ring badges?
A. Film
B. Thermoluminescence dosimetry (TLD)
C. Geiger-Mueller counter
D. Electrode

56. According to NCRP and NRC, a badge should be given to an individual:
A. When that individual has the potential to receive one-tenth of the applicable maximum permissible dose (MPD) for an adult, minor, or pregnant woman in a year
B. When that individual has the potential to receive half of the applicable MPD for an adult, minor, or pregnant woman in a year
C. When that individual has the potential to receive one-tenth of the applicable MPD for an adult, minor, or pregnant woman in a 6-month period
D. All individual who work in radiation department

1.6 Radiation Units (Questions)

57. Determine the dose (cGy) received by a patient's scar if the physicist decided to place a TLD on the scar during a treatment. TLD calibration dose is 50 cGy, patient reading is 80.5 nC, and the calibration reading is 32.7 nC.
A. 125 cGy
B. 20.3 cGy
C. 123 cGy
D. 52.5 cGy

58. Which of the following is the most accurate radiation monitoring device?
A. Film badge dosimeter
B. Direct reading pocket dosimeter (DRD)
C. Thermoluminescence dosimeter (TLD)
D. Ring badge dosimeter

59. Which of the following has recently been developed for occupational exposure monitoring?
A. Film badge dosimeter
B. Direct reading pocket dosimeter (DRD)
C. Thermoluminescence dosimeter (TLD)
D. Optically stimulated luminescence dosimeter (OSLD)

60. If you are at the dentist and radiographic images are required to be taken on you, where should you use your personal film badge?
A. At the collar inside the lead apron
B. At the collar outside the lead apron
C. At the waist inside the lead apron
D. No personal film badge to be used at all

61. The personal badge holder open window will determine:
A. Alpha particles
B. Beta particles
C. Photon beam energies
D. Gamma particles

62. Which of the following are advantages of personal film badges?
A. I, II, and III only
B. I and III only
C. II and IV only
D. IV only
E. All are correct
I. They provide a permanent record of dose.
II. They are able to distinguish between different energies of photons.
III. They can measure doses due to different types of radiation.
IV. No development or processing is needed to get the reading.

1.7 Atomic and Nuclear Structure (Answers)

Quiz-1 (Level 1)

1. **A** Units of mass are given in atomic mass units (amu). The conversion from kilograms (kg) to amu is given by 1 amu = 1.66×10^{-27} kg. Be careful because the other three answers are real. 1 amu = 931 MeV if we want to convert from amu to energy in MeV, so 1,862 MeV is equal to 2 amu; the unit of energy is Joule (J); the conversion from electron volts to Joules is given by 1 eV = 1.602×10^{-19} J; 0.511 MeV/c^2 is the rest mass of the electron.

2. **D** The conversion factor for changing from amu to MeV/c^2 is 1 amu = 931 MeV/c^2; neutron has a rest mass of 939 MeV/c^2, while proton has a rest mass of 938 MeV/c^2. The rest mass of an electron is 0.511 MeV/c^2.

3. **A** The proton has a charge of +1, 1.007277 amu, and a rest mass (in MeV/c^2) of 938. An electron has a charge of −1, 0.000549 amu, and a rest mass (in MeV/c^2) of 0.511; a neutron has 0 charge, 1.008665 amu, and a rest mass (in MeV/c^2) of 939, making the neutron slightly heavier than the proton.

4. **C** A nucleus does not contain electrons, so answers A and B are wrong. Also, positron is the antimatter of electron, which cannot be inside a nucleus. The nucleus of an atom is composed of protons and neutrons; these protons and neutrons are termed nucleons.

5. **B** Electromagnetic force makes charges that interact with each other; it can either attract (oppositely charged particles, like protons in the nucleus and electrons in the shell) or repel (like-charged particles); strong force binds protons and neutrons together to form the nucleus; weak force stabilizes particles through the process of radioactive decay; gravity is the force of attraction between anything that has mass. All four forces keep the atoms together, but electromagnetic force binds electrons to the atom.
Electrons do have gravitational interaction with the nucleus because both have a mass; however, gravitational force is about 36 times weaker than electromagnetic force, and hence C is incorrect.

6. **B** The binding energy of the electron is the amount of energy required to remove one of the electrons from the shell. The energy needed to remove an electron has to be equal or greater than the binding energy of that shell.

7. **C** From the nucleus outward, the shells are labeled, K, L, M, N, etc. K shell is the first shell closest to the nucleus and therefore has the greater binding energy; When the charge of the nucleus increases, the binding energy increases, which is also proportional to Z^2 (atomic number Z = # of protons or # of electrons).

1.7 Atomic and Nuclear Structure (Answers)   61

8. A The valence electrons are the electrons in the lowest energy level of an atom, and they determine the chemical properties of the atom. Shielding electrons are the electrons located in the levels between the nucleus and the valence electrons; they shield the valence electrons from the force of attraction applied by the nucleus. The effective nuclear charge is the charge experienced by the valence electrons after taking into account the number of shielding electrons that surround the nucleus. The nuclear diameter is the size of the nucleus of an atom, and it is estimated to be 10^{-13} cm.

9. C The maximum number of electrons allowed in an orbital shell is determined by the equation $2n^2$, where n represents the number of the energy level in question (K shell = 1, L shell = 2, etc.).
The formula (E^{kl}photon $= E_k - E_l$) is used to find the energy of a characteristic photon created when an L shell electron fills the vacancy created in the K shell due to an electron ejection/emission. $E = mc^2$ is the famous equivalence of mass and energy formula given by Einstein, where the energy of a physical system is numerically equal to the product of its mass and the speed of light square. $T_{1/2} = L_n 2/\lambda$ is the half-life formula, which is the period of time that a radionuclide takes to decay to half of its original value.

10. D The maximum number of electrons in the L shell is 8. This can be calculated using the formula $2n^2$ where n = 1 for the K shell, n = 2 for the L shell and n = 3 for the M shell, etc.

11. C In the periodic table, elements are represented as $^A_Z X$ where symbol A represents the mass number (equal to the number of protons plus the number of neutrons), X is the element's symbol (i.e., C for carbon), and Z is the atomic number which is the number of protons or number of electrons.

12. A The number of electrons equals the atomic number or Z of a neutral atom. Z symbolizes the number of protons or electrons, and the atomic symbol is X. The number of nucleons is equal to A which is the number of protons and neutrons. A photon is a quantum of electromagnetic energy, regarded as a discrete particle having zero mass, no electric charge, and an indefinitely long lifetime.

13. D The number of neutrons in an atom is the number of protons and neutrons (A = mass number) subtracted by the atomic number (Z = number of protons).

14. A The atomic number (Z) is the number of protons in an atom of an element, and it is located in a subscript; gold has 79, every atom of gold contains 79 protons in its nucleus, adding or removing protons from the nucleus of an atom creates a different element, and if a proton is removed from gold, it creates a new atom, in this case platinum, which has 78 protons in its nucleus. Atoms must have a balance between the protons (+) and electrons (−), so the number of electrons equals the number of protons; gold has 79 electrons. The number of neutrons in an atom is $A-Z$, in which A is the mass number or number of protons and neutrons, and it is located in the superscript; for gold $A = 197$. Thus the number of neutrons in gold is $197 - 79 = 118$; $Z = 79$. Remember the number of nucleons = mass number (A) which is the number of protons and neutrons in the nucleus. For any element number of protons = atomic number (Z), number of electrons = number of protons = atomic number (Z), and number of neutrons = mass number (A) − atomic number (Z).

15. B Mass is a property of a body that governs its acceleration when acted on by a force. Up to now, it is impossible to weigh a stationary electron; however, the mass of any object increases as its speed approaches the speed of light, so the rest mass of any object is found that way. The rest mass of an electron is equal to 0.511 (MeV/c^2); the rest mass of a proton is 938 (MeV/c^2), and the neutron rest mass is 939 (MeV/c^2). Remember, the rest mass of a neutron is slightly higher than the rest mass of the proton; the photon has no rest mass, but it has relativistic mass which is a function of the rest mass and the velocity of the object.

16. C The transfer of an electron from one energy level to another in an atom is called a transition. Atoms have all their electrons in the lowest allowable energy levels so they fill level K before L when in their ground state. Ionization occurs when an electron is removed or added to an atom which produces a transfer of energy. The closer the electrons are to the nucleus, the more tightly bound they are to the nucleus due to the attraction between the negative electrons and the positive nucleus; this is called the Coulomb or electromagnetic force.

17. B The maximum number of electrons in an orbit is given by the formula $2n^2$, where n is the orbit number; remember that the first and innermost orbit is the K (1) shell, then L (2), M (3), and N (4). The maximum number of electrons in the M shell is given by $2n^2 = 2 \times 3^2 = 18$.

18. C An atom is electrically neutral when it has the same number of protons and electrons, but if it is ionized, it may lose an electron and have a net positive charge resulting in formation of a positive ion or cation. However, if through ionization an atom captures an electron, it is said to have a net negatively charged, and it is called a negative ion. Characteristic radiation is produced when an electron leaves an inner shell and creates a vacancy, and an electron from an outer shell will fill this vacancy through a transition emitting a photon to conserve energy.

1.7 Atomic and Nuclear Structure (Answers)

19. D Atoms are classified based on different proportions of neutrons and protons. Isoto**p**es are atoms having the same number of **p**rotons in the nucleus, or the same atomic number, but different neutron numbers. Isoto**n**es are atoms whose nuclei have the same number of **n**eutrons but different numbers of protons, or different atomic number. Isobars are atoms having nuclei with the same number of nucleons, or mass number (A) but different number of protons, or different atomic number (Z); although isobars possess approximately equal masses, they differ in chemical properties. Isomers are identical atoms with the same mass number (A) and atomic number (Z) but different nuclear energy states or radioactive properties.

20. D $^{37}_{17}C, ^{39}_{19}P$, are isotones because these elements have the same number of neutrons 20, but a different number of protons. Answer A ($^{131m}_{54}Xe - ^{131}_{54}Xe$) is an isomer since both elements contain the same number of protons as well as neutrons; they only differ in their nuclear energy states (m stands for metastable state). Answer B ($^{76}_{32}Ce, ^{76}_{34}Se$) is an isobar because both elements have the same number of nucleons but different number of protons, and answer C ($^{12}_{6}C, ^{14}_{6}C$) is an isotope because both elements have the same atomic number (Z) but a different mass number (A).

Quiz-2 (Level 2)

1. B The 2p subshell belongs to the L shell ($n=2$), and each p subshell may hold 6 electrons, as long as $n \geq 2$. If $n=1$, which occurs for K shell, there is no 1p subshell since K shell only has 1s subshell.
The binding energies of subshells starting from maximum are 1s, 2s, 2p, 3s, 3p, 4s, 3d, 4p, etc. The numbers for subshells are determined by symmetry. In s subshell, 2 electrons are allowed; in p subshell, 6 electrons are allowed; in d subshell, 10 electrons are allowed. K shell has only 1 subshell, 1s; thus $K(n=1)$ shell contains at most 2 electrons; $L(n=2)$ shell has two subshells, 2s and 2p; thus the maximum number of electrons in L shell is $2+6=8$; $M(n=3)$ shell has three subshells, 3s, 3p, and 3d; thus it may contain $2+6+10=18$ electrons.

2. A Isotopes (refer to answer on Q 19 and 20)

3. B Isotones (refer to answer on Q 19 and 20)

4. C Isobars (refer to answer on Q 19 and 20)

5. D Isomers (refer to answer on Q 19 and 20)

6. A Isotopes (refer to answer on Q 19 and 20)

7. B Isotones (refer to answer on Q 19 and 20)

8. C Isobars (refer to answer on Q 19 and 20)

9. D Isomers (refer to answer on Q 19 and 20)

10. B Fission is the splitting of a large atom into two or more smaller stable nuclei producing great amount of energy (heat), radiation, and additional neutrons. The breakup can be accomplished if a neutron strikes the nucleus. Fusion is the opposite of fission, where light nuclei are combined or fused to create larger atoms and great amount of energy is produced. For fusion to occur, a high-density, high-temperature environment is required. Nuclei can lose excess energy during an isomeric decay by gamma emission where the nucleus releases excess energy by the emission of gamma rays from the nucleus or by internal conversion where the nucleus releases its energy by the emission of one of the orbital electrons from the atom.

11. C $c = \nu \lambda$ is the formula that establishes the relationship between wavelength (λ), frequency (ν), and velocity (c), where c is expressed in meter/second, λ in meters, and ν in cycles/second or hertz. $E = h\nu$ is the formula that establishes the amount of energy carried by a photon where E is the energy (Joules), h is the Planck's constant (6.62×10^{-34} j-s), and ν is the frequency (cycles/second). Answer B is the combined equation where E is expressed in electron volts (eV). Answer D is the rate of decay of a radioactive material or activity.

12. C The most stable atoms are the ones that have even numbers of protons and even numbers of neutrons, this is followed by atoms with even numbers of protons and odd numbers of neutrons, and atoms with odd numbers of protons and even numbers of neutrons are the least stable.

13. A Avogadro's number (N_A) refers to the ratio of the number of constituent particles in a sample to the amount of substance. By having this quantity every mole of a substance contains the same number of atoms. The smallest quantity of an element is an atom, the amount of energy required to remove an electron from an atom is the binding energy, and the number of electrons per unit cubic distance is the electron density.

14. D The accepted value of Avogadro's number (N_A) is 6.0228×10^{23} atoms per gram atomic weight. The speed of light is 3×10^8 m/s, 1 eV is equal to 1.602×10^{-19} C, and 1 amu = 1.66×10^{-27} kg.

1.7 Atomic and Nuclear Structure (Answers)

15. A Avogadro's number (N_A) can be used to calculate the number of atoms per gram, grams per atoms, or electrons per gram. The amount of energy is calculated by the equation $E=hv$, where h is the Planck's constant (6.62×10^{-23} J-s) and v is the frequency (cycles/second).

16. B To calculate the number of atoms/g, grams/atom, or number of electrons/g; the student must know Avogadro's number (N_A) value (6.0228×10^{23} atoms per gram atomic weight) and the atomic weight (A_w) of the material in question, in this case Cobalt ($A_w = 58.93$)
Apply the formula:
Number of atoms/g = N_A/A_w
Number of atoms/g = $6.0228 \times 10^{23}/58.93$
Number of atoms/g = 1.0220×10^{22}

17. C Number of atoms/g = N_A/A_w
Grams/atom = A_w/N_A
Number of electrons/g = $N_A \times Z/A_w$

18. D According to the atomic mass unit, the mass of a neutron is 1.00866 amu, the mass of an electron is 0.000548 amu, and the mass of a proton is 1.00727 amu; the photon does not have mass.

19. C The mass defect is defined as the difference in mass between an atom and the sum of the masses of its constituent particles; in other words, the mass of an atom is less than the mass of its individual constituents (proton, neutron, and electron). This is due to the fact that when the nucleus is formed, some mass is destroyed and converted into energy to keep the nucleons together. Every gram atomic weight of a substance contains the same number of atoms is the definition of Avogadro's number (N_A) value (6.0228×10^{23}). The propagation of energy through space or a material medium is the definition of radiation

20. E The electron is the only fundamental particle within the atom, so it cannot be broken into smaller particles. The electron can undergo collisions, has a mass (9.109389×10^{-31} kg), a charge (-1), and it spins around its axes creating a magnetic field. On the other hand, protons and neutrons are composed of combinations of the three quarks and the gluons.

21. B An atom is defined as the smallest component of an element having the chemical properties of that element. An atom consists of a nucleus containing neutrons and protons with electrons surrounding the nucleus. An element is a substance that consists of atoms with the same number of protons or same atomic number, the nucleus is the central part of an atom containing proton and neutrons, and protons and neutrons are composed of quarks.

22. B The configuration of the atom is called the Bohr model because Niels Bohr proposed this structure in 1913. The Bohr atom consists of a central nucleus which includes neutrons and protons surrounded by electrons that orbit around it. Niels Henrik David Bohr was a physicist who made great contributions to understanding atomic structure and quantum mechanics, for which he received the Nobel Prize in Physics in 1922. In 1896 Henri Becquerel discovered radioactivity, in 1895 Wilhelm Roentgen discovered X-ray and was awarded with the Nobel Prize in Physics in 1901, and Marie Curie and her husband Pierre Curie discovered the element Radium in 1898, and they received the Nobel Prize in Physics in 1903.

23. E All are correct. Ions are charged atoms where the number of electrons is different than the number of protons; they are named cations if the number of electrons is less than the number of protons and anions if the number of electrons exceeds the number of protons.

24. C All chemical atomic bonds involve sharing of electrons in the outer shell, so unstable atoms have excess or deficient of number of electrons in the outer shell, and they will become stable by bonding with another atom so that the outer shell has the amount of electrons required to be stable. A metallic bond is when an atom has a few electrons in the outer shell and tends to lose them to empty the shell. If an atom is deficient of a few electrons in the outer shell, it will look for another atom to bond with to fill the outer shell (nonmetal). This bond involves a sharing of the electrons between the bonding atoms and is called a covalent bond. An ionic bond occurs when a metal and nonmetal atom come together and one atom gives up an electron to the other atom, making a positive and a negative ion that bind together due to an electromagnetic attraction. Van der Waals bond is the attractions between atoms and differs from covalent and ionic bonding in that they are caused by correlations in the fluctuating polarizations of nearby particles.

25. D ^{137}Cs decomposes to a short life ^{137m}Ba by beta decay, so ^{137m}Ba is the daughter of ^{137}Cs, its half-life is 2.55 min, and ^{137}Cs half-life is 30 years. Both atoms possess the same mass number ($A = 137$) or total number of protons and neutrons. Remember, this is not to be confused with the atomic number (Z) or number of protons in the nucleus which identifies the chemical element. Additionally isotopes have the same atomic number but different number of neutrons, so these cannot be isotopes (they are isobars). ^{137}Cs has an atomic number (Z) of 55, while ^{137m}Ba has an atomic number (Z) of 56. ^{137}Cs is used for treatment of cancer as intracavitary brachytherapy.

Quiz-3 (Level 3)

1. **C** A relativistic particle always has larger kinetic energy than a nonrelativistic particle of the same type. An electron of a speed of 0.6c is relativistic.

2. **B** A meson is composed of a quark and an antiquark of different flavor. A is wrong, because a quark and an antiquark of the same flavor will annihilate.

3. **C** The cross section for neutrino interacting with matter is negligible, so the deposited dose is also negligible and does not need to be accounted for.

4. **D** Due to special relativity, as a particle approaches the speed of light, the mass of the particle increases and the time in a moving reference frame slows down. At speed of 0.999c, $t = t_0/(1-0.999^2)^{1/2}$; thus $t = 20 t_0$. No need to worry about the muon decay.

5. **B** A neutron has a structure, which contains 3 quarks (udd) and gluons. Those 3 quarks have their antiparticles, i.e., antiquarks. An antineutron is composed of 3 antiquarks.
   People used to think that neutron's antiparticle is itself in the time when antiparticles were discovered. However, this was because people had not found out that neutrons are made of quarks.

6. **A** There are three types of weak decays found in nature; each one is associated with a type of neutrino, plus their antiparticles. Therefore, there are six types of neutrinos in nature.

7. **A** Special relativity unifies electric interaction and magnetic interaction. In brief, a static magnetic field can be considered as a static electric field in another frame of reference.

8. **D** Gravity is the field that cannot be unified.

9. **D** In general, they are not exchangeable. Atomic bomb needs much higher purity fuel.

10. **B** In field theory, an interaction occurs through exchanging a particle. Interactions between protons or neutrons occur by exchanging mesons. Weak interactions occur by exchanging $W^{\pm}$ or neutral vector bosons.

11. **A** In the standard model, quarks are capable to have all interactions: strong, weak, and electromagnetic. Of course, quarks may have gravitational interaction because they have mass, but this is already known; thus it is not discussed in the standard model.

1.8 Radioactivity (Answers)

Quiz-1 (Level 1)

1. **C** In 1896 Henri Becquerel discovered radioactivity. In 1895 Wilhelm Roentgen discovered X-rays, and in 1898 Marie Curie and her husband Pierre Curie discovered the element Radium.

2. **A** Radioactivity is defined as the emission of radiation from unstable nuclei of element in the form of particles (e.g., alpha or beta particles), electromagnetic radiation, or both. Answer B is the definition of ionization radiation, C is the definition of linear energy transfer (LET), and D is the definition of activity.

3. **B** The number of atoms disintegrating per unit time is proportional to the number of radioactive atoms. Additionally, the average life or the mean life is the average lifetime for the decay of radioactive atoms. The activity per unit mass of a radionuclide is termed specific activity, and the time required for either the activity or the number of radioactive atoms to decay to half the initial value is termed half-life.

4. **D** $\tau = 1.44\, T_{1/2}$. Mean or average life is the average lifetime for the decay of radioactive atoms, where 1.44 is $1/\ln 2$ ($\ln(2) = 0.693$) and $T_{1/2}$ is the time required for either the activity or the number of radioactive atoms to decay to half the initial value.
   Remember: mean life τ is always longer than half-life $T_{1/2}$, and that is why there is a factor 1.44. Another formula to remember is that $\tau = 1/\lambda$.

5. **E** $N = N_0 e^{-\lambda t}$. It is impossible to know when a particular atom will disintegrate, but in a large group of atoms it is possible to calculate the amount that will disintegrate in a given time by the formula $N = N_0 e^{-\lambda t}$ (N is equal to the proportion of atoms that will disintegrate in a given time). N_0 = the initial number of radioactive atoms and e is the number base of the natural logarithm ($e = 2.718$). λ is a constant of proportionality or decay constant, and the − sign is used because decay is a negative (loss) concept ($\lambda = \ln 2 / T_{1/2}$). Finally, t represents the time of interest.

6. **B** $A = -\lambda N$ is the formula for remaining activity or the rate of decay of a radioactive material at time t.

7. **C** The time required for either the activity or the number of radioactive atoms to decay to half the initial value is given by the equation $T_{1/2} = 0.693/\lambda$, where $\ln(2)$ is the natural logarithm of 2 having a value of

1.8 Radioactivity (Answers)

0.693 and λ is the decay constant. It is important to recognize that after one half-life, the activity is ½ the initial value; after two half-lives, it is ¼, and so on. Thus, after n half-lives, the activity is reduced to $(1/2)^n$ of the initial activity.

8. **D** $\tau = 1/\lambda$ is similar to the equation $\tau = 1.44\, T_{1/2}$ explained in question 4 above.

9. **C** $T_{1/2} = \ln(2)/\lambda = T_{1/2} = 0.693/\lambda$ since $\ln(2) = 0.693$; for more explanation, see answer for Q 7 above.

10. **B** $A = A_0 e^{-\lambda t}$ or $A_n = A_0 \exp(-0.693 \times t/T_{1/2})$ is similar to formula $N = N_0 e^{-\lambda t}$, but expressed in terms of activity, where A is the activity remaining at time t and A_0 is the original activity, e is base natural log (approximately 2.718), λ the decay constant $= 0.693/T_{1/2}$ (where $T_{1/2}$ = half-life), and t is the amount of time elapsed from A_0 to A.

11. **F** Specific activity is the activity of a radionuclide per unit mass; its formula is $SA = \lambda(N_A/A_W)$ where SA = specific activity, λ is the decay constant or the disintegration rate, N_A is Avogadro's number (6.02×10^{23} atoms/g at. wt), and A_W is the atomic weight. The unit of SA is the curie/gram.

12. **G** According to Avogadro's law, every gram atomic weight of a substance contains the same number of atoms, so the formula Number of atoms/g $= N_A/A_w$ is used to calculate number of atoms per gram; equally the number of grams per atom can be calculated by gram/atom $= A_w/N_A$ or the electrons per gram, number of electrons/g $= N_A \times Z/A_W$.

13. **A** $\lambda = 0.693/T_{1/2}$ is used to calculate the decay constant for a radioisotope.

14. **D** Many radionuclide undergo transformation in which the original nuclide (parent) gives rise to a radioactive or stable nuclide (daughter). If the half-life of the daughter is slightly shorter than the half-life of the parent than transient equilibrium exists. In transient equilibrium, there is a point of maximum activity for the daughter that exceeds the activity of the parent. The $t_{max} = ((1.44 \times T_p T_d)/(T_p - T_d)) \times \ln(T_p/T_d)$. If half-life of the parent is much, much longer than half-life of the daughter, secular equilibrium is achieved where the daughter activity builds up and remains constant over time. Finally if the parent and daughter decay at their own respective half-lives, it is said that no equilibrium is established. When there is no equilibrium after some period of time, the parent is depleted and only the daughter remains. There is a rule of thumb that transient equilibrium is reached approximately $4(t_{1/2})$ of daughter and secular is established approximately $6(t_{1/2})$ of daughter.

Quiz-2 (Level 2)

1. **A.** Graph II: Secular equilibrium
    B. Graph I: Transient equilibrium
    C. Graph III: No equilibrium
    D. Graph IV: Proton depth dose distribution showing the Bragg peak.

2. **E** All answers are correct; radioactive nuclides with high atomic number (≥ 82) tend to decay by the emission of an alpha particle (2 protons and 2 neutrons; $^4_2$He); as a result, the atomic number is reduced by two and the mass number by four. Beta particle appears with the ejection of a positive electron (positron) or a negative electron (negatron) from the nucleus; it should be known that neither of these particles exists as such inside the nucleus but are created at the instant of the decay. In ß- decay, the atomic mass remains the same but the atomic number (number of protons) increases by one. In ß⁺ decay, the atomic mass remains the same but the atomic number decreases by one. Electron capture is an event in which one of the orbital electrons is captured by the nucleus, thus transforming a proton into a neutron, effectively decreasing the atomic number by one similar to ß⁺ decay. Finally, internal conversion means the nucleus can lose energy, and in this process the excess nuclear energy is passed on to one of the orbital electrons, which is then ejected from the atom. In internal conversion, there is no change in atomic number, and with the loss of the electron, the atom becomes ionized (+1 charge).

3. **A.** α = alpha particle
    B. β = beta particle
    C. β⁻ = negatron or negative electron
    D. β⁺ = positron or positive electron
    E. γ = gamma ray

4. **C** As can be seen in reaction C ($^A_Z X \rightarrow {}^{A-4}_{Z-2}Y + {}^4_2\text{He} + Q$) atomic number (Z) decreases by 2 and atomic mass (A) decreases by 4. This is a characteristic of alpha particle decay. $^4_2$He is a helium atom, and Q represents the total energy released in the process which is called disintegration energy. Answer A ($^A_Z X \rightarrow {}^A_{Z+1}Y + {}^0_{-1}\beta + v' + Q$) is a negatron emission (β⁻) where a neutron is converted into a proton, negatron, and antineutrino, Z increases by 1, but A remains the same. Answer B ($^A_Z X \rightarrow {}^A_{Z-1}Y + {}^0_1\beta + v + Q$) is a positron emission (β⁺) where a proton is converted into a neutron, positron, and neutrino and Z decreases by 1. Finally, answer D ($^A_Z X + {}^0_{-1}e \rightarrow {}^A_{Z-1}Y + v + Q$) is an electron capture process where one orbital electrons is captured by the nucleus transforming a proton into a neutron, similar to β⁺ decay.

1.8 Radioactivity (Answers)

5.
- **A.** V
- **B.** IV
- **C.** III
- **D.** I
- **E.** II

6. D All the answers are correct. The formula to calculate decay constant is $\lambda = 0.693/T_{1/2}$, where 0.693 is the natural logarithm of 2 (ln(2)); answers I and II are converted to hours. Answers I and III are using scientific notations which you must know and understand.

7. A The half-life is not always given for specific problems, especially for well-known radionuclides, so in order to know the decay constant, the half-life of the radionuclide in question needs to be known. ^{60}Co half-life is 5.26 years; ^{137}Cs half-life is 30 years. The decay constant formula is $\lambda = 0.693/T_{1/2}$, and after the math is done, ^{60}Co $\lambda = 0.1317$ per year versus ^{137}Cs $\lambda = 0.0231$ per year. The ^{60}Co decay constant is higher than the Cs-137 decay constant. A shorter half-life will have a larger decay constant.

8. C After n number of half-lives, the initial activity of a radionuclide decreases to ½ to the power of n or 0.5^n, where n is the number of half-lives. Answers II and III are correct. Remember, you must know the decimal equivalent, and answer II is the decimal equivalent of number III.

9. A As previously mentioned after n number of half-lives, the initial activity of a radionuclide will decrease to ½ to the power of n; in this case, for a radionuclide having an activity of 200 mCi to decay to 3.125 mCi, 6 half-lives are needed. $0.5^6 \times 200 = 3.125$, where 6 is the number of half-lives required to reduce 200–3.125 mCi. 200 is the initial activity. You can also verify your answer by dividing $200/2 = 100$ (1 $T_{1/2}$), $100/2 = 50$ (2 $T_{1/2}$), etc.

10. B For the activity in the future to be calculated, the formula of activity must be known ($A_n = A_0\, e^{-\lambda t}$); as you can see the decay constant (λ) is part of the activity formula, so the decay constant formula must be also known ($\lambda = 0.693/T_{1/2}$); finally, the question does not include the half-life of Au-198, so the half-life must be also known to find the λ. Au-198 $T_{1/2} = 2.7$ days.
The question includes *half-value layer* of Au-198; be careful, this is just to trick you so that you change half-life with half-value layer. With all that information, the activity of Au-198 can be calculated. Be organized.
Initial activity (A_0) = 15 mCi
Activity in 20 days (A_n) = ?
Half-value layer = 2.5, not needed

Half-life $(T_{1/2}) = 2.7$ days
$\lambda = 0.693/T_{1/2}$ $A_n = A_0 e^{-\lambda t}$
$\lambda = 0.693/2.7$ $A_n = 15 e^{-.2556 \times 20}$
$\lambda = 0.2556$ $A_n = 0.09036$ mCi
Answer A is the decay constant of gold $= 0.2556$ per day; $C = 2.8931$ mCi is if we plug $\lambda = 2.5$ instead of 0.2556 into activity formula which is found if the half-value layer is used for the calculation, and $D = 2,490$ mCi is the answer if we omit the negative sign during the activity calculation.

11. A There are several ways to solve this problem, and two possible methods can be found below. Method #1 is listed first and it is recommended. It might take a few more steps, so make sure you are organized.
Method #1: The question is asking about activity in the past. To know the activity in the past, the − sign must be omitted on the formula $(A_n = A_0 e^{-\lambda t})$ and replaced by $(A_n = A_0 e^{+\lambda t})$. Again the $T_{1/2}$ of I-125 must be known (59.6 days) to find the decay constant (λ). Be organized.
Initial activity $(A_0) = ?$
Activity in 10 days $(A_n) = 17.8095$ mCi
Half-life $(T_{1/2}) = 59.6$ days
$T = 10$ days
$\lambda = 0.693/T_{1/2}$ $A_0 = A_n e^{+\lambda t}$
$\lambda = 0.693/59.6$ $A_0 = 17.8095 \, e^{0.0116 \times 10}$
$\lambda = 0.0116$ $A_0 = 20$ mCi
Method #2: This question can also be interpreted as "In 10 days an I-125 source decays to 17.8095 mCi, find out the original activity."
All one needs to do is to find the ratio of decay in 10 days, given the half-life, so
$(0.5)^{10/59.6} = 0.89$
So the original activity $= 17.8095/0.89 = 20$ (mCi)
This method uses half-life directly, bypassing the decay constant. *In a timed exam, this method is highly recommended but in the end, choose the method that makes the most sense for you. Also, in a time crunch, eliminate the answers that are not possible like answer B as this activity is less than the required activity.*

12. C Be organized; the activity of both radionuclide will be equal at 9.15 days.
Rn-222   Au-198
$Ao = 10$ mCi $Ao = 5$ mCi
$\lambda = 1.8094 \times 10^{-1}$ $\lambda = 2.567 \times 10^{-1}$
$A_0 = A_n e^{-\lambda t}$ $A_0 = A_n e^{-\lambda t}$
$10 \times e^{-.18094 \times t} = 5 \times e^{-0.2567 \times t}$
$\ln(10) - 0.18094 \times t = \ln(5) - 0.2567 \times t$
$2.302 - 0.18094 \times t = 1.609 - 0.2567 \times t$
$2.302 - 1.609 = 0.18094 \times t - 0.2567 \times t$
$0.693 = 0.07576 \times t$
$T = 0.693/0.07576$
$T = 9.15$ days

1.8 Radioactivity (Answers)

13. B The mean or average life of any radionuclide is the average lifetime for the decay of radioactive atoms, and its formula is $\tau = 1.44 \times T_{1/2}$ or $\tau = 1/\lambda$, as mentioned previously. You must know the $T_{1/2}$ of the radionuclide because it is not always given. Remember: Co-60s $T_{1/2} = 5.26$ years. Again, the photon energy is not part of the formula, so be careful not to change the $T_{1/2}$ value by the energy given in the question.
$T_a = 1.44 \times T_{1/2}$
$T_a = 1.44 \times 5.26$
$T_a = 7.57$ years
Remember: the mean life has nothing to do with the γ-ray energy.

14. B A bombardment of a nucleus by α-particle with the subsequent emission of a neutron is written as the (α, n) reaction. The first letter, α, stands for the bombarding particle and the second one, n, stands for the ejected particle, in this case a neutron. Answer C is written as (p, α) reaction. Answer D is (p, d) reaction, where d stands for deuteron, a combination of a proton and a neutron ($^2_1$H).

15. D All are correct. A radionuclide is reduced over time after intake into the body by elimination by biological (λ_b) and by physical decay of the isotope (λ_p). The calculation for biological decay is identical to physical decay; you only need to know the biological half-life.

16. C Effective half-life is shorter than both physical and biological half-life ($T_{eff} = T_p \times T_b/T_p + T_b$). This makes sense as the combined effect of two decay processes will always result in a faster effective decay than one process on its own.

17. D Answers A and D are not correct since T_{eff} is always shorter than both T_p and T_b. Use the following formula to find the value of T_{eff}:
$1/T_{eff} = 1/T_p + 1/T_b$; this is the primitive formula, so $T_{eff} = T_p \times T_b/T_p + T_b$
$T_{eff} = T_7 \times T_{14}/T_7 + T_{14}$ $1/T_{eff} = 1/7 + 1/14$
$T_{eff} = 98/21$ $1/T_{eff} = 0.1428 + 0.0714$
$T_{eff} = 4.66$ h $1/T_{eff} = 0.2142$
                                              $T_{eff} = 1/0.2142 = 4.66$ h.

18. B $T_{eff} = T_p \times T_b/T_p + T_b$ or $1/T_{eff} = 1/T_p + 1/T_b$ is the formula used to calculate the T_{eff} or the fraction of a radionuclide eliminated per unit time by biological and physical processes. $T_a = 1.44 \times T_{1/2}$ is the formula used to calculate average or mean life or the average lifetime for the decay of radioactive atoms, and finally, the equation $A_0 = A_n e^{-\lambda t}$ is used to calculate activity or the rate of decay of a radionuclide. Remember all these formulas must be well known.

19. **B** It is possible to solve this using the formula $A_t = A_0 e^{-\lambda t}$ and then calculating the decay constant by $\lambda = -0.693/T\frac{1}{2}$, but this is very time consuming. Here is the suggested way (half-life of Ir-192 is 74.2 days):
$(0.5)^{X/74.2} = 0.995$, so
$X/74.2 = \ln(0.995)/\ln(0.5)$
Thus, $X = 74.2 \times \ln(0.995)/\ln(0.5) = 0.537$ (days)
A rule of thumb is that after 1 day an Ir-192 source will decay 1 %. Thus if it decays to 99.5 % of its original strength, i.e., decay 0.5 %, it is reasonable to estimate that it will take about half day, so answer (B) 0.537 days is correct.

20. **C** The decay constant is a statistical event process; in other words, it is impossible to know when a particular atom will disintegrate, but it is possible to know in a large collection of atoms the proportion that will disintegrate in a given time. Therefore, the number of atoms disintegrating per unit time is proportional to the number of radioactive atoms. Also, the decay constant symbol is λ and the decay constant is inversely proportional to half-life ($T_{1/2}$). Finally, remember that the half-life is the time required for the number of radioactive atoms to decay to half the initial value and not the decay constant.

21. **B** Electron capture decay is a result of a deficit of neutrons (low neutron to proton (n/p) ratio). The ratio is increased by converting a proton into a neutron. This can be done by capturing one of the orbital electrons by the nucleus transforming a proton into a neutron, often called K capture. This gives rise to characteristic X-ray with emission of Auger electrons. See question/answer 19 above. ß+ decay would result in the same increase in the n/p ration.

22. **A** In a decay process by internal conversion, the radionuclide has excess nuclear energy from the nucleus and passes it on to one orbital electron, which is then ejected from the atom and creates a vacancy which gives rise to characteristic X-ray with emission of Auger electrons. There is no change in atomic number and the resulting atom is an ion with a charge of +1 due to the loss of the electron.

23. **B** Both ß- decays, internal conversion and electron capture, give rise to emission of Auger electrons. Electron capture increases the n/p ratio by capturing one of the orbital electrons by the nucleus and transforms a proton into a neutron and gives rise to characteristic X-ray with emission of Auger electrons. Internal conversion occurs when a radionuclide passes the excess of nuclear energy on to one orbital electron, which is then ejected from the atom and creates a vacancy which gives rise to characteristic X-ray with emission of Auger electrons.

1.8 Radioactivity (Answers)

24. C Alpha particles (α) have the same nuclear structure of a $^4_2$He atom. During alpha decay, the atomic number (Z) decreases by 2, and atomic mass (A) decreases by 4 as the alpha particle is composed of two protons and two neutrons. ^{3}He is an isotope of helium, which is composed of 1 neutron and 2 protons.

25. A Radioactivity or rate of decay can be affected only by the atomic nucleus composition. Radioactivity is the process by which an atomic nucleus of an unstable atom losses energy by emitting energy and/or particles. There are some atoms that decay faster than others due to their composition.

26. C Radioactive decay is defined as the process by which an atomic nucleus of an unstable atom becomes more stable by emitting particles and/or electromagnetic radiation. Half-life ($T_{1/2}$) is the time necessary for a radioactive material to decay to 50 % of its original activity. Transmutation is the transformation of an element into another kind of element that takes place during radioactivity decay. Electron equilibrium is a condition in a high-energy photon beam where the number of electrons coming to rest equals the number of electrons being into motion by new photon interactions.

27. B Beta decay occurs when the neutron to proton ratio is too great or too small in the nucleus of an atom, so a neutron turns into a proton, or vice versa. Positron emission occurs during beta decay when the neutron to proton ratio is too small, so a proton turns into a neutron and the positron is emitted. Also, electron capture occurs when the neutron to proton ratio is too small, so the nucleus captures an electron which turns a proton into a neutron. Alpha decay (helium emission; remember an alpha particle is just a helium atom) occurs when the nucleus has too many protons and emits a helium nucleus. Finally, gamma decay occurs when the nucleus is in an excited energy state, so a photon called a gamma ray is emitted to lower the energy state.

28. C Beta decay is the process of radioactive decay in which an ejection of a positive or a negative electron from the nucleus occurs. A positron with a spectrum of energies is emitted in a beta plus (β$^+$) decay process in which positron-emitting nuclides have a deficit of neutrons. On the other hand, a negatron with a spectrum of energies is emitted in a beta minus (β$^-$) decay process in which the radionuclides have excessive number of neutrons. An alpha particle is emitted from radioactive nuclides with very high atomic numbers (typically greater than 82). Internal conversion occurs with the emission of a gamma (γ) ray from the nucleus to return the atom to a non-excited state.

1.9 Production of X-Ray (Answers)

Quiz-1 (Level 2)

1. **C** X-rays were discovered by Wilhelm Roentgen in 1895. A year after in 1896, Henri Becquerel discovered radioactivity. Marie and Pierre Curie discovered element Radium in 1898, and finally, the most remarkable scientific contribution of twentieth century was done by Albert Einstein, with the introduction of general theory of relativity in 1915–1916.

2. **A** The X-ray tube consists of a glass envelope to allow for the high vacuum inside the tube. The cathode (– charge) and anode (+ charge) are contained inside the evacuated tube. Answer VI is incorrect; a tissue compensator is used when irradiating an irregular surface. Examples of tissue compensators are bolus, wedges, and multiple treatment fields.

3. **C** All answers are correct except C because electrons are emitted from the cathode and are accelerated to the anode using an electric field. The cathode filaments are heated to produce electrons and a high voltage is applied between the anode and the cathode to accelerate the electrons. Since the cathode is negative and the anode is positive, electrons are accelerated toward the anode and strike the tungsten anode target to produce X-rays.

4. **B** The term thermionic emission refers to the emission of electrons by the heated tungsten filament and the particles are called thermions. The ratio of output energy emitted as X-ray to the input energy deposit by electrons is called efficiency of X-ray production. The region at the edge of a radiation beam where the dose rate changes rapidly as a function of distance from the beam axis is called the penumbra. Answer D describes ionization, where a neutral atom acquires a positive or a negative charge either by a removal or acquisition of an orbital electron.

5. **A** I, II, and III are correct; the target must have high atomic number and high melting point (3,370 °C). The high atomic number allows for more efficient X-ray production, and the high melting point is required as there is a lot of heat generated during the production of X-rays. Tungsten with $Z=74$ is preferred as the anode material.

6. **C** The efficiency of X-ray production depends on the atomic number (Z) or the number of protons or electrons in the target. X-rays are produced in a process called Bremsstrahlung (German for breaking or slowing down). The incoming electrons interact with the positively charged nucleus in the target which causes them to accelerate and change direction. As the elec-

1.9 Production of X-Ray (Answers)

trons accelerate, they release the X-rays. The higher the Z of the target, the more efficient is the Bremsstrahlung effect. Remember, the mass number (A) is the number of protons and neutrons, and it is not related to the efficiency of X-ray production.

7. **D** A rotating anode is used as well as oil, water, or air outside the glass envelope to help dissipate the heat from the anode. The target is actually angled, but this is to create the desired size of the focal spot. The added filtration is used to enrich the beam with higher-energy photons by absorbing the lower-energy ones that cannot be used for imaging. The cathode focusing cup is created to direct the electrons toward the anode so that they strike the target in a well-defined area.

8. Fig. 1.3.1

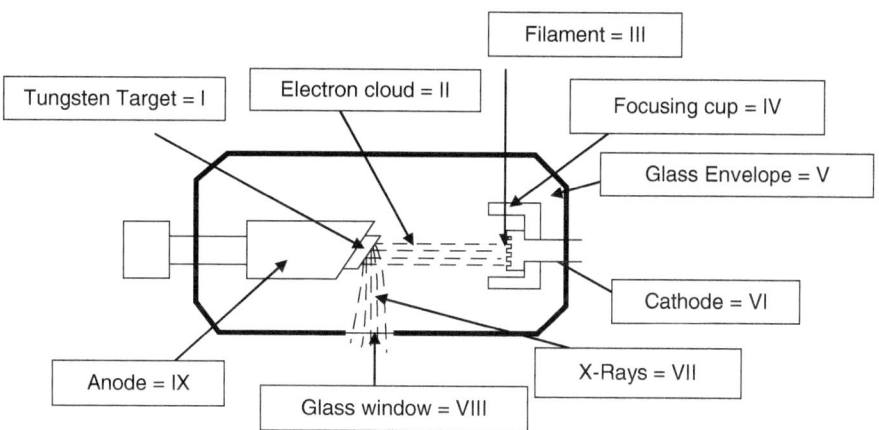

Fig. 1A.3.1

9.
- A. Anode (VI)
- B. Cathode (IV)
- C. Focusing cup (I)
- D. Filament (V)
- E. Glass window (III)
- F. X-rays (IX)
- G. Electron cloud (VIII)
- H. Tungsten target (VII)
- I. Glass envelope (II)
- J. Focal spot (X)

10. **D** Large focal spot is used in therapy machines where radiographic image quality is not the overriding concern. Diagnostic X-ray machines used both large and small focal spots, but mainly small due to the need of sharp radiographic images. The disadvantage of a small focal spot is the amount of heat generated per unit area, limiting beam current and exposure time. Stationary focal spots are used in dental or small portable units. There are two types of focal spots: small (up to 2 mm) and large (up to 7 mm).

11. **B** The target is angle about 30° in therapy machine, and the apparent focal spot size is 5×5–7×7 mm, whereas in diagnostic radiology the angle ranges from 6° to 17°, (usually 12°) and the apparent focal spot size is around 0.1×0.1–2×2 mm.

Fig. 1A.3.2

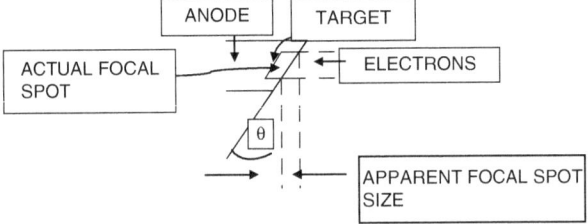

12. **C** Be organized. The apparent focal spot size is equal to the size of the actual focal spot times the sine of the target angle. Remember the apparent focal spot is never bigger than the actual focal spot.
    A = focal spot size = 2.5 mm
    θ = angle of target = 20°
    a = apparent focal spot
    a = A sin θ
    a = 2.5 sin 20
    a = 0.85 mm

13. **A** The function of the low-voltage circuit on an X-ray generator is to supply a heating current to the filament (low voltage, high current). On the other hand, to accelerate the electrons, a low-current, high-voltage electric field is required. The filament temperature controls the tube current, and the autotransformer and a rheostat provide a stepwise adjustment in voltage.

14. **A=** IV. Remember that the standard for electrical lines is alternating current which means that half the time the voltage is positive and the other half of the time the voltage is negative. When the voltage is negative, the anode will repel rather than attract electrons and therefore cannot generate X-rays.

1.9 Production of X-Ray (Answers)

B = V. With a half-wave rectification, when the voltage is negative, the rectifier blocks the electrical current. This is inefficient since the anode can only be used half of the time.

C = II. With full-wave rectification, when the voltage is negative, the polarity is reversed so the anode can remain positive at all times.

D = III. A transformer is used to change the voltage in an electrical circuit. In an X-ray generator a step-up transformer would be used to generate the high voltage to accelerate the electrons and a step-down transformer would be used to generate the high-current, low-voltage electric field for the filament. A simple transformer works by having a loop of conducting material. The incoming wire is wrapped around one side of the conducting material, and a second wire is wrapped around the other side. The ratio of the number of loops controls the voltage in and out of the transformer.

E = I

15. B The two types of X-rays are Bremsstrahlung X-rays and characteristic X-rays. Coherent scattering, photoelectric effect, Compton effect, pair production, and photo disintegration are types of interactions of photons (not electrons) with matter. Annihilation radiation is part of pair production process and results when a positron interacts with an electron.

16. E All answers are characteristics of Bremsstrahlung radiation. Also remember that Bremsstrahlung radiation is a continuous radiation spectrum, not a discrete or single energy. Each electron may have one or more Bremsstrahlung interactions.

17. B Transmission-type targets are used in megavoltage X-ray production (linear accelerators and sometimes betatrons and microtrons). This type of target allows electrons to produce an X-ray beam on the opposite side of the bombardment. Reflection (or scattering) targets are used on low-voltage X-ray tubes such as orthovoltage and superficial machines. Diagnostic X-rays are created on the same side of bombardment and due to the lower energy (kV range) are emitted around 90° from the direction of the incident electron. A flattening filter is not a target; it is located in the machine to make the beam intensity uniform across the field when inserted in the beam path. Filtration refers to the removal of low-energy photons when a filter is placed into the X-ray beam path.

18. C The energy loss per atom by electrons depends on the square of the atomic number. Thus the probability of Bremsstrahlung production varies with Z^2 of the target material where the higher the atomic number, the higher the probability of production of photons. However, the efficiency which remains constant of X-ray production depends on the first power of atomic number and the voltage applied to the tube. The efficiency of X-ray production increases by increasing the projected electron energy.

19. B Characteristic X-ray production is one of the two methods of X-ray production. The removal of an orbital electron in the K, L, or M shell by a direct hit of an incoming electron leaves the atom ionized. To fill this gap in the lower-energy shell, a higher-energy-level electron drops down emitting a characteristic X-ray whose energy is equal to the energy difference between the two electron shells. Remember that the photoelectric effect is an event in which a photon interacts with an atom and ejects one of the orbital electrons leaving the atom ionized. For Bremsstrahlung explanation see question 16 above. The Compton effect is a process where the photon interacts with an atomic electron. The electron receives some energy from the photon and is emitted at an angle while the photon with a reduced energy is scattered.

20. E All the answers are true about characteristic radiation. It is called characteristic radiation because the radiation produced is a characteristic of the element in the target which is dependent on the energy levels of the various electron shells between which the transitions take place.

21. B The formula to find energy of the photon when a transition takes place is $h\nu = E_k - E_L$, where E_k and E_L are the electron binding energies of the K and L shell, respectively. The other answers are multiplication, division, and addition, so be careful; all the formulas must be well known and take your time answering the question.
$h\nu = E_k - E_L$
$h\nu = 8.980 - 1.100$
$h\nu = 7.880$ keV

22. A. Illustration I. Bremsstrahlung process: a high-speed electron passes near the nucleus and undergoes a sudden deflection and acceleration. Part or all of its energy is dissociated from it and propagates in space as electromagnetic radiation.
  B. Illustration II. Characteristic radiation: An incident electron ejects an orbital electron leaving a vacancy. An outer orbital electron will fall down to fill the vacancy, and in doing so, a photon is created with an energy equal to the energy difference between the shells.
  C. Illustration VI. Coherent scattering: A photon passes near an orbital electron and sets it into an oscillation that re-irradiates the photon at the same frequency but at a different angle. No energy is transferred.
  D. Illustration III. Pair production: A photon with energy greater than 1.02 MeV interacts with the electromagnetic field of a nucleus and gives up all its energy by creating a negative electron (electron) and a positive electron (positron).

23. C The two types of filtration used in X-ray machine are inherent filtration and added filtration. Inherent filtration results from the glass and/or aluminum window that is required to maintain the vacuum in the X-ray tube. There is

1.9 Production of X-Ray (Answers)   81

no way to avoid this filtration or a vacuum would not be possible. Added filtration is used to "harden" the X-ray beam. Hardening is a process where the low-energy photons are removed leaving the higher-energy photons in the spectrum. Beam hardening removes the low-energy photons that do not have enough energy to penetrate through the body, increasing dose to the patient but not contributing to the image. A flattening filter makes the beam intensity uniform across the field when inserted in the beam path, and the magnetron is a device that produces microwaves. HVL refers to half-value layer which describes the quality of the X-ray beam.

24. **B** Inherent filtration refers to the change in X-ray spectrum from the absorption of photons when they pass through the X-ray tube housing (target, glass walls of the tube or a thin beryllium window), versus added filtration which is additional material added external to the tube so that the X-ray spectrum can be further modified. A flattening filter is used to harden the beam so that the beam intensity is uniform across the field and shielding against leakage radiation is a function of the treatment head and X-ray tube.

25. **C** As filtration is increased, lower-energy photons are absorbing leaving the beam with higher-energy photons. This effectively increases the average energy of the spectrum and provides greater penetrating power.

26. **B** One way to improve penetrating power of the beam is by adding filtration, since the added filtration absorbs lower-energy photons and increases average energy of the beam. On the downside, the overall intensity of the beam is lower so a higher tube current (more photons) is required to maintain the same image quality. The other method to increase the penetration is by increasing the voltage across the tube (kVp or kilovolt potential) which increases the overall energy of the photon spectrum. As discussed in prior questions, inherent filtration refers to the absorption of the photons when they pass through the target, glass walls of the tube, or a thin beryllium window. The mAs (milliampere seconds) is related to the beam current and number of photons produced which will affect image quality but not the penetration power of the beam.

27. **E** All the answers, kVp, mAs, distance, and filtration, can affect the X-ray emission spectrum. By increasing the kVp or voltage, the intensity of the beam is increased along with the maximum energy photons produced. Remember, as the photons are produced by Bremsstrahlung, the highest energy photons possible are equal to the energy of the incident electron which is dependent on the tube potential. The mAs is related to the number of photons produced. Basically, the mAs defines the exposure in terms of the beam current and time on. The longer the exposure and the higher the current, the more photons are produced. More photons means better image quality (less noise) but higher patient dose. Remember, there is always a

trade-off in imaging. The intensity of the X-ray spectrum is affected by the distance of the source to the image. The relationship between the intensity of X-rays produced at one distance is related to the intensity of X-rays at different distance by inverse square law. Finally, the filtration affects primarily the initial low-energy part of the spectrum and hardens the beam.

28. **D** The formula to approximate the mean or average energy of a photon spectrum is $E_{avg} = 1/3\ E_{max}$, where E_{avg} is the mean average and E_{max} is the maximum energy of the photon (dependent on the tube kVp). If you look at a typical Bremsstrahlung spectrum, the peak of the distribution falls around 1/3 of the max energy. $E = h\nu$ is the formula to find energy of a photon, where h is the physical constant called Planck's constant (6.62×10^{-34} J-s) and ν is the frequency of the photon.

29. **B** Remember that the maximum energy acquired by a photon is related to the potential across the tube (KVp), so it can have a maximum energy which equals to the kVp that is applied, in this case 110 kV. Again it is important to know the mean energy formula ($E_{avg} = 1/3\ E_{max}$).
$E_{avg} = 1/3\ E_{max}$
$E_{avg} = 1/3 \times 110$
$E_{avg} = 36.66$ kV

30. **C** Exposure is the measure of ionization produce per unit mass in air. The transmission of radiation through the edges of the collimator blocks is called the transmission penumbra and the bending magnet is used to bend the electron beam 90° or 270° from its original direction. Finally, the energy absorbed in a material per unit mass is the definition of absorbed dose.

31. **B** The X-ray tube has a housing which supports, insulates, and protects it. The X-ray tube is submerged in oil which provides heat conduction and electrical insulation.

32. **B** The cathode is the negative end of the X-ray tube, and it is composed of the filament and focusing cup. The filament is a tungsten wire that acts as the source of electrons that are generated through the process of thermionic emission when the filament is heated. Filaments are made from tungsten because of its high melting point (3,370 °C). The focusing cup helps control the electron cloud since the electrons repel each other and try to spread out. The focusing cup forces them to form a stream as they move toward the anode.

33. **C** The formula used to determine the heat unit of an X-ray machine is mA × kVp × time. Note: current × voltage is power and power × time is energy.

34. **A** The kilovoltage potential (kVp) determines the wavelength or energy of the X-ray beam; the higher the kVp selected, the higher the energy and of course the shorter the wavelength. mA controls the number of X-rays

1.9 Production of X-Ray (Answers) 83

produced at the cathode filament, and distance and time do not have any effect in determining the wavelength.

35. E All are correct. Additionally X-rays cannot be focused, they travel in straight lines and are exponentially attenuated by matter.

36. B X-rays are produced by the interaction of electrons with matter. The two types of interactions are collisional interactions with subsequent characteristic radiation production and radioactive interaction, which produces Bremsstrahlung radiation. Radioactive decay is the process by which the atomic nucleus of unstable atom becomes more stable by emitting particles and/or electromagnetic radiation. By definition, a photon emitted from the nucleus is a gamma (γ) ray, not an X-ray. The same goes for nuclear reactions where gamma rays are created in the nucleus.

37. A Electrons interact with electrons in the target and transfer momentum and energy through either elastic or inelastic collisions (or radioactive interactions). In an elastic collision, momentum and kinetic energy are conserved, and in an inelastic collision, momentum is conserved but kinetic energy is not conserved.

38. B The direction in which the X-ray beam is emitted from the target depends on the energy of the incoming electrons. At lower energies in the kV range, the emission is almost isotropic, meaning that there is an equal probability of being emitted in any direction, including right angles. At higher energies, such as linear accelerators which have MV energies, the X-rays are emitted from the target in about the same direction as the incoming electrons. On the other hand the beam direction also depends on X-ray target design. That is why in diagnostic energy X-ray beams, reflection or scattering targets are used so that the X-ray beam comes off the target unimpeded in directions useful for imaging. At higher energies, X-rays tend to leave the target in the same direction as the electrons entered so a transmission target is used.

39. E All must be present in order to produce X-rays. High-speed electrons are required and are produced using a high-voltage potential difference between the cathode and anode. A vacuum tube is needed so that the electrons travel at high speed without interacting with air or other molecules. When the electrons are stopped by the target (a means of deceleration), X-rays are produced.

40. A The function of the X-ray anode is to convert electronic energy into x-radiation through Bremsstrahlung and characteristic radiation, serve as the target surface for the high-voltage electrons, and also serve as the primary thermal conductor. The cathode is the source of electrons.

41. E All are correct

1.10 Interaction of Radiation with Matter (Answer)

Quiz-1 (Level 2)

1. **B** Ionization is the process by which a neutral atom acquires a positive or a negative charge. Excitation is the process by which an atom can absorb and re-irradiate energy. LET is the rate of energy loss per unit path length in a medium. The Bragg peak is a characteristic of heavy charged particles where dose is deposited approximately constantly with depth until near end of range where the dose peaks at a high value followed by a rapid falloff.

2. **A** Charge particles such as electrons, protons, and alpha particles are known as directly ionizing radiation because they have sufficient kinetic energy to produce ionization by collision as they penetrate matter. Indirectly ionizing radiation includes uncharged particles such as neutrons and photons because they liberate directly ionizing particles from matter when they interact with matter.

3. **A** The photoelectric effect, Compton effect, and pair production are interactions of a photon with matter. Coherent (Rayleigh) scattering, triplet production, and photonuclear interactions are also photon interactions, although less common. Characteristic X-ray production is a mechanism where a photon is produced when an electron fills an empty orbital location.

4. **D** The half-value layer (HVL) is the thickness of an absorber required to attenuate the intensity of the beam to half its original value. The energy absorption coefficient is the product of energy transfer coefficient and 1 minus the fraction of the energy of secondary charged particles that is lost to Bremsstrahlung in the material. The energy transfer coefficient is the fraction of photon energy transfer into kinetic energy of charge particles per unit thickness of absorber, and the attenuation coefficient is the fraction of photons removed per unit thickness.

5. **E** All are correct about heterogeneous photon beams.
   A heterogeneous beam means the beam is composed of many different photon energies, called a spectrum. The lower-energy X-rays compose the "softer" X-rays. "Softer" X-rays can be stopped by thinner layers of material. Thus, the first HVL for heterogeneous beam is thinner than the subsequent HVLs because these soft photons are removed, the beam hardens, and the penetrating power increases.

6. **A** HVL=$0.693/\mu$, where μ is the linear attenuation coefficient of the material of interest. The formula for decay constant is $\lambda=0.693/T_{1/2}$, and the formula of half-life of a radionuclide is $T_{1/2}=0.693/\lambda$. Again remember that all the formulas must be well known.

1.10 Interaction of Radiation with Matter (Answer)

7. E All of the answers are correct. The amount of photon attenuation by a material depends on the thickness or nature of the material in question, the energy of the incident photon (as the energy of the photon increases, the probability of interaction decreases, until at energies of a few MeV the value is roughly constant and then increases around 10 MeV), the linear attenuation coefficient (µ) of the material, and finally the density of the material in question.

8. B Coherent scattering, pair production, Compton scattering, and photoelectric effect are all types of interactions involving attenuation of photons. Additional interactions are triplet production and photonuclear disintegration which are only important at high photon energies. As discussed in prior questions, Bremsstrahlung and characteristic X-ray production are mechanisms by which X-rays are produced, and the half-value layer is a measurement of beam quality.

9. A In coherent scattering, the new photon has the same energy as the incoming photon but is scattered in a different direction. The photon (electromagnetic wave) passes near the electron and sets it into oscillation. The oscillating electron then re-irradiates the energy at the same frequency as the incident electromagnetic wave. No energy is converted into motion and no energy is absorbed in the medium.

10. C Coherent scattering is more probable in high atomic number materials and with photons of low energy. The process is only of academic interest in radiation therapy.

11. E All answers are the characteristics of the photoelectric effect.

12. C The photoelectric interaction is important for diagnostic imaging because it is the main method in which contrast is developed in radiographs. As the energy in diagnostic imaging is in the kV range, the probability of a photon undergoing a photoelectric interaction is proportional to Z^3. Therefore, the absorption in bone is much greater than in soft tissue.

13. A The probability of a photoelectric interaction depends on the atomic number (Z) and energy of the photon (E); the higher the Z of the material, the more likely the interaction, but the higher the energy of the photon, the less likely the interaction.

14. C During a Compton interaction, the photon interacts with an atomic electron as if the electron were a free electron. This means that the binding energy of the electron is much less than the energy of the incoming photon. In this interaction the electron receives some energy from the photon and is emitted at angle. The photons retains some if its energy and is emitted at another angle.

15. C II and IV are correct; because Compton interaction involves essentially free electrons, it is independent of atomic number (Z). Most materials except hydrogen can be considered as having approximately the same number of electrons per gram; thus, electron density is nearly the same for all materials. The energy of the incident photon must be large compared with the electron energy; thus, as the photon energy increases beyond the binding energy of the K electron, the Compton effect becomes more and more important. At the same time, the Compton effect also decreases with increasing photon energy around 10 MeV. Atomic mass (A) is independent of Compton interaction.

16. C Compton interactions depends primarily on the number of electrons per gram, and hydrogen has more electrons per gram than the rest of most materials. Therefore, hydrogen will attenuate more of the beam in Compton interactions.

17. B Because the rest mass energy of an electron is 0.51 MeV, a minimum energy of 1.02 MeV is required to create a pair of electrons (electron + positron). Thus, the threshold energy for the pair production process is 1.02 MeV.

18. E All the statements are correct about pair production. During pair production, the incoming photon interacts with the field of the nucleus and disappears. The result of this interaction is the electron and positron.

19. B If Compton photon makes a direct hit with the electron, the electron will travel forward 0° receiving the maximum energy, and the scattered photon will travel backward 180° left with the minimum energy. If a Compton photon makes a grazing hit with the electron, the electron will be emitted at right angles, and the scattered photon will go in the forward direction with almost no transfer of energy. If the photon is scattered at right angles (90°) to its original direction, it will have energy of 0.511 MeV. The most probably interaction for incoming photon with energy up to 50 keV is coherent scattering.

20. E All the statements are correct.

21. D Unlike photons, charged particles such as electrons, protons, and alpha particles interact with matter through ionization and excitation.

22. B The rate of kinetic energy loss per unit path length of the charged particle is called stopping power. The mass stopping power is the stopping power normalized by the density of the material. LET is the rate of energy loss per unit path length in collisions in which energy is locally absorbed. Activity (A) is the rate of decay of a radioactive sample, and the equation

1.10 Interaction of Radiation with Matter (Answer)

is $A(t) = A_0 e^{-\lambda t}$, where $A(t)$ is the activity remaining at time t, A_0 is the activity at time $t=0$, e is the mathematical constant 2.718, and λ is the decay constant.

23. B Stopping power caused by ionization interaction for charged particles is proportional to the square of the particle charge and inversely proportional to the square of its velocity. Thus, as the particle slows down, its rate of energy loss increases and so does the ionization to the medium. This is the reason for the Bragg peak.

24. A Paraffin wax and polyethylene are hydrogenous materials, meaning that they contain a lot of hydrogen. Therefore, I, II, and III are correct. The most efficient materials for absorbing neutrons are hydrogenous materials because energy transfer is very efficient if colliding particles have the same mass. Since a neutron and a proton (hydrogen atom) have approximately the same mass, the collisions efficiently reduce the energy of the incident neutrons. On the other hand, neutrons lose very little energy when colliding with a high-Z material such as lead since the neutron tends to scatter from the large nucleus rather than transfer energy.

25. B Because of the higher hydrogen content in fat, the dose absorbed is about 20 % higher than in muscle or bone. Remember that the most efficient absorber material for neutron beams is a hydrogenous material.

26. Energy range with its corresponding photon interactions
A. III. Coherent scattering (1–50 keV)
B. IV. Photoelectric effect (few eV to over 1 MeV in high atomic numbers elements)
C. I. Compton effect (150 keV to over 50 MeV)
D. II. Pair production (greater than 1.02 MeV)

27. A Electrons do not deposit dose with a Bragg peak because electrons have a relatively small mass and they suffer from multiple scattering and changes in direction. As consequence, the Bragg peak is not observed for electrons. Heavy charge particles like protons and alphas have a much larger mass and do not undergo multiple scatterings.

28. A In the process of ionization, the ejected electron is called a secondary electron or delta ray (δ) if it receives sufficient energy to produce an ionization track of its own.

29. E All of them. X-rays, gamma rays, (γ) and neutrons are indirectly ionizing because they liberate directly ionizing particles when they interact with matter. On the other hand, charged particles such as electrons, protons, and alpha (α) particles are known as directly ionizing radiation. Make sure to know all the particle symbols.

30. **A.** IV. Pair production
    B. II. Photoelectric effect
    C. I. Coherent scattering
    D. III. Compton effect

31. **A** From the longest to the shortest wavelength: radio wave (10^3 m), microwave (10^{-2} m), infrared (10^{-5} m), visible light (0.5×10^{-6} m), ultraviolet wave (10^{-8} m), X-rays (10^{-10} m), and gamma ray (10^{-12} m).

32. **C** Gamma ($>2 \times 10^{-14}$ J) rays have the highest photon energy followed by characteristic X-rays (2×10^{-17} to 2×10^{-14} J), ultraviolet light (5×10^{-19} to 2×10^{-17} J), and infrared light (2×10^{-22} to 3×10^{-19} J).
    Please note: clinical linear accelerator also generates X-rays, which could be as high as 50 MeV, higher than γ-rays. Only characteristic X-rays or diagnostic X-rays have lower energy than γ-rays. By definition, a gamma ray originates in the nucleus of an atom, while X-rays are created through characteristic radiation or Bremsstrahlung.

33. **A** Frequency is defined as the amount of times something happens within a given period of time. In the case of electromagnetic radiation, the frequency (hertz or Hz) is defined as the number of waves per second passing a given point or location. The wavelength is the distance covered by one cycle of wave. The higher the frequency, the shorter the wavelength and the higher the energy.

34. **C** The photoelectric effect and pair production do not produce scattered radiation when the photon interacts with the atom. Photoelectric effect emits characteristic X-rays, and there is also the possibility of emission of auger electrons. Pair production gives up all its energy in the process of creating a pair consisting of a negative electron and a positive electron. During Compton scattering, the electron receives some energy from the photon and is emitted at an angle, but the photon, with reduced energy, is scattered at an angle, too. During coherent scattering, a scattered X-ray with the same wavelength as the incident beam is produced.

35. **B** Coherent scattering can be also called classical, Thompson, elastic, or Rayleigh scattering, named after the British physicist Lord Rayleigh.

36. **E** All are properties of X-rays.

37. **C** As the wavelength of an X-ray decreases, frequency and energy both increase. Remember that X-rays and gamma rays contain short wavelength and high frequency and energy; on the other hand, radio waves have long wavelengths with low frequencies and energies.

38. B By increasing kVp, there will be more of the beam penetrating the tissue due to higher energy of the beam, so they interact more by Compton effect and less by the photoelectric effect. At higher kVps, more scatter will be produced which will increase image noise and reduce contrast

1.11 Treatment Machine Characteristics (Answers)

Quiz-1 (Level 2)

1.
A. IV: Grenz-ray therapy (less than 20 kV)
B. II   Contact therapy (40–50 kV)
C. III Superficial therapy (50–150 kV)
D. VI   Orthovoltage therapy (150–500 kV)
E. V   Supervoltage therapy (500–1,000 kV)
F. I   Megavoltage therapy (greater than 1 MV)
G. VII Van de Graff generator (typically at 2 MV)

2. **B** Contact therapy uses <2 cm SSD.
Superficial therapy uses 15–20 cm SSD.
Orthovoltage therapy uses 50 cm SSD.
Megavoltage therapy from 80 to 100 SSD.

3. **D** Grenz-ray therapy uses low penetration and can treat only shallow lesions.
Contact therapy can be used for tumors not any deeper than 1–2 mm.
Superficial therapy can treat up to 5 mm deep tumors.
Orthovoltage therapy can treat from 3 to 5 cm.

4. **B** The greatest limitation in using orthovoltage or deep therapy is the skin surface dose, which becomes large when adequate doses are to be delivered to deep tumors. Skin sparing is an advantage of megavoltage machines.

5.
A. IV   Microtron therapy (4–40 MeV)
B. I   Cyclotron therapy (15–50 MeV)
C. III Van de Graff generator (2–10 MeV)
D. V   Linear accelerator (4–25 MeV)
E. II   Teletherapy (Co-60: 1.25 MeV)

6. **B** High-energy electrons produced in a linear accelerator can be used to treat superficial tumors without the use of X-ray target and a flattening filter. If deep-seated tumors are needed to be treated, X-rays are produced by placing the target in the electron beam path and using a flattening filter if desired.

7. I. C Electron gun
   II. E Waveguide system
   III. B Modulator
   IV. F Accelerator tube
   V.   G Treatment head (straight beam)
   VI. A Power supply
   VII. D Magnetron or klystron
   VIII.H Treatment head (bent beam)

8. A. Power supply: V; provides direct current power to the modulator.
   B. Modulator: III; generates control pulse to the electron gun and the magnetron or klystron. The timing of these pulses is critical to the proper operation of the linear accelerator.
   C. Electron gun: I; provides a source of electrons.
   D. Magnetron or klystron: VI; generates and/or amplifies microwaves to accelerate the electrons through the waveguide.
   E. Waveguide system: II; microwaves generated from the magnetron or klystron are sent into the accelerator structure throughout this component.
   F. Accelerator tube: IV; electrons are accelerated to high energies in this component by the interaction with microwave radiation.
   G. Treatment head: VII; contains an X-ray target, scattering foil, flattening filter, ion chamber, fixed and movable collimator, and light localizer system.

9. D The record and verify section is used to control treatment parameters. The ionization chamber is a device that measures charge and is calibrated so that one monitor unit (MU) delivers 1 cGy with standard conditions (i.e., 100 cm SSD, D_{max}, 10×10 field). Calorimetry is a basic method of determining absorbed dose in a medium, and after electrons have been accelerated, they are redirected by beam handling section in the treatment head which includes the bending magnet, target, scattering foil, or flattening filter.

10. C The magnetron is a device that produces microwaves and the klystron amplifies microwaves. In the past magnetrons were limited by their output, but modern magnetrons can be used in high-energy linacs. Klystrons tend to be more efficient at producing high-energy microwaves. Magnetrons tend to be less expensive but have shorter life spans than klystrons.

11. A The two types of accelerator structure found in a linac are traveling waves and standing waves. Traveling waves accelerate electrons like a surfer on a wave, riding the wave down the accelerating tube. Standing waves accelerate the electrons but can be shortened as two traveling waves move in opposite directions producing a standing wave, meaning some sections never change polarity. These sections can be moved out of the beam, effectively shortening the length of the accelerating structure. An ion pump is a device that maintains a vacuum so that the electrons can be accelerated to high energies. The electron gun is not part of the accelerator structure but produces the initial electrons that will be accelerated down the structure.

1.11 Treatment Machine Characteristics (Answers)

12. Treatment head components
A. IV Flattening filter
B. VI Ion chamber
C. V Scattering foil
D. II X-ray target
E. III Primary collimator
F. VIII Electron applicator
G. VII Secondary collimator
H. I Bending magnet

13. B Electrons beams are bent at an appropriate 90° or 270° angle before striking the target; a chromatic 90° bending magnet or an achromatic 270° bending magnet is used. The benefit of the achromatic 270° magnet is that the electrons can be de-focused and refocused. During the defocusing, electrons that are either higher or lower energy can be filtered out of the beam, meaning the final beam is more uniform. Some bending magnets use a 135° bending system, called a slalom system, that can also filter out higher- or lower-energy electrons by de-focusing and refocusing.

14. A. VI Bending magnet: The electron beam is usually bent 90° or 270° from its original direction. The benefit of this is that the accelerating structure can be long, and this allows for easier delivery of the beam to the patient.

    B. IV Monitor chamber: monitor the dose rate, integrate dose, and monitor beam flatness and symmetry. This system is fed back into the linear accelerator, and if something is not correct, the linear accelerator will turn off.

    C. V X-ray target: produces a photon beam through the Bremsstrahlung process.

    D. III Flattening filter: reduces the intensity of the forward peaked dose in the center of the field to produce dose uniformity across the radiation field at a specified depth. With modern linacs, some treatments, especially small fields, are done without the flattening filter. This is not a problem as long as the planning system can model the peaked beam. Additionally, much higher dose rates can be delivered without any extra contamination in the beam.

    E. VIII Fix primary collimator: defines the X-ray beam.

    F. VII Electron cone: used in electron mode to collimate electron beams since they scatter readily in air.

    G. I Movable X-ray collimator: consists of two pairs of lead or tungsten blocks (jaws) which provide a rectangular opening.

    H. IX Light localizing system: It is congruent with the radiation field and is used in the alignment of the radiation beam and the treatment field marked on the patient's skin surface.

I. II Scattering foil: spreads the narrow electron beam and causes a fairly uniform electron distribution across the beam.

15. B The flattening filter and X-ray target are moved aside when the linear accelerator is in the electron mode. Remember that X-ray target is used to produce photons which are not needed in the electron mode, and flattening filter reduces the intensity of the forward peaked dose in the center of the field to produce dose uniformity across the radiation field at a specified depth. The scattering foils are used instead in electron mode so that the 3-mm-diameter electron beam can be properly spread and flattened causing a uniform electron distribution across the beam. An electron cone is also used in electron mode to collimate electron beam once it exits the head of the machine as electrons scatter much more readily in air than photons. The ion chamber is always in the beam path to monitor the dose rate, integrate dose, and monitor the beam flatness and symmetry.

16. A The scattering foil is moved in front of the electron beam by a rotating carrousel. The flattening filter and X-ray target are moved away. The ion chamber always stays in the beam path.

17. B Ion chambers are made of low-Z materials like aluminum or plastic so that the beam is not perturbed. Tungsten and lead should be eliminated quickly in this case as these are obviously incorrect.

18. B The correct path of the beam when a linac accelerator is on the X-ray mode is bending magnet, X-ray target, primary collimator, flattening filter, monitor chamber, and secondary collimators. The correct path of the beam when a linac accelerator is on the electron mode is answer C: bending magnet, primary collimator, scattering foils, monitor chamber, secondary collimator, electron applicator, and cutout. Remember on an X-ray mode the target and the flattening filter are needed, while on electron mode both are moved away and the scattering foil is used instead.

19. B The secondary collimator uses two jaws which provide a rectangular opening from 0×0 to the maximum field size of 40×40 cm at the isocenter. Some specialized linear accelerators like those used for stereotactic therapy might not have that large of a field size.

20. D The isocenter is the point of intersection of the collimator axis and the axis of rotation of the gantry. The secondary collimator is used to collimate the beam, the SSD is the distance from the source to patient's surface, and a wiggler point is an instrument used to determine the tolerance of the isocenter motion.

1.11 Treatment Machine Characteristics (Answers)

21. A The main disadvantages of a betatron are the low dose rates and small field sizes. Two advantages of a microtron generator over linac accelerator are easy energy selection and simplicity. Time errors and wide penumbra are disadvantages of radioisotope machines like Co-60 teletherapy machines.

22. B A microtron is an electron accelerator that combines the principles of both the linear accelerator and the cyclotron. Like a cyclotron, there are circular magnets that create a permanent, static magnetic field perpendicular to the electron path. Unlike a cyclotron, a linear accelerator is used to accelerate the electrons rather than changing the polarity of the magnets. The acceleration is done once per rotation of the electron. As the velocity of the electron increases, the radius of the electron path increases. The desired energy can be obtained by extracting the beam at that particular radius. A betatron is a device that accelerates electrons in a circular orbit using a varying magnetic and electric field with an accelerating tube shaped like a hollow doughnut. A cyclotron is a charged particle accelerator mainly used for nuclear physics research and works by accelerating particles in a circular path by changing the polarity of two large "D"-shaped magnets. A teletherapy machine is a device that uses radioisotopes to treat at extended distances.

23. C Even though Radium-226 and Cesium-137 have been used for radionuclide external beam radiotherapy, the most appropriate radionuclide for external beam radiotherapy is Cobalt-60. The reason for this is the energy of Co-60 is about 1.25 MeV (almost equal probability of photons of 1.17 and 1.33 MeV). Cs-137 has an energy of about 662 keV, and Ra-226 has an average energy of about 800 keV. Iridium-192 is used for on HDR treatment and has an average energy of about 380 keV. For better depth dose and skin sparing, higher energy is advantageous for teletherapy.

24. B Cobalt-60 is produced by irradiating stable ^{59}Co with neutrons in a nuclear reactor. High-energy neutrons are created by bombarding deuterons or protons against beryllium target in a deuterium tritium (D-T) generator, cyclotron, or linear accelerator. Protons and other heavy ions can be created in a cyclotron or linear accelerator.

25. D Only IV is true; Co-60 decays to ^{60}Ni with emission of electrons of 0.32 MeV and two photons of energy 1.17 and 1.33 MeV. The half-life of Co-60 is 5.26 years, the average photon energy is 1.25 MeV, and (exposure rate constant) Γ (R-cm^2/mCi-h) is 13.07. The half-life for Cs-137 $T_{1/2}$ is 30 years and Ra-226 has (exposure rate constant) Γ (R-cm^2/mCi-h) of 8.25. You should know the $T_{1/2}$, (exposure rate constant) Γ, photon energy, and half-value layer for each common radionuclide.

26. **E** All of the statements are advantages of Co-60 over Ra-226 and Cs-137.

27. **B** The geometric penumbra associated with Co-60 is due to the finite size of the source. Transmission penumbra is due to irradiated photons transmitted through the edge of the collimator block.

28. **B** Every 5.26 years the radioactivity of Cobalt-60 is reduced by 50 % ($T_{1/2}$). This continual drop in output requires a correction for this decay of about 1.09 % per month in all patient treatment calculations.
5.26 years = 63.12 months, so the percentage of decay per month is:
$1-(0.5)^{1/63.12} = 1 - 0.989 = 0.0109 = 1.09 \%$

29. **E** All the answers are mechanisms used to move the Co-60 source from the off to on position.

30. **B** Due to the large size of a Cobalt source, typically 1–2 cm, the penumbra or unsharp edge of the beam is larger than that of the beam from a linear accelerator, which has a smaller focal point.

31. **C** Transmission penumbra can be minimized if the collimator blocks are shaped so that the inner surface of the blocks remains parallel to the edge of the beam. If the inner surface of the blocks is made parallel to the central axis of the beam, the radiation will pass through the inner edges resulting in transmission penumbra. Using larger collimator openings will result in more penumbra because of greater obliquity of the rays at the inner edges of the blocks.

Fig. 1A.5.1

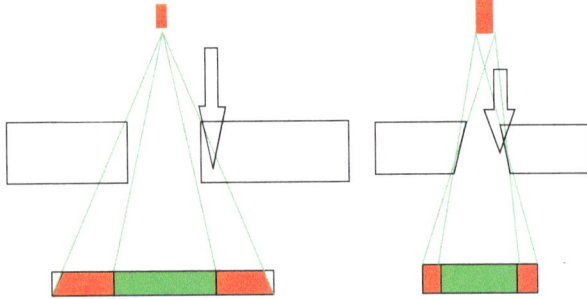

32. **A.** Graph IV; electron depth dose curve illustrating the practical range (R_p) which is the depth of the point where the tangent to the descending linear portion of the curve intersects the extrapolated background and (R_{50}) which is the depth at which the dose is 50 % of the maximum dose.

1.11 Treatment Machine Characteristics (Answers)

Fig. 1A.5.2

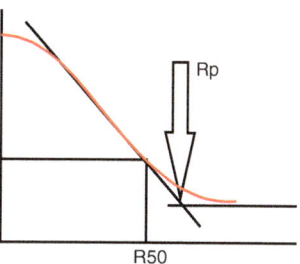

- **B.** Graph I; transmission penumbra is the region irradiated by photons which are transmitted through the edge of the collimator.
- **C.** Graph III; geometry of two adjacent beams to calculate the gap of the skin surface.
- **D.** Graph II; geometric penumbra which is associated with finite size of the source.

33. C Geometric penumbra formula:
$P_d = s\,(SSD + d - SDD)/SDD$, where s is source diameter, SSD is source to surface distance, d is depth, and SDD is the source to diaphragm distance. Answer A, $A/P = a \times b/2(a+b)$, is the formula used to calculate equivalent field parameters where a is field width and b is field length. In answer B, $H = (\mu_{tissue} - \mu_{water}/\mu_{water})$ 1,000 refers to housefield number formula where μ is the linear attenuation coefficient. In answer D, gap $= 0.5 L_1 \times d/SSD_1 + 0.5 L_2 \times d/SSD_2$ is the gap formula when two adjacent fields are separated on the surface, L is ½ of field, d is the junction at depth, and SSD is source to surface distance.

34. E All the answers are correct about penumbra.

35. C Geometric penumbra is independent of field size; for answers A, B, and D, refer to question 35 explanation.

36. A. Physical penumbra width encompasses both geometric and transmission penumbra. It is the lateral distance between two specified isodose curves, usually the 80 and 20 % lines at a specified depth. Trimmer bars are heavy metal bars used in Co-60 machines to attenuate the beam in the penumbra region. The penumbra is not eliminated but reduced since the SDD is increased with the trimmers extended.

37. C As mentioned earlier, Penumbra formula is $P_d = s\,(SSD + d - SDD)/SDD$.
$S = 1.5$ cm
$SSD = 90$ cm
$d = 10$ cm
$SDD = 20$ cm
$P_d = s\,(SSD + d - SDD)/SDD$
$P_d = 1.5\,(90 + 10 - 20)/20$
$P_d = 6$ cm

38. A The high cost of the machine, low dose rates, and beam contamination are the major disadvantages of proton therapy. One of the advantages is the sharper penumbra region.

39. A All of them are characteristics of proton therapy but the MAJOR advantage is the Bragg peak, where dose is deposited approximately constantly with depth until near end of range where the dose peaks at a high value followed by a rapid falloff. This means that there is no exit dose when treating with protons. Proton dose distributions also have a very sharp penumbra region. Range modulation changes the depth of the Bragg peak to ensure that it falls within the tumor. Finally proton uses energies in the range of 150–250 MeV.

40. E Orthovoltage X-ray units are usually set at 50 cm SSD with a potential energy range from 150 to 500 kV. The maximum dose usually occurs close to the skin surface, and because of this they are used to treat lesions NO deeper than 2–3 cm or else the skin dose will be too high.

41. B Task group No. 224 is used for proton machine QA. This task group was approved on 1/17/2012, and the main objective is to develop uniform and comprehensive QA procedures for proton radiotherapy machines. Task group No.185 is based on clinical commissioning of proton therapy machines, and its role is to provide clinical commissioning guidance for scattered/collimated uniform scanning and modulated scanning beam delivery systems. Task group No.202 reviewed the relevant published literature with regard to physical uncertainties and correlated them with different planning and delivery techniques, and Task group No.140 focused on absolute calibration of light power and fluence rate for photo dynamic therapy (PDT).

Quiz-2 (Level 3)

1. C A klystron is a microwave amplifier. The larger the magnitude of the microwaves, the energy of the electrons can be increased.

2. B First of all, commissioning data is the baseline for QA. Once commissioning is completed, many of these measurements cannot be obtained again as the accelerator could in theory change over time. Therefore, it is imperative that the commissioned data be comprehensive and well documented so if there is a machine parameter change in the future, the initial value can easily be found. Next, the beam model in the planning system provided by the vendor needs to be tweaked to fit this particular linear accelerator; thus the commissioning data is put into TPS for tweaking the beam model. Finally, tests are run to ensure that the doses calculated in the planning system match those being delivered at the linac. For Eclipse, the dose calculation

algorithm is AAA (analytical anisotropic algorithm), for ADAC system the algorithm is CCC (collapsed cone convolution), etc.

Commissioning data cannot be directly used for dose calculation; hence the beam is modeled in the planning system. This is done because the calculation time would be extremely long if every data point was used rather than a single modeled equation.

3. **C** Unlike a Co-60 teletherapy machine, a linac delivered radiation in pulses, not in a continuous beam. It would be impossible to generate enough power to be able to generate a continuous beam, and therefore there is a duty cycle. The duty cycle refers to the percentage of time that the linac is actually delivering radiation. A rule of thumb is that the linac is delivering microsecond pulses of radiation that are spaced milliseconds apart. By stringing together many of these pulses, the linac can produce a beam of radiation. This is also the reason that the linac cannot be stopped based on the time the beam is on like Co-60, but rather the monitor unit (MU) determines when to turn the beam off.

4. **A** The waveguide needs extremely high current to deliver X-rays of high dose rate, and most of this energy converts into heat instead of photons. To effectively dissipate energy, in addition to water cooling system, the linear accelerator is turned on and off periodically with a fast switch, thus to keep a very low working duty (~0.1 %) to allow heat dissipation.

    The thyratron is a high-voltage switch of 250–300 Hz, with duration of 4 μs of "on" time in each cycle of 3–4 ms. Therefore ~99.9 % in a second the linac is actually off. Remember the rule of thumb: microsecond pulses spaced milliseconds apart.

    The thyratron is a component of pulse forming network (PFN), providing stable HV pulses to fire the linac electron gun, and microwave amplifier (klystron or magnetron). The timing of these pulses between the electron gun and klystron/magnetron is critical to proper functioning of the linac.

5. **A** In standing wave (SW) accelerators, coupling cavities cannot accelerate electrons because the voltage inside those cavities is zero. This is due to the fact that there are two identical waves but in opposite directions. This means that the cavities that fall on the nodes of the wave always have zero charge. Thus they can be put shifted off-axis in the waveguide and hence significantly save the space.

6. **A** Beam loading is the simplest method for switching high energy to low energy in a traveling wave (TW) waveguide. During beam loading, the electron gun current is increased which produces a larger clump of electrons to be accelerated. Due to the larger mass of this clump, the electrons cannot be accelerated as efficiently and therefore result in a lower energy. An energy switch is typically used in a SW.

7. **D** For standing wave (SW) waveguide, beam loading is not suitable because it only provides a narrow range of energy variation, beyond which the energy spectrum will rapidly degrade.

   The best method is to use a non-contact energy switch at a coupling cavity to the second portion of the waveguide. In this method only one-side coupling cavity is used (remember coupling cavities are at both side of waveguide).

   There are other methods, such as single-side cavity shorting method, as well as double-side cavity shorting. Those methods do not use non-contact switch and are not preferred. The principle behind this method is to "de-phase" the standing wave in part of the SW to lower the efficiency of the waveguide which results in a lower energy.

8. **B** AFC = automatic frequency controller

   An AFC is used for magnetrons only, because the magnetron is less stable than a klystron due to changes that can result from heating and other factors. If the frequency is not optimized, this may have negative influence on waveguide operation.

   In general, AFC is a feedback circuit to the magnetron. The magnetron frequency is sampled and then sent to two resonance cavities, which are tuned slightly below or above the desired frequency. The output of those two cavities are sampled, amplified, rectified, and then compared in the comparator. If the frequency in the magnetron is correct, the output is null; if not (higher or lower), the output of those two cavities will be quite different. This two-cavity setup is more sensitive than a simple comparator between sampled values to a fixed value.

   The output signal from AFC is used to control the magnetron tuner drive to move to the right direction for frequency adjustment.

   The frequency of the cavities is tunable by a probe drive controlled by frequency selector. The AFC is for the initial adjustment of frequency.

   The phase shifter is also a feedback circuit used for fine adjustment of the frequency, whereas the AFC performs the initial (coarse) frequency adjustment. Since the frequency may change the velocity of electrons, a very small change of velocity actually reveals the phase difference between the input and output of waveguide.

   The hardware is a length of dielectric material (mounted onto a ceramic rod), which is held parallel to the long axis of the transmission waveguide.

   The AFC and phase shifter are used together for frequency tuning, but only for magnetron-powered TW-type linear accelerator.

9. **A** The only difference in hardware between diode gun and triode gun is that triode gun has an extra control grid for beam current control. By applying a voltage to the grid, the number and energy of the electrons can be controlled.

It is necessary to ensure that all the electrons have the same energy, and this can be performed by a triode-gun system. In this setup it is possible that the microwave and electron pulses are not in the same phase, whereas in a diode-gun system this is impossible. In reality, the microwave is "filled" into the waveguide first, and then electron pulses are injected; thus all the pulses are accelerated the same way, i.e., to have the same energy.

For each 4-μs pulse, the SW in the accelerator waveguide takes 1 μs to reach its maximum. All electrons will have the same energy ONLY when the SW is in maximum amplitude.

This can be achieved by using a triode gun and waiting 1 μs until the SW is ready then injecting electrons into the waveguide. Thus, the real time interval for a pulse is 3 μs (of 4 μs), which is characteristic of SW accelerator. Due to the specifit timing required for the electron injection, a diode gun cannot be used for a SW accelerator.

10. A The method to change energies for electron modes is quite different from X-ray modes in TW and SW linear accelerator.

e-beam energy for a traveling wave (TW) accelerator

Relatively small change in frequency may produce wide variations in electron energy.

The relative position of the electron bunch at the wave front of a microwave (e.g., the phase) is actually quite important for the eventual energy of electrons as the wave-front position of the electron bunch determines how strong the electric field is, and hence the electron bunch "feels" the strength of the field.

By adjusting the relative phase, that is, by injecting the electrons at a different time point in the wave, the efficiency of the system drops rapidly. The drop in efficiency is because e-beams need 2 orders of magnitude less power than X-rays (no energy loss in target or flattening filter).

(To change frequency, please see note for AFC and phase shifter, the answer for question 50.)

e-beam energy for standing wave (SW) accelerator

For SW accelerator, electron energies can be changed by either changing the wave amplitude or by changing the frequency phase, or both.

Remember, the energy for X-rays can be changed by a non-contact energy switch, which as a result changes the electric field of the second portion of the waveguide.

11. A Normally 250–300 Hz. Remember that 1 Hz is one cycle per second.

12. B 4 μs in 4-ms cycle.

13. B The circulator (normally 4-port) lies in the microwave transmission waveguide between klystron and accelerator waveguide. A typical klystron-driven machine is a SW accelerator.

The circulator allows *one-way passing of microwaves*. The main function is to restrict the reflecting microwave from the accelerator waveguide from entering back into the klystron.

The reflected microwave is absorbed in a port where there is a water load (cooling). In addition, a shunt tee (a "T" shape splitter) inside the circulator is used to provide fine control of power fed into the waveguide. To prevent arcing (electrical breakdown of a gas) in the transmission waveguide, the waveguide is filled with pressurized SF_6 gas which is very stable and is an excellent electrical insulator.

14. **D**   The triode electron gun is able to control the timing of the electron cloud release to be in the correct phase with the microwave.

15. **D**   The thyratron is a fast on/off high-voltage switch; thus it is filled with gas working as insulator. 1 atm = 760 mmHg = 760 Torr.

1.12   Radiation Units (Answers)

Quiz-1 (Level 2)

1. **C**   The SI unit for mass is the kilogram (kg), for time is the second (s), for electrical current is the ampere (A) and for length is the meter (m). Remember that all quantities and units must be well known.

2. **B**   Only I and III are correct; the SI unit of force is Newton (N), the SI unit of frequency is hertz (Hz), the SI unit of power of work is the watt (W), and the SI unit of energy is the Joule (J)

3. **D**   Power is actually equal to energy (E)/time (t). The other formulas are all correct: Velocity (v) = distance (d)/time (t), Acceleration (a) = velocity (v)/time (t), and Force (F) = mass (m) × acceleration (a). Also remember that for photons energy (E) = frequency (h) × wavelength (υ).

4.
A. IV   Electric resistance (R) – SI unit is Ohm (Ω)
B. I   Charge (Q) – SI unit is Coulomb (C)
C. III Capacitance (C) – SI unit is Farad (F)
D. II   Electric potential – SI unit is volt (V)

5.   Electrical unit formulas.
A. IV   Resistance (R) = Electric potential (V)/current (I)
B. I   Charge (Q) = Current (I) × time (t)
C. III Capacitance (C) = Charge (Q)/electric potential (V)
D. II   Electric potential (V) = Energy (E)/charge (Q)

1.12 Radiation Units (Answers)

6.

A. III The SI unit for activity is the Becquerel (Bq), which is equal to 1 decay per second. The curie (Ci) is also a unit of activity and 1 Ci is equal to 3.7×10^{10} Bq.

B. I The SI unit for absorbed dose is the Gray (Gy). The non-SI unit is the rad. 1 Gy = 100 rads.

C. II The SI unit for exposure is C kg^{-1}, also called the roentgen (R).

D. I The SI unit for KERMA is also the Gray (Gy).

A Sievert (Sv) is the SI unit of dose equivalent (H) and the non-SI unit is the rem. 1 Sv = 100 rem. To convert from Gy to Sv, you multiply by a radiation weighting factor (or quality factor) that accounts for how effective a particular type of radiation is at cell killing.

7. B Absorbed dose is defined as energy absorbed from all ionizing radiations per unit mass of a material. Energy loss by electrons per unit path length of a material is the definition of stopping power and exposure is defined as the charge liberated by ionization radiation per unit mass in air. Finally, activity is defined as the rate of decay of a radioactive material per unit time.

8. A Only I, II, and II are correct. Wheras absorbed dose is applicable to all ionizing radiation, exposure can only be used for X-rays and gamma rays lower than ~3 MeV. Additionally, absorbed dose is applicable even in areas where electronic equilibrium does not exist (exposure cannot be measured for photons that have an energy greater than about 3 MeV). Finally, absorbed dose is directly related to radiation effects or measure of the biological effects produced by ionizing radiation, while exposure is only defined in air.

9. E All the answers are correct.

10. B Ionization in AIR is measured by the unit of roentgen, which is the unit for exposure. Absorbed dose is a measurement of biological effect in a particular material and specific activity measures the activity per unit mass of a radionuclide. The radiobiological effect (RBE) describes the efficiency in which a particular type of radiation evokes a certain biological effect.

11. A The unit for KERMA is the same as for dose, J/kg, the SI unit is the Gy, and its non-SI unit is rad.

12. A I, II, and III are definitions of kinetic energy released per unit mass (KERMA). Answer D refers to absorbed dose which is the quantity of energy released for all types of ionizing radiation.

13. E All are correct. Additionally, the thermoluminescent detector (TLD) detector (or optically stimulated luminescent dosimeter (OSL) or film) should always be turned to face the source of radiation.

14. C Film badges will be issued to users of 20 mCi or more of gamma- or beta-emitting radionuclides, and ring badges will be issued to users of 5 mCi or more of gamma- or beta-emitting radionuclides.

15. B The film is contained inside the badge which incorporates a series of filters to determine the quality of the radiation. Radiation of different energies would be attenuated to a different extent by various types of absorbers, and the same quantity of radiation incident on the badge will produce a different degree of darkening under each filter. Remember that the dose equivalent is determined from the absorbed dose multiplied by a radiation weighting factor.

16. A The f-factor is the roentgen-to-rad conversion factor. The roentgen is a measure of exposure which is a measure of ionization in air. Absorbed dose is a measure of energy released in a material; therefore I, II, and III are all correct. It is a good idea to remember that the f-factor is greater for high-Z materials and low-energy photons.

17. C The f-factor is a function of the composition of the medium and the photon energy and is defined as $D_{med} = X(R) \times f_{med}$.
D_{med} = Dose to bone?
$X(R)$ = exposure = 30 R
f_{med} = f-factor = 6.17 cGy/R (bone)
Formula
$D_{med} = X(R) \times f_{med}$
$D_{med} = 30 \times 6.17$ cGy/R
$D_{med} = 185.1$ cGy

18. B The f-factor's constant for air is 0.876 cGy/R (rad/R). ln(2) is the natural logarithm of 2 having a value of 0.693. ln(2) is used to find half-life, decay constant, HVL, etc. of a radioactive substance, and 0.511 MeV is the rest mass of an electron.

19. E All are disadvantages of films.

20. E All are correct.

21. B Radiation absorbed dose when measured on a film is related to the degree of blackening of the film created by the metallic silver, which is not affected by the fixer. The film base is coated with an emulsion containing very small crystals of silver bromide; when film is exposed, a chemical change takes place within the crystals to form a latent image. After development, the affected crystals are reduced to metallic silver (blackening of the film); the unaffected granules are removed by the fixing solution.

1.12 Radiation Units (Answers)   103

22. A The optical density of the film is measured by a densitometer which works by shining a bright light through the film and measuring the transmitted light. An extrapolation chamber is a special ionization chamber for measuring surface dose, an electrometer is a device used to measure the charge collected in an ionization chamber, and a TLD is a dosimeter that emits light proportional to the absorbed dose when heated.

23. E All are advantages of radiochromic films. Radiochromic films are replacing radiographic films in many institutions because there is no need to maintain a developer.

24. D The most frequently used TLD material for clinical dosimetry is lithium fluoride (LIF), although other phosphors can be used too.

25. B OD = log (I_0/I_t), where I_0 is the amount of light collected without film and I_t is the amount of light transmitted through the film.

26. E All are correct.

27. C Radiochromic films' response depends on temperature, not on humidity, pressure, or chemical, physical, and/or thermal processing. Radiographic film response depends on chemical processing.

28. E All the answers are correct. Radiochromic films are almost tissue equivalent with an effective Z of 6–6.5.

29. B Film badges need to be worn correctly so that the dose that they receive accurately represents the dose the wearer receives. Whole body badges are worn on the body between the neck and the waist, often on the belt or a shirt pocket.

30. B A control badge is issued with each group of film badges to determine the background radiation exposure to the shipment of film badges and also will serve to evaluate any exposures to the shipment during transit.

31. A LET stands for linear energy transfer. It is the energy absorbed per unit distance of ionizing particles passing through a material (e.g., MeV/cm). LET is very important in biological effectiveness of radiations.

32. Instruments that provide an absolute measurement do not need a calibration factor to determine dose. Those that provide a relative measurement need a calibration factor or they require a reference measurement to compare against.
A. II. The ion chamber is a relative dosimeter. Its exposure is calibrated against a free-air ion chamber or a standard cavity chamber, under conditions of electronic equilibrium.

B. II. A film is a relative dosimeter. A film suffers from several potential errors such as changes in processing conditions, interfilm emulsion differences, and artifacts caused by air pockets adjacent to the film, so absolute dosimetry with a film is impractical.
C. I. A calorimetry dosimeter is an absolute dose measurement.
D. II. A TLD is a relative dosimeter.
E. II. A diode is a good relative dosimeter due to its high sensitivity and quick response as well as excellent reproducibility, stability, and small size.

33. B The most commonly used radiochromic films for dosimetry are GafChromic HD-810 and double-layer GafChromic MD-55-2.

34. C Only II and IV are correct. A radiochromic film consists of ultrathin colorless, radiosensitive leuco dye bonded onto a 100-μm-thick mylar base. Other varieties include thin layers of radiosensitive dye sandwiched between two pieces of polyester base. Radiographic films is composed of a transparent film base (cellulose acetate or polyester resin) coated with an emulsion containing small crystals of silver bromide. During development of the radiographic film, the exposed crystals are reduced to metallic silver.

35. D In the megavoltage range of photon energies, films have been used to measure isodose curves with acceptable accuracy of ±3 %.

36. B Thermoluminescence dosimetry (TLD) refers to energy recovered as visible light when crystalline materials are heated or release visible photons by thermal emission. In a TLD (and OSLD), there are impurities that are trapped in the crystal. When the TLD is irradiated, the ionized electrons gain energy and are moved up into the conduction band from the valence band. When these electrons give up their energy, they want to drop back to the valence band, but they get trapped by the impurities in the crystal. In a TLD, the way to release these trapped electrons is by heating. Once heated, the electrons can leave the trap and return to the valence band. When they do this, visible light is emitted. By using a photomultiplier tube (PMT), the visible light is detected, and this can be converted into a dose. For OSLDs, instead of using heat to release the trapped electrons, light of a certain wavelength is used. The freed electrons emit light at a different wavelength that can be detected.

37. E All of them are correct. Both TLDs and OSLDs are robust and can be made very small to be placed where they are needed.

38. A A photomultiplier tube (PMT) is used to measure visible light emitted from some crystal lattice. The PMT converts the visible light into an electric signal that can be used to make an image or measure dose. A thermistor is a device that changes resistance with temperature which is needed for calorimetry. A spectrophotometry measures the change in molar amount of Fe^{2+} contained

in a Fricke dosimeter which uses the change in chemical properties to measure dose. A densitometer is used to measure the optical density when the film is irradiated and processed.

39. B Radiographic density is a measurement of degree of film darkening. It is the logarithm of the intensity of light incident on the film (I_0) and the intensity of light transmitted through the film (I_t). Useful densities in diagnostic radiology range from about 0.2 to about 4. The optical density formula is $D = \log(I_0/I_t)$. Using that equation, it can be seen that a density reading of 3 is the result of 0.1 % of transmitted light reaching the far side of the film. $I_0 = 100\%$, and $I_t = 0.1\%$
$D = \log(I_0/I_t)$
$D = \log(100/0.1)$
$D = 3$

40. C The relationship between film density and relative exposure is offered in an H and D (Hurter and Driffield) curve which contains three regions. The first region is the toe, and it is associated with relatively low exposures and corresponds to low density portions of an image. The second part is the shoulder which corresponds to the upper portion of the curve in which the slope decreases with increasing exposure due to the reduced ability of the film to transfer contrast in areas that receive relatively high exposures. Finally, there is the linear region between the toe and the shoulder where the curve is relatively straight and very steep because the highest level of contrast is produced. The H-D curve can be used to do relative dosimetry for patient-specific QA tests in radiation therapy.

41. B The most recent recommended protocol by the AAPM for calibration parameters of megavoltage beams is TG-51. This protocol was introduced by the AAPM in 1999 and replaced the TG-21 protocol. The TRS-398 protocol was published by the IAEA in 2000 and supersedes the previous IAEA TRS-277 protocol.

42. E All are major changes from TG-21.

43. B According to the TG-51 protocol, electrons are calibrated in water (in cm) at R_{50} or percent depth dose at 50 % of broad beam. Photons are calibrated in water at 10 cm depth, 10×10 cm² field at the surface of a water phantom, typically at an SSD of 100 cm. TG-51 does not discuss neutron or proton dosimetry.

44. A Disadvantages of diode detectors include temperature, directional, and energy dependence; also damage to the diode occurs at each use due to radiation. As the manufacturing process for diodes improves, the radiation damage is not that big of a concern.

45. A Only I, II, and III are correct. Silicon diodes are well suited for relative measurements but are not recommended for absolute measurements.

46. D Diodes are far more sensitive than ion chambers because the energy to produce an electron-hole pair in Si is 3.5 eV for diodes versus 34 eV to produce an ion pair in air for ion chambers. Also, the density of Si is 1,800 times that of air. Thus, a diode can provide an adequate signal even with a small collecting volume. At the same time, diodes have a much higher energy dependence than ion chambers because of these differences.

47. B Heat is the method used in calorimetry to determine the absorbed dose in the medium. Calorimetry is based on the principle that energy absorbed in a medium appears as heat energy, while a small amount may appear in the form of a chemical change. Ferrous sulfate (Fricke) dosimeters are the most precise dosimeter used to measure absorbed dose in a patient using a chemical reaction.

48. B The TG-51 protocol provides step-by-step implementation of linac photon and electron calibration. Photons are calibrated using an ionization chamber in water at a depth of 10 cm with a field size of 10×10 cm^2 at 100 SSD.

49. C Absorbed dose is energy absorbed from all ionizing radiations per unit mass of materials, its SI unit is Gray (Gy), and the old unit is RAD; Becquerel (Bq) is the SI unit of activity and curie (Ci) is its unit; the SI unit of exposure is C kg^{-1}, and its unit is the roentgen.

50. B A pocket dosimeter is used to provide an immediate reading from exposure to X-ray or gamma rays. It can be reusable but it cannot provide a permanent record. In order to get a reading from a TLD, the crystal needs to be heated, the signal from the photomultiplier tube (PMT) must be processed and then the result can be converted to a dose. Silicon diodes are very sensitive, respond instantly, and are very small. The film badge uses radiographic film which consists of a transparent film base coated with an emulsion containing silver bromide. To obtain a dose, the film must be developed.

51. B Linear energy transfer (LET) is defined as the energy absorbed per unit distance of ionizing particle passing through a material (KeV/μm). Stopping power (S) is defined as the amount of energy lost by a charged particle per unit distance as it travels. The attenuation coefficient (μ) is the probability per unit length that an interaction will occur that removes a particular photon from the beam, and absorption is the process whereby energy is taken out of a beam by a material and kept within that material.

52. A Half-life is the time necessary for a radioactive material to decay to 50 % of its original activity. Decay is the process by which a radioactive element

1.12 Radiation Units (Answers)

moves toward stability, governed by a characteristic half-life. Excitation is the raising of an electron to higher energy level and half-value layer (HVL) is the thickness of a given material needed to reduce the intensity of a photon beam to 50 % of its initial value (HVL=0.693/μ).

53. B TLDs have recently replaced film badges as the most common type of personnel monitor found in a medical environment because it is inexpensive compared to others. Another reason for this is the elimination of the film processors. Some badges use radiochromic film.

54. C The two disadvantages of using film badges are that one has to wait until the results are reported by the commercial vendor and the other is the energy dependence exhibited by film. For example, a film exposed to 1 cGy of 140 kVp X-ray will be darker upon development than a film exposed to 1 cGy of Co-60 gamma rays due to the film absorbing more energy at 140 kVp because of the increased occurance of the photoelectric effect for kV photons rather than MV photons which tend to interact through Compton Scattering. Filters are used to reduce this effect and determine the quality of radiation that the exposure resulted from. Film badges are inexpensive and can be reread to confirm a reported exposure.

55. B Ring badges typically use TLD chips instead of a piece of radiographic film; film is used on film badges. A Geiger-Mueller counter is a type of ion chamber that is very sensitive to detect radiation but cannot quantify the amount or type of radiation.

56. A According to NCRP and NRC, a badge should be given to an individual when that individual has the POTENTIAL to receive one-tenth of the applicable MPD for an adult, minor, or pregnant woman in a year. Not all individuals who work in radiation department have to wear a radiation badge depending on the type of work they do.

57. C First collect all the data.
Dose in cGy=?
TLD calibration dose=50 cGy
Patient reading=80.5 nC
Calibration reading=32.7 nC
Formula
Remember that the ratio of the calibration is the same as the ratio to the reading.
This means: (Calibration dose/Calibration reading)=(Patient dose/Patient reading).
Dose to patient cGy=Calibration dose×patient reading/calibration reading
Dose to patient cGy=50 cGy×80.5 nC/32.7 nC
Dose to patient=123 cGy

58. C A thermoluminescent dosimeter (TLD) is considered to be the most accurate radiation monitoring device.

59. D Optically stimulated luminescence dosimeter (OSLD) has recently been developed for dosimetry. It is more sensitive than a film badge or TLD, it uses aluminum oxide to record radiation, results can be read up to a year following exposure, and it is available for use on torso and finger due to its small size.

60. D The personal film badge should never be used outside working area. Radiation workers should not wear their film badges during medical X-ray procedures because the badge is for monitoring only OCCUPATIONAL exposure. Exposures from medical and dental procedures and background radiation exposure are excluded from your occupational dose.

61. B The badge holder contains an open window to determine radiation exposure due to beta particles which can be shielded by a thin amount of material. Typically one is not concerned about external alpha exposure as the range of alpha particles in tissues is very short. Alpha particles that are inhaled or ingested are a significant concern because they have a very high RBE and LET.

62. A Film badges provide a permanent record, can distinguish between different energies of photons, and can measure doses due to different types of radiation. The major disadvantage is that it must be developed to get the reading which is time consuming. Also heat can affect the film and exposures of less than 20 millirem of gamma radiation cannot be accurately measured.

Dose Calculation Methods

Contents

2.1	Dose Calculation (Questions)	110
2.2	Applied Mathematics (Questions)	133
2.3	External Beam Calculations (Questions)	144
2.4	Effects of Beam-Modifying Devices (Questions)	145
2.5	Irregular Field Calculations (Questions)	148
2.6	Special Calculations (Questions)	155
2.7	Manual Corrections for Tissue Inhomogeneities (Questions)	162
2.8	Dose Calculation (Answers)	164
2.9	Applied Mathematics (Answers)	180
2.10	External Beam Calculations (Answers)	199
2.11	Effects of Beam-Modifying Devices (Answers)	200
2.12	Irregular Field Calculations (Answers)	204
2.13	Special Calculations (Answers)	212
2.14	Manual Corrections for Tissue Inhomogeneity (Answers)	219

As a dosimetrist, the basic skill is dose calculations. There are two essential categories for dose calculations: correction-based methods and model-based methods.

Correction-based methods use basic dose calculation methods based on PDD or TMR tables and then are corrected for other factors such as wedge, field size, distance, depth, inhomogeneity, etc. The main advantages for correction-based methods are that they are direct, fast, and easy to check and can be done manually. Most of the secondary MU calculation software, either commercial or customized, is correction based. However, correction-based methods can only calculate a single-point dose per calculation, which is inconvenient for volume dose calculations.

Model-based methods have become the standard dose calculation algorithm in modern treatment planning systems (TPS). Model-based methods are more accurate than correction-based methods since they consider more factors such as photon and

© Springer International Publishing Switzerland 2015
W. Amestoy, *Review of Medical Dosimetry: A Study Guide*,
DOI 10.1007/978-3-319-13626-4_2

electron scattering, secondary particle generation, and beam hardening, among others. A Monte Carlo simulation (MC) is considered as the most precise model-based method. Other well-known model-based methods include the pencil beam algorithm (PBA), the collapsed-cone convolution (CCC) by ADAC/Pinnacle, and the analytical anisotropic algorithm (AAA) by Eclipse/Varian. Model-based methods can be time consuming, but modern computing and variance reduction methods have reduced the calculation burden. The standard dose calculation algorithms in commercial TPSs calculate volume dose in which there are hundreds of points.

Most of the exam questions on dose calculations are for correction-based methods. It would be difficult to use a model-based algorithm to calculate dose on a written exam; therefore, CMD candidates only need to know the concepts and principles of model-based methods.

2.1 Dose Calculation (Questions)

Quiz 1 (Level 2)

1. Basic dosimetry measurements are usually performed in a water phantom because:
   A. I, II, and III only
   B. I and III only
   C. II and IV only
   D. IV only
   E. All are correct
   I. Water approximates the radiation absorption and scattering properties of muscle and soft tissues.
   II. Water is universally available with reproducible radiation properties.
   III. Water is tissue equivalent.
   IV. Water has a high Z.

2. Which of the following phantom materials is/are frequently used for radiation dosimetry?
   A. I, II, and III only
   B. I and III only
   C. II and IV only
   D. IV only
   E. All are correct
   I. Lucite
   II. Tungsten
   III. Polystyrene
   IV. Graphite

2.1 Dose Calculation (Questions)

3. A phantom with materials that simulate various body tissues like muscle, bone, lung, and air cavities is called:
A. Homogeneous phantoms
B. Anthropomorphic phantoms
C. Solid water phantoms
D. Wood phantoms

4. The variation of absorbed dose in a patient or phantom depends on:
A. I, II, and III only
B. I and III only
C. II and IV only
D. IV only
E. All are correct
I. Beam energy
II. Depth
III. Field size and collimator
IV. Distance from source

5. The percentage of the absorbed dose at any depth d to the absorbed dose at a fixed reference depth d_0 along the central axis of the beam is the definition of:
A. Mayneord F Factor
B. Percentage depth dose
C. Tissue-air ratio
D. Tissue-phantom ratio

6. Which of the following statements is/are true?
A. I, II, and III only
B. I and III only
C. II and IV only
D. IV only
E. All are correct
I. PDD beyond Dmax increases with beam energy.
II. PDD decreases with depth beyond the Dmax.
III. PDD increases with increasing field size.
IV. PDD increases with increases SSD.

7. The region between the surface and the point of maximum dose is called:
A. Skin-sparing effect
B. Dmax
C. Dose buildup region
D. Penumbra

8. Match the following quality photons with its corresponding depth dose distribution.
A. 25 MV (IV)
B. 4 MV (II)
C. 10 MV (III)
D. 60Co (I)

Fig. 2.1.1

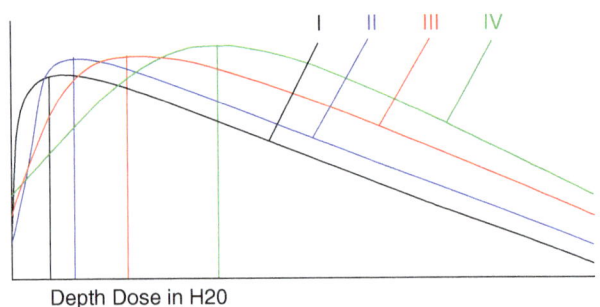

Depth Dose in H20

9. The projection, on a plane perpendicular to the beam axis, of the distal end of the collimator as seen from the front center of the source is the definition of:
A. Source-to-surface distance
B. Source-to-axis distance
C. Dosimetric or physical field size
D. Geometric field size

10. Which of the following statements is/are true?
A. I, II, and III only
B. I and III only
C. II and IV only
D. IV only
E. All are correct
I. Rectangular field is equivalent to a square field if they have the same area/perimeter (A/P).
II. Sterling developed the rule-of-thumb method for equating rectangular and square fields.
III. Clarkson's method includes irregular field dose calculations.
IV. As the field size increases, PDD increases.

11. Which of the following formulas is/are used to calculate equivalent square?
A. I, II, and III only
B. I and III only
C. II and IV only
D. IV only
E. All are correct
I. $r = 4/\sqrt{\pi} \times A/P$
II. $ESF = 4 \times A/P$
III. $A/P = a/4$ or $A/P = a \times b/2(a+b)$
IV. $ESF = 2(L \times W)/L + W$

2.1 Dose Calculation (Questions)

12. The equivalent square formula can be used with:
A. Circular-shaped fields
B. Irregular-shaped fields
C. Rectangular-shaped fields
D. Triangular-shaped fields

13. A PDD needs to be found for an equivalent square of a rectangular tangential breast field of 20 cm by 14 cm. Which of the following answers is the equivalent square of the above RT breast tangent field?
A. 23.33×23.33
B. 41.11×41.11
C. 16.47×16.47
D. 4.11×4.11

14. What is the A/P of 10×25 cm field?
A. 35.7
B. 3.57
C. 125
D. 17.5

15. Which of the following statements is/are true?
A. I, II, and III only
B. I and III only
C. II and IV only
D. IV only
E. All are correct
I. PDD data for radiation therapy beams are usually tabulated for square fields.
II. As the field size increase, the contribution of the scattered radiation to the absorbed dose increases.
III. The increase in PDD caused by increase in field size depends on beam quality.
IV. The field size dependence of PDD is less pronounced for the higher-energy than for the lower-energy beams.

16. A rectangular field is equivalent to a square field if:
A. Both have the same area/perimeter (A/P).
B. Both have different area/perimeter (A/P).
C. The rectangular is twice as bigger as the square.
D. Both have the same isocenter.

17. Match the following answers using a rectangular field of 25×5 cm.
A. Area
B. Perimeter
C. Area/perimeter (A/P)
D. Equivalent square
I. 60
II. 125
III. 8.33
IV. 2.083

18. Match the following statements. There can be more than one answer for each letter:
A. Energy increases.
B. Depth increases.
C. Field size increases.
D. SSD increases.
I. PDD increases.
II. PDD decreases.
III. PDD remains the same.

19. The increase in PDD with an increase in SSD can be found by:
A. Mayneord F factor formula
B. Equivalent square formula
C. Inverse square formula
D. Tissue-air ratio formula

20. Which of the following is the Mayneord F factor formula?
A. $F = [(SSD2 - dm)/(SSD1 - dm) \times (SSD1 - d)/(SSD2 - d)]2$
B. $F = [(SSD1 + dm)/(SSD1 + dm) \times (SSD2 + d)/(SSD2 + d)]2$
C. $F = [(d + dm)/(SSD1 + dm) \times (d + d)/(SSD2 + dm)]2$
D. $F = [(SSD_2 + d_m)/(SSD_1 + d_m) \times (SSD_1 + d)/(SSD_2 + d)]^2$

21. A CNS single spine field was calculated from C3 to S1 using 100 cm SSD at a depth of 5 cm, the PDD was determine to be 80 %, and the Dmax depth was 0.5 cm. After plan revision, the physician decided to include the entire sacrum. What is the new PDD if the field was changed from 100–120 SSD?
A. 1.0144
B. 81.2 %
C. 80.6 %
D. 75.5 %

22. Which of the following field size has the highest PDD for the same beam energy at the same depth?
A. I, II, and III only
B. I and III only
C. II and IV only
D. IV only
E. All are correct
I. 20×4
II. 12×6
III. 6.7×6.7
IV. 8×8

23. At a lung-tissue interface, the dose is affected primary by:
A. Attenuation of the primary beam
B. Scatter
C. Mass attenuation coefficient
D. Heterogeneity correction

2.1 Dose Calculation (Questions)

24. One method for correcting tissue inhomogeneities and use to remove the SSD dependence is:
A. SAR
B. Clarkson's method
C. TAR
D. TMR

I do not like this question. It is introducing two very different concepts of TAR, and the answer does not fully explain them. I would remove this question. The important point about the SSD independence of TAR is addressed in a few questions.

25. The TAR is calculated by finding:
A. The ratio of dose at depth in phantom to dose at a specified reference depth in phantom
B. The ratio of dose at depth in phantom to dose in free space at the same point
C. The ratio of dose at depth in phantom to dose at a depth of maximum dose in phantom
D. The ratio of dose at maximum dose in phantom to dose in free space at the same point

26. TAR depends on:
A. I, II, and III only
B. I and III only
C. II and IV only
D. IV only
E. All are correct
I. Field size
II. Depth
III. Energy
IV. SSD

27. The difference between TAR and BSF is:
A. TAR is defined at Dmax only, and BSF is defined at any depth.
B. TAR is defined at any depth, and BSF is defined at Dmax only.
C. TAR and BSF are measured at a point in air.
D. TAR and BSF are independent of distance.

28. TAR increases as:
A. I, II, and III only
B. I and III only
C. II and IV only
D. IV only
E. All are correct
I. Energy increases.
II. Depth decreases.
III. Field size increases.
IV. Field size decreases.

29. Determine the treatment time to deliver 150 cGy (rad) at the center of rotation of an arc treatment where the dose rate in free space at SAD is 80.5 cGy/min and the average TAR is 0.550.
A. 3 min
B. 3.39 cGy/min
C. 3.39 min
D. 5 min

30. Which of the following statements about scatter-air ratio (SAR) is/are true?
A. I, II, and III only
B. I and III only
C. II and IV only
D. IV only
E. All are correct
I. SAR is defined as the ratio of the scattered dose at a given point in the phantom to the dose in free space at the same point.
II. SAR is used for the purpose of calculating scattered dose in the medium.
III. SAR in the phantom is equal to the total dose minus the primary dose at that point.
IV. SAR is the difference between the TAR for a given field and the TAR for the 0×0 field.

31. SAR depends on:
A. I, II, and III only
B. I and III only
C. II and IV only
D. IV only
E. All are correct
I. Beam energy
II. Depth
III. Field size
IV. SSD

32. The SAR formula is:
A. $SAR = TAR_{(d, rd)} + TAR_{(d, 0)}$
B. $SAR = TAR_{(d, rd)} - TAR_{(d, 0)}$
C. $SAR = TAR_{(d, rd)} / TAR_{(d, 0)}$
D. $SAR = TAR_{(d, rd)} \times TAR_{(d, 0)}$

33. Match the correct name with the corresponding diagram.
A. TMR
B. PDD
C. SAR
D. TAR
E. TPR
F. Off-axis ratio
G. BSF

2.1 Dose Calculation (Questions)

Fig. 2.1.2

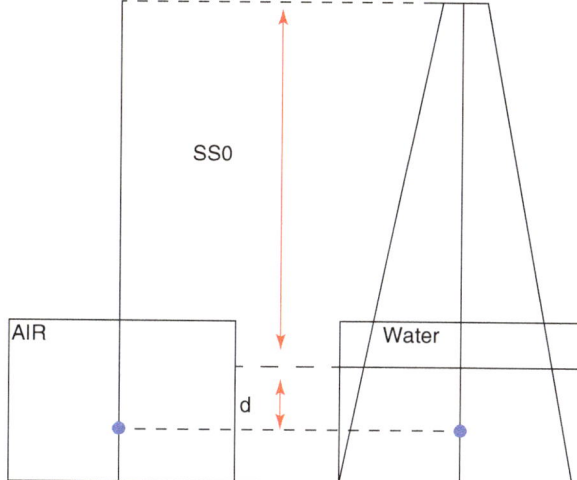

Fig. 2.1.3

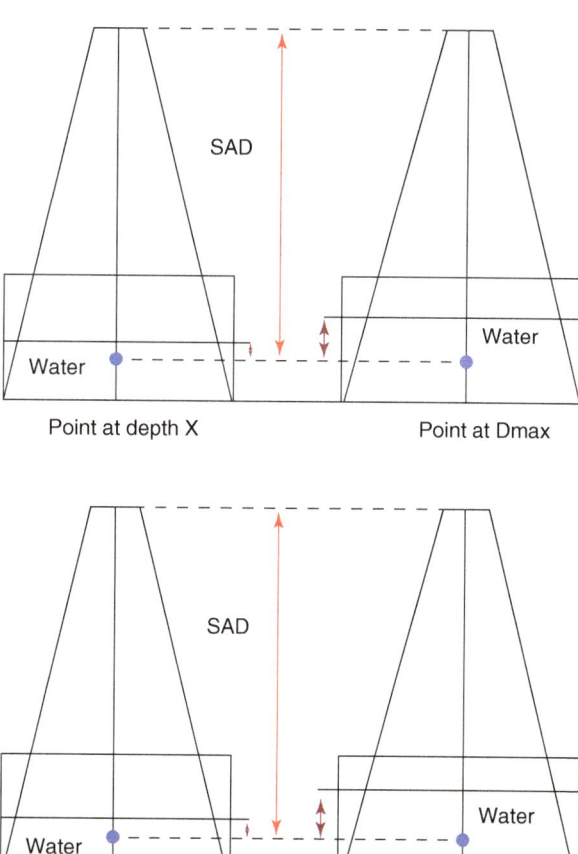

Fig. 2.1.4

Fig. 2.1.5

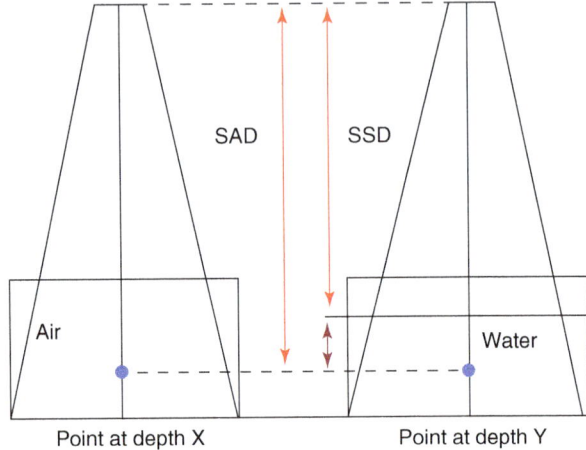

Fig. 2.1.6

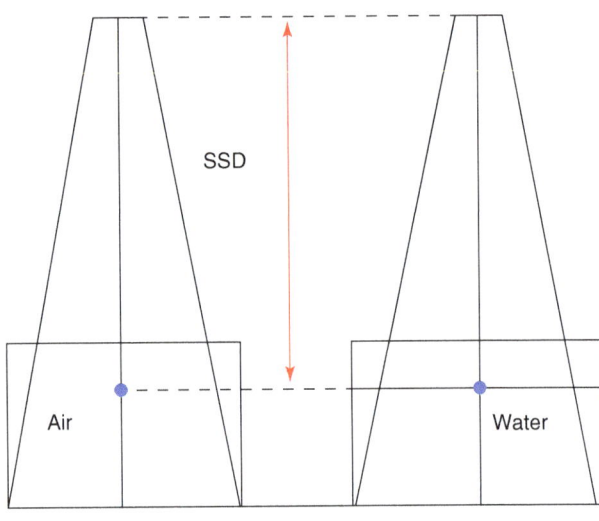

2.1 Dose Calculation (Questions)

Fig. 2.1.7

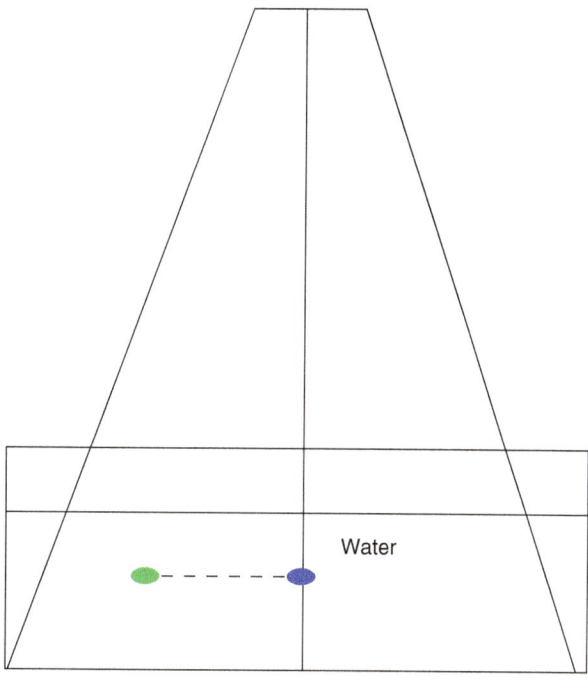

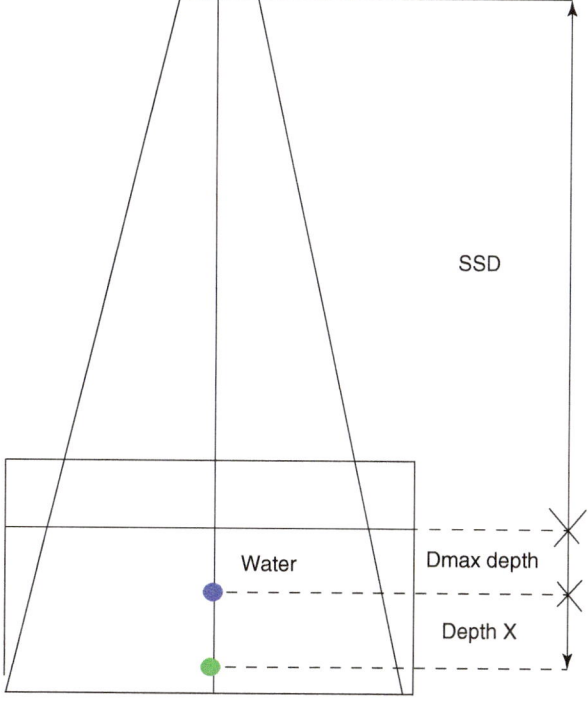

Fig. 2.1.8

34. An irregular field is:
A. I, II, and III only
B. I and III only
C. II and IV only
D. IV only
E. All are correct
I. Any rectangular or circular field
II. Any blocked or rectangular field
III. Any square and rectangular field
IV. Any field other than the rectangular, square, or circular field

35. Which of the following data is/are used in the calculation of Clarkson's method?
A. I, II, and III only
B. I and III only
C. II and IV only
D. IV only
E. All are correct
I. SAR
II. PDD
III. TAR $_{(0)}$
IV. TMR

36. TAR at Dmax is equal to:
A. PDD
B. BSF
C. TPR
D. SAR

37. The interrelationship between TAR and PDD is:
A. TAR = BSF × PDD/inverse square
B. TAR = PDD × BSF × inverse square
C. PDD = TAR × inverse square
D. TAR = TMR × BSF/inverse square

38. Limitations of PDD and TAR include:
A. I, II, and III only
B. I and III only
C. II and IV only
D. IV only
E. All are correct
I. PDD depends on SSD only.
II. PDD depends on SAD only.
III. TAR cannot be used on higher-energy photons.
IV. TAR cannot be used on lower energies such as ^{60}Co.

2.1 Dose Calculation (Questions)

39. The dose to a point in the medium may be calculated using:
A. Primary and scattered radiation
B. Compton and pair production
C. Scatter and neutron radiation
D. Photoelectric and coherent scatter

40. Effective primary dose is:
A. Dose due to the primary photons only
B. Dose scatters produced by the patient
C. Dose scatters produced by the collimating system
D. Dose due to primary photons as well as those scattered from the collimating system

41. The most commonly used beam-modifying device is:
A. Flattening filter
B. The anode
C. Bending magnet
D. A wedge

42. A wedge angle refers to:
A. The angle between the central axes of the two beams
B. The angle of the isodose tilt at Dmax
C. The angle through which an isodose curve is tilted at the central axis of the beam at a specified depth
D. The physical degree angle of the wedge

43. Which of the following wedge types should be avoided in the medial tangent of a breast treatment?
A. I, II, and III
B. I and III only
C. II and IV only
D. IV only
E. All are correct
I. Dynamic wedge
II. Asymmetric wedge
III. Universal wedge
IV. Physical wedge

44. Physical wedge should be avoided, if possible, in the medial field of a tangent breast treatment:
A. Because physical wedge can fall and harm the patient
B. Because physical wedge produces scatter which affect the contralateral breast
C. Because the physical wedge is too close to the patient
D. Because wedge factor is difficult to calculate on the medial tangent

45. What happens to the wedge angle or tilt of the isodose curve as depth is increased?
A. Increases
B. Decreases
C. Stays the same
D. Depth has no effect on the isodose curve

46. The wedge transmission factor expresses:
A. The ratio of the dose rate at Dmax with and without the wedge
B. The ratio of the dose rate on the central axis at specified depth with and without the wedge
C. The dose rate on the central axis with the wedge
D. The dose rate at Dmax with the wedge on in-out position

47. The thicker end of a wedge is called:
A. The toe
B. The heel
C. The compensator
D. The grow

48. Wedges are typically used:
A. I, II, and III
B. I and III only
C. II and IV only
D. IV only
E. All are correct
I. On sloped surfaces such as AP chest fields
II. On tangential breast treatments
III. On lateral larynx treatments
IV. On a PA lumbar spine

49. Which of the following wedges is designed so that the central axis thickness remains constant and the center of the wedge is fixed in the center of the beam for all field sizes?
A. Dynamic wedge
B. Universal wedge
C. Asymmetric wedge
D. Individualized wedge

50. Which of the following definitions are true?
A. I, II, and III only
B. I and III only
C. II and IV only
D. IV only
E. All are correct

2.1 Dose Calculation (Questions)

I. Output of a machine is defined as the dose delivered at a specified point in the beam, at a specified distance from the target, and in a specified medium.
II. Absorbed dose in the irradiated medium is the energy absorbed per unit mass.
III. Maximum dose or Dmax is obtained at the depth where electron equilibrium is reached.
IV. The buildup region is the region between the surface and Dmax.

51. Which of the following is/are true about half-value layer (HVL)?
A. I, II, and III only
B. I and III only
C. II and IV only
D. IV only
E. All are correct
I. The HVL is the thickness of the material that reduces the intensity of the beam to half (50 %) its original value.
II. The HVL expresses the penetration, quality, or hardness of a beam.
III. If the HVL of a given beam is 5 mm Cu, inserting 5 mm Cu in the beam path will reduce its intensity to half of its original value.
IV. The HVL is related to the linear attenuation coefficient (μ) by the equation (HVL = 0.693/μ).

52. Which of the following is/are true about dose rate?
A. I, II, and III only
B. I and III only
C. II and IV only
D. IV only
E. All are correct
A. Dose rate increases with increasing field size.
B. Dose rate decreases with increasing field size.
C. Dose rate varies inversely proportional with the square of the distance from the source.
D. Dose rate increases as distance from the source increase.

53. Which of the following materials is used for the measurement of HVL?
A. Aluminum (Al), Cerrobend, or tin (Sn)
B. Aluminum (Al), copper (Cu), or tungsten
C. Lipowitz, copper (Cu), or tin (Sn)
D. Aluminum (Al), copper (Cu), or tin (Sn)

54. For a monoenergetic beam:
A. $HVL_1 > HVL_2$
B. $HVL_1 < HVL_2$
C. $HVL_1 = HVL_2$
D. $HVL_1 \leq HVL_2$

55. For a polyenergetic beam:
A. $HVL_1 > HVL_2$
B. $HVL_1 < HVL_2$
C. $HVL_1 = HVL_2$
D. $HVL_1 \leq HVL_2$

56. For monoenergetic photon beams, the linear attenuation coefficiency formula is:
A. $HVL \times 0.693$
B. $0.693/HVL$
C. $\lambda = -0.693/T\frac{1}{2}$
D. $T_a = 1.44 \times T_{1/2}$

57. If the linear attenuation coefficient for a 23 MV photon beam is 0.046 mm^{-1} lead, what is the HVL thickness?
A. 0.03 mm lead
B. 15 mm lead
C. 0.066 mm lead
D. 10 mm lead

58. Match the following definitions.
A. Tissue maximum ratio (TMR)
B. Tissue-phantom ratio (TPR)
C. Backscatter factor (BSF)
D. Scatter-air ratio (SAR)
I. The ratio of dose at a specified point in tissue or in a phantom to the dose at the same distance in the beam at a reference depth
II. The ratio of the dose at a specified point in tissue or in a phantom to the dose at the same point when it is at the depth of maximum dose
III. Scattered dose at a given point in a medium to the dose in air at the same point
IV. The ratio of dose on the central axis at Dmax to the dose at the same point in air or free space

59. TMR is a special case of:
A. TPR
B. SAR
C. SMR
D. Backscatter factor

60. Which of the following statements is/are true?
A. I, II, and III only
B. I and III only
C. II and IV only
D. IV only
E. All are correct

2.1 Dose Calculation (Questions)

I. The difference between SAR and SMR is that SMR reference point is at Dmax only versus SAR reference point is at any given point.
II. The difference between TAR and TMR is that TMR reference point is at Dmax only versus TAR reference point is at any given point.
III. SAR and TAR are independent of distance.
IV. SAR and SMR are mainly used in calculation of scattered dose in a phantom or tissue.

61. Methods of inhomogeneity corrections for photon beams are:
A. I, II, and III only
B. I and III only
C. II and IV only
D. IV only
E. All are correct
I. TAR
II. Effective SSD method
III. Isodose shift method
IV. Coefficient of equivalent thickness

62. How many HVLs are required to reduce a photon beam of 320 mR/h to 5 mR/h?
A. 5 HVLs
B. 7 HVLs
C. 6 HVLs
D. 12 HVLs

63. How many TVLs are required to reduce a photon beam of 4,000 mR/min to 4 mR/min?
A. 3 HVLs
B. 5 HVLs
C. 7 HVLs
D. 12 HVLs

64. Match the beams with its corresponding characteristics (monoenergetic or polyenergetic beam).
A. Photon beam from a diagnostic or therapeutic device
B. Electron beam
C. Gamma rays
D. Characteristic x-rays
I. Monoenergetic beam
II. Polyenergetic beam

65. Match the following reduction and/or increase of dose from each photon beam energy due to the presence of bone or healthy lung in the irradiated area.
A. 3 mm Cu
B. 60Co
C. 4 MV
D. 10 MV
E. 20 MV

I. 2 %/cm increase in dose beyond healthy lung
II. −3 % reduction of dose beyond bone or 4 %/cm increase in dose beyond healthy lung
III. −3.5 % reduction of dose beyond bone or 3.5–5/cm % increase in dose beyond healthy lung
IV. −2 % reduction of dose beyond bone
V. −7 % reduction of dose beyond bone or 10 %/cm increase in dose beyond healthy lung

66. A test has been conducted with a material having a HVL of 3.5 cm. What will be the transmission of the beam through the same material with a thickness of 10.5 cm?
A. 0.0007
B. 0.125
C. 0.088
D. 0.795

67. After 10 HVLs, the intensity of the beam is reduced by:
A. $I = I_0(0.1)^{10}$
B. $I = I_0(0.5)^{10}$
C. $I^{10} = I_0(0.5)$
D. $I = I_0(10)^{10}$

68. The collimator scatter factor (Sc):
A. I, II, and III only
B. I and III only
C. II and IV only
D. IV only
E. All are correct
I. Is commonly called the output factor.
II. Is the ratio of the output in air for a given field to that for a reference field.
III. As the field size increased, Sc or output factor increases.
IV. Is the ratio of the output in the tissue for a given field to that for a reference field.

69. The phantom scatter factor (Sp):
A. I, II, and III only
B. I and III only
C. II and IV only
D. IV only
E. All are correct
I. Takes into account the change in scatter radiation originating in the phantom at a reference depth as the field size is changed.
II. Is the ratio of the dose rate for a given field at a reference depth to the dose rate at the same depth for the reference field size, with the same collimator opening.
III. Is related to changes in the volume of the phantom irradiated for a fixed collimator opening.
IV. If backscatter factors can be measured, Sp at Dmax may be defined as the ratio of BSF for the given field to that for the reference field.

2.1 Dose Calculation (Questions)

70. Clarkson's method is used to calculate:
A. Circular fields
B. Irregular fields
C. Rectangular fields
D. Square fields

71. The relationship between TMR and TAR is:
A. $TMR_{(d, rd)} = BSF_{(rd)}/TAR_{(d, rd)}$
B. $TMR_{(d, rd)} = BSF_{(rd)} \times TAR_{(d, rd)}$
C. $TMR_{(d, rd)} = TAR_{(d, rd)}/BSF_{(rd)}$
D. $TMR_{(d, rd)} = SAR_{(rd)}/TAR_{(d, rd)}$

72. Scatter-maximum ratio (SMR):
A. I, II, and III only
B. I and III only
C. II and IV only
D. IV only
E. All are correct
I. Is the quantity designated specifically for the calculation of scattered dose in a medium
II. Is the ratio of the scattered dose at a given point in the phantom to the effective primary dose at the same point at Dmax
III. Is related to SAR
IV. Is the ratio of the scattered dose at a given point in the phantom to the effective primary dose at any point

73. Which of the following statements is/are true about the backscatter factor?
A. I, II, and III only
B. I and III only
C. II and IV only
D. IV only
E. All are correct
I. BSF is independent of SSD.
II. BSF depends on energy and the field size.
III. BSF and TAR at Dmax are the same.
IV. BSF is much lower for megavoltage beams than lower-energy beams.

74. Match the formulas with their corresponding definitions.
A. PDD
B. TMR
C. TAR
D. TPR
E. BSF
F. Output
G. SAR
H. Absorbed dose
I. Collimator scatter factor (Sc)
J. Phantom scatter factor (Sp)
K. SMR

I. Ratio of dose at depth in a phantom to dose at a depth of Dmax in a phantom. $TAR_{(d, rd)}/BSF_{(rd)}$. Dose in tissue/dose in phantom at Dmax
II. Percentage of the absorbed dose at any depth d to the absorbed dose at a fixed reference depth d_0, along the central axis of the beam
III. Ratio of dose at depth in phantom to dose in free space at the same point. BSF×PDD/inverse square. Dose in tissue/dose in air
IV. Ratio of dose at maximum dose in phantom to dose in free space at the same point or tissue-air ratio at the depth of maximum dose on central axis of the beam. Dose at Dmax/dose in free space
V. Ratio of dose at depth in phantom to dose at a specified reference depth in phantom. Dose in tissue/dose in phantom at reference depth
VI. Dose delivered at a specified point in the beam, at a specified distance from the target, and in a specified medium
VII. Energy absorbed in a material per unit mass
VIII. Ratio of scattered dose at a given point in the phantom to the dose in free space at the same point. $TAR_{(d, rd)} - TAR_{(d, 0)}$
IX. Ratio of the output in air for a given field to that for a reference field. Also called the output factor. $D_{fs}(r)/D_{fs}(ref)$
X. Ratio of the scattered dose at a given point in the phantom to the effective primary dose at the same point at Dmax
XI. Ratio of the dose rate for a given field at a reference depth to the dose rate at the same depth for the reference field size, with the same collimator opening

75. The dose on a fixed SAD technique is usually normalized at:
A. The surface of the patient
B. The isocenter
C. At Dmax
D. The tissue surrounding the target

76. Which of the following statements is/are true?
A. I, II, and III only
B. I and III only
C. II and IV only
D. IV only
E. All are correct
I. The SAD technique is also known as an isocentric technique.
II. The axis of rotation of the machine is the isocenter.
III. Small errors in SSD are balanced out using an opposing field.
IV. SAD technique is inferior to an SSD technique.

77. Which of the following methods are used in calculating the dose in an SAD technique?
A. I, II, and III only
B. I and III only
C. II and IV only
D. IV only
E. All are correct

2.1 Dose Calculation (Questions)

  I. TAR and dose rate in air
 II. PDD
III. TPR and TMR
IV. Clarkson's method

78. Which of the following is/are correct about the isocenter?
A. I, II, and III only
B. I and III only
C. II and IV only
D. IV only
E. All are correct
  I. Refers to a point in space that is the same distance from the source for all gantry angles.
 II. Is the intersection of the collimator axis and the axis of rotation.
III. Linacs have the isocenter typically at 80 or 100 cm.
IV. The isocenter is fixed and cannot be changed.

79. The dose on a fixed SSD technique is usually normalized at:
A. The surface of the patient
B. The isocenter
C. At Dmax
D. The tissue surrounding the target

80. Which of the following statements is/are true about SSD?
A. I, II, and III only
B. I and III only
C. II and IV only
D. IV only
E. All are correct
  I. SSD is patient specific.
 II. Field size is defined on the patient's skin on an SSD setup.
III. SSD is a non-isocentric technique.
IV. SSD calculation uses the PDD method.

81. If an SAD technique is used for treatment, the SAD is equal to:
A. SSD − depth
B. SSD + depth
C. SSD/depth
D. SSD × depth

82. Machines are usually calibrated:
A. To deliver 1 cGy per monitor unit (MU) at 100 cm SSD, the reference depth, for a maximum open field 40 × 40 cm
B. To deliver 1 cGy per monitor unit (MU) at 100 cm SSD, the reference depth, for a reference field size 10 × 10 cm
C. To deliver 1 cGy per monitor unit (MU) at 100 cm SSD, the reference depth, for a reference field size, usually 10 × 10 cm
D. To deliver 100 cGy per monitor unit (MU) at 100 cm SAD, for a reference field size, usually 10 × 10 cm

83. An isodose line is defined as:
A. A line passing through points of equal dose representing a percentage of dose at a reference point
B. A region near the edge of the field margin where the dose falls rapidly
C. A tilting of the isodose lines from their standard position
D. A line passing through points of different dose and representing percentage of dose at a reference point

84. A number of isodose curves depicted in 10 % increments is a function of:
A. Isodose line
B. Isodose chart
C. DVH
D. BEV

85. The light source, which coincides with the beam, is aligned to match:
A. 100 % isodose line
B. 75 % isodose line
C. 50 % isodose line
D. 25 % isodose line

86. Geometric field size is defined as:
A. The intersection of the 50 % isodose line and the surface
B. The intersection of the collimator axis and the axis of rotation
C. The region between the surface and maximum dose or Dmax
D. Region near the edge of the field margin, where the dose falls rapidly

87. The size of the penumbra depends on:
A. I, II, and III only
B. I and III only
C. II and IV only
D. IV only
E. All are correct
I. Size of the radiation source
II. Source-to-collimator distance (SCD)
III. Source-to-skin distance (SSD)
IV. Depth of penumbra calculation

88. Which of the following statements is/are true?
A. I, II, and III only
B. I and III only
C. II and IV only
D. IV only
E. All are correct

2.1 Dose Calculation (Questions)

I. Isodose chart for a Co^{60} machine dose decreases away from the central axis near the surface.
II. Isodose chart for a linac machine dose increases away from the central axis near the surface.
III. Increased dose away from the central axis near the surface is due to overflattening of the beam at shallow depths.
IV. The flattening filter reduces the dose along the central axis and produces a flat beam at a specified depth, usually 10 cm.

89. Which of the following statements is/are true?
A. I, II, and III only
B. I and III only
C. II and IV only
D. IV only
E. All are correct

I. For an SSD technique, dose at Dmax is usually normalized to 100 %.
II. For an SAD technique, dose at isocenter is usually normalized at 100 %.
III. Dose profile displays relative doses across a field or across a treatment plan consisting of multiple beams.
IV. A beam's eye view shows the beam in a plane perpendicular to the central axis.

90. Match the following wedge types with its corresponding characteristic.
A. Dynamic wedge
B. Universal wedge
C. Asymmetric wedge
D. Individualized wedge

I. Wedge of a given angle that is fixed in the beam and serves all beam widths up to a designated limit.
II. Multiple wedges are required for each isodose tilt and are typically used in Co-60 beams. This wedge is mounted so that the thin edge of the wedge coincides with the edge of the light field.
III. Wedge effect can be produced by driving one of the secondary collimator jaws across the field.
IV. A wedge is mounted such that one can use an asymmetric jaw to block half the treatment field and utilize the wedging effect for the other open half.

91. The angle of the sloping isodose curve on a dynamic wedge is determined by:
A. The speed with which the gantry moves
B. The dose rate
C. The speed with which the collimator jaw moves
D. The amount of monitor units delivered

92. What is the distance in cm that a block or wedge should be placed away from the patient skin?
A. At least 10 cm away from the skin.
B. It could be placed as close as 1 cm away from the skin.
C. The distance is not important.
D. At least 15 cm away from the skin.

93. A wedge is usually constructed of:
A. I, II, and III
B. I and III only
C. II and IV only
D. IV only
E. All are correct
I. Lead
II. Steel
III. Copper
IV. Tungsten

94. Which of the following statements is/are true about a dynamic wedge?
A. I, II, and III
B. I and III only
C. II and IV only
D. IV only
E. All are correct
I. Can be produced by driving one of the collimator jaws across the field
II. Can generate different wedge angles
III. Has different transmission factors as a function of field size
IV. Has a sharper penumbra

95. Which of the following techniques can be used to create the junction between the cranial field and the upper spine field for craniospinal irradiation?
A. I, II, and III
B. I and III only
C. II and IV only
D. IV only
E. All are correct
I. Using a gap on the skin
II. Using independent jaws or half-beam block
III. Using collimator and couch angles
IV. Positioning the patient in a Trendelenburg or decubitus position

96. The advantage of using independent table and collimator angles to match the craniospinal fields is:
A. I, II, and III
B. I and III only
C. II and IV only
D. IV only
E. All are correct

I. Field matching is achieved with no overlap between the cranial and spine fields at any depth.
II. Patient's comfort and reproducibility are better.
III. The independent jaw can be conveniently used to move the craniospinal junction line caudally to smooth out the junction dose distribution.
IV. The independent jaw can be conveniently used to move the craniospinal junction line cephalic to smooth out the junction dose distribution.

97. Which of the following is/are true about field matching?
A. I, II, and III
B. I and III only
C. II and IV only
D. IV only
E. All are correct

I. The site of the field matching should not contain tumor or a critically sensitive organ.
II. For deep-seated tumors, the fields may be separated on the skin surface.
III. The line of field matching must be de drawn at each treatment session on the basis of the first treated fraction.
IV. The field-matching technique must be verified by actual isodose distributions before it is adopted for general clinical use.

98. What will be the outcome of the HVL if a machine is assigned a HVL of 3 mm Cu, but the engineer accidentally inserts a 3.5 mm Cu HVL filter?
A. HVL will decrease.
B. HVL will increase.
C. HVL will remain unchanged.
D. HVL will increase at extended SSDs only.

99. The International Commission on Radiological Units and Measurements (ICRU) recommends that dose delivered to a tumor to be:
A. Within 5.0 % of the prescribed dose
B. Within 8.0 % of the prescribed dose
C. Within 10.0 % of the prescribed dose
D. Within 15.0 % of the prescribed dose

2.2 Applied Mathematics (Questions)

Quiz 1 (Level 1)

1. Match the following problems with its corresponding answer.

A. $15^5 \times 10^3$ I. 3

B. $1.5 \times 12^{10} \times 2.5 \times 10^7$ II. 8,000

C. 20^3 III. 4.5^{17}

D. $\sqrt{25}$ IV. 4

E. $\sqrt[3]{27}$ V. 759,375,000

F. $\sqrt{16}$ VI. 5

2. Match the following metric system with its corresponding equivalent.

A. 10^{12} I. 0.1

B. 10^{3} II. 1000

C. 10^{-9} III. 0.000 000 001

D. 10^{1} IV. 1 000 000 000 000

E. 10^{-6} V. 0.000 001

3. Match the following metric system with its corresponding equivalent.

A. 10^{-6} Pico

B. 10^{-2} Centi

C. 10^{-12} Mega

D. 10^{6} Micro

E. 10^{9} Giga

4. Match the following metric system with its corresponding equivalent.

A. 10^{15} One thousandth

B. 10^{2} One tenth

C. 10^{-1} One quadrillionth

D. 10^{-3} One hundred

E. 10^{12} One trillion

5. Match the following problems with its corresponding hot or cold doses.

A. Rx = 30 Gy: 15 % of 30 Gy   I. 0.40

B. Rx = 40 Gy: 95 % of 40 Gy   II. 32.4 Gy

C. Rx = 46 Gy: 90 % of 36 Gy   III. 15

D. Rx – 30 Gy: 10 % hot spot   IV. 0.05

E. Rx = 30 Gy: 10 % reduction from 30 Gy   V. 33 Gy

F. Rx = 60 Gy: What % of 60 Gy is 9 Gy?   VI. 38 Gy

G. Decimal equivalent of 40 %   VII. 0.50

H. Decimal equivalent of 50 %   VIII. 27 Gy

I. Decimal equivalent of 5 %   IX. 4.5 Gy

2.2 Applied Mathematics (Questions)

6. An ENT plan was given to the dosimetrist. The Rx is 60 Gy, and the dose goal states that 95 % of the PTV should receive 100 % of the Rx dose and no more than 115 % of the Rx dose is accepted. Also, 107 % of the Rx dose should cover less than 10 % of the volume, and 110 % of the Rx dose should cover less than 5 % of the volume. Which of the following answer is correct?
   A. V95 % = 60 Gy; max dose = 69 Gy; V10 % = 42 Gy; V5 % = 6.6 Gy
   B. V95 % = 60 Gy; max dose = 96 Gy; V10 % = 66 Gy; V5 % = 64.2 Gy
   C. V95 % = 66 Gy; max dose = 96 Gy; V10 % = 64.2 Gy; V5 % = 66 Gy
   D. V95 % = 60 Gy; max dose = 69 Gy; V10 % = 64.2 Gy; V5 % = 66 Gy

7. Match the following with its corresponding answer.
   A. $\sin 20°$ I. 84.3
   B. $\cos 30°$ II. 0.34
   C. $\tan 50°$ III. 0.40
   D. $\sin^{-1} 0.10$ IV. 36
   E. $\cos^{-1} 0.5$ V. 60
   F. $\tan^{-1} 10°$ VI. 0.87
   G. $\sin 25° + \cos 20°$ VII. 5.7
   H. $\tan^{-1} 0.15 + \cos^{-1} 0.10$ VIII. 1.19
   I. $\sin^{-1} 0.8 - \tan^{-1} 0.3$ IX. 92.8

8. Match the following with its corresponding answer.
   A. e^3 I. 0.00001
   B. $Ln(30)$ II. 20
   C. $Log(150)$ III. 2.18
   D. 10^{17} IV. 3.40
   E. 10^{-5} V. 10,000,000

9. Convert the following.
   A. 100 Gy to cGy   I. 1.2
   B. 10 cGy to Gy   II. 3,000
   C. 120 rad to Gy   III. 10,000
   D. 30 Gy to rad   IV. 0.1

10. Convert the following meter, cm, mm, inches, feet, °F, and °C and match to the corresponding number.

    A. 10 m to cm   I. 30
    B. 550 cm to meters   II. 0.3937
    C. 120 cm to mm   III. 8
    D. 300 mm to cm   IV. 24.8
    E. 15 in. to cm   V. 38.1
    F. 10 mm to inches   VI. 240
    G. 20 ft to inches   VII. 1,000
    H. 46.5 °F to °C   VIII. 1,200
    I. −4 °C to °F   IX. 5.5

11. A PA field is clinically set up at 70 SSD using 20×25 cm on the skin, but the whole treatment area is not included, and the SSD needs to be extended to 95 cm. What is the new field size on the skin at 95 cm SSD?
    A. 34×27 cm
    B. 27×34 cm
    C. 332.5×266 cm
    D. 45×50 cm

12. A femur is set up AP/PA to cover a prosthesis that lies 10 cm from the anterior surface and 5 cm from the posterior surface. Assume that this means the separation is 15 cm and the treatment is 100 cm SAD with the isocenter placed on the prosthesis. Both AP/PA fields are 30×7 cm. What is the field size on the anterior and posterior skin?
    A. AP=28.5×6.65 cm; PA=27×6.3 cm
    B. AP=6.65×6.3 cm; PA=28.5×2.7 cm
    C. AP=27×6.3 cm; PA=28.5×6.65 cm
    D. AP=10×15.3 cm; PA=25×7 cm

13. A tumor 10 cm deep needs to be treated using 100 cm SSD, 25×20 cm field size on the tumor. If a 1 cm bolus is placed on the skin what will be the new field size on the tumor?
    A. 25×20 cm
    B. 20.45×16.36 cm
    C. 22.5×18 cm
    D. 30.5×24.4 cm

14. Calculate the SSD required if a TBI patient needs to be set up using at least 1 cm flash on a patient who is 5 ft and 7 in. tall by 18 in. wide, but the maximum field size at machine isocenter (100 cm) is 40×11.5 cm.
    A. 170.5 cm SSD
    B. 174 cm SSD

2.2 Applied Mathematics (Questions)

C. 432.5 cm SSD
D. 400 cm SSD

15. A treatment setup is done at 100 SSD using a 110 mm × 150 mm on the skin, what is the field size 25 in. below the surface where the tumor lies?
A. 125 mm × 187.5 mm
B. 179.3 mm × 245.25 mm
C. 179.3 cm × 245.25 cm
D. 125 cm × 187.5 cm

16. Calculate the magnification factor to construct a block if the field size at 100 cm SAD is 13 × 15 cm and the image projection on the film is 15.6 × 18 cm.
A. 0.833
B. 28.6
C. 2.6
D. 1.2

17. An HDR cylinder measuring 12 × 2 cm is placed in the patient's vagina at a depth of 5 cm. The patient is set up at 80 cm SSD, and the film is placed at 130 cm from the source. Calculate the size of the cylinder image on the film along with the magnification factor.
A. 18.4 cm × 3.05 cm image size and 1.5 magnification
B. 18.4 cm × 3.05 cm image size and 0.65 magnification
C. 19.5 cm × 3.25 cm image size and 1.5 magnification
D. 920 cm × 5,525 cm image size and 1.5 magnification

18. Calculate the size of the field on a film if the field size on the skin measures 20 × 15 cm and the magnification factor is 1.45.
A. 21.7 × 29 cm
B. 29 × 21.75 cm
C. 21.45 × 16.45 cm
D. 13.8 × 10.34 cm

19. Which of the following statements is/are correct about patient anatomical orientation using Cartesian coordinates in radiation therapy?
A. I, II, and III
B. I and III only
C. II and IV only
D. IV only
E. All are correct
I. $+Y$ direction corresponds to the superior or cephalic location.
II. $+X$ direction corresponds to the LT side of patient.
III. $+Z$ direction corresponds to the anterior aspect of the patient.
IV. $-Z$ direction corresponds to the posterior aspect of the patient.

20. A CT scan was performed on a patient, and the umbilicus was selected as the user origin (0, 0, 0). On the day of the simulation, the right posterior lung lobe was selected as the isocenter which is 15 cm superior, 10 cm right, and 5 cm posterior from the user origin. What will be the coordinates if the patient needs to be moved to the isocenter from the user origin so that the AP film can be taken (patient supine, head toward gantry)?
   A. X=+15 cm, Y=+10 cm, Z=+5 cm
   B. X=+10 cm, Y=+15 cm, Z=−5 cm
   C. X=−10 cm, Y=+15 cm, Z=−5 cm
   D. X=+15 cm, Y=10 cm, Z=−5 cm

21. A patient's right calf needs to be treated with an electron field, so the patient is positioned prone, feet toward gantry. If the user origin (0, 0, 0) is at the umbilicus, what direction would the patient have to be shifted to position the isocenter near the right calf?
   A. +X, +Y, +Z
   B. −X, +Y, +Z
   C. −X, +Y, −Z
   D. +X, −Y, −Z

22. Explain the location of the isocenter in reference to a patient who is supine, head toward gantry, and the Cartesian coordinates are (−12, 20, 6).
   A. X right, Y caudal, Z posterior
   B. X left, Y cephalic, Z posterior
   C. X right, Y caudal, Z anterior
   D. X right, Y cephalic, Z posterior

23. How is the sine of an angle defined?
   A. The ratio of the length of the side adjacent to the angle to the length of the hypotenuse
   B. The ratio of the length of the side opposite of the angle to the length of the adjacent side
   C. The ratio of the length of the side opposite the angle to the length of the hypotenuse
   D. The length of the side opposite the right angle

24. Which of the following equations is/are correct?
   A. I, II, and III
   B. I and III only
   C. II and IV only
   D. IV only
   E. All are correct
   I. Sin $(X°)$ = opposite/hypotenuse
   II. Tan $(X°)$ = opposite/adjacent
   III. Cos $(X°)$ = adjacent/hypotenuse
   IV. Cos $(X°)$ = hypotenuse/adjacent

2.2 Applied Mathematics (Questions)

25. Which of the following equations is/are used when calculating collimator and couch angles in a craniospinal irradiation?
    A. I, II, and III
    B. I and III only
    C. II and IV only
    D. IV only
    E. All are correct
    I. $\theta_{couch} = \arctan (1/2 \, L \times 1/SSD)$
    II. $\theta_{coll} = \arctan (1/2 \, L \times 1/SSD)$
    III. $\theta_{coll} = \arctan (1/2 \, L \times 1/SAD)$
    IV. $\theta_{couch} = \arctan (1/2 \, L \times 1/SAD)$

Quiz 2 (Level 2)

1. Calculate the cranial field collimator angle needed to match the divergence from the PA spine field for a craniospinal treatment where the upper spine field is 36 cm × 8 cm at 100 cm SSD and the brain field is 14 cm long by 21 cm wide at midplane (100 cm SAD).
    A. 0.18°
    B. 79.7°
    C. 10.2°
    D. 15°

2. Calculate the couch angle needed on the lateral cranial field to match the divergence with the upper PA spine field on a craniospinal treatment where the upper spine field length is 40 cm × 10 cm at 100 cm SSD and the cranial field is 16 cm long by 22 cm wide at midplane (100 cm SAD).
    A. 12.5°
    B. 4.57°
    C. 0.08°
    D. 7.5°

3. Calculate the cranial field couch angle needed to match a PA spine divergence on a craniospinal treatment where the upper spine field is 30 cm × 5 cm, the lower spine field is 18 cm × 15 cm at 100 cm SSD, and the lateral cranial fields are 18 cm × 20 cm at isocenter. The SSD is 93 cm, and the separation of the patient's head is 14 cm.
    A. 5.14°
    B. 4.57°
    C. 5.48°
    D. 0.15°

4. From the following table, calculate the TMR to be used in a patient with a 10 MV photon beam, 12×12 cm² field size at a depth of 3.5 cm.

Table 2.2.1

Depth (cm)	4×4 cm	8×8 cm	12×12 cm
1.0	0.854	0.874	0.888
3.0	1.000	1.000	1.000
4.0	0.992	0.993	0.993
6.0	0.930	0.937	0.941

A. 0.003
B. 1.496
C. 0.996
D. 0.496

5. From the following table, calculate the scatter-maximum ratio to be used in a patient with a 10 MV photon beam, 8×8 cm² field size at a depth of 10.6 cm.

Table 2.2.2

Depth (cm)	4×4 cm	8×8 cm	12×12 cm
6.0	0.048	0.056	0.060
10.0	0.055	0.074	0.085
12.0	0.0.56	0.080	0.094
16.0	0.055	0.086	0.106

A. 0.077
B. 0.076
C. 0.925
D. 0.003

6. From the following table, calculate the PDD to be used for a patient using a 10 MV photon beam, a 7×7 cm² field size at a depth of 21 cm.

Table 2.2.3

Depth (cm)	6×6 cm	8×8 cm	10×10 cm
1.0	89.0	90.0	91.0
20.0	43.9	45.0	45.9
22.0	39.8	41	41.9
30	26.9	28	28.9

A. 41.8
B. 43.0
C. 4.05
D. 42.4

2.2 Applied Mathematics (Questions)

7. From the following helmet brain field, calculate the effective equivalent square.

Fig. 2.2.1

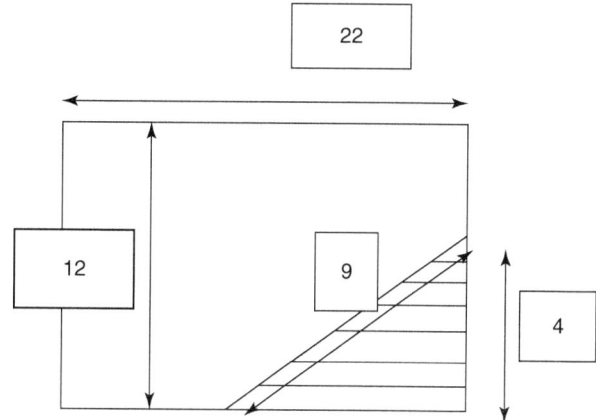

A. 14.9 cm²
B. 14.3 cm²
C. 2.5 cm²
D. 16 cm²

8. From the following hemi-pelvic field, calculate the effective equivalent square.

Fig. 2.2.2

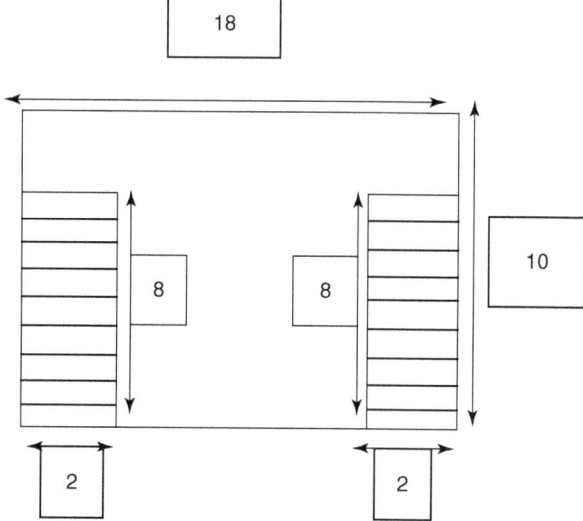

A. 16.07 cm²
B. 11.54 cm²
C. 12.59 cm²
D. 13.87 cm²

9. From the following helmet brain field, calculate the effective equivalent square.

Fig. 2.2.3

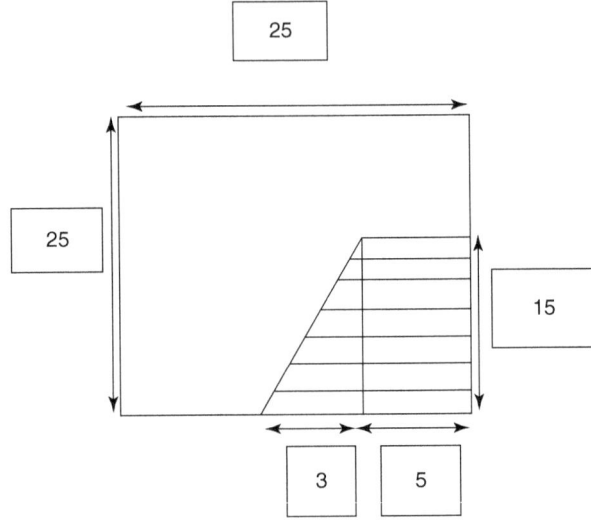

A. 24.54 cm²
B. 23.45 cm²
C. 22.96 cm²
D. 26.87 cm²

10. From the following hemi-pelvic field, calculate the effective equivalent square.

Fig. 2.2.4

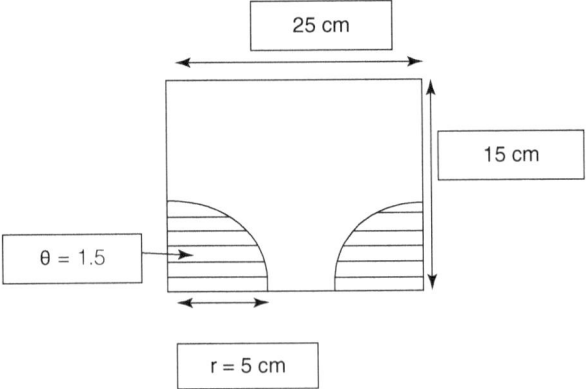

A. 16.63 cm²
B. 17.72 cm²
C. 56.25 cm²
D. 20.65 cm²

2.2 Applied Mathematics (Questions)

11. What percentage of the original dose rate is the new dose rate if the distance from the source is increased from 100 to 120 cm?
A. 83.33 %
B. 144.44 %
C. 69.44 %
D. 122.22 %

12. A dosimetrist calculated the delivered dose from a beam covering the right femur at a distance of 100 cm SSD, 40 cm × 10 cm, to be 3,000 cGy. The physician decided to cover past the knee joint, so the SSD had to be extended to a distance of 130 cm. Which will be the new intensity and the new field size if no change is made to the original plan?
A. 1,775 cGy, field size 13 cm × 52 cm
B. 1,775 cGy, field size 52 cm × 13 cm
C. 5,070 cGy, field size 52 cm × 13 cm
D. 1,775 cGy, field size 67.6 cm × 16.9 cm

13. A photon beam was calculated to deliver 300 cGy daily at 120 cm SSD to treat a surface lesion. If the patient thickness is 50 cm, what is the daily dose the patient received at midplane (assume no attenuation)?
A. 192 cGy
B. 363 cGy
C. 438 cGy
D. 205 cGy

14. Calculate the distance that the patient was treated if the patient received 50 cGy when the prescribed dose was 120 cGy at 75 cm.
A. 13,500 cm
B. 116 cm
C. 180 cm
D. 53 cm

15. Calculate the dose delivered at 50 cm in 45 s if the machine is programed to deliver 100 cGy at 80 cm in 2 min.
A. 14.6 cGy
B. 39 cGy
C. 140.6 cGy
D. 120 cGy

16. Which of the following field size has the greater TMR?
A. 18 × 2 cm
B. 20 × 6 cm
C. 30 × 14 cm
D. 30 × 12 cm

17. Calculate the collimator rotation required to align a 20×20 cm cranial field isocentric at 100 cm SAD with an adjacent PA spine field which is 40 cm in length at 100 cm SSD.
A. 21.8°
B. 11.3°
C. 78.7°
D. 15.2°

2.3 External Beam Calculations (Questions)

Quiz 1 (Level 2)

1. Calculate the MU setting for an electron beam cheek treatment if the output for that particular cutout is measured to be 0.972 cGy/MU at Dmax and the physician wants to prescribe a dose of 250 cGy to the 85 % isodose line (IDL).
A. 206 MU
B. 303 MU
C. 286 MU
D. 257 MU

2. A tumor at a depth of 3–4 cm is best treated with:
A. 6 MeV
B. 9 MeV
C. 12 MeV
D. 18 MeV

3. Calculate the maximum practical range (Rp) of a 12 MeV electron if a tumor is to be treated with a dose of 250 cGy for 30 fractions.
A. 3 cm
B. 6 cm
C. 8 cm
D. 10 cm

4. Calculate the therapeutic range of a 16 MeV electron if a tumor is to be treated with a dose of 250 cGy for 30 fractions.
A. 1.5 cm
B. 3 cm
C. 4 cm
D. 5 cm

5. Calculate the depth of the 50 % IDL of a 12 MeV electron if a tumor is to be treated with a dose of 180 cGy for 35 fractions.
A. 2.57 cm
B. 3.86 cm
C. 5.15 cm
D. 6.86 cm

2.4 Effects of Beam-Modifying Devices (Questions)

6. Which beam energy is used if the 50 % IDL covers a 7 cm depth?
   A. 4 MeV beam
   B. 6 MeV beam
   C. 9 MeV beam
   D. 16 MeV beam

7. Calculate the correction to an ionization chamber reading ($P_{t,p}$) if the treatment room temperature is 21 °C and the pressure is 772 mm mercury (mmHg).
   A. 1.980
   B. 0.987
   C. 0.980
   D. 0.012

8. What will be the effect on the chamber reading for a given exposure if the temperature in the room decreases by 10 % and the pressure increase by 10 %?
   A. Approximately 10 % decrease
   B. Approximately 10 % increase
   C. Approximately 5 % increase
   D. Approximately 25 % decrease

9. Calculate the MUs required to deliver 250 cGy to the 90 % IDL if the breast electron cutout has an output of 1.07 cGy/MU at Dmax.
   A. 260 MU
   B. 234 MU
   C. 241 MU
   D. 268 MU

2.4 Effects of Beam-Modifying Devices (Questions)

Quiz 1 (Level 2)

1. Calculate the HVL if a material with a linear attenuation coefficient of 0.35 mm^{-1} is placed in the beam path.
   A. 1.04 mm
   B. 0.24 mm
   C. 1.98 mm
   D. 0.50 mm

2. Calculate the thickness of a copper needed to attenuate the beam intensity to half of its initial value if its linear attenuation coefficient is 0.40 mm^{-1}.
   A. 1.73 mm
   B. 0.57 mm
   C. 1.09 mm
   D. 0.27 mm

3. Calculate the linear attenuation coefficient of an aluminum material placed in the beam path if the HVL of the material is 1.5 mm.
A. 1.03 mm−1
B. 0.46 mm^{-1}
C. 2.16 mm^{-1}
D. 2.19 mm^{-1}

4. Calculate the transmission if a lead block measuring 2.5 cm thickness with a 10 mm HVL is used to block the esophagus on a patient at 100 SAD.
A. 18 %
B. 0.069 %
C. 80 %
D. 6 %

5. If a the beam quality of a particular machine was measured to have a HVL of 2.5 mm tin (Sn), what will be approximately the percentage of the radiation beam transmitted through 15 mm tin (Sn)?
A. 1.56 %
B. 0.89 %
C. 98.44 %
D. 0.015 %

6. From the following transmission data table, select the Al filter to provide 2 HVLs of shielding.

	Al filter (mm)	Reading (R/min)
A.	0	30
B.	1	20
C.	2	15
D.	3	7.5

7. Calculate the homogeneity coefficient (HC) of a beam if first HVL is 0.40 mm Cu and the second HVL is 0.86 mm Cu.
A. 0.465
B. 0.344
C. 1.260
D. 0.460

2.4 Effects of Beam-Modifying Devices (Questions)

8. Calculate the wedge factor if the output of a beam is 0.700 cGy/MU without the wedge and 0.350 cGy/MU with the wedge.
A. 2.000
B. 0.500
C. 1.050
D. 0.350

9. What percentage of the beam is attenuated if a wedge is placed in the beam path and the wedge factor is calculated to be 0.624?
A. 62.4 %
B. 37.6 %
C. 6.24 %
D. 0.376 %

10. Calculate the wedge factor if a beam is measured and the result reveals 65 % transmission with a wedge in place.
A. 0.650
B. 0.350
C. 1.857
D. 0.538

11. Calculate the hinge angle used in order to get the most homogeneous dose distribution in a wedged pair technique if 45° wedges are used.
A. 157.5°
B. 67.5°
C. 90°
D. 315°

12. Calculate the wedge angle used in order to get the most homogeneous dose distribution in a wedged pair technique if the hinge angle is 120°.
A. 60°
B. 45°
C. 30°
D. 15°

13. What would be the wedge angle used to get the most homogeneous dose distribution if two oblique fields were planned 50° apart?
A. 60°
B. 45°
C. 30°
D. 15°

14. What is the wedge angle (in degree) used to get the most homogeneous dose distribution for the following beam arrangement?

Fig. 2.4.1

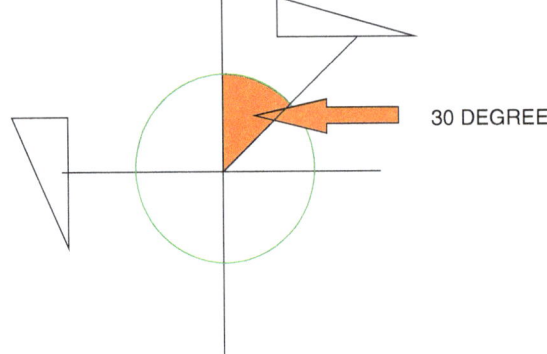

A. 60°
B. 45°
C. 30°
D. 15°

15. Calculate the MU setting with a wedge in place if the wedge transmission factor is 0.640 and the MU setting for a field without wedge is 300 MU.
A. 469 MU
B. 192 MU
C. 364 MU
D. 300.6 MU

16. A tongue and groove is used in MLC design to:
A. Reduce interleaf leakage
B. Correct for lack of divergence
C. Change the beam into a broad, clinically useful beam
D. Tilt the isodose lines through a specific angle

2.5 Irregular Field Calculations (Questions)

Quiz 1 (Level 2)

1. What is the dose rate (cGy/min) a patient received in a cobalt 60 machine if the plan was done using 120 cGy/min at 80 SAD, but the patient was placed at 100 SAD?
A. 96 cGy/min
B. 76.8 cGy/min
C. 150 cGy/min
D. 100 cGy/min

2.5 Irregular Field Calculations (Questions)

2. A PA 6 MV photon beam at 100 cm SSD was used in a T3–L5 spine plan prescribed to a depth of 4.5 cm where the cord lies. At this depth, the PDD=65 %. The physician decided to include up to T1 in the field, but the field length was already at the maximum of 40 cm so the patient had to be moved to 110 cm SSD. Calculate the new percentage depth dose (PDD).
   A. 1.001 %
   B. 53.7 %
   C. 65.1 %
   D. 71.5 %

3. Calculate the backscatter factor if a 6 MV linear accelerator has a dose rate in air of 100 cGy at 100 cm SAD and at the same point (distance) in the patient measures 150 cGy.
   A. 1.50
   B. 0.66
   C. 150
   D. 3.45

4. Calculate the output for a beam that delivers 300 cGy to Dmax when 375 MUs are delivered.
   A. 1.250
   B. 0.800
   C. 75
   D. 80

5. Calculate the dose rate if a Co-60 machine delivers 400 cGy in 3 min.
   A. 403 cGy/min
   B. 0.007 cGy/min
   C. 1,200 cGy/min
   D. 133 cGy/min

6. Calculate the output at Dmax using 120 cm SSD if a 6 MV linear accelerator beam is calibrated to deliver 1.2 cGy/MU at Dmax at 100 cm SSD.
   A. 0.837 cGy/mu
   B. 0.833 cGy/mu
   C. 1.000 cGy/mu
   D. 1.440 cGy/mu

7. Calculate the MUs required to treat a patient whose dose is 180 cGy to the 84 % IDL and the output factor is 0.970 cGy/MU.
   A. 156 MU
   B. 186 MU
   C. 221 MU
   D. 147 MU

8. Calculate the dose from a four-field box delivered to the 75 % isodose line if 50 Gy was prescribed to the 100 % isodose line.
A. 3,750 cGy
B. 37.50 cGy
C. 66.6 cGy
D. 150 cGy

9. Calculate the prescribed dose if a dosimetrist evaluates a three-field rectum plan and concludes that the max dose in the plan is 277.5 cGy given to the 111 % IDL.
A. 111 cGy
B. 30.52 cGy
C. 308 cGy
D. 250 cGy

10. A plan was calculated to deliver 180 cGy daily with 195 MUs to an AP femur field at 100 cm SSD. What would be the new MU setting if the physician wants the same prescription dose but decided to include 3 more cm of the femur by changing the SSD to 120 cm?
A. 163 MU
B. 135 MU
C. 281 MU
D. 234 MU

11. A 10 MV plan was calculated to deliver 200 cGy daily using 250 MUs to a shoulder at 100 cm SSD (20×20 field size at a depth of 9 cm). The PDD is 78 %, and Dmax is 2.5 cm. What is the new PDD at a depth of 9 cm if the physician decided to treat at 115 cm SSD so that part of the ulna is included in the field?
A. 103 %
B. 78.0 %
C. 79.1 %
D. 89.7 %

12. What would be the dose to Dmax if an electron plan is prescribing 250 cGy to the 85 % IDL?
A. 294 cGy
B. 213 cGy
C. 300 cGy
D. 165 cGy

2.5 Irregular Field Calculations (Questions)

13. Calculate the MU needed to deliver 150 cGy to the 85 % IDL using 12 MeV electrons. The treatment unit is calibrated to deliver 1 cGy per MU at Dmax for the prescribed field size.
    A. 128 MU
    B. 176 MU
    C. 149 MU
    D. 160 MU

14. Calculate the dose received by a patient if the output was 0.875 cGy/MU and the calculated MU was 195, but the machine broke and only delivered 105 MU instead.
    A. 91.8 cGy
    B. 171 cGy
    C. 79.2 cGy
    D. 120 cGy

15. Calculate the time setting for AP/PA field to deliver a mediastinum treatment using a cobalt-60 unit with a prescription dose of 250 cGy at midplane when the patient separation is 20 cm. Both fields are equally weighted using a field size of 20×20 cm. The field size factor (FSF) for this field is 1.07. The dose rate for a 10×10 field side is 115 cGy/min at Dmax, and the PDD is 0.556 at 10 cm depth.
    A. 1 min 30 s
    B. 2 min 36 s
    C. 1 min 49 s
    D. 1 min 82 s

16. Calculate the MU needed to deliver a prostate treatment using a 354° arc technique if the average TMR is known to be 0.570 and the prescription dose to the isocenter is 180 cGy.
    A. 621 MU
    B. 354 MU
    C. 103 MU
    D. 316 MU

17. Calculate the MU/degree in a 300° arc technique if the average TMR is known to be 0.570 for a prescription dose to the isocenter of 250 cGy. The beam uses 351 MU.
    A. 1.17 MU/degree
    B. 0.002 MU/degree
    C. 1.2 MU/degree
    D. 0.71 MU/degree

18. Use the following table to answer the following two questions. Calculate the MUs needed to deliver 250 cGy at a depth of 7, 100 cm SSD. The field size is 15×15 cm, the energy is 10 MV, and there is a single PA beam.

Table 2.5.1

Depth/PDD	6×6 cm	15×15 cm	20×20 cm
5 cm	91.8	92.3	92.5
7 cm	83.2	84.5	84.9
10 cm	71.8	74	74.7
Output Dmax (cGy/MU)			
100 cm SSD	0.972	1.034	1.053
100 cm SAD	1.025	1.072	1.094

A. 286 MU
B. 242 MU
C. 276 MU
D. 218 MU

19. Use the table from the previous question to calculate the dose (cGy) received at 7 cm if the prescription dose from a single PA 10 MV photon beam was 180 cGy to a depth of 5 cm, 100 SSD, with a 20×20 cm field size.
A. 197 cGy
B. 165 cGy
C. 152 cGy
D. 213 cGy

20. Calculate the max dose to a PA spine which is treated at 100 SSD, 10 MV, field size 12×12 at a depth of 6 cm, PDD 0.881 to a prescribed dose of 300 cGy daily.
A. 341 cGy
B. 264 cGy
C. 357 cGy
D. 300 cGy

21. What will be the percentage change in PDD if a patient is planed with 10 MV using an SSD of 110 cm at a prescription depth of 15 cm, but the physician changes the treatment area to be extended 4 cm and the SSD now is set to 120 cm?
A. 1.6 % increase
B. 0.9 % increase
C. 1.6 % decrease
D. No change in PPD

2.5 Irregular Field Calculations (Questions)

22. Calculate the total MU per treatment if a three-field rectum plan is calculated with a prescription dose to the isocenter of 60 cGy per field, equally weighted, 10 MV beams. All the fields use wedges with a wedge factor of 0.730. The machine output factor is 0.950 cGy/MU at Dmax, the TMR is 0.753 at the prescription depth, and the field size factor (FSF) is 1.036 for these fields.
    A. 60 MU
    B. 333 MU
    C. 32 MU
    D. 111 MU

23. A physician reviews a plan but wants the skin to receive a higher dose. Which of the following energies should the dosimetrist select so that the skin has the highest dose?
    A. 10 MV photon
    B. 10 MeV electron
    C. 23 MV photon
    D. 18 MeV electron

24. What is the thickness required of lead eye shields to stop a 6 MeV electron that is used to treat the nose at 100 SSD?
    A. 12 mm
    B. 18 mm
    C. 3 mm
    D. 23 mm

25. From the following table, calculate the MU setting per beam to deliver 300 cGy to the isocenter using 6 MV, parallel-opposed brain fields. The patient separation is 14 cm and the field size is 20×20 cm.

Table 2.5.2

Depth/TMR	5×5 cm	15×15 cm	20×20 cm
4 cm	0.952	0.965	0.967
7 cm	0.857	0.892	0.904
14 cm	0.651	0.724	0.743
Output at Dmax (cGy/MU)			
100 cm SSD	0.972	1.034	1.053
100 cm SAD	1.025	1.072	1.094

A. 152 MU
B. 303 MU
C. 369 MU
D. 184 MU

26. Calculate the MU setting for each 10 MV beam if a total of 250 cGy is to be delivered at a depth of 15 cm using a 12×12 cm field size, from parallel-opposed brain fields. The patient has been set up at 100 cm SAD.
TMR = (12×12 cm at depth of 15 cm) = 0.731
Output factor at 100 cm SAD = 1.023 cGy/MU
Backscatter factor (BSF) 12×12 = 1.035
PDD = (12×12 cm at depth of 15 cm) = 58.5 %
Output factor at 100 cm SSD = 1.000 cGy/MU
A. 97 MU
B. 33 MU
C. 323 MU
D. 167 MU

27. The correct formula to calculate the fractional weighted contribution for two opposed fields (RT and LT lateral) is:
A. RT lateral fractional weight = RT/(RT−LT); LT lateral fractional weight = LT/(LT−RT)
B. RT lateral fractional weight = (RT−RT)/LT; LT lateral fractional weight = (LT−RT)/LT
C. RT lateral fractional weight = RT/(RT+LT); LT lateral fractional weight = LT/(LT+RT)
D. RT lateral fractional weight = RT×(RT−LT); LT lateral fractional weight = LT×(LT−RT)

28. Calculate the fractional contribution to the AP/PA lung treatment if the AP/PA fields are weighted 2:1.
A. AP = 0.333; PA = 0.667
B. AP = 0.667; PA = 0.333
C. AP = 6; PA = 3
D. AP = 0.667; PA = 1

29. Calculate the dose received by each field if a patient is treated using opposed fields AP/PA RT hip weighted 2:1 at the isocenter for a daily dose of 250 cGy.
A. AP: 125 cGy, PA: 125 cGy
B. AP: 200 cGy, PA: 50 cGy
C. AP: 170 cGy, PA: 80 cGy
D. AP: 167 cGy, PA: 83 cGy

30. Calculate the dose received by each field if a patient is treated using opposed lateral fields RT/LT larynx weighted 3:1 at the isocenter for a daily dose of 180 cGy.
A. RT: 45 cGy, LT: 135 cGy
B. RT: 135 cGy, LT: 135 cGy
C. RT: 179 cGy, LT: 45 cGy
D. RT: 150 cGy, LT: 30 cGy

2.6 Special Calculations (Questions)

31. Calculate the dose received by each field if a patient is planned using three-field rectum technique, PA/RT/LT lateral weighted 3:2:1 at the isocenter for a daily dose of 200 cGy.
    A. PA: 78 cGy, RT: 68 cGy, LT: 54 cGy
    B. PA: 33 cGy, RT: 67 cGy, LT: 100 cGy
    C. PA: 100 cGy, RT: 67 cGy, LT: 33 cGy
    D. PA: 200 cGy, RT: 1 cGy, LT: 1 cGy

2.6 Special Calculations (Questions)

Quiz 1 (Level 2)

1. Calculate the off-axis ratio or factor to be used if the tumor lies 10 cm deep and 6 cm lateral from the central axis. PDD at a depth of 10 cm along the central axis is 93.5 %, whereas the PDD 6 cm lateral where the tumor lies is 87.3 %.
    A. 1.071
    B. 0.933
    C. 6.200
    D. 0.816

2. Calculate the off-axis ratio to be included in the treatment calculation using the following 10 MV PDD table if the patient's separation is 20 cm and a tumor is located midplane, but 5 cm to the right of the central axis. The PDD on tumor is 62.3 % using an 11×11 cm field size with an SSD of 82 cm.

Table 2.6.1

Depth	6×6 cm	10×10 cm	12×12 cm	20×20 cm
5.0 cm	91.8	92.1	92.2	92.5
10 cm	71.8	73	73.5	74.7
20 cm	43.9	45.9	46.7	48.8

    A. 0.85
    B. 1.34
    C. 1.17
    D. 0.74

3. Calculate the penumbra width in a spine field where the source size is 1.5 cm and the patient is treated at 100 cm SSD using a source-to-collimator distance of 75 cm.
    A. 3.50 cm
    B. 0.50 cm
    C. 2.00 cm
    D. 1.125 cm

4. Calculate the penumbra width needed in a spine field lying 5 cm from the skin using a source size of 2 cm and the patient is treated at 80 cm SSD with a source-to-collimator distance of 52 cm. The field size is 25×8 cm.
A. 4.88 cm
B. 0.19 cm
C. 1.27 cm
D. 0.13 cm

5. Calculate a craniospinal field gap if the thoracic spine field measures 38×8 cm at 100 SSD and the lumbosacral field measures 20×30 cm at 105 SSD and the fields are matched at a depth of 7 cm.
A. 1.99 cm
B. 1.33 cm
C. 0.66 cm
D. 0.67 cm

6. Calculate the skin gap required if fields A/B are parallel-opposed fields having a length of 25 cm, and fields C/D are also parallel-opposed fields having a length of 15 cm, and all fields are treated at midplane, 100 cm SSD. Patient thickness is 20 cm.
A. 1.25 cm skin gap
B. 2 cm skin gap
C. 0.75 cm skin gap
D. 0.50 cm skin gap

7. A patient is treated with two parallel-opposed fields to the T and L spine adjacent to each other (field 1 A: AP, B: PA; field 2 C: AP, D: PA). Field 1 skin gap is 1.25 cm and field 2 skin gap is 0.75 cm; both are treated at a midplane depth of 10, 100 cm SSD. What will be the new gap required to eliminate the field overlap on the cord at a depth of 35 cm from the anterior surface?
A. 1.25 cm skin gap
B. 0.75 cm skin gap
C. 3.25 cm skin gap
D. 2 cm skin gap
    This question is very confusing. Maybe a diagram would help. Additionally, if the midplane depth is 10 cm, the separation would be 20 cm, so how can the cord be 35 cm from the anterior surface?

8. Two fields are planned to intersect at a depth of 5 cm. Calculate the skin separation (gap) necessary for a 25×25 cm and a 15×15 cm fields using 100 cm SSD.
A. 2.00 cm skin gap
B. 0.38 cm skin gap
C. 0.63 cm skin gap
D. 1.01 cm skin gap

2.6 Special Calculations (Questions)

9. What would be the depth needed to calculate the exit dose if a patient is to be planed using a PA spine, max dose of 300 cGy at 2.5 cm depth? The patient thickness is 25 cm.
A. 15 cm depth
B. 12.5 cm depth
C. 22.5 cm depth
D. 25 cm depth

10. An opposed 6 MV AP/PA isocentric abdominal plan is calculated using a 20×20 cm field size. The patient separation is 40 cm with a daily dose of 180 cGy. 195 MUs are delivered each day and a total of 35 fractions will be delivered. The patient is treated for 30 fractions, and the separation is reduced by 4 cm due to weight loss. Approximately what will be the new MU correction for the final 5 fractions, if the separation changed from 40 to 36 cm?
A. 23 MU
B. 171 MU
C. 189 MU
D. 218 MU

11. Calculate the max dose from a 6 MV PA spine field treated at 100 cm SSD with a field size of 15×15 cm at a depth of 7 cm. The PDD at 7 cm is 80.3 % and the daily dose is 250 cGy.
A. 330 cGy
B. 201 cGy
C. 311 cGy
D. 200 cGy

12. From the following table, calculate the total MU setting per fraction if a RT lower leg using parallel-opposed, isocentric fields. The patient separation is 12 cm, and the field size is 12×12 cm. The fractional dose to isocenter is 180 cGy.

Table 2.6.2

Depth	1.5 cm	4 cm	6 cm	8 cm	12 cm
PDD (%)	100	91	83.9	75.7	61.5
TMR	1.000	0.963	0.919	0.865	0.756

Output	1.031 cGy/MU at 100 cm SSD, Dmax
Output	1.075 cGy/MU at 100 cm SAD, Dmax

A. 182 MU
B. 190 MU
C. 231 MU
D. 152 MU

13. Use the following table to answer the next two questions. First, calculate the entrance dose from the AP beam if a RT shoulder is treated with parallel-opposed fields using an isocentric technique. The patient separation is 8 cm, the field size is 12×12 cm, and the dose to the isocenter is 300 cGy.

Table 2.6.3

Depth	1.5 cm	4 cm	6 cm	8 cm	12 cm
PDD (%)	100	91	83.9	75.7	61.5
TMR	1.000	0.963	0.919	0.865	0.756

Output	1.031 cGy/MU at 100 cm SSD, Dmax
Output	1.075 cGy/MU at 100 cm SAD, Dmax

A. 136.2 cGy
B. 195.5 cGy
C. 160.4 cGy
D. 146.5 cGy

14. From the previous table, calculate the exit dose to the opposite Dmax for the AP beam for the same treatment as in the previous question.
A. 120.5 cGy
B. 143.1 cGy
C. 163.5 cGy
D. 138.9 cGy

15. From the following table, calculate the global max dose if a RT hip is treated with parallel-opposed isocentric fields with the isocenter at midplane. The patient separation is 12 cm, the field size is 12×12 cm, and the daily dose to isocenter is 300 cGy.

Table 2.6.4

Depth	1.5 cm	4 cm	6 cm	10.5 cm	12 cm	14.5 cm
PDD (%)	100	91	83.9	75.7	61.5	55.6
TMR	1.000	0.963	0.919	0.865	0.756	0.709

Output	1.031 cGy/MU at 100 cm SSD, dmax
Output	1.075 cGy/MU at 100 cm SAD, dmax

A. 315.8 cGy
B. 304.4 cGy
C. 178.9 cGy
D. 298.2 cGy

16. Use the following table to calculate the total dose received at midplane on the right femur. The prescription point in this case is midplane in the right hip where the separation is 16 cm. The dose to the prescription point is 300 cGy per fraction delivered in 10 fractions. The treatment field also covers the right femur which only has a separation of 8 cm. Ignoring the off-axis ratio, the dose to midplane in the right femur is:

Table 2.6.5

Depth	1.5 cm	4 cm	6 cm	8 cm	16 cm
PDD (%)	100	91	83.9	75.7	61.5
TMR	1.000	0.963	0.919	0.865	0.756

A. 2,695 cGy
B. 333.9 cGy
C. 3,340 cGy
D. 3,433 cGy

17. A patient is treated to the left hip using a 6 MV, 12×12 cm field size. The prescription dose is 250 cGy to midplane with an SSD of 92.5 cm. The separation is 15 cm, and the TMR is 0.685 at a depth of 7.5 cm. Calculate the new TMR if the SSD is changed to 100 cm.
A. 0.685
B. 0.814
C. 0.484
D. 0.772

18. A left breast plan is calculated to deliver 200 cGy daily for 25 fractions to the isocenter. The plan reveals a hot spot of 108 %. How hot does the plan become if the physician decides to renormalize it to the 90 % IDL to the isocenter?
A. 108 %
B. 120 %
C. 83 %
D. 140 %

19. From the following table, calculate the MU setting to deliver 200 cGy to 7.5 cm using a 10 MV beam with a field size of 25×25 cm field size at 100 SSD?

Table 2.6.6

	FS	6×6 cm	10×10 cm	15×15 cm	20×20 cm	30×30 cm
PDD	2 cm	98.0	98.0	99.0	99.0	99.5
	5 cm	91.8	92.1	92.3	92.5	92.7
	10 cm	71.8	73.0	74.0	74.7	75.7
	15 cm	56.2	57.9	59.3	60.4	61.8
	18 cm	48.5	50.4	52.0	53.1	54.8
TMR	2 cm	0.970	0.970	0.980	0.980	0.985
	5 cm	0.963	0.966	0.968	0.970	0.972
	10 cm	0.824	0.838	0.850	0.858	0.869
	15 cm	0.701	0.723	0.741	0.753	0.772
	18 cm	0.634	0.659	0.680	0.695	0.717
Output at 2 cm, SSD 100 cm	cGy/MU	1.030	1.045	1.063	1.070	1.085
Output at 2 cm, SAD 100 cm	cGy/MU	1.042	1.051	1.072	1.089	1.120

- A. 215 MU
- B. 195 MU
- C. 221 MU
- D. 200 MU

20. Calculate the maximum tissue dose using the previous table if the dose delivered to 7.5 cm is 200 cGy using a 10 MV beam with a field size of 25×25 cm at 100 cm SSD.
- A. 214 cGy
- B. 238 cGy
- C. 200 cGy
- D. 157 cGy

21. Calculate the MU per field to deliver a total of 200 cGy at midline if parallel-opposed brain fields are used. Both fields are 20×20 cm with output factors of 1.089. The TMR at 10 cm depth is 0.863 and the SSD is 90 cm. There is also a small block covering the face (tray factor of 0.980).
- A. 215 MU
- B. 218 MU
- C. 94 MU
- D. 109 MU

2.6 Special Calculations (Questions)

22. Calculate the exit dose at depth of 15 cm using the table from Question 19 if the dose is 200 cGy using a 10 MV beam prescribed to a depth of 7.5 cm. The field size is 25×25 cm and the SSD is 100 cm.
A. 145.6 cGy
B. 127.3 cGy
C. 56.70 cGy
D. 274.7 cGy

23. Calculate the total dose at Dmax if a dose of 200 cGy is prescribed to midline using parallel-opposed brain fields. The field sizes are 20×20 cm with output factors of 1.089 and a TMR of 0.858 at 10 cm. The SSD for both fields is 90 cm with a small block covering the face (tray factor of 0.980).
A. 136.9 cGy
B. 69.9 cGy
C. 206.8 cGy
D. 230.2 cGy

24. Refer to Table 2.6.6 Question 19. Calculate the MUs required to deliver 90 cGy to a depth of 5 cm for an AP shoulder treatment with a field size of 15×15 cm setup at 100 cm SSD using a corner block to block the humeral head (tray factor=0.93). Also, calculate the MUs required if the treatment has the same parameters but is changed to a 100 SAD treatment with the isocenter at 5 cm depth?
A. 84 MU SSD, 102 MU SAD
B. 93 MU SSD, 99 MU SAD
C. 99 MU SSD, 93 MU SAD
D. 102 MU SSD, 95 MU SAD

25. An abdominal treatment technique was delivered using two equally weighted 30° wedged fields (transmission factor of 0.82) with a hinge angle of 120° for a total of 244 MU delivering 200 cGy to the isocenter. What is the dose at isocenter if the therapist forgot to insert one of the wedges and the patient was treated?
A. 364 cGy
B. 182 cGy
C. 100 cGy
D. 222 cGy

26. A patient is receiving 250 cGy/fx to a depth of 5 cm from a single spine field at 100 SSD. What will be the dose received at 5 cm depth if the optical distance indicator (ODI) is misread and the therapist set up the patient at 100 cm SSD when in reality it is 115 cm SSD?
A. 189 cGy
B. 217 cGy
C. 330 cGy
D. 200 cGy

27. Calculate the fractional dose to the esophagus which is at a depth of 5 cm from the posterior (PDD at 5 cm = 85 %) if a C spine is treated to 180 cGy per fraction with a single PA field to a depth of 3 cm (PDD at 3 cm = 95 %). The field size is 10×4 cm at 100 SSD, and the output of the machine is 180 cGy/min at Dmax.
   A. 201 cGy
   B. 161 cGy
   C. 153 cGy
   D. 180 cGy

2.7 Manual Corrections for Tissue Inhomogeneities (Questions)

Quiz 1 (Level 2)

1. How many cm of the lung is equivalent to 1 cm of water or tissue?
   A. 5 cm
   B. 3 cm
   C. 2 cm
   D. 10 cm

2. An AP mantle field was planned to deliver 250 cGy to a depth of 18 cm. There is 12 cm of the lung along the central axis. If this original plan was calculated without correcting for the lung density, what would the approximate dose actually delivered to the isocenter be before a second plan was recalculated using heterogeneity corrections to account for the lung?
   A. 200 cGy
   B. 300 cGy
   C. 244 cGy
   D. 175 cGy

3. Calculate the effective depth used to plan a patient's treatment that has 5 cm of tissue from the skin to the center of the leg where a 3 cm titanium metal rod replaced the bone. From the bone to the back of the leg, there is additional 7 cm tissue for a total separation of 15 cm.
   A. 9 cm tissue
   B. 15 cm tissue
   C. 16.5 cm tissue
   D. 20 cm tissue

2.7 Manual Corrections for Tissue Inhomogeneities (Questions)

4. Calculate the skin dose using the following 12 MeV PDD table if a dose of 250 cGy is delivered to a tumor at a depth of 4 cm from the skin and 1 cm bolus is used.

Table 2.7.1

Depth	0	1	2	3	4	5	6
PDD	90	95	98	100	80	60	10

A. 417 cGy
B. 396 cGy
C. 277 cGy
D. 225 cGy

5. Which of the following is the practical range of a 16 MeV electron beam?
A. 3 cm
B. 6 cm
C. 8 cm
D. 11.5

6. The 90 % depth dose of a 16 MeV occurs at:
A. 2 cm
B. 4 cm
C. 5 cm
D. 8 cm

7. Which of the following lead cutout thickness will be optimal to adequately stop a 12 MeV electron beam?
A. 6 mm lead thickness cutout
B. 6 cm lead thickness cutout
C. 8 mm lead thickness cutout
D. 4 mm lead thickness cutout

8. Which of the following Cerrobend cutout thickness will be optimal to adequately stop an electron beam using 12 MeV energy?
A. 6 mm Cerrobend thickness cutout
B. 7.2 mm Cerrobend thickness cutout
C. 8 mm Cerrobend thickness cutout
D. 4.5 mm Cerrobend thickness cutout

2.8 Dose Calculation (Answers)

Quiz 1 (Level 2)

1. **A** Only I, II, and III are correct. The effective Z of water is close to that of tissue.

2. **B** The phantom materials that are frequently used for radiation dosimetry are Lucite and polystyrene because of their tissue equivalent. They have almost the same effective atomic number, number of electrons per gram, and mass density of water (and tissue). Tungsten is used as target material for x-ray production because of its high Z value. Graphite also has an effective Z similar to water, but it is brittle and difficult to shape into a useful phantom. Graphite is most commonly used wall material of a thimble ionization chamber.

3. **B** Anthropomorphic phantoms have sections that simulate various body tissues like muscle, bone, lung, and air cavities. One such commercially available phantom is known as Alderson RANDO Phantom. Homogeneous phantoms have the same material throughout the entire phantom and are usually made of water-equivalent materials like solid water. Solid water is manufactured to be as close to water equivalent as possible (Lucite is less expensive but deviates a bit more from true water equivalence). Wood phantoms are not commonly used.

4. **E** All are correct; the variation of absorbed dose in a patient or phantom depends on the beam energy or the penetrating power of the beam, the depth where the calculation is required, the field size and collimator setting, the distance from source to the calculation point, and also the density or material of body or phantom.

5. **B** Percentage depth dose is defined as the percentage of the absorbed dose at any depth d to the absorbed dose at a fixed reference depth d_0, along the central axis of the beam. The Mayneord F Factor is used to calculate the PDD curve at a new SSD. The tissue-air ratio is the ratio of dose at depth in the phantom to dose in free space at the same point, and tissue-phantom ratio is the ratio of the dose at depth d in a phantom to dose at a specified reference depth in the phantom.

6. **E** All are correct; PDD beyond Dmax increases with beam energy because higher-energy beams have greater penetrating power and thus deliver a higher percentage depth dose. PDD decreases with depth beyond the Dmax because there is a buildup region at depths shallower than Dmax and then the photons experience exponential attenuation so the PDD decreases. PDD increases with increasing field size because of the contribution of scattered radiation into the center of the field. PDD increases with increased SSD because of the effect of the inverse square law.

2.8 Dose Calculation (Answers)

7. **C** The region between the surface and the point of maximum dose is called the dose buildup region. The skin-sparing effect refers to surface dose receiving less absorbed dose because the electrons that are created at the surface have a range that causes them to deposit dose downstream, not at the surface where they are formed. Dmax is the depth at the central axis where electronic equilibrium is reached. It is also the depth of the peak absorbed dose. Finally, penumbra is the region of rapid dose falloff at the edges of the beam, normally the distance from the 80 to 20 % isodose line at Dmax.

8. **A.** 25 MV: (IV)
   B. 4 MV: (II)
   C. 10 MV: (III)
   D. ^{60}Co: (I)
   Remember, as energy increases, PDD increases and Dmax increases.

9. **D** Geometric field size is the projection, on a plane perpendicular to the beam axis, of the distal end of the collimator as seen from the front center of the source. This usually corresponds to the field defined by the light localizer. Source-to-surface distance (SSD) is the distance from the source to the surface of the patient or phantom. The source-to-axis distance (SAD) is the distance from the source to the axis of gantry rotation, and dosimetric or physical field size refers to the field size defined by a given isodose curve at a particular depth, usually the 50 % isodose line.

10. **E** All the statements are correct; a rectangular field is equivalent to a square field if they have the same area/perimeter (A/P), Sterling developed the rule-of-thumb method for equating rectangular and square fields, and Clarkson's method includes irregular fields dose calculations. As previously mentioned, as the field size increases, PDD increases due to the production of scatter radiation at larger field sizes.

11. **C** The formulas used to calculate equivalent square are ESF = $2(L \times W)/L+W$ or ESF = $4 \times A/P$, where A is the area and P is the perimeter. $A/P = a \times b/2(a+b)$ is the area/perimeter of a rectangle and $A/P = a/4$ is the area/perimeter of a square. The ESF is calculated by equating the A/P of a square to the A/P of a rectangle. The radii of an equivalent circle may be obtained by the relationship $r = 4/\sqrt{\pi} \times A/P$.

12. **C** Equivalent square formula can be used with rectangular-shaped fields only; it does not apply to circular- or irregular-shaped fields.
    This type of question is extremely common in real clinics, so it would be very useful to remember the following formula, which is directly derived from the equivalent A/P relationship.
    Given the dimension A and B of a rectangular field, the length for the equivalent square field is $L = 2AB/(A+B)$.

13. **C** The equivalent square of a rectangle of length 20 cm and width 14 cm is 16.47×16.47. Answer D is the *A/P* ratio of the rectangle 20×14 cm.

   ESF=2(L×W)/L+W   or ESF=4×A/P
   ESF=2(20×14)/20+14   ESF=4×280/68
   ESF=16.47   ESF=16.47

14. **B** Remember the right equation of A/P of a rectangular field.
   A/P=a×b/2(a+b)
   A/P=10×25/2(10+25)
   A/P=3.57

15. **E** All the answers are correct; PDD data for radiation therapy beams are usually tabulated for a square field which is why we use equivalent square formula to find equivalent square fields having the same PDD. As the field size increases, the contribution of the scattered radiation to the absorbed dose increases, and the increase in PDD caused by increase in field size depends on beam quality. The field size dependence of PDD is less pronounced for the higher-energy than for the lower-energy beam because higher-energy photons are scattered more predominantly in the forward direction rather than laterally.

16. **A** A simple rule-of-thumb method developed by Sterling states that a rectangular field is equivalent to a square field if they have the same area/perimeter (A/P).

Fig. 2A.1.1

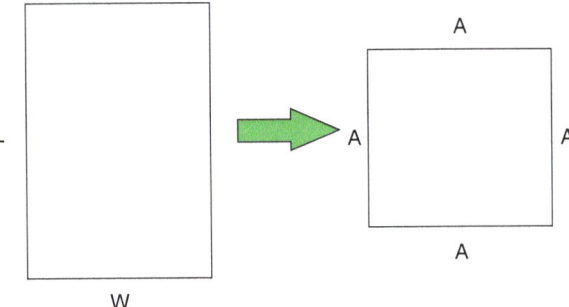

17. First, all the formulas must be well known:
   - **A.** II Area of 25×5 cm
     A−L×W
     A=25×5
     A=125
   - **B.** I Perimeter of 25×5 cm
     P=L+W+L+W
     P=25+5+25+5
     P=60

2.8 Dose Calculation (Answers)

    C. IV Area/perimeter (A/P) of 25×5 cm, a = width and b = length
            $A/P = 25 \times 5/2(25+5)$
            $A/P = 2.083$
    D. III Equivalent square of 25×5 cm
            $ESF = 2(L \times W)/L + W$ or $ESF = 4 \times A/P$
            $ESF = 2(25 \times 5)/25 + 5$ or $ESF = 4 \times 125/60$
            $ESF = 8.33$ or $ESF = 8.33$

18. **A.** I Energy increases; PDD increases due to greater penetrating power.
      B. II Depth increases; PDD decreases due to attenuation of the photon beam.
      C. I Field size increases; PDD increases due to increased scatter.
      D. I SSD increases; PDD increases due to inverse square law.

19. **A** The increase in PDD with an increase in SSD can be found by the Mayneord F factor formula which will be discussed further in the next question. PDD data for radiation therapy beams are usually tabulated for a square field which is why we use the equivalent square formula to find equivalent square fields having the same PDD. The inverse square formula is used to find the dose rate or intensity of the beam if the distance from the source needs to be changed because the intensity of the beam is inversely proportional to the square of the distances from the source. Finally, the tissue-air ratio formula is a method used to calculate dose for an SAD treatment technique. TAR is defined as the dose at a depth d in a phantom to the dose in free space at the same point

20. **D** The Mayneord F factor formula is
      $F = [(SSD_2 + d_m)/(SSD_1 + d_m) \times (SSD_1 + d)/(SSD_2 + d)]^2$
      where
      SSD_1 = original source-to-skin distance
      SSD_2 = new source-to-skin distance
      d = depth
      d_m = Dmax or depth of maximum dose

21. **B** Whenever a new PDD is to be determined because of a change on SSD, the Mayneord F factor formula must be applied.
      Rule of thumb for F factor: F factor is *always larger than 1.0* when the SDD is extended because as SSD increases, PDD increases. This can help eliminate extra incorrect answers.
      To do this calculation, be organized. First, collect all the information, write the formula, make sure the information collected can be plugged into the formula, discard any additional information, calculate, and verify that the answer makes sense.
      F = Mayneord F factor
      SSD_1 = 100 SSD
      SSD_2 = 120 SSD

Dmax = 0.5 cm
Depth $(d) = 5$ cm
$PDD_1 = 80\%$
$F = [(SSD_2 + d_m)/(SSD_1 + d_m) \times (SSD_1 + d)/(SSD_2 + d)]^2$
$F = [(120 + 0.5)/(100 + 0.5) \times (100 + 5)/(120 + 5)]^2$
$F = 1.0144$
New PDD = F * PDD = 1.0144 * 80 %
New PDD = 81.2 %

New PDD at 120 SSD is 81.2; it does make sense because the PPD increased with an increase in SSD. Answers A and D are discarded since the PPD must be greater than 80.

22. **D** As field size increases, PDD increases due to the increase in scatter radiation. Even though the equivalent square of 12×6 is 8×8, the 8×8 has more scatter and increases PDD because some parts of the 12×6 field size are farther from the central axis.

23. **B** Tissue inhomogeneities are volumes within the patient that have nonuniform tissue densities. These inhomogeneities alter the dose distribution due to attenuation and scatter differences in the various mediums. At any interface or near an inhomogeneity, the dose is affected primarily by scatter, while beyond the inhomogeneity; the dose is affected mainly by attenuation of the primary beam. The mass attenuation coefficient is a measure of the probability of energy absorption through various photon interactions, and it is affected by a combination of absorption and scatter. Heterogeneity corrections are modifications in the dose calculation algorithm to account for nonuniform tissue densities or inhomogeneities within the patient.

24. **C** TAR is a method for correcting tissue inhomogeneities, and it is used to remove the SSD dependence, SAR is used to calculate scattered dose in the medium, Clarkson's method is used to calculate irregular field, and TMR is the ratio of dose at depth in a phantom to dose at a depth of Dmax in a phantom.

25. **B** TAR = dose at depth in phantom to dose in free space at the same point.
 TPR = dose at depth in phantom to dose at a specified reference depth in phantom.
 TMR = dose at depth in phantom to dose at a depth of maximum dose in phantom.
 BSF = dose at maximum dose in phantom to dose in free space at the same point (basically the TAR at Dmax).

26. **A** TAR depends on field size, energy, and depth but is independent of SSD. The concept of TAR was introduced when treatments became more complex and were delivered from multiple angles. This made treating with constant SSD difficult as the patient is not round nor is the tumor always centered in the patient.

2.8 Dose Calculation (Answers)

27. B The different between TAR and BSF is that TAR is defined at any depth versus BSF is defined only at Dmax. Both are measured at a point in air and are independent of distance.

28. A As energy of the beam and field size increase, more scatter is produced, so TAR increases; as depth increases, there is less scatter so TAR decreases. The TAR and PDD behave in a similar fashion (besides the SSD independence of TAR) so if you can remember the rules for one, you can remember the rules for the other.

29. C TAR can be used for dose calculations in SAD treatments such as rotation or arc therapy where the SSD changes at every angle. Rather than converting the PDD for every angle, the TAR can be used to simplify the calculation due to the SSD independence. It is important to note that there is a slight SSD dependence, but in the clinical treatment range, the dependence is <2 %. In this case, average TAR is given, but if a table is given for each angle including depth along the radius and TAR, simply add all TARs and divide the sum by the total number of angles given to find the average TAR. As always, be organized, collect all the information, write the formula, and calculate.
Dose to be delivered at isocenter = 150 cGy.
Dose rate in free space = 80.5 cGy/min.
Average TAR = 0.550.
- Dose to be delivered at iso = dose in free space at isocenter/TAR.
- Dose to be delivered at iso = 150 cGy/0.550.
- Dose to be delivered at iso = 272.7 cGy (because the dose is being delivered to the tissue and not free space, the dose at iso must be higher than 150 cGy to account for the attenuation in the tissue).
- Treatment time = dose to be delivered at isocenter/dose rate in free space at isocenter.
- Treatment time = 272.7 cGy/80.5 cGy/min.
- Treatment time = 3.39 min.

30. E All statements about SAR are true.

31. A Scatter-air ratio is similar to the TAR in that it depends on beam energy, depth, and field size and it is independent of the treatment distance or source-to-surface distance.

32. B The scatter-air ratio formula is
$SAR = TAR_{(d, rd)} - TAR_{(d, 0)}$
where d is dose, rd is a given field size with scatter + primary beam, and 0 represents a 0×0 field size or primary component of the beam only.

33. A. (Fig. 2.1.3) Tissue maximum ratio (TMR). TMR is a special case of the tissue-phantom ratio (TPR) where the reference depth is chosen to be at Dmax. TMR is the ratio of the dose at a specified point in tissue or in a phantom to the dose at the same point when it is at the depth of maximum dose. TMR = dose in the tissue/dose in phantom (Dmax).
   B. (Fig. 2.1.8) Percent depth dose (PDD) is the absorbed dose at a given depth expressed as a percentage of the absorbed dose at a reference depth, usually taken to be Dmax, on the central axis of the field. The formula is PDD = absorbed dose at a given depth/absorbed dose at Dmax × 100 %. This is affected by energy, field size, SSD, and composition of the irradiated medium.
   C. (Fig. 2.1.2) Scatter-air ratio (SAR) is the ratio of the scattered dose at a given point in a medium to the dose in air at the same point. The SAR, like the TAR, is independent of the treatment distance but depends on energy, field size, and depth. SAR (D, FS) = TAR (D, FS) – TAR (D, 0) where D is depth and FS is the field size.
   D. (Fig. 2.1.5) Tissue-air ratio (TAR) is the ratio of the dose at a given point in a medium (water) to the dose *at the same point* in free space (air). TAR = dose in tissue/dose in air. TAR depends on depth and field size at that depth but is *independent of distance* (<2 % in the clinical ranges).
   E. (Fig. 2.1.4) Tissue-phantom ratio (TPR) is the ratio of dose at a specified point in the tissue or in a phantom to the dose at the same distance in the beam at a reference depth. TPR = dose in tissue/dose in phantom (ref. depth). The reference can be any depth that the user wants.
   F. (Fig. 2.1.7) The off-axis ratio (OAR) is used to calculate the dose at points away from the central axis and is the ratio of dose along the central axis at the depth under consideration to the dose off the central axis of the beam at the same depth and at the appropriate distance away from the central axis. OAR = dose at the off-axis point/dose on the central axis.
   G. (Fig. 2.1.6) Backscatter factor (BSF) is the ratio of dose on the central axis at Dmax to the dose at the same point in air or free space. BSF is also independent of SSD but depends on the energy and the field size. Remember that BSF and TAR at Dmax are the same.

34. D Any field other than the rectangular, square, or circular field may be termed an irregular field.

35. B The data used in the calculation of Clarkson's methods are SAR which is used to calculate the scatter dose and TAR $_{(0)}$ use to calculate the primary beam. Clarkson's method is used to calculate the dose to a point in an irregular field and is based on the principle that the scattered and primary components of the beam can be calculated independently.

36. B TAR at Dmax is equal to BSF, remember BSF is simply the tissue-air ratio at the depth of maximum dose on central axis of the beam, and it is defined as the ratio of the dose on central axis at the depth of maximum dose to the dose at the same point in free space. The PDD is the quotient, expressed as a percentage, of the absorbed dose at any depth to the absorbed dose at a fixed

reference depth, along the central axis of the beam. The TPR is the ratio of the dose at a given point in phantom to the dose at the same point at a fixed reference depth, and the SAR is defined as the ratio of the scattered dose at a given point in the phantom to the dose in free space at the same point.

37. A TAR = BSF × PDD/inverse square.

38. B PDD depends on source-to-surface distance, which makes this quantity unsuitable for isocentric techniques. TAR cannot be used with higher-energy photons as it requires measurement of dose in free space which is difficult due to the larger dose buildup region.

39. A The dose to a point in the medium may be calculated using both the primary and scattered radiation components. The primary is a contribution of photons emitted from the source, and the scattered photons are a result of the interactions in the collimator and phantom. Photoelectric, coherent scatter, Compton scattering, pair production, and photo disintegration are the five major types of interactions of photons with matter.

40. D Effective primary dose is the dose due to primary photons as well as those scattered from the collimating system only. The effective primary dose is introduced because for megavoltage photon beams, it is reasonably accurate to consider collimator scatter as part of the primary beam so that the phantom scatter could be calculated separately.

41. D The most commonly used beam-modifying device is a wedge. There are different kinds of wedges: physical wedges that are placed in the beam, universal wedges that stay in the beam for a certain percentage of the beam, and dynamic wedges that are created by moving one of the jaws across the treatment field. The wedges are made of dense materials such as lead, steel, or tungsten which attenuate the beam progressively across the field. A flattening filter is placed in the path of the raw photon beam so that it can be flattened for clinically use. The anode is a tungsten target used for production of x-rays, and the bending magnet is used in the gantry head to bend the electron beam from its original direction to allow for more efficient delivery.

42. C A wedge angle refers to the angle through which an isodose curve is tilted at the central axis of the beam at a specified depth. The angle between the central axes of two beams is called the hinge angle, and the physical degree angle of the wedge (15, 30, 45, or 60) does not necessarily represent the wedge angle.

43. D Physical wedges are usually made of lead or other high Z material which produce scatter on the contralateral breast. This is one of the downsides of a physical wedge. An advantage is they can be placed in any orientation so the MLC can be used to shape the field in the most efficient manner. Both universal and dynamic wedges are fixed in their relationship to the MLC.

44. B Physical wedge should be avoided, if possible, in the medial field of a tangent breast treatment because physical wedge produce scatter which affect the contralateral breast.

45. B The wedge angle or tilt of the isodose curve decreases at greater depth because of the increased effect of scattered radiation.

46. B The wedge transmission factor expresses the ratio of the dose rate on the central axis at a specified depth with and without the wedge. Any device placed in the beam path must be accounted for by increasing the number of MUs, or the correct dose will not be delivered. Some commercial isodose charts are normalized with the wedge transmission factor included, in those cases, the isodose line at Dmax along the central axis represents the wedge transmission factor, and no transmission factor should be used in cases like this.

47. B The thicker part of the physical wedge is called the heel, and it is the area of the wedge where attenuation is needed the most. The heel part is placed where tissue deficit exists so that the isodose line can be more homogeneous. The thinner part of the wedge is called the toe. A compensator can also be used to account for a tissue deficit.

48. A Isodose lines are shapeless when a beam enters an irregular surface causing dose nonuniformities throughout the treatment area. Wedges are typically used in cases where hot spots need to be reduced such as on lateral larynx treatments where hot spots are generated anteriorly due to the thinner separation. Also, uneven surfaces such as the chest and breast require wedges to even out the dose through the treatment region. A PA lumbar spine field usually does not require the use of a wedge because it is a flat surface.

49. B A universal wedge is designed so that the central axis thickness remains constant (meaning there is only one wedge in the head of the machine) and that the center of the wedge is fixed in the center of the beam for all field sizes. To change the wedge angle, the universal wedge is left in the field for a certain portion of the beam and is then removed for the remaining portion of the beam. This allows for the creation of any wedge angle.

50. E All definitions are correct; the output of a machine is defined as the dose delivered at a specified point in the beam, at a specified distance from the target, and in a specified medium. Absorbed dose in the irradiated medium is the energy absorbed in a material per unit mass; this requires knowledge of the composition of the irradiated material, geometric relationship with the

2.8 Dose Calculation (Answers)

beam and the size of the irradiated field. Maximum dose or Dmax is obtained at the depth where electron equilibrium is reached, and finally, the buildup region is the region between the surface and maximum dose or Dmax.

51. E All are correct; the half-value layer (HVL) is the thickness of the material that reduces the intensity of the beam to half (50 %) its original value, and also it expresses the penetration, quality, or hardness of a beam. If the HVL of a given beam is 5 mm Cu, inserting 5 mm Cu in the beam path will reduce its intensity to half of its original value, and the half-value layer or thickness is related to the linear attenuation coefficient (μ) by the equation (HVL = .693/μ).

52. B I and III only; dose rate increases with increasing field size due to scatter within the irradiated volume. Dose rate increases more rapidly in smaller fields, and as the field size becomes larger (20 × 20 cm), the increase in dose rate stabilizes and remains practically unchanged. Also, dose rate varies inversely with the square of the distance from the source.

53. D The materials used for the measurement of HVL are aluminum (Al) used for low-energy machines, copper (Cu) used for orthovoltage, or tin (Sn) used for high-energy machines. Lipowitz metal, also known as Cerrobend, is used in the construction of treatment blocks as it has a low melting point so it can easily be shaped. Tungsten is used as target material as well as for the construction of the MLC.

54. C For a monoenergetic beam, $HVL_1 = HVL_2 = HVL_3$.

55. B For a polyenergetic beam, $HVL_1 < HVL_2$ due to hardening of the beam. HVL_1 absorbs many of the low-energy photons effectively increasing the energy of the beam before the HVL_2.

56. B For monoenergetic photon beams, the linear attenuation coefficiency formula is $\mu = 0.693/HVL$. $\lambda = -0.693/T\frac{1}{2}$ is the constant decay formula, and $T_a = 1.44 \times T_{1/2}$ is the mean or average life formula of a radionuclide.

57. B Half-value layer is related to the linear attenuation coefficient (μ) by the equation HVL = 0.693/μ, so if μ is given (0.046 mm^{-1}) and 0.693 is constant, just calculate the HVL thickness from the formula.
$\mu = 0.046$
Constant = 0.693
HVL = ?
HVL = 0.693/μ
HVL = 0.693/0.046
HVL = 15 mm lead

58. A II. Tissue maximum ratio (TMR) is defined as the ratio of the dose at a specified point in the tissue or in a phantom to the dose at the same point when it is at the depth of maximum dose.
B. I. Tissue-phantom ratio (TPR) is defined as the ratio of dose at a specified point in the tissue or in a phantom to the dose at the same distance in the beam at a reference depth.
C. IV. Backscatter factor (BSF) is defined as the ratio of dose on the central axis at Dmax to the dose at the same point in air or free space.
D. III. Scatter-air ratio (SAR) is defined as the scattered dose at a given point in a medium to the dose in air at the same point.

59. A TMR is a special case of TPR where the reference depth is chosen to be at Dmax.

60. E All the statements are correct. The difference between SAR and SMR is that SMR reference point is at Dmax only versus SAR reference point is at any given point, the difference between TAR and TMR is that TMR reference point is at Dmax only versus TAR reference point is at any given point, SAR and TAR are independent of distance, and SAR and SMR are mainly used in calculation of scattered dose in a phantom or tissue.

61. B Methods of inhomogeneity corrections for photon beams are TAR and isodose shift method. Coefficient of equivalent thickness (CET) is used in inhomogeneity corrections for electron beam only, and the effective SSD method is used when corrections for surface irregularities are needed.

62. C 6 HVLs are required to reduce the intensity of a photon of 320 mR/h to 5 mR/h
$I = I_0(0.5)^n$
$I = 5$ mR/h
$I_0 =$ initial intensity $= 320$ mR/h
$N = \#$ of HVL?
$320 \times (0.5)^6 = 5$ mR/h

63. A The tenth-value layer (TVL) is the thickness of material required to attenuate a beam of radiation to one tenth of its original intensity. This is used as well as half-value layer (HVL) to denote the quality of the beam and depends on the beam quality, beam energy, and the amount of filtration at the source. The tenth-value layer (TVL) formula is TVL = $\log_e 10/\mu$ or $I = I_0(0.1)^n$ where I_0 is the initial intensity, $\log_e 10 = 2.3$, n is the

2.8 Dose Calculation (Answers)

number of TVL needed, and the linear attenuation coefficient (μ) is a constant that describes the unique properties of a material in question with a unit of cm^{-1}.
$I = I_0(0.1)^n$
$I = 10$ mR/min
$I_0 =$ initial intensity $= 4,000$ mR/min
$N = $ # of TVL?
$4,000 \times (0.1)^n = 4$ mR/min
$4,000 \times (0.1)^3 = 4$ mR/min

64. **A.** II. Photon beams are polyenergetic.
B. II. Electron beams are polyenergetic.
C. I. Gamma rays are monoenergetic.
D. I. Characteristic x-rays are monoenergetic (for a specific element and transition).

65. The presence of bone in the kilovoltage range results in an increased absorption due to photoelectric interactions, but this is not observed in the megavoltage range as Compton scatter dominates and the electron density for the bone and soft tissue is very similar. The presence of healthy lung creates overdose beyond this area due to decreased attenuation caused by the low density of the lung.
A. V. A 3 mm Cu beam will see a -7 % reduction of dose beyond bone or 10 %/cm increase in dose beyond healthy lung.
B. III. A ^{60}Co beam will see a -3.5 % reduction of dose beyond bone or 3.5–5/cm % increase in dose beyond healthy lung.
C. II. A 4 MV beam will see a 3 % reduction of dose beyond bone or 4 %/cm increase in dose beyond healthy lung.
D. IV. A 10 MV beam will see a -2 % reduction of dose beyond bone.
E. I. A 20 MV beam will see a 2 %/cm increase in dose beyond healthy lung.

66. B
HVL $= 3.5$ cm, and material thickness $= 10.5$ cm, so
$10.5/3.5 = 3$ HVLs (10.5 cm of material will have 3 HVLs).
Since the beam will be reduced 50 % of the dose for each HVL, then the transmission is $(1/2)^n$, n being the number of HVL.
Transmission $= (1/2)^3$
Transmission $= 0.125$ (or 12.5 %)

67. B After 10 HVLs, the intensity of the beam is reduced by $I = I_0(0.5)^{10}$. The formula $I = I_0(0.1)^n$ is used for tenth-value layer (TVL) calculations.

68. A I, II, and III only are true about collimator scatter factor (Sc); Sc is commonly called the output factor, and it is defined as the ratio of the output in air for a given field to that for a reference field. Finally, as field size increased, Sc or output factor increases due to an increase in collimator scatter. Normally these measurements of Sc are done at the SAD.

69. E All are correct. The phantom scatter factor (Sp) takes into account the change in scatter radiation originating in the phantom at a reference depth as the field size is changed. Sp is the ratio of the dose rate for a given field at a reference depth to the dose rate at the same depth for the reference field size, with the same collimator opening, and also is related to changes in the volume of the phantom irradiated for a fixed collimator opening. If a backscatter factor can be measured, Sp at Dmax may be defined as the ratio of BSF for the given field to that for the reference field.

70. B Clarkson's method is used to calculate irregular fields; circular, rectangular, and square fields are not considered irregular fields.

71. C $TMR_{(d, rd)} = TAR_{(d, rd)} / BSF_{(rd)}$

72. A I, II, and III only. Scatter-maximum ratio (SMR) is the quantity designated specifically for the calculation of scattered dose in a medium, and it is defined as the ratio of the scattered dose at a given point in the phantom to the effective primary dose at the same point at Dmax.

73. E All statements about BSF are correct. BSF is independent of SSD and only depends on energy and the field size. BSF and TAR at Dmax are the same, and BSF is much lower for megavoltage beams than lower-energy beams.

74. A   II.   PDD = percentage of the absorbed dose at any depth d to the absorbed dose at a fixed reference depth d_0, along the central axis of the beam.

    B.   I.   TMR = ratio of dose at depth in a phantom to dose at a depth of Dmax in a phantom. $TAR_{(d, rd)}/BSF_{(rd)}$. Dose in tissue/dose in phantom at Dmax

    C.   III.   TAR = ratio of dose at depth in phantom to dose in free space at the same point. BSF × PDD/inverse square. Dose in tissue/dose in air

    D.   V.   TPR = ratio of dose at depth in phantom to dose at a specified reference depth in phantom. Dose in tissue/dose in phantom at reference depth

    E.   IV.   BSF = ratio of dose at maximum dose in phantom to dose in free space at the same point or tissue-air ratio at the depth of maximum dose on central axis of the beam. Dose at Dmax/dose in free space

    F.   VI.   Output = dose delivered at a specified point in the beam, at a specified distance from the target, and in a specified medium

    G.   VIII.   SAR = ratio of scattered dose at a given point in the phantom to the dose in free space at the same point. $TAR_{(d, rd)} - TAR_{(d, 0)}$

    H.   VII.   Absorbed dose = energy absorbed in a material per unit mass.

2.8 Dose Calculation (Answers)

I.	IX.	Collimator scatter factor (Sc) = ratio of the output in air for a given field to that for a reference field. Also called the output factor. $D_{fs}(r)/D_{fs}(\text{ref})$
J.	XI.	Phantom scatter factor (Sp) = ratio of the dose rate for a given field at a reference depth to the dose rate at the same depth for the reference field size, with the same collimator opening
K.	X.	SMR = ratio of the scattered dose at a given point in the phantom to the effective primary dose at the same point at Dmax

75. B The dose on a fixed SAD technique is usually normalized at the isocenter which will be at a fixed distance from the source. Normalizing at Dmax is difficult as beams are coming in from multiple angles because the SSD will change.

76. A Only I, II, and III are correct; the SAD technique is also known as an isocentric technique, and the axis of rotation of the machine is the isocenter, and small errors in SSD are balanced out using an opposing field. When treating with multiple beams, the SAD technique is superior to an SSD technique because the patient only needs to be positioned one time.

77. B The method used in calculating the dose in an SAD technique are TAR and dose rate in air or TPR and TMR because these methods are independent of distance. PDD is used in an SSD technique, and Clarkson's method is used for calculation of irregular fields.

78. E Isocenter refers to a point in space that is the same distance from the source for all gantry angles, it is also the intersection of the collimator axis and the axis of rotation, linacs have the isocenter typically at 80 or 100 cm, and the isocenter is fixed and cannot be changed.

79. C The dose on a fixed SSD technique is usually normalized at Dmax.

80. E All statements are correct; SSD is patient specific because it does not exist until patient is present on the couch. Field size is defined on the patient's skin, SSD is a non-isocenter technique, and SSD calculation uses the PDD method.

81. B SAD = SSD + depth.

82. C Machines are usually calibrated to deliver 1 cGy per monitor unit (MU) at 100 cm SSD, the reference depth, for a reference field size, usually 10 × 10 cm.

83. A. An isodose line is a line passing through points of EQUAL dose representing a percentage of doses at a reference point. The region near the edge of the field margin where the dose falls rapidly is called the penumbra, and the tilting of the isodose lines from their standard position is the wedge angle created when a wedge-shaped material is inserted into the beam path.

84. B. A number of isodose curves depicted in 10 % increments are a function of isodose chart. A DVH is a graph that provides quantitative information with regard to how much dose is absorbed in how much volume and also summarizes the entire dose distribution into a single curve for each anatomic structure of interest. A beam's eye view (BEV) displays the segmented target and normal structures in a plane perpendicular to the central axis of the beam used to shape the beam appropriately.

85. C The light source, which coincides with the beam, is aligned to match the 50 % isodose line.

86. A Geometric field size is defined as the intersection of the 50 % isodose line and the surface. Part of the isocenter definition is the intersection of the collimator axis and the axis of rotation, and the region between the surface and maximum dose or Dmax is called the buildup region. The region near the edge of the field margin, where the dose falls rapidly, is the definition of penumbra.

87. E The size of the penumbra depends on the size of the radiation source (source size increases, penumbra increases), the source-to-collimator distance (SCD) or source-to-diaphragm distance (SDD) (if SDD decreases, penumbra increases), the source-to-skin distance (SSD) (if SSD increases, penumbra increases), and depth of penumbra calculation (if depth increases, penumbra increases).

88. E All the statements are correct; isodose lines for Co^{60} machines decrease as one moves away from the central axis near the surface, and for linacs, isodose lines increase as one moves away from the central axis near the surface. Due to the lower-dose rate with Co^{60}, the beam cannot be flattened as much. For linacs, the increasing dose away from the central axis near the surface is due to overflattening of the beam at shallow depths which results in a flat beam at a certain depth (more photons scatter into the central part of the beam and some photons scatter out of the beam at the edges as the depth increases which results in a beam with "horns" near the surface and a flat beam at depth). This shape results because the flattening filter reduces the dose along the central axis and produces a flat beam at a specified depth, usually 10 cm.

89. E All the statements are correct. For an SSD technique, dose is usually normalized at Dmax. For an SAD technique, dose is usually normalized at isocenter. A dose profile displays relative dose across a field or across a treatment plan consisting of multiple beams. A beam's eye view shows the beam in a plane perpendicular to the central axis.

90. A III. Dynamic wedge: wedge effect can be produced by driving one of the secondary collimator jaws across the field with the beam on. This creates the wedged isodose distribution.

2.8 Dose Calculation (Answers)   179

    B.   I.   Universal wedge: wedge of a given angle that is fixed in the beam and serves all beam widths up to a designated limit.
    C.   IV.   Asymmetric wedge: a wedge is mounted such that one can use an asymmetric jaw to block half the treatment field and utilize the wedging effect for the other open half.
    D.   II.   Individualized wedge: multiple wedges are required for each isodose tilt and are typically used in Co-60 beams. This wedge is mounted so that the thin edge of the wedge coincides with the edge of the light field.

91. C   The angle of the sloping isodose curve on a dynamic wedge is determined by the speed with which the collimator jaw moves. In an enhanced dynamic wedge, not only is the jaw speed varied, but the dose rate is varied as well.

92. D   A block or wedge should be placed at least 15 cm away from the patient's skin so that the skin-sparing effect is not lost due to low-energy contaminants caused by the wedge or block. Remember that any device placed in the beam will generate additional electrons and particles that add contamination to the beam as the photons interact in that device. The farther that the device is placed from the skin, the contamination dose is reduced.

93. A   A wedge is usually constructed of a high Z material such as lead, steel, copper, or tungsten.

94. E   All the answers are correct about dynamic wedges. By varying the collimator speed, different wedge angles can be generated. Because the wedge is formed by moving the collimator jaw, which is located inside the treatment head, the dynamic wedge has a sharper penumbra.

95. A   The junction between the cranial and the upper spine field for craniospinal irradiation is a crucial aspect of the treatment because if there is overlap, a hot spot in the cord could cause paralysis and if there is a large gap, a cold spot could allow for a recurrence. The important concept to remember is that if a normal beam arrangement is used and the fields are matched on the surface, there will be divergence of each beam into the other at depth. To prevent this, one can leave a gap on the skin with the inferior border meeting at a point midway on the posterior neck surface, the collimator jaw can be used to create a half-beam block which eliminates beam divergence, or collimator and couch angles can be used to match the divergence of the beams to prevent overlap. The matching of the beam divergence with collimator and table angles is the most commonly used technique. The half-beam block technique is simpler but limits the field size that can be used.

96. B   The advantage of using independent table and collimator angles to match the craniospinal field divergence is that field matching is achieved with no overlaps between the cranial and spine fields at any depth. Additionally, the jaws can be conveniently used to move the craniospinal junction line caudally to smooth out the junctional dose distribution in a procedure called feathering. Feathering is typically done three times during the treatment, and the junction is usually shifted about 1 cm each time. Feathering is another technique to reduce the possibility of a hot or cold spot at the junction.

97. **E** All statements are correct. The site of the field matching should not contain tumor or a critically sensitive organ so that the tumor is not over- or underdosed. For superficial tumors at the junction site, the fields should not be separated because a cold spot on the tumor will increase the risk for recurrence. For deep-seated tumors, the fields may be separated on the skin surface so that the junction point lies at the midline due to the divergence of the fields at depth. The line of field matching must be drawn at each treatment session on the basis of the first treated fraction to verify positioning. The field-matching technique must be verified by actual isodose distributions in the planning system before it is adopted for general clinical use to ensure there are not hot or cold spots.

98. **B** If a machine is assigned a HVL of 3 mm Cu, but the engineer inserts by mistake a 3.5 mm Cu HVL filter, the HVL will increase due to hardening of the beam because more low-energy photons will be removed from the beam. This means that the penetration of the beam will be higher and the assumed dose will be lower than what is actually be delivered especially if the prescription point is deep.

99. **A** The International Commission on Radiological Units and Measurements (ICRU) recommends that dose delivered to a tumor to be within 5.0 % of the prescribed dose (and also within 5 mm spatially). There are many components of a linac so that means the tolerance on each specific component must be much tighter than the overall goal.

2.9 Applied Mathematics (Answers)

Quiz 1 (Level 1)

1. A. V. $15^5 \times 10^3 = 759{,}375{,}000$
   B. III. $1.5 \times 12^{10} \times 2.5 \times 10^7 = 4.5^{17}$
   C. II. $20^3 = 8{,}000$
   D. VI. $\sqrt{25} = 5$
   E. I. $\sqrt[3]{27} = 3$
   F. IV. $\sqrt{16} = 4$

2.9 Applied Mathematics (Answers)

2–4.

Factor	Exponent	Prefix	
1 000 000 000 000	10^{12}	Tera	One trillion
1 000 000 000	10^{9}	Giga	One billion
1000 000	10^{6}	Mega	One million
1 000	10^{3}	Kilo	One thousand
100	10^{2}	Hecto	One hundred
10	10^{1}	Deka	Ten
0.1	10^{-1}	Deci	One tenth
0.01	10^{-2}	Centi	One hundredth
0.001	10^{-3}	Milli	One thousandth
0.000 001	10^{-6}	Micro	One millionth
0.000 000 001	10^{-9}	Nano	One billionth
0.000 000 000 001	10^{-12}	Pico	One trillionth
0.000 000 000 000 001	10^{-15}	Femto	One quadrillionth
0.000 000 000 000 000 001	10^{-18}	Atto	One quintillionth

5. An important calculation done by dosimetrists, physicists, and physician is %s.
   - A. IX. Rx = 30 Gy: 15 % of 30 Gy = 4.5 Gy
   - B. VI. Rx = 40 Gy: 95 % of 40 Gy = 38 Gy
   - C. II. Rx = 46 Gy: 90 % of 36 Gy = 2.4 Gy
   - D. V. Rx = 30 Gy: 10 % hot spot = 33 Gy
   - E. VIII. Rx = 30 Gy: 10 % reduction from 30 Gy = 27 Gy
   - F. III. Rx = 60 Gy: What % of 60 Gy is 9 Gy = 15 %
   - G. I. Decimal equivalent of 40 % = 0.40
   - H. VII. Decimal equivalent of 50 % = 0.50
   - I. IV. Decimal equivalent of 5 % = 0.05

6. D With a Rx to 60 Gy, 95 % of the PTV should receive 100 % of the Rx (60 Gy). This means that the V95% must equal 60 Gy. The max dose is 115 % of the Rx dose so the maximum dose accepted is 69 Gy (60 × 1.15). Also 107 % of the Rx dose (64.2 Gy) should be less than 10 % of the volume, and 110 % of the Rx dose (66 Gy) should be less than 5 % of the volume. This means that the V10 % = 64.2 Gy and the V5 % = 66 Gy.

7. A. II.   Sin 20° = 0.34
B. VI.   Cos 30° = 0.87
C. VIII. Tan 50° = 1.19
D. VII. sin⁻¹ 0.10 = 5.7
E. V.   cos⁻¹ 0.5 = 60
F. I.   tan⁻¹ 10° = 84.3
G. III. sin 25° + cos 20° = 0.40
H. IX.   tan⁻¹ 0.15 + cos⁻¹ 0.10 = 92.8
I. IV.   sin⁻¹ 0.8 − tan⁻¹ 0.3 = 36

8. A. II. $e^3 = 20$
B. IV.   Ln (30) = 3.40
C. III. Log (150) = 2.18
D. V. $10^7 = 10,000,000$
E. I. $10^{-5} = 0.00001$

9. Remember that 1 Gy = 100 cGy = 100 rad.
A. III. 100 Gy = 10,000 cGy
B. IV.   10 cGy = 0.1 Gy
C. I.   120 rad = 1.2 Gy
D. II.   30 Gy = 3,000 rad

10. Do not forget that:
1 m = 100 cm
1 cm = 10 mm
1 cm = 0.3937 in.
1 in. = 2.54 cm
1 ft v 12 in.
1 ft = 30.48 cm
Conversion formula from °F to °C:
$C = (F − 32) \times 5/9$
Conversion formula from °C to °F:
$F = (C \times 9/5) + 32$
A. VII.   10 m = 1,000 cm
B. IX.   550 cm = 5.5 m
C. VIII. 120 cm = 1,200 mm
D. I.   300 mm = 30 cm
E. V.   15 in. = 38.1 cm
F. II.   10 mm − 0.3937 in.
G. VI.   20 ft 240 in.
H. III.   40 °F = 8 °C
I. IV.   −4 °C = 24.8 °F

11. B If a PA field is clinically set up at 70 SSD using 20×25 cm, but the whole area is not included and the SSD needs to be extended to 95 cm, cross multiplication can be used to find the answer. Remember the field size divergence will increase as SSD is extended so the answer must be bigger than 20×25.

2.9 Applied Mathematics (Answers)

Fig. 2.2A.1

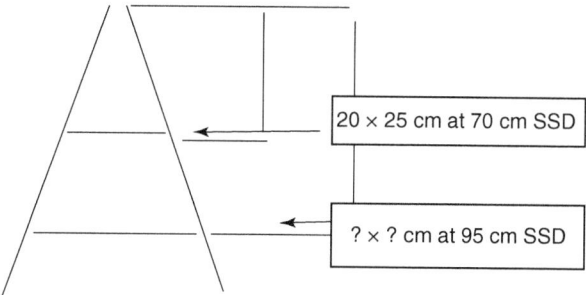

The easy way to solve is to set up ratios that relate the known parameters to the unknown:
$20/70 = X/95$.
–Solve for X.
$X = 95 \text{ SSD} \times 20/70 = 27$ cm
–Repeat for the other dimension: $25/70 = X/95$.
$X = 95 \text{ cm SSD} \times 25/70 = 34$ cm

12. **C** If a femur is set up AP/PA to cover the prosthesis that lies 10 cm from the anterior surface and 5 cm from the posterior surface, remember that the field size for an SAD setup is defined at isocenter which is at 100 cm. Since the SSD will be less than 100 cm, the projected field size on the skin must be less than the field size at isocenter. By setting up ratios, the field size on the anterior skin will be 27×6.3 cm and on the posterior skin will be 28.5×6.65 cm. Remember to directly relate the know quantities to the unknown quantities. The AP SSD will be 90 cm and the posterior SSD will be 95 cm.

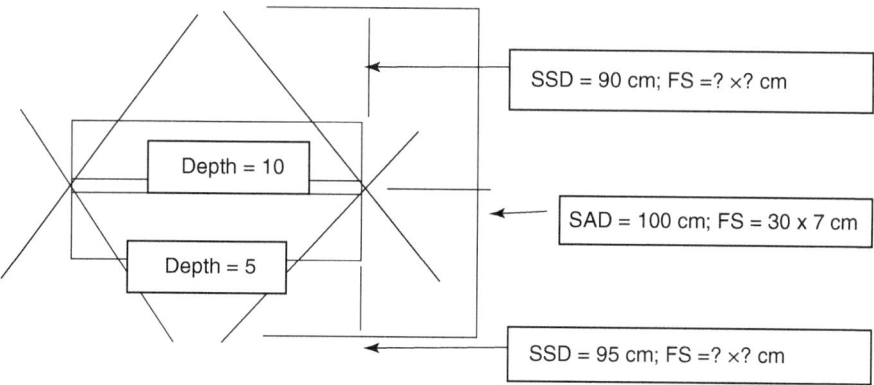

Fig. 2.2A.2

AP: $30/100 = X/90$
–Solve for X
$X = 90 \text{ cm SSD} \times 30/100 = 27$ cm
$-7/100 = X/90$
$X = 90 \text{ cm SSD} \times 7/100 = 6.3$ cm

PA: $30/100 = X/95$
—Solve for X
$X = 95\ SSD \times 30/100 = 28.5$ cm
$-7/100 = X/95$
$X = 95\ SSD \times 7/100 = 6.65$ cm

13. **A** If a tumor is 10 cm deep, it needs to be treated using a 25×20 cm field size on the tumor with a source-to-skin distance of 100 cm. If a 1 cm bolus is placed on the skin, the new field size on the tumor will be the same since the geometry never changed or distance from the source to the tumor never changed. Be careful because if the physician prescribed the dose to be 100 cm source-to-surface distance, the field size would change because the new source-to-skin distance would be 101 cm and the tumor would be at a depth of 11 cm.

14. **C** A conversion from feet and inches to cm must be done first:

1 ft = 30.48 cm	1 in. = 2.54 cm
5 ft = X cm	7 in. = X cm
X = 5 ft. × 30.48 cm/1 ft.	X = 7 in × 2.54 cm/1 in
X = 152.40 cm	X = 17.78 cm
	1 in. = 2.54 cm
	18 in. = X
	X = 18 in × 2.54 cm/1 in
	X = 45.72 cm

    5 ft and 7 in. = 170.18 cm tall and 18 in. = 45.72 cm wide
    Field size = 170.18 × 46 cm + 2 cm flash (1 cm on each side)
    Field size = 173 × 48 cm approximately

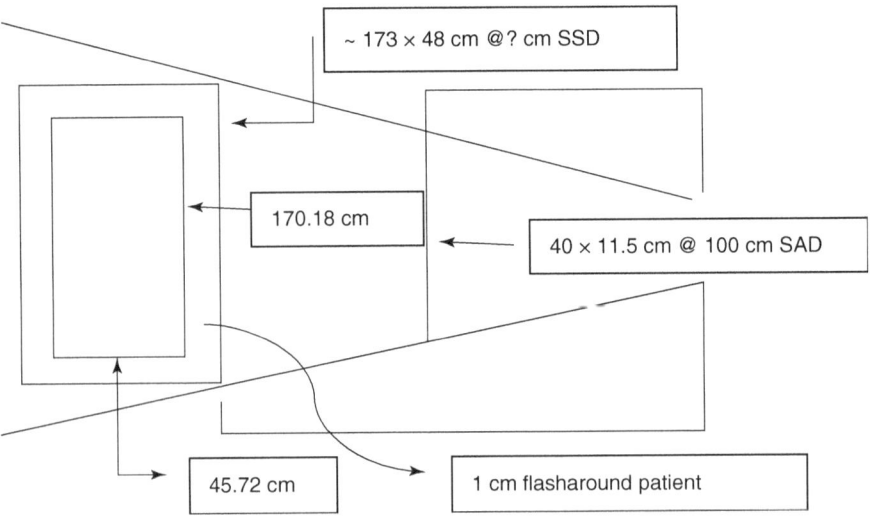

Fig. 2.2A.4

40 cm at 100 SAD	11.5 cm at 100 SAD
40/100 = 173/X	11.5/100 = 48/X
X = 173 × 100/40	X = 48 × 100/11.5
X = 432.5 cm SSD	X = 417.4 cm SSD

In this case, we are limited by the vertical field size. Even though we have enough coverage at 417.4 cm for the lateral field size, we need at least 432.5 cm for the vertical dimension. Therefore, the SSD has to be 432.5 cm.

15. B If a treatment setup is done at 100 cm SSD using a 110×150 mm on the skin, the field size 25 in. (63.5 cm) below the surface where the tumor lies is 179.3×245.25 mm.

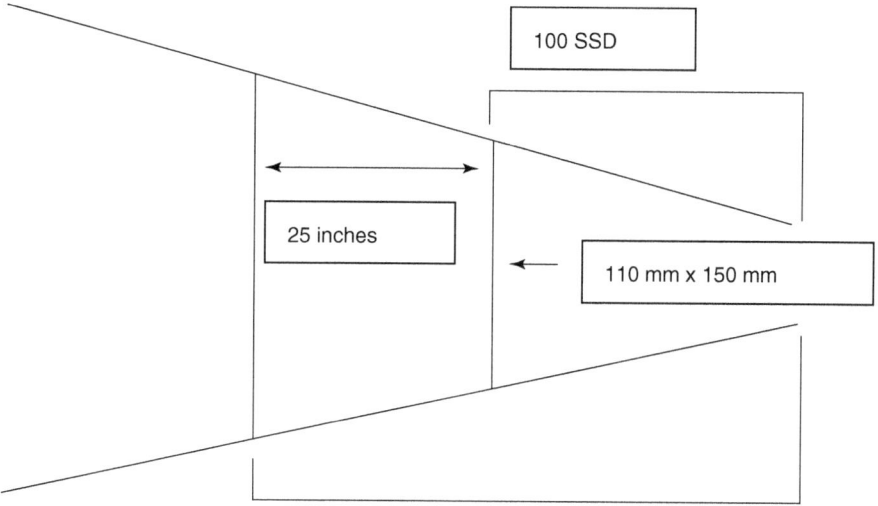

Fig. 2.2A.5

1 in. = 2.54 cm
25 in. = X
X = 25 in 2.54 cm/1 in
X = 63.5 cm
So we need to calculate the field size at 25 in. +100 cm SSD = 163.5 cm.

100 SSD = 110 mm	100 SSD = 150 mm
110/100 = X/163.5	150/100 = X/163.5
X = 163.5 × 110/100	X = 163.5 × 150/100
X = 179.3 mm	X = 245.25 mm

16. D The magnification factor (MF) is the ratio of the image size to the object size: image size/object size. To calculate the MF uses in the construction of a block if the field size at SAD is 13×15 cm and the image projection on the film is 15.6×18 cm, the following steps can be used:

Fig. 2.2A.6

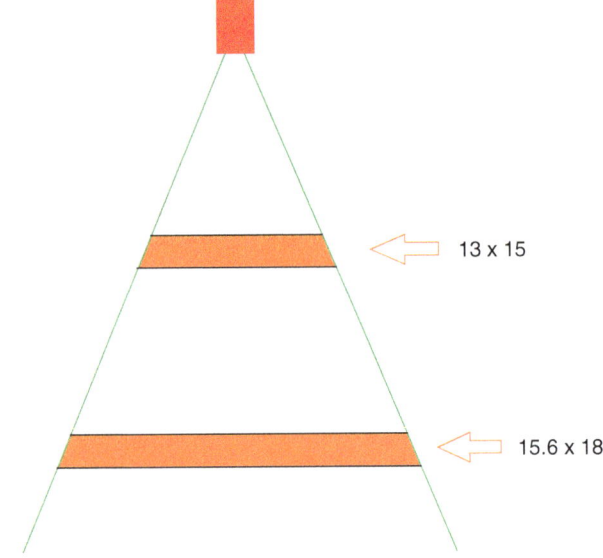

MF = field size on the film (or image size)/field size setting (or object size)
MF = 15.6/13 = 1.2
MF = 18/15 = 1.2

17. A The image size of the cylinder on the film will be 18.4×3.05 cm with a magnification factor of 1.5.

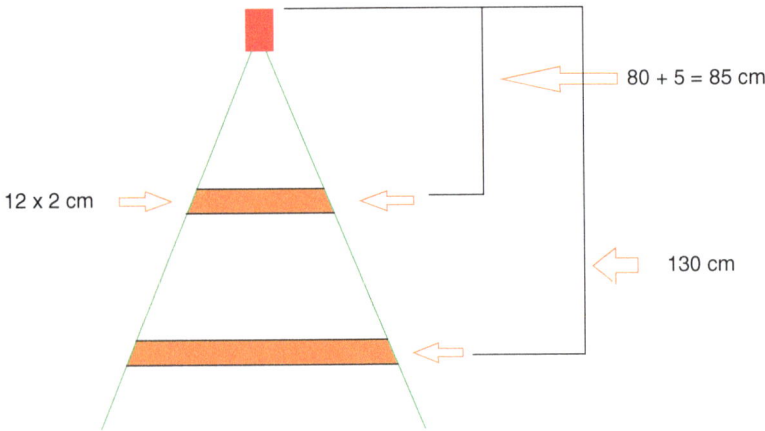

Fig. 2.2A.7

2.9 Applied Mathematics (Answers)

Set up ratios:

Object: 12 cm at 85 cm	2 cm at 85 cm
Image: X cm at 130 cm	X cm at 130 cm
$12/85 = X/130$	$2/85 = X/130$
$X = 18.4$ cm	$X = 3.05$ cm

Use magnification factor formula. Remember that the image size is always going to be larger than the object since the object must be in between the source and image:
MF = image size/object size
MF = 18.4/12 = 1.5
MF = 3.05/2 = 1.5

18. B Be organized:
Image size = ?
Field size = 20 × 15 cm
Magnification factor = 1.45
MF = image size/object size (field size in this case)
Image size = field size × MF
Image size = 20 cm × 1.45 = 29 cm
Image size = 15 cm × 1.45 = 21.75 cm
Image size (or the field size as seen on the film) = 29 × 21.75 cm

19. E All statements are correct in terms of *radiation therapy*. Be careful because in some diagnostic imaging, the Z-axis represents the superior/inferior direction with the Y-axis representing the anterior/posterior direction.
X-axis represent patient $-X$ = right, $+X$ = left
Y-axis represent patient $-Y$ = inferior, $+Y$ = superior
Z-axis represent patient $-Z$ = posterior, $+Z$ = anterior
Cartesian coordinate system:

Fig. 2.2A.8

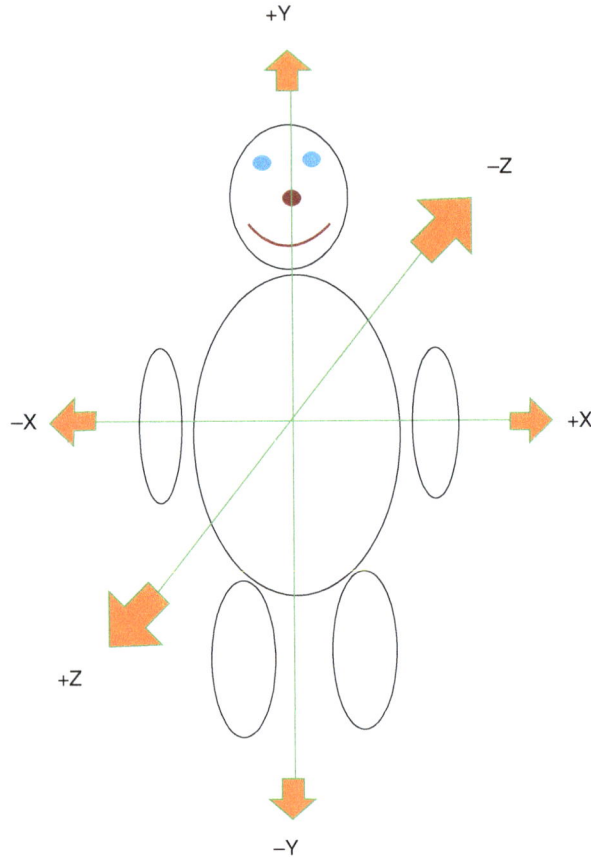

20. **C** Umbilicus user origin (0, 0, 0). Shift (15 superior, 10 lateral, 5 posterior) the patient supine head toward gantry. Remember superior/inferior=Y; right/left lateral=X; and anterior/posterior=Z. Refers to diagram in answer 19. $X=-10$ cm, $Y=+15$ cm, $Z=-5$ cm

21. **B** The right calf is the back portion of the lower leg. If the umbilicus is the user origin (0, 0, 0), since the patient is prone, feet toward gantry, the shift needs to be superior ($+Y$) to the leg. The superior direction is flipped because the patient is feet first rather than head first which is standard. The right leg will still be on the right because not only is the patient feet first (reversed from the standard) but the patient is prone which is also reversed from the standard supine position. The combination of the two result in the right side still being the right side ($-X$). The posterior aspect of the patients becomes the anterior coordinate because the patient is prone ($+Z$). Remember that the correct order of the coordinates is X, Y, and Z.

22. **D** Patient supine, head toward gantry; Cartesian coordinates are ($-12, 20, 6$) $-X$ right, $+Y$ cephalic (superior), $+Z$ posterior

2.9 Applied Mathematics (Answers)

23. C There are many ways to remember the trigonometric identities, but one simple way is the acronym SOH-CAH-TOA. In this acronym, the first letter represents the identity; the second and third represent the ratio of the triangle's sides as shown below:
Sin (A) = $o$pposite/$h$ypotenuse = a/h
Cos (A) = $a$djacent/$h$ypotenuse = b/h
Tan (A) = $o$pposite/$a$djacent = a/b

Fig. 2.2A.9

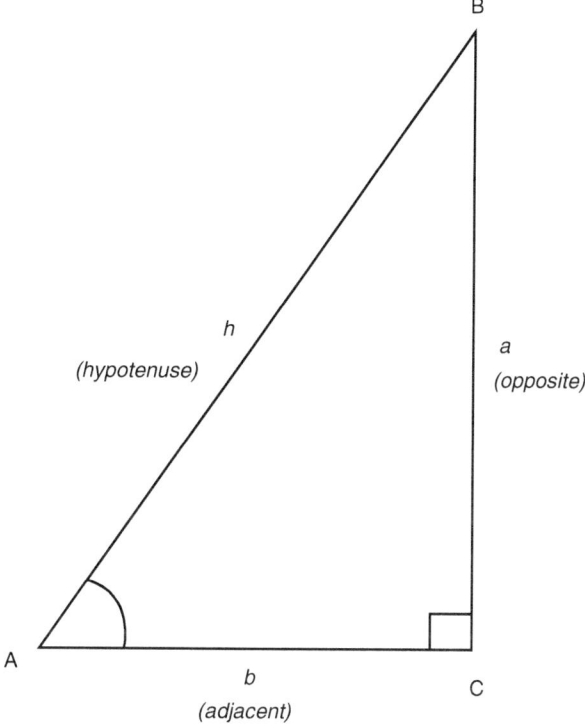

24. A Sine, cosine, and tangent formulas are trigonometric functions used to relate the angles of a triangle to the length of the side of the triangle. Remember SOH-CAH-TOA.
Sin $(X°)$ = opposite/hypotenuse
Cos $(X°)$ = adjacent/hypotenuse
Tan $(X°)$ = opposite/adjacent

25. C Remember that a radiation beam can be treated like a right triangle with one side being equal to the SSD and the other being equal to half the field size at that SSD. Using trig identities, the collimator or couch angle needed to match the divergence of the beam can be calculated. The student not only must know the formula but should select the correct one. A quick reminder is when calculating brain field collimator angle, use PA upper spine field SSD and length because we are concerned of divergence of the spine field into the cranial field. On the other hand, when calculating cranial field couch angle, the lateral cranial field length and SAD (if isocentric treatment setup) should be used as we are concerned of the cranial field divergence into the spine field.

Quiz 2 (Level 2)

1. **C** When you see a question for a craniospinal case, you can most likely count on having to use a trigonometric identity to solve the problem. The cranial field collimator angle must be chosen to match the divergence of the upper PA spine field. The only information needed to solve this is the upper spine field length and SSD, and the other information is extra. Be organized and collect the necessary data.
Cranial field collimator angle = ?
PA upper spine field = 36×8 cm at 100 cm SSD
Cranial field = 14×21 cm at 100 cm SAD
Remember that to make a right triangle, you only need half of the spine field's length: ½ of PA upper spine length = 36/2 = 18
This length is now the side of the triangle opposite to the angle you need to solve.
The side of the triangle adjacent to the angle of interest is equal to the SSD of the PA field = 100 cm.
Remember that the first number on a field size is the length and the second the width. The PA field length is the one diverging into the cranial field so the width is not necessary for this calculation.
Remember your trigonometric identities:
We know the opposite and adjacent side lengths; therefore, we can use the tangent to relate everything together (SOH-CAH-TOA).
Tan (θ_{coll}) = opposite/adjacent or arc tan $(1/2\ L_1 \times 1/SSD)$
Tan (θ_{coll}) = 18/100
Tan (θ_{coll}) = 0.18
$Tan^{-1}\ (\theta_{coll})$ = 10.2°

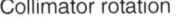
Collimator rotation

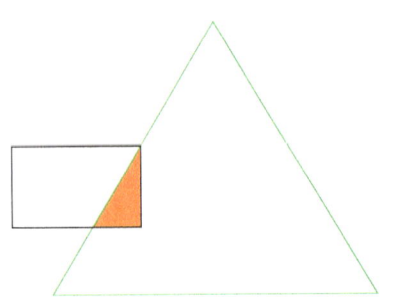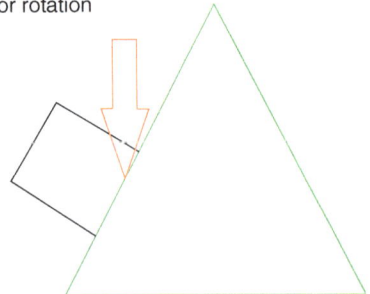

Fig. 2.2A.10

2.9 Applied Mathematics (Answers)

2. B This problem is solved in the same manner as the previous question only; this time we are concerned about the divergence of the cranial field into the spine field. Therefore, the cranial couch angle depends on the divergence of the cranial field so we need those dimensions and SSD this time. Be organized and collect the necessary data.
Cranial field couch angle = ?
PA upper spine field = 40 × 10 cm at 100 cm SSD
Brain field = 16 × 22 cm at 100 cm SAD
Just as before, the opposite side = ½ of the cranial field length = 16/2 = 8 cm
The adjacent side = cranial SAD = 100 cm
Remember that the first number on a field size is the length and the second the width. The collimator angle we calculated previously takes care of the divergence for the spine into the cranial field so the spine field parameters are extra information.
Based on trigonometric functions:
Tan (θ_{couch}) = opposite/adjacent or arc tan $(1/2 L_2 \times 1/SAD)$
Tan (θ_{couch}) = 8/100
Tan (θ_{couch}) = 0.08
Tan^{-1} (θ_{couch}) = 4.57°

Fig. 2.2A.11

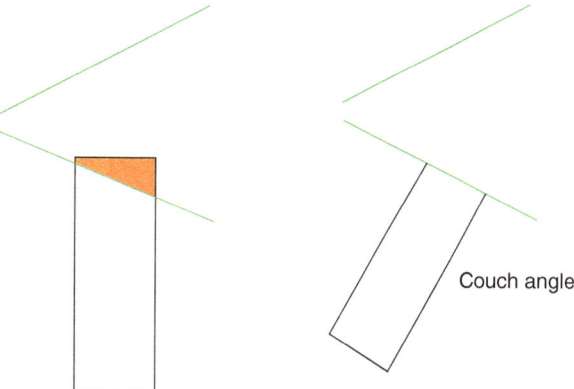

Couch angle

3. A It is very important to read the question, collect the appropriate information, and discard the extra information before working on the problem. We want to solve for the couch angle to account for cranial field divergence into the upper spine field. Therefore, we only need information about the cranial field. All spine field information can be discarded. Next, we need to set up our right triangle. Remember that the opposite side from the angle of interest is half the length of the cranial field. The adjacent side is the SAD. Be careful here because an SSD is given. Since the SSD is 93 cm and the separation is 14 cm, we can figure out the SAD as it is not given.

Cranial θ_{couch} = arc Tan (1/2 brain length × 1/brain field SAD)
Cranial θ_{couch} = ?
Cranial field length = 18 cm
Cranial SAD = ?
Patient separation = 14 cm
Cranial field SSD = 93 cm
Cranial SAD = patient separation/2 + SSD
Cranial SAD = 14/2 + 93 cm
Cranial SAD = 7 + 93 = 100 cm SAD
Cranial θ_{couch} = arc tan (1/2 L × 1/SAD)
Cranial θ_{couch} = arc tan (9 × 1/100)
Cranial θ_{couch} = arc tan^{-1} 0.09
Cranial θ_{couch} = 5.14°

4. **C** The TMR to be used in a patient with a 10 MV beam, 12 × 12 cm field size at a depth of 3.5 cm is 0.996.

Table 2.2A.1

Depth (cm)	4 × 4 cm	8 × 8 cm	12 × 12 cm
1.0	0.854	0.874	0.888
3.0	1.000	1.000	1.000
4.0	0.992	0.993	0.993
6.0	0.930	0.937	0.941

This is a simple linear interpolation problem. Just use the values in red chosen to match the correct field size, add them, and divide by two. This can be done because 3.5 is halfway between 3.0 and 4.0 cm.
(1.000 + 0.993)/2 = 0.996

5. **B** The scatter-maximum ratio to be used in a patient with a 10 MV photon beam, 8 × 8 cm field size at a depth of 10.6 cm is 0.076.

Table 2.2A.2

Depth (cm)	4 × 4 cm	8 × 8 cm	12 × 12 cm
6.0	0.048	0.056	0.060
10.0	0.055	0.074	0.085
12.0	0.0.56	0.080	0.094
16.0	0.055	0.086	0.106

Because 10.6 cm is not halfway between 10 and 12, this linear interpolation problem must be treated differently.
First, find the difference between the depths 10 and 10.6 and 12 and 10.6 cm:
10.6 − 10 = 0.6 cm
12 − 10 = 2 cm
Now divide both:

0.6/2 = 0.30
Second, do the same for the SMR and find the difference between 0.080 and 0.074:
0.080 − 0.074 = 0.006
Now multiply 0.006 by 0.30:
0.006 × 0.30 = 0.0018
Then, add this value to the lower SMR:
0.0018 + 0.074 = 0.076
If you prefer to memorize an equation for linear interpolation, the following can be used. In this case, you know the three depths; we will call the x_1, x_2, and x_3. x_2 is the depth of 10.6 cm. We also know the SMRs which we can call y_1, y_2, and y_3. Here, we do not know y_2. To solve for y_2, use the following equation:
$y_2 = (((x_2−x_1) \times (y_3−y_1))/(x_3−x_1)) + y_1$

6. **D** The PDD to be used is 42.4 %.

Table 2.2A.3

Depth (cm)	6×6 cm	8×8 cm	10×10 cm
1.0	89.0	90.0	91.0
20.0	43.9	45.0	45.9
22.0	39.8	41.0	41.9
30	26.9	28	28.9

This is a dual problem where you have to interpolate two times as 21 falls between 20 and 22 and the field size of 7×7 falls between the 6 and 8 cm field sizes. Luckily in this case, each parameter is halfway between the known parameters so a simple average can be used for both values.
First, find the PDD at 21 cm for the 6×6 cm² field:
(43.9 + 39.8)/2 = 41.8 %
Second, find the PDD at 21 cm for the 8×8 cm² field:
(45 + 41)/2 = 43 %
Finally, average both PDDs to interpolate between 6 and 8 cm fields:
(41.8 + 43)/2 = 42.4 %

7. **A** It is very common to use the MLC or a block on a conformal field to protect critical structures. The following diagram shows a brain field blocking the eyes, face, mouth and jaw while treating a whole brain to cervical vertebrae C2. To determine the amount of scatter, the effective equivalent square needs to be known. This is a two-in-one problem where the student faces a rectangle and a triangle. In this case, the Eff Eq² is 14.9 cm².

Fig. 2.2A.11

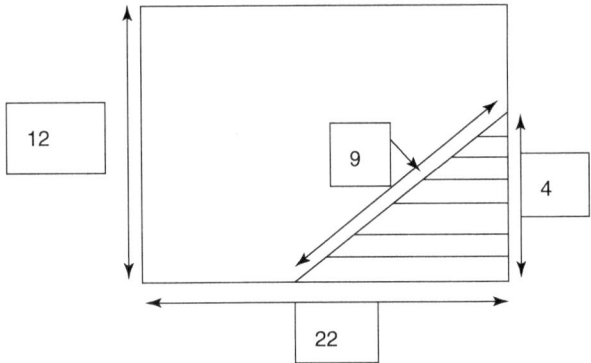

First, find the equivalent square of the open collimator 12×22 cm:
Formula for equivalent square = 4 A/P (A is area and P is perimeter)
Formula for equivalent square = $2 \times L \times W / L + W$
$Eq^2 = 2 \times 22 \times 12/22 + 12$ cm
$Eq^2 = 15.5$ cm²
Second, find the area of the triangle or blocked area:
Triangle area = ½ × b × h (b is base length and h is the vertical height)
Block area = ½ × b × h
Block area = ½ × 9 × 4 cm
Block area = 18 cm²
Third, find the square root of the open field Eq^2 minus the blocked area:
Eff $Eq^2 = \sqrt{(15.5 \times 15.5) - 18}$
Eff $Eq^2 = 14.9$ cm²

8. B The following field is blocking the femoral heads and femur while treating a L2 spine and pelvic area. To determine the amount of scatter, the effective equivalent square needs to be known. As before, this is a two-in-one

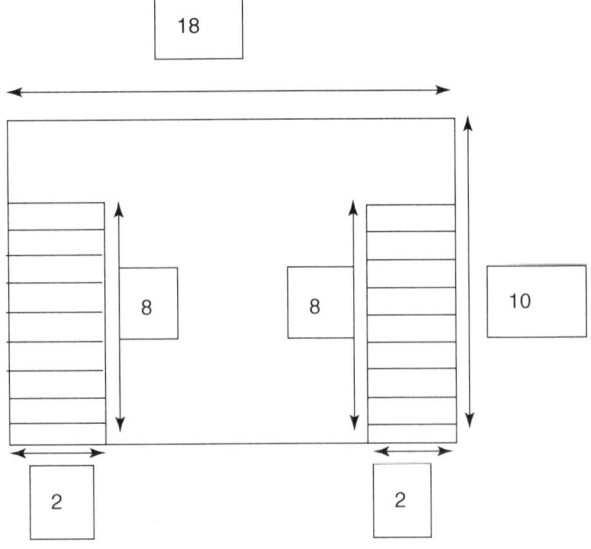

Fig. 2.2A.11

2.9 Applied Mathematics (Answers)

problem where the student has the field (big rectangle) and two smaller blocked rectangles on each side. In this case, the Eff Eq² is 11.54 cm².
First, find the equivalent square of the open collimator 10×18 cm:
Eq² = 4 A/P (A is area and P is perimeter)
Eq² = 2×L×W/L+W
Eq² = 2×10×18/10+18
Eq² = 12.85 cm²
Second, find the area of both small rectangles or block area:
Area of rectangle = W×h (W is the width and h the height)
Area of rectangle = W×h
Area of rectangle = 2×8
Area of rectangle = 16 cm
Because both rectangles are similar, multiply the area by 2:
Total Block area = 16×2 = 32 cm²
Third, find the square root of the open field Eq² minus the block area:
Eff Eq² = √(12.85×12.85) − 32
Eff Eq² = 11.54 cm²

9. C This is a three-in-one problem where the student has a rectangular field with a block, similar to before, but here, the block is not a simple triangle or rectangle. Here, a combination of a square and triangle is used. Remember this problem because for many situations, complex shapes are just made up of a bunch of simple shapes. Draw some lines to break up the complex shape into simple shapes and calculate the areas. In this case, the Eff Eq² is 22.96 cm².

Fig. 2.2A.14

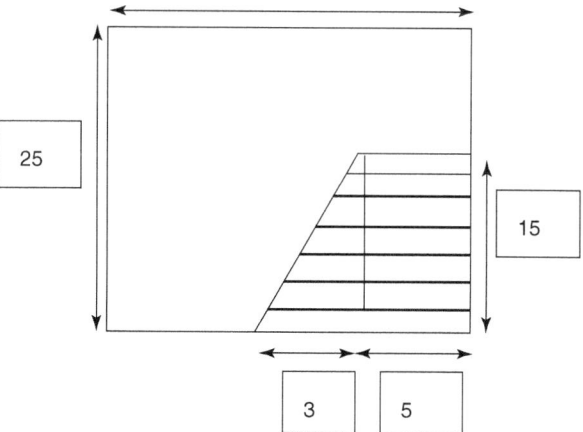

First, find the equivalent square of the open collimator 25×25 cm².
Since the open field is a square:
Eq² = 25 cm²
Second, find the area of the triangle or block 1 area:
Triangle formula = ½×b×h (b is base and h is the vertical height)
Block 1 area = ½×b×h
Block 1 area = ½×3×15 cm

Triangle block 1 area = 22.5 cm²
Third, find the area of the rectangle or block 2 areas:
Area of rectangle = $W \times h$ (W is the width and h is the height)
Area of rectangle = $W \times h$
Area of rectangle = 5×15 cm
Area of rectangle = 75 cm²
Add both triangle and rectangle areas to calculate total block area:
Total block area = 22.5 + 75 cm = 97.5 cm²
Finally, find the square root of the open field Eq² minus the block area:
Eff Eq² = $\sqrt{(25 \times 25) - 97.5}$
Eff Eq² = 22.96 cm²

10. **B** The following field is blocking the femoral heads. In this case, the Eff Eq² is 17.72 cm².

Fig. 2.2A.15

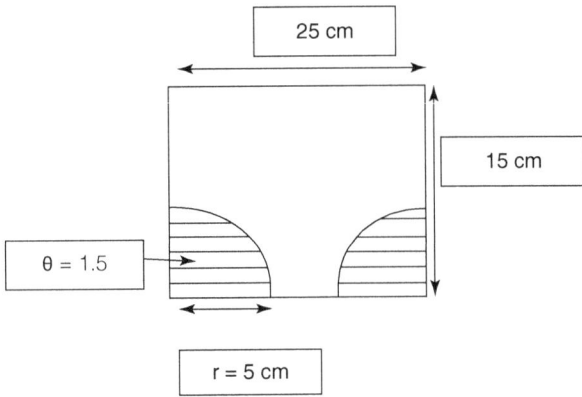

First, find the equivalent square of the open collimator 25×15 cm:
Eq² = 4 A/P (A is area and P is perimeter)
Eq² = $2 \times L \times W/L + W$
Eq² = $2 \times 25 \times 15/25 + 15$ cm
Eq² = 18.75 cm²
Second, find the area of both small block sectors:
Area of sector = ½ $r^2\theta$ (r is the radius and θ is the angle of radians)
Area of sector = ½ $5^2 \times 1.5$
Area of sector = 18.75 cm²
Because both sectors are similar, multiply the area by 2:
Block area = $18.75 \times 2 = 37.5$ cm²
Third, find the square root of the open field Eq² minus the block area:
Eff Eq² = $\sqrt{(18.75 \times 18.75) - 37.5}$ cm
Eff Eq² = 17.72 cm²
If you did not remember the area of a sector formula, you could approximate each block as a quarter of a circle. Remember that the area of a circle is $\pi \times r^2$. Here, the area would be about 78.5 cm². One quarter of this is

2.9 Applied Mathematics (Answers)

19.62 cm² which is close to our calculated value of 18.75 cm². On an exam, this would probably get you close enough to the correct answer.

11. C When the intensity of the beam or dose rate needs to be calculated because of a change in distance or vice versa, the inverse square law must be used. The inverse square law states that as the distance from the source increases, the intensity decreases by the distance squared. The percentage change in dose rate if the distance is increased from 100 to 120 cm is:

Inverse square formula:
$I_1/I_2 = [D_2/D_1]^2$
$1/X = [120/100]^2$
$1/X = 14,400/10,000$
$X = 10,000 \times 1/14,400$
New dose rate $= 0.6944 = 69.44\,\%$ of the original

After an inverse square question is answered, the student must quickly verify the answer by knowing that if distance increased, the dose rate or intensity must have decreased. In this question, the distance increased from 100 to 120 cm so the answer must be less than 100 %, which 69.44 %.

12. B This question involves both the inverse square law and geometry. The new dose if plan is not modified will be 1,775 cGy and the new field size is 52×13 cm.

Be organized and collect the data:
Distance 1 = 100 cm
Distance 2 = 130 cm
Dose 1 = 3,000 cGy
Dose 2 = ?
Field size (FS) 1 = 40×10 cm
Field size (FS) 2 = ?

Inverse square formula	Similar triangle geometry
$I_1/I_2 = [D_2/D_1]^2$	$FS_1/FS_2 = D_1/D_2$
$3,000/X = [130/100]^2$	$40/X = 100/130$ (ratio of side lengths)
$3,000/X = 16,900/10,000$	$X = 130 \times 40/100$
$X = 10,000/3,000 \times 16,900$	$X = 52$ cm
$X = 1,775$ cGy	$FS_1/FS_2 = D_1/D_2$
	$10/X = 100/130$
	$X = 130 \times 10/100$
	$X = 13$ cm

Remember, if the distance increases, the dose rate, output factor, and beam intensity will decrease, but the field size will increase.

13. D Since attenuation is not accounted for, this question only involves the inverse square law. Be organized and collect the data:
$I_1 = 300$ cGy
$I_2 = X$

$D_1 = 120$ cm SSD
$D_2 =$ if the patient's thickness is 50 cm, ½ of 50 cm is 25 cm.
25 cm + 120 cm = 145 cm
Inverse square formula:
$I_1/I_2 = [D_2/D_1]^2$
$300/X = [145/120]^2$
$1/X = 21,025/14,400$
$X = 14,400 \times 300/21,025$
Daily dose at 145 cm = 205.46 cm (without attenuation)

14. B This question involves inverse square law. Be organized and collect the data:
$I_1 = 120$ cGy
$I_2 = 50$ cGy
$D_1 = 75$ cm
$D_2 = X$
Inverse square formula:
$I_1/I_2 = [D_2/D_1]^2$
$120/50 = [X/75]^2$
$120/50 = X^2/5,625$
$X^2 = 120 \times 5,625/50$
$X^2 = 13,500$
$X = \sqrt{13,500}$
Distance $_2 = 116$ cm
Again, if the dose decreased from 120 to 50 cGy, the distance must have increased.

15. A This question involves inverse square law and a direct proportionality. Be organized and collect the data:
$Dose_2 = X$
$Distance_2 = 50$ cm
$Time_2 = 45$ s
$Dose_1 = 100$ cGy
$Distance_1 = 80$ cm
$Time_1 = 2$ min $= 120$ s
Inverse square formula:

$I_1/I_2 = [D_2/D_1]^2$	120 s – 39 cGy
$100/X = [80/50]^2$	45 s – X
$100/X = 6,400/2,500$	$X = 45 \times 39/120$
$X = 2,500 \times 100/6,400$	$X = 14.6$ cGy
$X = 39$ cGy	

You could also convert to a dose rate of 50 cGy per minute at 80 cm and then use the inverse square law to calculate the new dose rate at 50 cm. This dose rate would be higher. Using this new dose rate, you could multiply by the time of 45 s.

2.10 External Beam Calculations (Answers)

16. C The equivalent field sizes of the following fields are:
18×2=4×4
20×6=9×9
30×14=18×18
30×12=16×16
The larger the field size, the larger the TMR.

17. B Remember, the cranial field collimator angle depends on the divergence of the upper PA spine field. The only two pieces of information needed are the upper spine field length and SSD. Be organized and collect the necessary data:
Cranial field collimator angle=?
PA upper spine field=40 cm long at 100 cm SSD
Opposite side=½ of PA upper spine length=40/2=20 cm
Adjacent side=PA spine SSD=100 cm
Based on trigonometric functions (SOH-CAH-TOA):
Tan (θ_{coll})=opposite/adjacent or arc tan $(1/2\ L_1 \times 1/SSD)$
Tan (θ_{coll})=20/100
Tan (θ_{coll})=0.20
Tan^{-1} (θ_{coll})=11.3°

2.10 External Beam Calculations (Answers)

Quiz 1 (Level 2)

1. B MU=dose/(output at Dmax×PDD/100)
MU=250/(0.972×85/100)
MU=302.6

2. C The rule of thumb states that electrons treat to a depth in cm of approximately energy (MeV)/3 to energy (MeV)/4. The reason for this will be explained in the following questions.

3. B The practical range of an electron is defined as the extrapolation of the descending part of an electron PDD curve. The rule of thumb states that the practical range of an electron is energy (MeV)/2 or around 2 MeV/cm. The 2 MeV/cm is the average energy lost by an electron as it travels through the tissue. The dose received by the tumor is independent of the practical range, so for a 12 MeV electron the practical range is 6 cm. The practical range is useful to know where the electrons will stop depositing dose.

4. D The rule of thumb states that the therapeutic range (or 90 % IDL) of an electron is around energy (MeV)/3. The dose received by the tumor is independent to this range, so for a 16 MeV electron the therapeutic range (or 90 % IDL) is about 5 cm.

5. **C** The rule of thumb states that the 50 % IDL of an electron is approximately energy (MeV)/2.33. Again, the dose received by the tumor is independent of this range, so for a 12 MeV electron the 50 % IDL is around 5.15 cm depth.

6. **D** Remember that the rule of thumb states that the 50 % IDL of an electron is energy (MeV)/2.33. Therefore, a beam with the 50 % IDL at a depth of 7 cm depth is around 16 MeV since $7 \times 2.33 = 16.3$ MeV.

7. **C** In the United States, the calibration laboratories (National Institute of Standards and Technology (NIST) and Accredited Dose Calibration Laboratories (ADCLs)) provide chamber calibration factors for standard environmental conditions of temperature $T_0 = 22$ °C and pressure $P_0 = 760$ mmHg. The formula used to correct for nonstandard temperature and pressure conditions ($C_{t,p}$) is
$C_{T,P} = (760/P)(273.2 + T/273.2 + 22)$.
Entering our values:
$C_{T,P} = (760/772)(273.2 + 21/273.2 + 22)$
$C_{T,P} = (0.984)(294.2/295.2)$
$C_{T,P} = 0.980$

8. **A** Most ion chambers are unsealed, so the density of air in the chamber volume (V) depends on the atmospheric conditions due to the ideal gas law (PV = nRT). If the temperature of the room decreases and/or the pressure increases, the volume of air in the chamber will decrease, and the chamber reading will decrease.

9. **A** MU = dose/fx/(output × (PDD/100))
MU = 250 cGy/(1.07 × (90/100))
MU = 260

2.11 Effects of Beam-Modifying Devices (Answers)

Quiz 1 (Level 2)

1. **C** The formula to calculate HVL is:
HVL = 0.693/μ
HVL = 0.693/0.35
HVL = 1.98 mm

2. **A** HVL is the thickness of a given material needed to reduce the intensity of a photon beam to 50 % of its initial value or the thickness required for a particular material to cut the beam's intensity in half. So this question is asking about HVL of copper.
The formula to calculate HVL is:
HVL = 0.693/μ
HVL = 0.693/0.40
HVL = 1.73 mm

2.11 Effects of Beam-Modifying Devices (Answers)

3. B Linear attenuation coefficient (μ) represents the probability per unit thickness of a material that any one photon will be attenuated.
The formula to calculate μ is:
μ = 0.693/HVL
μ = 0.693/1.5 mm
μ = 0.46 mm^{-1}

4. D The ratio of the initial beam intensity to the intensity of the beam after passing through the material is called the transmission. So if a lead block measuring 2.5 cm thickness with a HVL of 10 mm is inserted in the beam path, then the transmission factor is 0.062 %. The SAD is not taken in consideration since the transmission is a factor of intensity and thickness of the material and not distance dependent.
To solve the problem, we need to determine how many HVLs of material are present. If the block measures 2.5 cm and the HVL is 10 mm:
2.5 cm = 25 mm
25 mm/10 mm = 2.5 HVLs
Transmission = $(0.5)^{2.5}$
Transmission = 0.177 = 17.7 %
This means that about 82 % of the beam was attenuated in the material. This value also makes sense because 2 HVLs will reduce the beam to 25 % of the original and 3 HVLs will reduce the beam to 12.5 %. Therefore, 2.5 HVLs will reduce the beam somewhere in between these values.

5. A If a beam has a HVL of 2.5 mm tin (Sn), the approximate percentage of the radiation beam transmitted through a 15 mm tin (Sn) will be around 1.56 %. Remember, each HVL will decrease the intensity by a factor of ½ or 50 %, so
15 mm Sn/2.5 mm Sn = 6 HVL
$(0.5)^6$ = 0.01563 × 100% = 1.56 %

6. D The first HVL will decrease the intensity by 50 %, so if the intensity with no filter was 30 R/min, then it would be 15 R/min after 1 HVL. Following a second HVL, the reading would be ½ of 15, which is 7.5 R/min.

7. A The ratio of the first to the second HVL is sometimes used as a second method of describing x-ray beams. Hence, a beam may be characterized by the combination of its first HVL and also the ratio of the first to the second HVL. This is called the homogeneity coefficient (HC).
Homogeneity coefficient formula:
HC = 1st HVL/2nd HVL
HC = 0.40/0.86
HC = 0.465

8. B A wedge is a device made of high Z materials (brass, lead, or steel) that has the general shape of an inclined plane so that the isodose curve can be tilted at specific depths. The quality of the beam or output is decreased when a wedge is inserted in the beam path due to attenuation. When calculations

are done, this attenuation due to wedge placement must be taken into account. The ratio of doses with and without wedge at a point in phantom along the central axis of the beam is called the wedge transmission factor or the wedge factor.
Wedge factor formula:
WF = dose with wedge/dose without wedge
WF = 0.350/0.700
WF = 0.500

9. **A** The wedge transmission factor or the wedge factor is the ratio of doses with and without wedge at a point in phantom along the central axis of the beam. This means that the wedge factor represents the amount of attenuation of the wedge in the beam. If the wedge factor is 0.624, then 62.4 % of the beam was attenuated and 37.6 % was transmitted.

10. **B** If there is a 65 % transmission of the beam with a wedge in place, that means that 35 % of the beam is attenuated by the wedge. Therefore, the wedge factor is 0.350.

11. **C** Hinge angle is the angle between the central rays of the two beams.

Fig. 2A.4.1

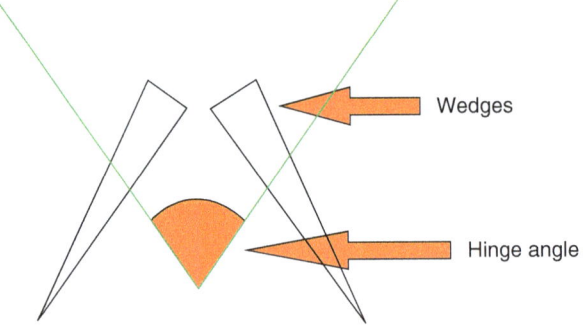

Hinge angle formula:
Hinge angle = 180° − (2 × wedge angle)
Hinge angle = 180° − (2 × 45°)
Hinge angle = 180° − 90°
Hinge angle = 90°
In order to get the most homogeneous plan, if 45° wedges are used, then a 90° hinge angle should be used, meaning the beams should be orthogonal to each other.

12. **C** The angle to which a specific isodose line is bent is also the name of the wedge and is called the wedge angle.
Wedge angle formula:
Wedge angle = 90° − (0.5 × hinge angle)
Wedge angle = 90° − (0.5 × 120°)

2.11 Effects of Beam-Modifying Devices (Answers)

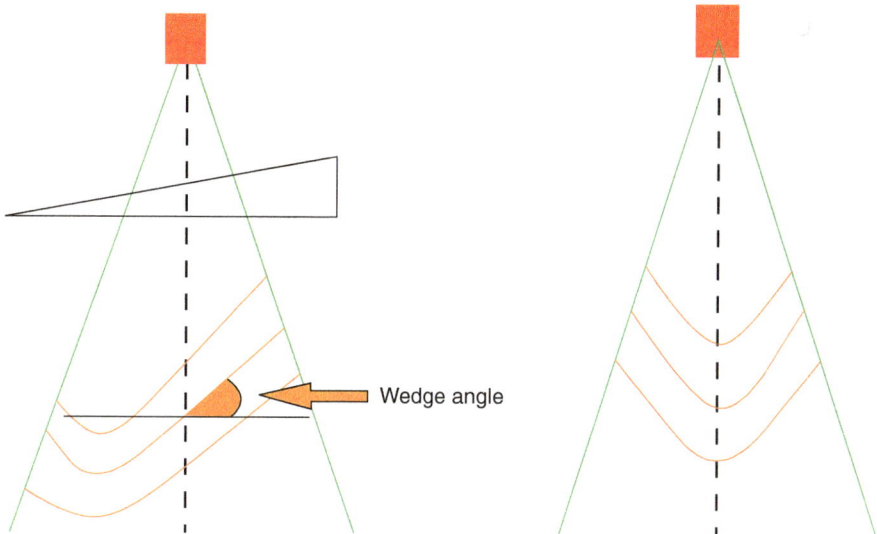

Fig. 2A.4.2

Wedge angle = 90° − 60°
Wedge angle = 30°
In order to get the most homogeneous plan, if 120° hinge angle is used, then a 30° wedge angle should be used.
Another substitute wedge angle formula is:
Wedge angle = 90° − (hinge angle/2)

13. D If two oblique fields were planned at 150° apart (hinge angle is 150°), then the wedge angle is:
Wedge angle formula:
Wedge angle = 90° − (0.5 × hinge angle)
Wedge angle = 90° − (0.5 × 150°)
Wedge angle = 90° − 75°
Wedge angle = 15°

14. C Based on the diagram, the hinge angle is about 90 + 30 = 120. The wedge angle is:
Wedge angle formula:
Wedge angle = 90° − (0.5 × hinge angle)
Wedge angle = 90° − (0.5 × 120°)
Wedge angle = 90° − 60°
Wedge angle = 30°

15. A MU = field without wedge MU/wedge factor
MU = 300/0.640
MU = 469 MU
Remember that the MUs must be higher with the wedge because something is placed in the beam path which attenuates the beam and decreases the dose.

16. **A** A MLC is designed with a tongue and groove to reduce interleaf leakages between adjacent leaves in MLC. The diagram below shows a cut away view of a typical MLC and the arrows indicate the direction of the beam. To correct for divergence, most leaves have a rounded tip which provides a uniform penumbra across the entire field. The flattening filter used in the machine is a device that changes the pencil beam into a broad, clinically useful beam. A flattening filter is thicker at the center and commonly made of lead, steel, copper, brass, or similar materials. Finally, a wedge is a compensator used to distort the isodose distribution by tilting it through a specific angle.

Fig. 2A.4.3

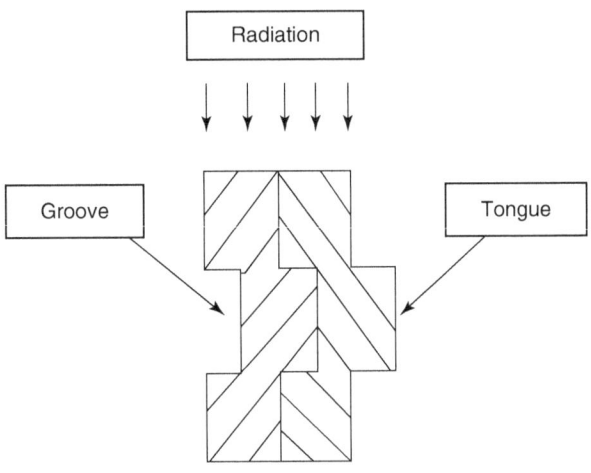

2.12 Irregular Field Calculations (Answers)

Quiz 1 (Level 2)

1. **B** Remember that dose rate for a given energy and field size varies inversely with the square of the distance from the source.
   This problem is solved using inverse square law formula:
   Inverse square formula:
   $I_1/I_2 = [D_2/D_1]^2$
   120 cGy/min/I_2 = [100 cm SAD/80 cm SAD]^2
   120/I_2 = 10,000/6,400
   I_2 = 120×6,400/10,000
   I_2 = 76.8 cGy/min

2. **C** The ratio between Dmax dose and dose at specific depth is defined as PDD. If the distance is changed, then the PDD will change (distance increased, PDD increased). Whenever there is a change in distance and

a new PDD needs to be calculated, the Mayneord F Factor formula can be used to determine the new PDD. As you can see the Dmax is not given, but the energy is, so you must know the approximate Dmax of each energy. Co-60 = 0.5 cm, 4 MV = 1 cm, 6 MV = 1.5 cm, 10 MV = 2.5 cm, 15 MV = 3 cm, 20 MV = 3.5 cm, 25 MV = 4 cm, 34 MV = 5 cm.
Collect all the data:
Dmax of 6 MV = 1.5 cm
$SSD_1 = 100$ cm
Depth = 4.5 cm
$PDD_1 = 65\%$
$SSD_2 = 110$ cm
$PDD_2 = ?$
Mayneord F factor formula:
$F = [(SSD_2 + Dmax/SSD_1 + Dmax) \times (SSD_1 + d/SSD_2 + d)]^2$
$F = [(110 + 1.5/100 + 1.5) \times (100 + 4.5/110 + 4.5)]^2$
$F = [(111.5/101.5) \times (104.5/114.5)]^2$
$F = [(1.098) \times (0.912)]^2$
$F = 1.001^2$
$F = 1.002$
New PDD = 0.650×1.002
New PDD = 0.651 or 65.1 %
Important to remember: as energy increases, PDD increases; as depth increases, PPD decreases; as field size increases, PDD increases; and as SSD increases, PDD increases.

3. A Remember that the ratio of the dose at a point at depth in a phantom or patient including backscatter to the dose at the same point in air without backscatter is the backscatter factor (BSF) and is defined as:
BSF = dose at phantom (Dmax of depth)/dose in air at same depth
BSF = 150 cGy/100 cGy
BSF = 1.50
Also remember that the BSF is a special case of TAR where the depth is Dmax.

4. B When calculating output or dose rate and dose and MU are given, the dose rate formula must be used:
Dose rate = dose/MU
Dose rate = 300 cGy/375 MU
Dose rate = 0.800 cGy/MU

5. D When calculating output or dose rate and dose and MU or time is given, the dose rate formula must be used:
Dose rate = Dose/time
Dose rate = 400 cGy/3 min
Dose rate = 133 cGy/min

6. **A** When the output at new distance needs to be calculated, the inverse square formula is used. Remember that 6 MV Dmax is 1.5 cm, so this needs to be added to both SSDs.
Inverse square formula:
$I_1/I_2 = [D_2/D_1]^2$
$1.20/X = [121.5/101.5]^2$
$1.20/X = 14,762/10,302$
$X = 0.837$ cGy/mu

7. **C** Dose rate = dose/MU, so MU = dose/dose rate, but this is if 100 % isodose line is selected. The question stays that the physician selected the 84 % IDL, so the output factor must be adjusted to the selected IDL:
MU = dose/(dose rate × IDL)
MU = 180 cGy/(0.970 × 0.84)
MU = 221

8. **A** Be organized, and collect the data:
75 % IDL = ?
Prescription dose = 50 Gy to 100 % IDL
75/100 × 50 = 37.5 Gy
Be careful with the units on this question. The answers are in cGy, but the question was in units of Gy.

9. **D** The question simple states that the plan is hot by 111 % and the result is 277.5 cGy; remember that the prescription dose must be smaller than 277.5 by 1.11 so
277.5 cGy/1.11 = 250 cGy
Or (100/111) × 277.5 cGy = 250 cGy
So, 111 % of 250 cGy is 277.5 cGy

10. **C** First, since the dose and MU are given, the output can be found:
Output at 100 cm SSD = dose/MU
Output at 100 cm SSD = 180 cGy/195 MU
Output at 100 cm SSD = 0.923 cGy/MU
Second, find the output at 120 cm SSD using inverse square law formula:
$I_1/I_2 = (D_2/D_1)^2$
$0.923/I_2 = (120/100)^2$
$0.923/I_2 = (14,400/10,000)$
$I_2 = 10,000 \times 0.923/14,400$
$I_2 = 0.641$ cGy/MU
Output at 120 SSD = 0.641 cGy/MU
Finally, the MU needed to give 180 cGy at 120 cm SSD can be found using the output at 120 SSD:
180 cGy/0.641 cGy/MU = 281 MU

2.12 Irregular Field Calculations (Answers)

11. C Before starting any problem, carefully analyze the question. As you can see, you are asked to find a new distance using a prior PDD. PDD with a new distance can be solved using the Mayneord F factor formula. As the distance increased, be aware that your answer must also increase because as distance increases, PDD increases.
Collect all the data:
Dmax of 10 $X = 2.5$ cm
$SSD_1 = 100$ cm
Depth $= 9$ cm
$PDD_1 = 78$ %
$SSD_2 = 115$ cm
$PDD_2 = ?$
Mayneord F factor formula:
$F = [(SSD_2 + Dmax/SSD_1 + Dmax) \times (SSD_1 + d/SSD_2 + d)]^2$
$F = [(115 + 2.5/100 + 2.5) \times (100 + 9/115 + 9)]^2$
$F = [(117.5/102.5) \times (109/124)]^2$
$F = [(1.146) \times (0.879)]^2$
$F = 1.007^2$
$F = 1.014$
New PDD $= 0.780 \times 1.014$
New PDD $= 0.791$ or 79.1 %
Important: as energy increases, PDD increases; as depth increases, PPD decreases; as field size increases, PDD increases; and as SSD increases, PDD increases.

12. A This is a simple question. Remember that Dmax = dose/prescription isodose line, so:
Dmax $= 250$ cGy/0.85
Dmax $= 294$ cGy

13. B Remember the MU formula, and include all the factors where the output is (denominator):
MU = dose/output
MU $= 150$ cGy/(0.85 × 1 cGy)
MU $= 176$

14. A Since the MU given was only 105 MU and the output is 0.875 cGy/MU, then the delivered dose can be calculated:
Dose = MU given × output
Dose $= 105$ MU × 0.875 cGy/MU
Dose delivered $= 91.8$ cGy
Not included in the question, but we can also calculate the original dose the patient was supposed to receive:
Dose = MU × output

Dose = 195 MU × 0.875 cGy/MU
Dose = 171 cGy
Now that both doses are known, we can also calculate the dose not delivered:
Dose not delivered = 171 cGy − 91.8 cGy
Dose not delivered = 79.2 cGy
The patient can have a treatment completion of 79.2 cGy so that the whole dose is delivered.

15. **C** Collect the data:
Rx dose = 250 cGy to midplane
Patient separation = 20 cm/2 = 10 cm depth
FSF 20 × 20 cm = 1.07
Dose rate = 115 cGy/min
PDD at 10 cm = 0.556
Remember the MU (or time) formula. The goal of this formula is to take the calibrated, known dose rate for the standard field size, SSD, etc. and convert it to the current treatment parameters. The dose always goes in the numerator, and the output and all conversion factors go in the denominator.
Time = dose/(dose rate (or output) × FSF × PDD)
Time = 125 cGy per field/(115 cGy/min × 1.07 × 0.556)
Time = 1.82 min
Time = 1 min 49 s
Remember that the 1.07 is to convert the standard output to the current field size. Also be careful to change the dose from 250 to 125 cGy per field since the field arrangement is AP/PA and half the dose will be delivered from each since they are equally weighted.

16. **D** Again the formula for MU must be used:
MU = dose/average TMR
MU = 180 cGy/0.570
MU = 316 MU
Remember that PDD is used for SSD calculations and TMR is used for SAD calculations. Because this is an arc, we can assume that an isocentric technique is being used.

17. **B** If the MU is known as well as the number of degrees of rotation, just divide the MU by the total degrees in the arc. All other information is extraneous in this problem.
MU/degree = MU/degrees in the arc
MU/degree = 351 MU/300°
MU/degree = 1.17 MU per each degree

18. **A** Remember the MU formula, and include all the correct factors in the denominator:
MU = dose at depth/(output at Dmax and correct SSD × (PDD/100))
MU = 250 cGy/1.034 × 84.5/100
MU = 286

2.12 Irregular Field Calculations (Answers)

19. B Collect all data before starting the calculation. The question asked to calculate dose at depth 7 cm when the prescription dose was to a depth of 5 cm. If PDDs at both depths are given, just find the ratio and multiply by the Rx dose:
Dose at 7 cm = PDD at 7 cm/PDD at 5 cm × prescription dose
Dose at 7 cm = 0.845/0.923 × 180 cGy
Dose at 7 cm = 165 cGy
Finally, analyze the answer. Dose at 7 cm should be less than dose at 5 cm. The max dose will be at Dmax at 2.5 cm, and this dose can be calculated in the same manner.

20. A For a single field, the maximum dose is always the dose at Dmax, in this case at 2.5 cm because we are using 10 MV. Now we have the PDD at a depth of 6 cm, and by finding the ratio of the PDD at 2.5 cm depth to the PDD at 6 cm depth and multiplying by the prescription dose, we can calculate the max dose:
Max dose = (PDD at 2.5 cm/PDD at 6 cm) × prescription dose
Max dose = (1.000/0.881) × 300 cGy
Max dose = 341 cGy

21. A In order to find the percentage change in PDD when the SSD is changed, the Mayneord F factor formula must be used:
Mayneord F factor formula:
$F = [(SSD_2 + Dmax/SSD_1 + Dmax) \times (SSD_1 + d/SSD_2 + d)]^2$
$F = [(120 + 2.5/110 + 2.5)^2 \times (110 + 15/120 + 15)]^2$
$F = [(122.5/112.5)^2 \times (125/135)]^2$
New PDD = Old PDD × 1.016
New PDD = 1.000 × 1.016
New PDD = 1.016 or 101.6 %
Important: as energy increases, PDD increases; as depth increases, PPD decreases; as field size increases, PDD increases; and as SSD increases, PDD increases.

22. B MU = Rx dose/(output × WF × TMR × FSF)
MU = 60 cGy/(0.950 cGy/MU × 0.730 × 0.753 × 1.036)
MU = 111 MU per field × 3 fields
MU = 333 MU
The tricky part about this question is that the prescription dose is given per field so you need to multiply by the number of fields. Sometimes, the total dose will be given and you must calculate the MU per field.

23. D Electrons deliver higher skin dose than photons due to the fact that photons are indirectly ionizing radiation so the electron created at the surface have kinetic energy and tend to deposit dose downstream. Electrons are directly ionizing and therefore deposit dose right at the surface. The higher the electron energy, the higher the skin dose. The opposite is true for photons. The higher the energy, the lower the surface dose.

24. **C** In water or tissue, electrons lose energy at approximately 2 MeV per cm traveled. In lead, this can be approximated as 2 MeV per mm traveled. Therefore, a 6 MeV electron will be stopped by approximately 3 cm of water or 3 mm of lead.

25. **A** MU = dose at depth/(output at Dmax and correct SAD × TMR)
MU = 150 cGy/(1.094 cGy/MU × 0.904)
MU = 152
Remember that SSD treatments use PDD and SAD treatments use TMR.

26. **D** MU = dose per beam/(output × TMR)
MU = 125 cGy/(1.023 cGy/MU × 0.731)
MU = 167
Remember that PDD is only used for SSD setups and should not be included for SAD setups. Secondly, watch out for the BSF. The BSF can be used for SAD calculations but only if TARs are given. If TMRs are given, use the TMR only. TMR = TAR/BSF so they are interchangeable, but using TMR makes for an easier calculation. Also, the question asks for the per beam MU although the total dose for both fields is given. Be careful!

27. **C** For most opposed beams, the dose can be delivered with equal beam weights, especially if the prescription point is midplane. Sometimes adjustments to dose distributions are needed and can be accomplished by assigning different weightings to the beams. An example might be a spinal treatment where more weight from the PA beam can optimize the dose distribution. The correct fractional contribution for a RT and LT lateral field arrangement is found by RT Lat contribution = RT weighting/(RT weighting + LT weighting); LT Lat contribution = LT weighting/(LT weighting + RT weighting).

28. **B.** Fractional contribution from AP field:
AP = AP/(AP + PA)
AP = 2/(2 + 1)
AP = 2/3
AP = 0.667
Fractional contribution from PA field:
PA = PA/(AP + PA)
PA = 1/(2 + 1)
PA = 1/3
PA = 0.333

29. **D** Fractional contribution from AP field:
AP = AP/(AP + PA)
AP = 2/(2 + 1)
AP = 2/3
AP = 0.667
AP = 0.667 × 250 cGy
AP = 167 cGy
Fractional contribution from PA field:
PA = PA/(AP + PA)

2.12 Irregular Field Calculations (Answers)

PA = 1/(2+1)
PA = 1/3
PA = 0.333
PA = 0.333 × 250 cGy
PA = 83 cGy
Remember to always check your answer:
AP = 167 cGy + PA = 83 cGy = 250 cGy total

30. B Fractional contribution from RT field:
RT = RT/(RT + LT)
RT = 3/(3+1)
RT = 3/4
RT = 0.750
RT = 0.750 × 180 cGy
RT = 135 cGy
Fractional contribution from LT field:
LT = LT/(RT + LT)
LT = 1/(3+1)
LT = 1/4
LT = 0.250
LT = 0.250 × 180 cGy
LT = 45 cGy
Remember to always check your answer:
RT = 135 cGy + LT = 45 cGy = 180 cGy total

31. C Fractional contribution from PA field:
PA = PA/(PA + RT + LT)
RT = 3/(3+2+1)
RT = 3/6
RT = 0.500
RT = 0.500 × 200 cGy
RT = 100 cGy
Fractional contribution from RT field:
RT = RT/(PA + RT + LT)
RT = 2/(3+2+1)
RT = 2/6
RT = 0.333
RT = 0.333 × 200 cGy
RT = 67 cGy
Fractional contribution from LT field:
LT = LT/(PA + RT + LT)
LT = 1/(3+2+1)
LT = 1/6
LT = 0.166
LT = 0.166 × 200 cGy
LT = 33 cGy
Remember to always check your answer:
PA = 100 cGy, RT = 67 cGy, LT = 33 cGy, total = 200 cGy

2.13 Special Calculations (Answers)

Quiz 1 (Level 2)

1. **B** The student is not always given the off-axis ration (OAR) to be used in a calculation, so if this is the case, the OAR needs to be determined. The OAR factor is defined as the ratio of the dose at any point on a dose profile to the dose at the central ray on that profile and describes the uniformity and symmetry of the beam. The deeper you go in the phantom, the more uniform and symmetric the beam becomes due to increased scatter.
   OAR = PDD at the off-axis point/PDD on the central axis
   OAR = 87.3/93.5
   OAR = 0.933

2. **C** The OAR factor is defined as the ratio of the dose at any point on a dose profile to the dose at the central ray on that.
   It is very important to know the formula so that the correct data can be obtained and the rest discarded.
   OAR = ?
   Depth = 10 cm, because treatment is midplane
   PPD on the tumor = 62.3 %
   PDD at central axis, 10 cm depth, 11×11 cm field size = 73.25. Linear interpolation needs to be done.
   OAR formula:
   OAR = PDD at the off-axis point/PDD on the central axis
   OAR = 73.25/62.3
   OAR = 1.17

3. **B** Penumbra is the region at the edge of a radiation beam, over which the dose rate changes rapidly as a function of distance from the beam axis. It is typically defined as the distance between the 80 and 20 % isodose lines at the edge of the field. The formula is:
   P = penumbra
   S = source size
   SCD or SDD = source-to-collimator or diaphragm distance
   Remember that if depth is not given, use 0 cm.
   P = S (SSD + d − SCD)/SCD
   P = 1.5 (100 + 0 − 75)/75
   P = 1.5 (100−75)/75
   P = 0.50 cm

4. **C** Remember the formula for calculating the penumbra:
   P = penumbra
   S = source size
   SCD or SDD = source-to-collimator or diaphragm distance

2.13 Special Calculations (Answers)

d = depth

It is important to know all your formulas so that the correct information is used and the rest discarded.

P = s (SSD + d − SDD)/SDD
P = 2 (80 + 5 − 52)/52
P = 2 (33)/52
P = 1.27 cm

5. A

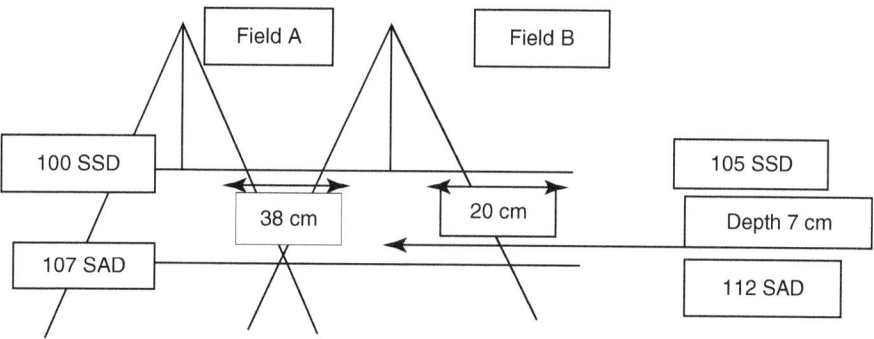

Fig. 2A.6.1

The gap calculation is important because it ensures that the patient is being set up properly on the table. If the gap is incorrect, the match will not be correct, and this could result in a hot or cold spot in the treatment.

The formulas below can all be calculated using ratios formed using similar triangles. Remember that similar triangles are triangles that share two common angles. For radiation therapy, we can break beams down into right triangles, meaning they have a right, or 90° angle. To form a similar triangle, you therefore only need one more common angle. The second common angle can be found by using the vertical angles, which are angles that are opposite each other when two lines cross. Once similar triangles are found, just set up ratios that match the same sides together. If three lengths are known, the fourth can always be calculated with similar triangles.

Gap formula:

Field A gap = ½ $L_1 \times d$/SSD$_1$ Field B gap = ½ $L_2 \times d$/SSD$_2$

Field A gap = 19 × 7/100 cm   Field B gap = 10 × 7/105 cm

Field A gap = 1.33 cm   Field B gap = 0.66 cm

Total separation (gap) on the surface is:
Skin gap = field A gap + field B gap
Skin gap = 1.33 cm + 0.66 cm
Skin gap = 1.99 cm

6. **B** Gap formula:
    Fields A/B = ½ $L_1 \times d/SSD_1$
    Fields A/B = 0.5 × 25 × 10/100
    Fields A/B = 1.25 cm
    Fields B/C = ½ $L_2 \times d/SSD_2$
    Fields B/C = 0.5 × 15 × 10/100
    Fields B/C = 0.75 cm
    Total separation (gap) on the surface is:
    Skin gap = field A/B + field C/D
    Skin gap = 1.25 cm + 0.75 cm
    Skin gap = 2 cm

7. **C** For this exercise, first subtract both gaps to get the maximum length of all the field overlaps (ΔS):
    Field 1 gap = 1.25 cm
    Field 2 gap = 0.75 cm
    Δ fields = fields 1 − field 2
    Δ fields = 1.25 cm − 0.75 cm
    Δ fields = 0.50 cm
    Second, all field overlaps must be zero, so that there is no hot spot at the spine.
    $\Delta S = 0.50$ cm
    d' = depth of the cord from the anterior surface
    d = midline depth
    $\Delta S' = \Delta S \times (d' - d)/d$
    $\Delta S' = 0.5 \times (35 - 10)/10$
    $\Delta S' = 1.25$ cm
    New gap required = field 1 gap + field 2 gap + $\Delta S'$
    New gap required = 1.25 cm + 0.75 cm + 1.25 cm
    New gap required = 3.25 cm

8. **D**

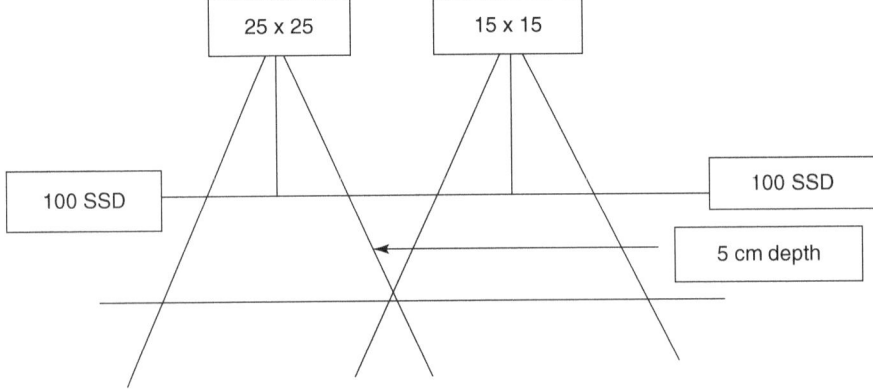

Fig. 2A.6.2

2.13 Special Calculations (Answers)

Gap formula:

Field A = ½ $L_1 \times d$/SSD$_1$ Field B = ½ $L_2 \times d$/SSD$_2$

Field A = 12.5 × 5/100   Field B = 7.5 × 5/100

Field A = 0.63 cm   Field A = 0.38 cm

Total separation (gap) on the surface is:
Skin gap = field A + field B
Skin gap = 0.63 cm + 0.38 cm
Skin gap = 1.01 cm

9. D

10. B The attenuation of a 6 MV is about 3 % per cm in water or tissue, so if the patient lost 4 cm, then there will be approximately 12 % attenuation difference. A 10 MV attenuation is about 2.5 % per cm in water or tissue.
New MU = 12% of 195 = 23
New MU = 195 − 23 = 171

11. C Remember that the maximum dose is delivered at Dmax where the PDD is 100 %. Just take the ratio of the PDD at the prescription depth to the Dmax depth:
Max dose = dose at depth/(PDD at depth/100)
Max dose = 250 cGy/(80.3/100)
Max dose = 311 cGy

12. A MU formula:
MU = (dose/fraction)/(output (SAD) × TMR at iso)
MU = 180 cGy/1.075 cGy/MU × 0.919
MU = 182

13. C To calculate the entrance dose, an inverse square law must be used as well as the ratio between the TMR at Dmax versus at depth. The Dmax dose from the AP beam is found by using the ratio of the TMR at the prescription point and at Dmax. To get the entrance dose, the inverse square law must be used to convert the dose at Dmax to the entrance dose:
Dmax dose = AP field dose × (TMR at 1.5/TMR at 4 cm) × (Dmax to source distance/SSD)^2
Entrance dose = AP field dose × (1.000/0.963) × (97.5/96)^2
Entrance dose = 150 cGy × (1.000/0.963) × (97.5/96)^2
Entrance dose = 150 cGy × 1.038 × 1.03
Entrance dose = 160.4 cGy

14. **D** To calculate the exit dose, an inverse square law must be used as well as the ratio between the exit TMR at Dmax versus at exit depth:
Exit dose = AP field dose × (TMR at 6.5/TMR at 4 cm) × (opposite Dmax to source distance/exit to source distance)^2
Exit dose = AP field dose × (0.919/0.963) × (102.5/104)^2
Exit dose = 150 cGy × (0.954) × (0.986)^2
Exit dose = 150 cGy × 0.954 × 0.971
Exit dose = 138.9 cGy

15. **B** Remember that the global max dose along the central axis is at Dmax. The total Dmax is composed of the entrance dose from one beam at Dmax + the exit dose from the opposite beam; thus, both of these doses must be calculated and then summed. Unlike the previous question, we are not trying to solve the actual entrance and exit dose as we know the global max dose will occur at Dmax. Therefore, we only need to use the ratio of TMRs for both beams to calculate the contribution of each beam to the total dose.
Entrance dose (dose to Dmax from AP beam) = AP field dose × (TMR at 1.5/TMR at 6 cm)
Entrance dose = 150 cGy × (1.000/0.919) entrance dose = 150 cGy × 1.088
Entrance dose = 163.2 cGy
Exit dose (dose to same Dmax point but from the PA beam) = PA field dose × (TMR at 10.5/TMR at 6 cm) Exit dose = 150 cGy × (0.865/0.919)
Exit dose = 150 cGy × 0.941
Exit dose = 141.2 cGy
Total dose at Dmax = 163.2 cGy + 141.2 cGy
Total dose at Dmax = 304.4 cGy

16. **C** If off-axis ratio is ignored, then the TMR ratio must be found and multiplied by the total dose.
Total RT hip dose at midplane = axis dose × (TMR at 4 cm/TMR at 8 cm)
Total RT hip dose at midplane = 3,000 cGy × (0.963/0.865)
Total RT hip dose at midplane = 3,340 cGy

17. **A** TMR is the most commonly used patient attenuation factor, and it is defined as the ratio of the dose at a given point in phantom to the dose at the same point at the reference depth of maximum dose. TMR is based on the assumption that the fractional scatter contribution to the depth dose at a point is independent of the divergence of the beam and depends only on the field size at the point and the depth of the overlying tissue making TMR practically independent of SSD for clinically relevant distances.

18. **B** If the plan is renormalized to 90 % IDL, then 108/90 % = 120 %. The total plan dose was 200 cGy × 25 fractions = 5,000 cGy, and the original plan was 108 % hot. This meant the maximum dose was 5,000 cGy × 1.08 = 5,400 cGy. With the renormalization, the plan now has a maximum dose of 6,000 cGy (5,000 cGy × 1.20), and the isocenter is receiving 5,556 cGy (5,000 cGy/0.9).

2.13 Special Calculations (Answers)

19. C First, linear interpolation must be used so that the correct PDD and output are selected for a 7.5 cm depth and a 25×25 cm field size:
(74.7+92.5)/2=83.6
(92.7+75.7)/2=84.2
(83.6+84.2)/2=83.9
Output at 2 cm, SSD 100 cm for 25×25=(1.070+1.085)/2=1.077

Table 2.A.6.1

Field size	20×20	25×25	30×30
PDD at 5	92.5		92.7
PDD at 7.5	83.6	83.9	84.2
PDD at 10	74.7		75.7

MU=(dose/fx)/(output cGy/MU at SSD×PDD at 7.5 cm/100)
MU=200/(1.077×83.9/100)
MU=221

20. B The maximum tissue dose from a single field is always to dose at Dmax. To calculate this dose, it is the ratio of the dose at Dmax to the dose at depth times the prescribed dose.
Maximum dose=(prescribed dose/fx)×(PDD at Dmax/PDD at 7.5 cm)
Maximum dose=200 (1.000/0.839)
Maximum dose=238.4 cGy
Use linear interpolation to solve for the PDD at 7.5 cm and the correct field size. Remember that the dose at Dmax must be larger than the dose at depth for a single field.

21. D MU=(dose/fx)/[(output in cGy/MU at SAD)×TMR×TF]
MU=100 cGy/1.089 cGy/MU×0.858×0.980
MU=109
Remember that half the dose is delivered from each field.

22. A Interpolation must be used to find the correct PDD at depth 7.5 and 15 cm for a 25×25 cm field size.
The exit dose at a depth of 15 cm is simply the ratio of PDDs at a depth of 15–7.5 cm.
Exit dose at 15 cm=dose×(PDD at depth 15, 25×25/PDD at depth 7.5, 25×25)
Exit dose at 15 cm=200×(61.1/83.9)
Exit dose at 15 cm=145.6 cGy

23. C Remember that total dose at Dmax=right lateral entrance dose at Dmax+left lateral exit dose at the same Dmax point.
Collect all the data:
Depth at midline=10 cm
Depth to Dmax=2 cm (10 MV)

Depth to exit point = 20 cm − 2 cm = 18 cm
Distance to midline = 100 cm
Entrance dose at Dmax = dose at 10 cm from one field × (TMR at Dmax/TMR at 10 cm)
Entrance dose at Dmax = 100 cGy (1.0/0.863)
Entrance dose at Dmax = 100 cGy × 1.1587
Entrance dose at Dmax = 115.9 cGy
Exit dose = dose at 10 cm from one field × (TMR at 18 cm/TMR at 10 cm)
exit dose = 100 cGy (0.695/0.863)
Exit dose = 100 cGy × 0.805
Exit dose = 80.5 cGy
Total dose at Dmax = 115.9 cGy + 80.5 cGy
Total dose at Dmax = 196.4 cGy
Notice that the dose here is actually a little lower than the midplane dose. This is because two fields were used. As more fields are added, you can deliver a higher dose to isocenter and have a lower dose at Dmax. The more beams added, the more conformal the plan. The downside of adding more beams is that the size of the low-dose region increases. This means that the integral dose, or total dose deposited in the patient, might actually increase even though the global maximum dose is lower.

24. C Remember that that PDDs are used for SSD treatment calculations and TMR is used for SAD calculations. Be careful when selecting the parameters to be used:
MU SSD setup = (dose/fx)/(cGy/MU at SSD × TF × PDD/100)
MU SSD setup = 90 cGy/(1.063 cGy/MU × 0.93 × (92.3/100))
MU SSD setup = 99
MU SAD setup = (dose/fx)/(cGy/MU at SAD × TF × TMR)
MU SAD setup = 90/1.072 × 0.93 × 0.968
MU SAD setup = 93
The SAD setup needs fewer MUs as the distance to the prescription point is only 100 cm versus 105 cm for the SSD setup.

25. D The hinge angle is only a distraction here. Remember that the wedge transmission factor is defined as the dose with wedges/dose without wedges, so let us separate and calculate both fields first:
Field 1 dose = 200 cGy/2 = 100 cGy
Since the plan was calculated and delivered using the WF already, the dose from field 1 is unchanged at 100 cGy.
Field 2 = 200 cGy total/2 = 100 cGy
This field was calculated with the wedge, but the treatment was delivered without the wedge so the delivered dose must be higher than planned. If the wedge transmission factor is 0.82, then the dose with wedges = dose open field × WF
Dose with wedges = dose without wedge × 0.82
Dose without wedges = dose with wedge/0.82
Field 2 dose without wedges = 100 cGy/0.82

Field dose without wedges = 122 cGy
Total dose deliver = 100 cGy + 122 cGy
Total dose deliver = 222 cGy
Not only did this patient receive a higher dose than expected, but the removal of the wedge also shifted the isodose lines so the delivered plan did not match the plan calculated and approved in the planning system.

26. A The inverse square law must be used to find the new dose at extended SSD. As the SSD was increased, the dose must decrease.
$I_1/I_2 = (SSD_2/SSD_1)^2$
$250/I_2 = (115/100)^2$
$I_2 = 189$ cGy

27. B Dose to the esophagus = dose (PDD at 5 cm/PDD at 3 cm)
Dose to the esophagus = 180 cGy (85/95)
Dose to the esophagus = 161 cGy

2.14 Manual Corrections for Tissue Inhomogeneity (Answers)

Quiz 1 (Level 2)

1. B 3 cm of lung is equivalent to 1 cm tissue (water). The mass density (g/cm^3) of lung is approximately 0.3 g/cm^3. Bone has a bone mass density between 1.7 and 2.0 g/cm^3, fat has a mass density of 0.92 g/cm^3, and water has a mass density 1.00 g/cm^3.

2. B Tissue inhomogeneities are volumes within the patient that have nonuniform tissue densities playing an important role in planning. The physical depth of the prescription point in the fields is 18 cm, or 6 cm tissue +12 cm of lung. The effective depth is less than that because the density of lung is lower than tissue. Three centimeters of lung is approximately equal to 1 cm of tissue, so the total effective path length is 6 cm of tissue +4 cm of equivalent tissue = 10 cm total. This is 8 cm less than 18 cm, and a 10 MV is attenuated at about 2.5 % per cm. Therefore, if a correction for lung is not used, there will be an overdose of 2.5×8 = 20 %. This means the actual deliver dose would have been 250 cGy × 1.20 = 300 cGy. The physicist created a second plan and reduced the MUs by 20 % so that there would not be an overdose to the patient.

3. C The effective path length is used for heterogeneity corrections calculations. In order to calculate the appropriate TAR for each material, the water-equivalent path length must be determined. This is the thickness of water that will provide the identical attenuation of the actual beam path. See the figure bellow.

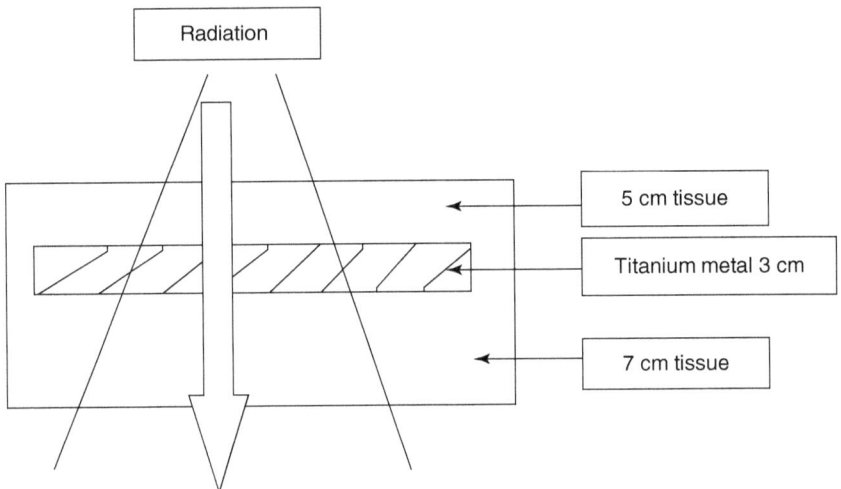

Fig. 2A.7.1

Physical depth = 5 cm tissue + 3 cm titanium + 7 cm of tissue = 15 cm
Effective depth = 12 cm tissue + 3 cm titanium (titanium density/water density)
Titanium density is approximately 4.507 g/cm^3.
Effective path length = 12 cm tissue + 4.507 cm of tissue equivalent titanium
Effective path length = 16.5 cm tissue

4. **B** Since the prescription depth is 4 cm from the skin and there is 1 cm bolus, the prescription point is at a depth of 5 cm. The dose at the surface is the ratio of the PDD at 5 cm (0.60) to the PDD at 1 cm (0.95):
Dose at the skin (1 cm) = 250 cGy × (95/60)
Dose at the skin = 396 cGy

5. **C** The practical range of an electron beam is ½ its energy (MeV), so the practical range of a 16 MeV electron energy is 8 cm.

6. **C** The 90 % depth dose takes place at about 1/3 of the electron energy (MeV).

7. **A** As a rule of thumb, MeV/2 or half of the energy should be the lead cutout thickness in mm to stop the energy in question, so a 12 MeV energy will be stop using a 6 mm lead thickness cutout.

8. **B** As a rule of thumb, MeV/2 or half of the energy should be the lead cutout thickness in mm to stop the energy in question. For a 12 MeV beam, a 6 mm lead cutout should be sufficient. If Cerrobend is used in the construction of the cutout instead of lead, 20 % is added to the cutout thickness in question, so 12 MeV energy will be stopped using 6 mm × 1.20 = 7.2 mm thick Cerrobend cutout.

Treatment Planning and Treatment Planning System (TPS)

Contents

3.1	Isodose Curve Parameters and Isodose Distributions (Questions)	222
3.2	Electron Beam Dose Distributions (Questions)	236
3.3	IMRT and VMAT (Questions)	246
3.4	Special Procedures and SRS (Questions)	251
3.5	Nuclear Medicine Therapy (Questions)	266
3.6	Isodose Curve Parameters and Isodose Distributions (Answers)	268
3.7	Electron Beam Dose Distributions (Answers)	281
3.8	IMRT and VMAT (Answers)	288
3.9	Special Procedures and SRS (Answers)	291
3.10	Nuclear Medicine Therapy (Answers)	301

Treatment planning is the central task for dosimetrists and is also a very important task for medical physicists. Planning skill and experience are the major standards in the job market for dosimetrists.

Readers are expected to be very familiar with TPS tools (e.g., contouring, BEV, wedges, EDW, MLC, bolus, blocks, IDLs, DVH, etc.), case-specific skills, optimization skills, and dose calculation algorithms (correction-based, model-based), as well as the principles standing behind those tools.

Intensity-modulated radiotherapy (IMRT) was developed after 3-dimensional conformal radiation therapy (3D-CRT) had been popularly applied. The primary goal for IMRT was to spare dose to normal tissue and hence significantly reduce normal tissue complication probability (NTCP). The implementation of IMRT was the key reason that the field of medical physics and dosimetry has been booming since the 1990s.

3.1 Isodose Curve Parameters and Isodose Distributions (Questions)

Quiz 1 (Level 2)

1. A plot of the volume of a given structure receiving a certain dose or higher as a function of dose is the definition of?
   A. Differential DVH
   B. Cumulative integral DVH
   C. Dose volume histogram (DVH)
   D. Beam's eye view

2. Which of the following about dose volume histograms (DVH) are correct?
   A. I, II, and III.
   B. I and III only.
   C. II and IV only.
   D. IV only.
   E. All are correct.
   I. Provide quantitative information with regard to how much dose is absorbed in how much volume
   II. Are a great tool for evaluating a given plan or comparing competing plans
   III. Summarize the entire dose distribution into a single curve for each anatomic structure of interest
   IV. Display the area where hot spot is located

3. Which of the following about isodose charts are correct?
   A. I, II, and III.
   B. I and III only.
   C. II and IV only.
   D. IV only.
   E. All are correct.
   I. Consist of a family of isodose curves.
   II. Isodose curves are usually drawn for equal increments of percent depth dose.
   III. Have lines that represent equal percentage depth dose for a particular field size and SSD at a specific plane in the tissue.
   IV. Give you specific hot spot location.

3.1 Isodose Curve Parameters and Isodose Distributions (Questions)

4. Which of the following are correct according to the following DVH?
A. I, II, and III.
B. I and III only.
C. II and IV only.
D. IV only.
E. All are correct.

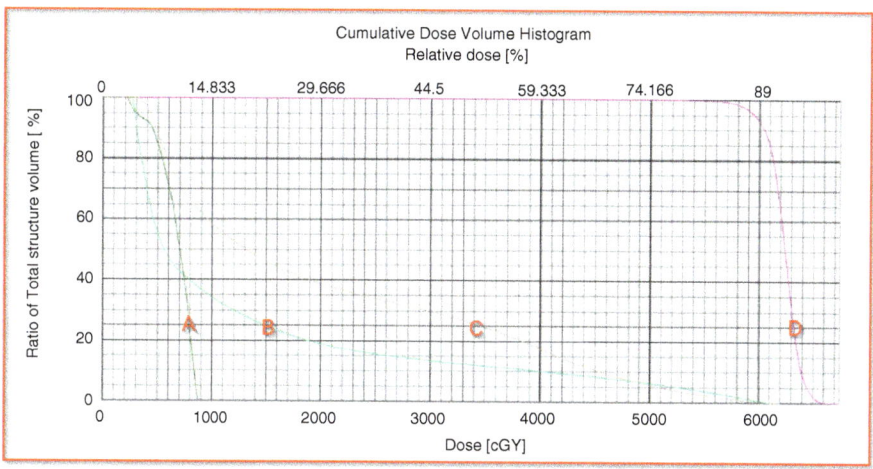

Fig. 3.1.1 Courtesy of the University of Miami, Sylvester Cancer Center

I. Line A, max dose is approximately 9 Gy.
II. Line B, V20 Gy <20 % was achieved.
III. Line C, 30 % of the volume receives at least 30 Gy.
IV. Line D, Rx dose of 60 Gy (>95 % coverage) was not achieved.

5. Based on the following graph, line B represents the oral cavity and the prescription dose is 60 Gy to a head and neck area. What percentage of the oral cavity received more than the prescribed dose (V60 Gy)?

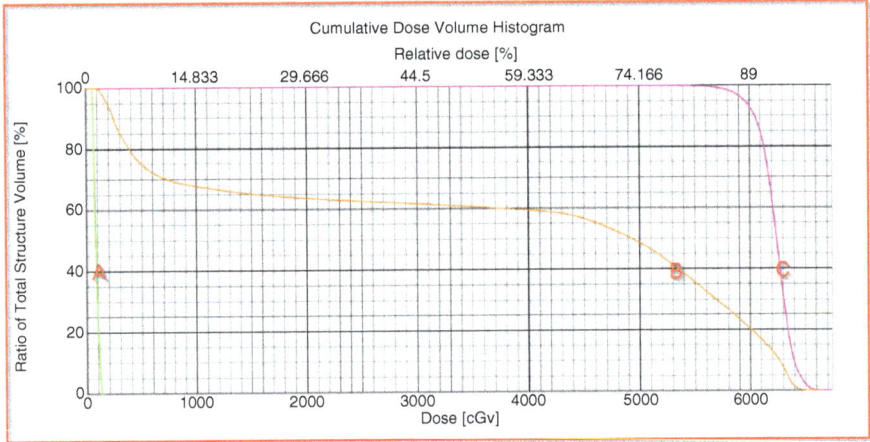

Fig. 3.1.2 Courtesy of the University of Miami, Sylvester Cancer Center

A. 0 %
B. 20 %
C. 70 %
D. 96 %

6. Which of the following dose volume histogram (DVH) has been found to be more useful and more commonly used?
A. Differential
B. Cumulative
C. Isodose curve
D. Beam's eye view

7. Which of the following scenarios will not include a DVH?
A. 3D conformal planning
B. IMRT planning
C. IMRT ARC planning
D. Electron clinical setup

3.1 Isodose Curve Parameters and Isodose Distributions (Questions) 225

8. Which of the following plans should contain a dose volume histogram (DVH) of the PTV and organs at risk?
A. I, II, and III.
B. I and III only.
C. II and IV only.
D. IV only.
E. All are correct.
I. 3D conformal planning
II. HDR breast planning
III. IMRT planning
IV. Electron planning

9. Which of the following isodose lines (IDLs) typically represent the field edge or border?
A. 100 % isodose line
B. 75 % isodose line
C. 50 % isodose line
D. Cannot be identified

10. Which of the following statements are true?
A. I, II, and III.
B. I and III only.
C. II and IV only.
D. IV only.
E. All are correct.
I. When a composite plan is done, it is essential that the doses contributed by each plan be added together and a composite isodose distribution be displayed.
II. When a composite plan is done, just the current plan isodose distribution is needed to be displayed on the contour and DVH.
III. Isodose charts are produced by measuring the dose distribution in a water phantom.
IV. A DVH is the only way to analyze a plan.

11. In general, the ideal DVH for a treatment target like a PTV is?
A. I, II, and III.
B. I and III only.
C. II and IV only.
D. IV only.
E. All are correct.
I. 95 % of the volume to receive 100 % of the prescribed dose.
II. 50 % of the volume to receive 100 % of the prescribed dose.
III. 5 % of the volume should not receive more than 110 % of the prescribed dose.
IV. 5 % of the volume should receive more than 110 % of the prescribed dose.

12. Which of the following about isodose curves are correct?
A. I, II, and III.
B. I and III only.
C. II and IV only.
D. IV only.
E. All are correct.
I. They are lines passing through points of equal dose.
II. They are expressed as a percentage of the dose at a reference point.
III. They represent levels of absorbed dose.
IV. They represent the hot spot location.

13. The depth dose values of the isodose curves are typically normalized:
A. I, II, and III.
B. II and III only.
C. II and IV only.
D. IV only.
E. All are correct.
I. At 50 % of the prescribed dose
II. At the point of the central axis
III. At the point of maximum dose in any area of the field
IV. At a fixed distance along the central axis in the irradiated medium

14. Which of the following statements are true?
A. The dose at depth is greatest on the central axis of the beam and gradually decreases toward the edges of the beam.
B. The dose at any depth is lower on the central axis of the beam and gradually increases toward the edges of the beam.
C. Near the field edges, the dose rate increases rapidly as a function of lateral distance from the beam axis.
D. Isodose curves at specified depth are not of concern when defined physical penumbra.

15. Horns are?
A. I, II, and III.
B. I and III only.
C. II and IV only.
D. IV only.
E. All are correct.
I. High-dose areas near the surface in the periphery of the field
II. Low-dose areas near the surface in the periphery of the field
III. Are created by the flattening filter
IV. Are created by the scatter in the body

3.1 Isodose Curve Parameters and Isodose Distributions (Questions)

16. Which of the following statements is/are true?
A. I, II, and III.
B. I and III only.
C. II and IV only.
D. IV only.
E. All are correct.
I. The field size is defined as the medial distance between the 50 % isodose lines at a reference depth.
II. The field size is defined as the lateral distance between the 50 % isodose lines at a reference depth.
III. The field-defining light is made to coincide with the 100 % isodose line of the radiation beam projected on a plane perpendicular to the beam axis.
IV. The field-defining light is made to coincide with the 50 % isodose line of the radiation beam projected on a plane perpendicular to the beam axis.

17. The following graph represents the:
A. Isodose chart
B. Isodose distribution
C. Dose volume histogram
D. Beam profile

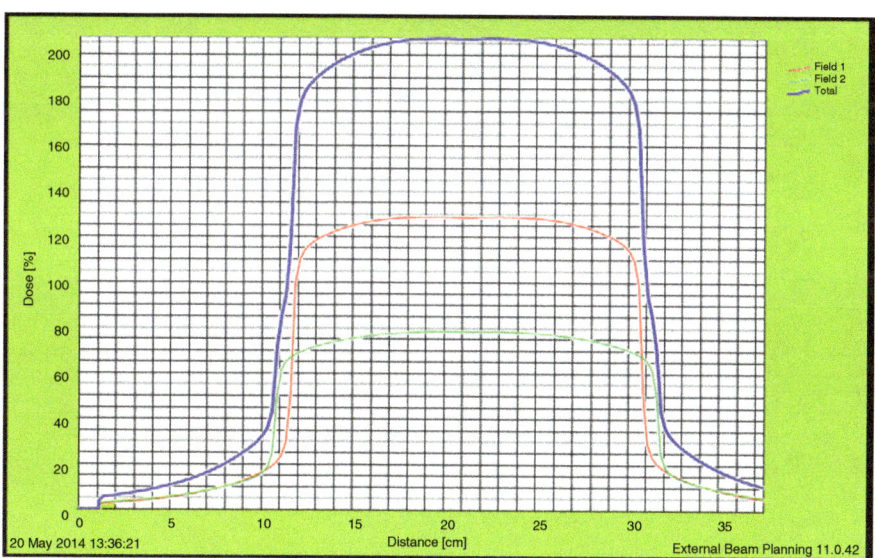

Fig. 3.1.3 Courtesy of the University of Miami, Sylvester Cancer Center

18. Which of the following parameters affect the isodose distribution?
A. I, II, and III.
B. I and III only.
C. II and IV only.
D. IV only.
E. All are correct.
I. Beam energy
II. Source size, SSD, and SDD
III. Collimation
IV. Field size

19. Which of the following statements are true?
A. I, II, and III.
B. I and III only.
C. II and IV only.
D. IV only.
E. All are correct.
I. The depth of a given isodose curve increases with beam quality or energy.
II. Lower-energy beams cause the isodose curves outside the field to bulge out.
III. The isodose curves outside the primary beam are greatly distended in the case of orthovoltage radiation.
IV. The isodose curves outside the primary beam are minimized for megavoltage beams as a result of predominantly forward scattering.

20. Which of the following has the greatest influence in determining the shape of the isodose curves?
A. Field size
B. Flattening filter
C. Source-to-skin distance (SSD)
D. Beam energy

21. The function of the flattening filter is?
A. To reduce the penumbra of a therapy beam
B. To measure and verify precise amounts of radiation to the patient
C. To make the beam intensity distribution relatively uniform across the field
D. To power high-energy linear accelerators

22. The most commonly used isodose beam-modifying device is?
A. Block
B. Wedge
C. Cut out
D. Bolus

23. Which of the following are correct about wedges?
A. I, II, and III.
B. I and III only.
C. II and IV only.
D. IV only.
E. All are correct.
I. Tilt the isodose curves toward the thin end of the wedge.
II. Tilt the isodose curves toward the thicker end of the wedge.
III. The degree of tilt depends on the slope of the wedge filter.
IV. The degree of tilt depends on the position of the wedge (RT, LT, in or out).

24. Match the following dose volume histogram.
A. Differential DVH displayed in absolute dose
B. Cumulative DVH displayed in absolute dose
C. Cumulative DVH displayed in absolute volume
I.

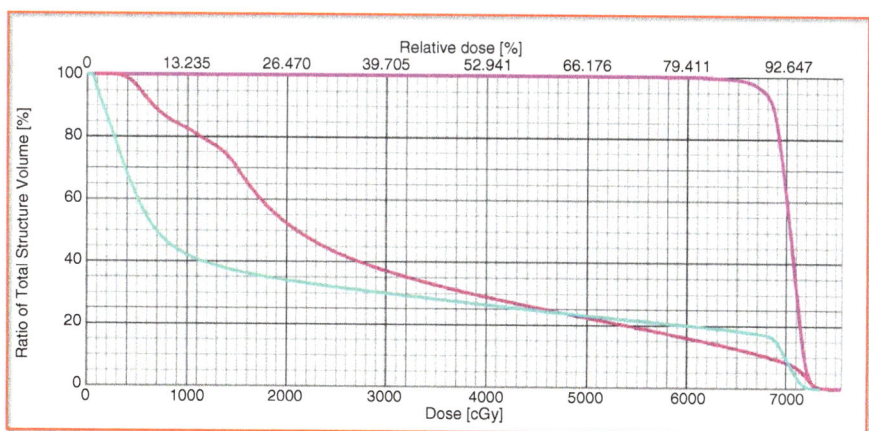

Fig. 3.1.4 Courtesy of the University of Miami, Sylvester Cancer Center

II.

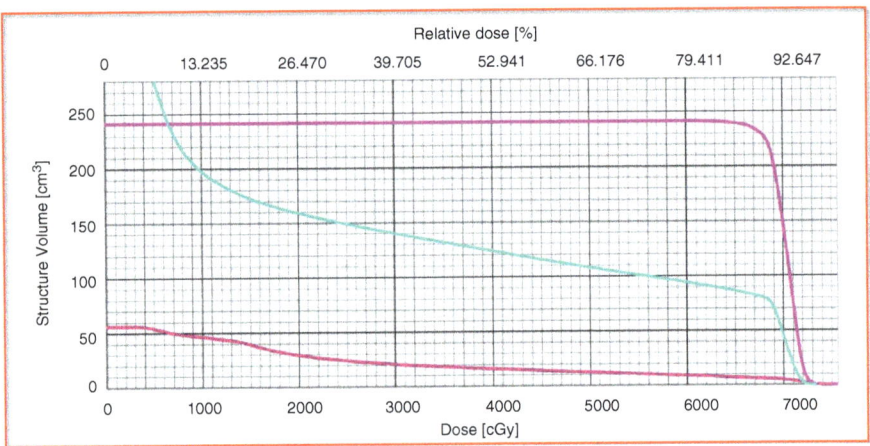

Fig. 3.1.5 Courtesy of the University of Miami, Sylvester Cancer Center

III.

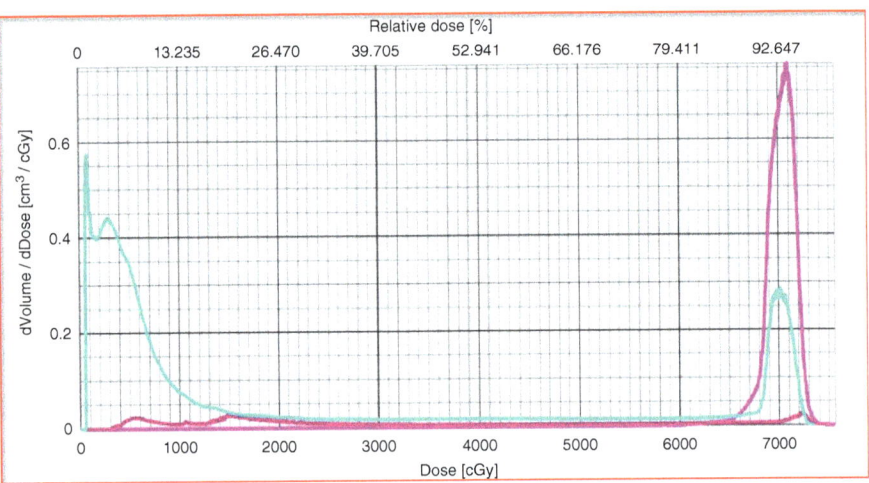

Fig. 3.1.6 Courtesy of the University of Miami, Sylvester Cancer Center

25. Which of the following DVHs is used to evaluate a particular volume for a critical structure?
   A. Differential DVH displayed in absolute dose
   B. Cumulative DVH displayed in absolute dose
   C. Cumulative DVH displayed in absolute volume

3.1 Isodose Curve Parameters and Isodose Distributions (Questions)

26. The advantages of parallel opposed fields are?
A. I, II, and III.
B. I and III only.
C. II and IV only.
D. IV only.
E. All are correct.
I. Simplicity and reproducibility of the setup
II. More homogeneous dose to the tumor than a single field
III. Less chances of geometrical miss
IV. Excessive dose to normal tissues and critical organs above and below the tumor

27. The isodose uniformity distribution depends on?
A. I, II, and III.
B. I and III only.
C. II and IV only.
D. IV only.
E. All are correct.
I. Patient thickness
II. Beam energy
III. Beam flatness
IV. Correct weighting

28. Which of the following dose is used by NIST and/or an ADCL?
A. Absolute dose
B. Integral dose
C. Relative dose
D. Radiation dose

29. Some strategies used to maximize dose to the tumor while minimizing dose to surrounding tissue are?
A. I, II, and III.
B. I and III only.
C. II and IV only.
D. IV only.
E. All are correct.
I. Increasing the number of fields
II. Selecting appropriate beam direction
III. Adjusting beam weights
IV. Using appropriate beam energy

30. What is an isocentric treatment technique?
A. I, II, and III.
B. I and III only.
C. II and IV only.
D. IV only.
E. All are correct.
I. It consists of placing the isocenter of the machine at a depth within the patient and directing the beams from different directions.
II. The distance of the source from the isocenter (SAD) remains constant irrespective of the beam direction.
III. Source-to-skin distance (SSD) may change, depending on the beam direction and shape of the patient contour.
IV. Isocenter is the point of intersection of the collimator axis and the gantry axis of rotation.

31. For an isocentric treatment technique, the source-to-skin distance is?
A. SSD = SAD − d
B. SSD = SAD + d
C. SSD = SAD/d
D. SSD = SAD × d

32. The lateral distance between two specified isodose curves at specified depth is used to estimate?
A. Tissue lateral effect
B. Transmission penumbra
C. Physical penumbra
D. Beam profile

33. Outside the geometric limits of the beam and the penumbra, the dose variation is the result of?
A. I, II, and III.
B. I and III only.
C. II and IV only.
D. IV only.
E. All are correct.
I. Side scatter from the field
II. Lateral scatter from the medium
III. Leakage and scatter from the collimator
IV. Leakage from the head of the machine

3.1 Isodose Curve Parameters and Isodose Distributions (Questions)

34. Isodose charts can be measured by means of?
A. I, II, and III.
B. I and III only.
C. II and IV only.
D. IV only.
E. All are correct.
I. Ion chambers
II. Solid-state detectors
III. Radiographic films
IV. Calorimeter

35. The ionization chamber used for isodose measurements should?
A. I, II, and III.
B. I and III only.
C. II and IV only.
D. IV only.
E. All are correct.
I. Be small (sensitive volume, less than 15 mm long and inside diameter of 5 mm or less)
II. Be energy dependent
III. Be energy independent
IV. Be as big as possible to cover the beam

36. When using a wedge pair technique:
A. I, II, and III.
B. I and III only.
C. II and IV only.
D. IV only.
E. All are correct.
I. The high-dose region (hot spot) is moved to the thick end of the wedges (heel).
II. The high-dose region (hot spot) is moved to the thin end of the wedges (toe).
III. The high-dose region (hot spot) decreases with field size and wedge angle.
IV. The high-dose region (hot spot) increases with field size and wedge angle.

37. Which of the following techniques can be used to obtain an acceptable uniform dose distribution?
A. I, II, and III.
B. I and III only.
C. II and IV only.
D. IV only.
E. All are correct.
I. Wedge pair
II. Field in field
III. Open field and wedged field combinations
IV. Open field and block MLC field combinations

38. The treatment planning process is based on?
A. I, II, and III.
B. I and III only.
C. II and IV only.
D. IV only.
E. All are correct.
I. Pathology
II. Staging
III. Diagnostic exams
IV. Karnofsky score

39. Which of the following organizations established or proposed a general dose specification system to be adopted universally?
A. International Commission on Radiation Units and Measurements (ICRU)
B. Nuclear Regulatory Commission (NRC)
C. National Council on Radiation Protection and Measurements (NCRP)
D. Atomic Energy Commission (AEC)

40. The gross tumor volume (GTV):
A. Is the tumor(s) if present and any other tissue with presumed tumor or microscopic disease
B. Is the extent and location of the visible tumor only
C. Compensates for internal physiological movements and variation in size, shape, and position of the CTV
D. Includes the CTV and setup margin for patient movement and setup uncertainties

3.1 Isodose Curve Parameters and Isodose Distributions (Questions)

41. Which of the following statement(s) are true?
A. I, II, and III.
B. I and III only.
C. II and IV only.
D. IV only.
E. All are correct.
I. Delineation of CTV assumes that there are no tumor cells outside this volume.
II. Delineation of the GTV is possible if the tumor is visible, palpable, or demonstrable through imaging.
III. The margin around CTV in any direction must be large enough to compensate for internal movements as well as patient motion and setup uncertainties.
IV. GTV can be defined if the tumor has been surgically removed by outlining the tumor bed.

42. Which of the following are correct about planning organ at risk (OAR)?
A. I, II, and III.
B. I and III only.
C. II and IV only.
D. IV only.
E. All are correct.
I. It needs adequate protection.
II. All organs at risk need the same margins.
III. It may need margins to compensate for its movements, internal, as well as setup.
IV. It is not of importance if abutting the PTV.

43. Which of the following are correct about treatment volumes?
A. I, II, and III.
B. I and III only.
C. II and IV only.
D. IV only.
E. All are correct
I. It is larger than the planning target volume.
II. It is a margin added to the target volume to allow for limitations of treatment technique.
III. It depends on a particular treatment technique.
IV. It is larger than the irradiated volume.

44. The highest dose in the target area that covers a minimum of 2 cm^2 is called:
A. Hot spot
B. Mean target dose
C. Maximum target dose
D. Modal target dose

45. The reference point used to record target dose recommended by the ICRU:
A. I, II, and III.
B. I and III only.
C. II and IV only.
D. IV only.
E. All are correct.
I. Should represent dose throughout the PTV
II. Should be selected where the dose can be accurately calculated
III. Should not lie in the penumbra region
IV. Should lie where steep dose gradient is

46. The reference point used to record target dose recommended by the ICRU for parallel opposed, unequally weighted beams:
A. Should be specified at the center of rotation in the principal plane
B. Should be on the central axis midway between the beam entrances
C. Should be specified on the central axis placed within the PTV
D. Should be at the intersection of the central axes of the beams placed within the PTV

47. Which of the following detectors is possibly traceable by NIST and/or ADCL?
A. Ion chamber
B. Radiochromic film
C. Silicon detector
D. TLD

3.2 Electron Beam Dose Distributions (Questions)

Quiz 1 (Level 2)

1. Electron dose rate and isodose distribution depend on?
A. I, II, and III.
B. I and III only.
C. II and IV only.
D. IV only.
E. All are correct.
I. Electron energy
II. Specific linear accelerator
III. Secondary blocks
IV. Field size

3.2 Electron Beam Dose Distributions (Questions)

2. The PDD for electron beams is uniform within the first few cm in tissue followed by a rapid falloff of dose. The depth at which this rapid falloff of dose is located depends on?
A. Electron cutout
B. Electron field size
C. Electron cone
D. Electron energy

3. What electron energy in MeV should be selected if a tumor is located at 4 cm depth?
A. 6 MeV electron energy
B. 9 MeV electron energy
C. 12 MeV electron energy
D. 16 MeV electron energy

4. The most clinically useful energy range for electrons is?
A. 12–24 MeV
B. 6–12 MeV
C. 6–20 MeV
D. 16–20 MeV

5. Electron treatment can be used for all of the following except?
A. Boost dose to nodes
B. Skin and lip lesions
C. Chest wall/breast irradiation
D. Prostate irradiation

6. Electrons interact with atoms through?
A. I, II, and III.
B. I and III only.
C. II and IV only.
D. IV only.
E. All are correct.
I. Inelastic collisions with atomic electrons
II. Inelastic collisions with nuclei
III. Elastic collisions with atomic electrons
IV. Elastic collisions with nuclei

7. The rate of electron energy loss depends primarily on:
A. Electron density of the medium
B. Type of cutout used
C. Electron energy
D. Type of collision

8. The rate of energy loss per gram per cm squared (stopping power) is greater for?
A. I, II, and III.
B. I and III only.
C. II and IV only.
D. IV only.
E. All are correct.
I. High atomic number materials
II. Low atomic number materials
III. High-Z materials
IV. Low-Z materials

9. The energy loss rate of electrons per cm in water is roughly about?
A. 3 MeV/cm of water
B. 2 MeV/cm of water
C. 1 MeV/cm of water
D. 2 KeV/cm of water

10. For bremsstrahlung photon creation, the rate of energy loss in electron beam per cm is proportional to?
A. I, II, and III.
B. I and III only.
C. II and IV only.
D. IV only.
E. All are correct.
I. Electron energy
II. Electron mass
III. Square of the atomic number (Z2)
IV. Rest mass of an electron (0.511 MeV)

11. The electron scattering power varies?
A. I, II, and III.
B. I and III only.
C. II and IV only.
D. IV only.
E. All are correct.
I. Inversely as the electron mass
II. Approximately as the square of the atomic number (Z2)
III. Approximately as the square of the kinetic energy
IV. Inversely as the square of the kinetic energy

12. The practical electron range is defined as?
A. The depth of the point where the tangent to the descending linear portion of the curve intersects the extrapolated background
B. The depth at which the dose is 50 % of the maximum dose

C. A point in space that is the same distance from the source for all gantry angles
D. The thickness of the material that reduces the intensity of the beam to half (50 %) its original value

13. As electron beam energy increases:
A. I, II, and III.
B. I and III only.
C. II and IV only.
D. IV only.
E. All are correct.
I. Dose increases
II. Surface penumbra decreases
III. Penumbra at depth increases
IV. Surface penumbra increases

14. What will be the correct energy if a physician asks the dosimetrist that he/she would like to prescribe an electron treatment at a depth of 3 cm using 90 % depth dose?
A. 6 MeV
B. 9 MeV
C. 12 MeV
D. 16 MeV

15. Which of the following energies generates the highest surface dose or less skin sparing?
A. 6 MeV
B. 9 MeV
C. 12 MeV
D. 16 MeV

16. Superficial tumors are best treated with:
A. Photon treatments
B. Electron treatments
C. Proton treatments
D. CyberKnife treatments

17. The most useful treatment depth or therapeutic range of electrons is given by:
A. 50 % depth dose
B. 90 % depth dose
C. 100 % depth dose
D. 25 % depth dose

18. If the treatment depth on an electron is in doubt, the dosimetrist should:
A. Use a bigger cutout.
B. Use a bigger cone size.
C. Use higher electron energy.
D. Treatment depth is not important.

19. Which of the following statements are true?
A. I, II, and III.
B. I and III only.
C. II and IV only.
D. IV only.
E. All are correct.
I. The skin-sparing effect with clinical electron beams is only modest or nonexistent.
II. Percent surface dose for electrons increases with energy.
III. At lower energies, the electrons are scattered more easily and through larger angles.
IV. The ratio of surface dose to maximum dose is less for the lower-energy electrons than for the higher-energy electrons.

20. Uniformity or flatness of the electron beam is usually specified:
A. I, II, and III.
B. I and III only.
C. II and IV only.
D. IV only.
E. All are correct.
I. In a plane perpendicular to the beam axis
II. Horizontal to the beam axis
III. At the depth of the 95 % isodose beyond the depth of dose maximum
IV. At Dmax

21. Which of the following statements are true?
A. I, II, and III.
B. I and III only.
C. II and IV only.
D. IV only.
E. All are correct.
I. The symmetry of electron beam is the comparison of a dose profile on one side of the central axis to that on the other.
II. AAPM recommends that the cross-beam profile in the reference plane should not differ more than 2 % at any pair of points located symmetrically on opposite sides of the central axis.
III. AAPM recommends that the variation in dose relative to the dose at the central axis should not exceed ±5 % over an area confined within lines 2 cm inside the geometric edge of fields equal to or larger than 10 × 10 cm.
IV. Scattering foils widen the electron beam as well as give a uniform dose distribution across the treatment field.

22. Acceptable field flatness and symmetry on an electron beam can be obtained:
A. I, II, and III.
B. I and III only.

3.2 Electron Beam Dose Distributions (Questions)

C. II and IV only.
D. IV only.
E. All are correct.
I. Using the MLC
II. Using proper design of beam scatterers
III. Using cones close to the skin
IV. Using proper beam-defining collimators

23. An electron beam emanates from:
A. The physical source
B. A virtual point
C. The target
D. The cutout

24. The tail of the electron depth-dose curve at the point where it becomes straight is due to:
A. Photoelectric effect interactions of electrons with the collimator system
B. Bremsstrahlung interactions of electrons with the collimator system
C. Bremsstrahlung interactions of electrons with the target
D. Bremsstrahlung interactions of electrons with the patient

25. Which of the following electron fields has the highest PDD?
A. I only.
B. II only.
C. III only.
D. IV only.
E. All have the same PDD.
I. 10×10 cm
II. 10×15 cm
III. 10×20 cm
IV. 20×20 cm

26. In an electron treatment, energy should be selected based on:
A. I, II, and III.
B. I and III only.
C. II and IV only.
D. IV only.
E. All are correct.
I. Depth of target volume
II. Minimum target dose required
III. Clinically acceptable dose to critical organs
IV. Field size used

27. Electron beam obliquity tends to:
A. I, II, and III.
B. I and III only.
C. II and IV only.
D. IV only.
E. All are correct.
I. Increase side scatter at Dmax
II. Decrease the depth of penetration
III. Shift Dmax toward the surface
IV. Shift Dmax away from the surface

28. For a large and uniform slab, the dose distribution for an electron beam beyond an inhomogeneity can be corrected by using:
A. TAR method
B. Effective SSD method
C. Isodose shift method
D. Coefficient equivalent thickness (CET) method

29. Bolus is often used in electron beam therapy to:
A. I, II, and III.
B. I and III only.
C. II and IV only.
D. IV only.
E. All are correct.
I. Flatten out an irregular surface
II. Reduce the penetration of the electrons in parts of the field
III. Increase the surface dose
IV. Increase the depth-dose

30. Some bolus materials used for radiation treatment are:
A. I, II, and III.
B. I and III only.
C. II and IV only.
D. IV only.
E. All are correct.
I. Paraffin wax
II. Polystyrene
III. Lucite
IV. Superflab

31. A plate of low atomic number material used on the patient's skin to reduce the energy of an electron beam is known as?
A. Accelerators
B. Decelerators
C. Compensators
D. Wedges

3.2 Electron Beam Dose Distributions (Questions)   243

32. Bolus should conform to the patient's surface as much as possible. Large air gaps between the absorber and the surface would result in:
A. I, II, and III.
B. I and III only.
C. II and IV only.
D. IV only.
E. All are correct.
I. Reduction in dose
II. Increase in dose
III. Scattering of electrons outside the field
IV. Scattering of electrons inside the field

33. When an electron field is abutted at the surface with a photon field?
A. I, II, and III.
B. I and III only.
C. II and IV only.
D. IV only.
E. All are correct.
I. Hot spot develops on the side of the electron field.
II. Hot spot develops on the side of the photon field.
III. Cold spot develops on the side of the photon field.
IV. Cold spot develops on the side of the electron field.

34. Field shaping can be accomplished in electron beam therapy by using?
A. MLC
B. Cones
C. Cutout
D. Wedges

35. Adequate cutout transmission for an electron beam treatment is?
A. ≤5 % transmission
B. >5 % transmission
C. ±10 % of the given dose
D. ±15 % of the given dose

36. What is the required thickness of a lead cutout for electron energies less than 10 MeV in order to keep an acceptable transmission or reduce the dose to an acceptable value to critical structures?
A. I, II, and III.
B. I and III only.
C. II and IV only.
D. IV only.
E. All are correct.
I. 5 mm thickness of lead
II. 5 cm thickness of lead
III. 6 mm thickness of Cerrobend
IV. 5 cm thickness of lead

37. The required thickness of Cerrobend is approximately?
A. 50 % greater than that of pure lead
B. 30 % greater than that of pure lead
C. 20 % greater than that of pure lead
D. Equal to that of pure lead

38. As a rule of thumb, the minimum thickness of lead required for blocking of electrons in mm is given by?
A. Electron energy in MeV/4
B. Electron energy in MeV/2
C. Electron energy in MeV × 2
D. Electron energy in MeV + 4

39. Which of the following treatments often require internal shielding?
A. I, II, and III.
B. I and III only.
C. II and IV only.
D. IV only.
E. All are correct.
I. Lip treatments
II. Buccal mucosa
III. Eyelid lesions
IV. Stoma lesions

40. Which of the following cases have the most substantial change of dose due to electron backscatter?
A. Lung tissue interface
B. Shielding shape
C. Tissue-lead interface
D. Bone tissue interface

41. To dissipate the effect of electron backscatter (a bremsstrahlung) on an internal lead, shield is recommended to?
A. I, II, and III.
B. I and III only.
C. II and IV only.
D. IV only.
E. All are correct.
I. Use a low atomic number absorber between the lead shield and the preceding tissue surface.
II. Use aluminum sheath around any lead used for internal shielding.
III. Use dental acrylic around any oral shielding.
IV. Use an internal cutout of size bigger than 3 cm always.

3.2 Electron Beam Dose Distributions (Questions)

42. The physician wants to treat the lower lip which measures 2 cm thick using a 9 MeV electron beam. What is the thickness of lead required in order to protect the structures beyond the lips?
A. 2 mm
B. 2.5 cm
C. 2.5 mm
D. 4.5 cm

43. A superficial tumor along a curved surface such as the chest wall or ribs is better treated with?
A. Multiple abutting electron fields
B. Electron arc therapy
C. Rapid arc photon therapy
D. Pseudo-arc technique

44. What energies are most used for total skin irradiation?
A. 9–12 MeV.
B. 12–23 MeV.
C. 2–9 MeV.
D. All energy can be used.

45. Which of the following algorithms is commonly used for electron beam treatment?
A. AAA algorithms
B. Pencil beam algorithms
C. Convolution superimposition algorithms
D. Monte Carlo algorithms

46. Provided that the radiation oncologist accepts the rounded edges of the treatment volume at depth, which of the following diameter applicators should be appropriate if a 12 MeV beam is used?
A. 4 cm
B. 6 cm
C. 10 cm
D. 15 cm

3.3 IMRT and VMAT (Questions)

Quiz 1 (Level 2)

1. Rotational therapy is best suited:
A. I, II, and III.
B. I and III only.
C. II and IV only.
D. IV only.
E. All are correct.
I. For lateral tumors
II. For large tumor volumes
III. For external surface tumors
IV. For small, deep-seated tumors

2. Advantages of inverse treatment planning (IMRT) over standard forward planning include:
A. I, II, and III.
B. I and III only.
C. II and IV only.
D. IV only.
E. All are correct.
I. Improved dose homogeneity inside the target volume
II. Increase speed and lesser complexity of the proposed solution
III. A quantitative introduction of cost functions, often incorporating dose volume constraints and biological functions
IV. Adjustment of the optimal treatment planning to the actual dose delivery technique

3. Delivery of IMRT treatments can be accomplished via:
A. I, II, and III.
B. I and III only.
C. II and IV only.
D. IV only.
E. All are correct.
I. Segmented MLC mode (SMLC)
II. Dynamic MLC mode (DMLC)
III. Intensity-modulated arc therapy (IMAT)
IV. Synchronized MLC mode (SYMLC)

4. Which of the following IMRT treatment modes is referred to as sliding window mode?
A. Segmented MLC mode (SMLC)
B. Dynamic MLC mode (DMLC)

C. Intensity-modulated arc therapy (IMAT)
D. Synchronize MLC mode (SYMLC)

5. IMRT stands for:
A. Intensity-multiple radiation therapy
B. Intensity-modulated rotational therapy
C. Intensity-modulated radiation therapy
D. Irregular-modulated radiation therapy

6. IMRT refers to:
A. Radiation therapy technique in which nonuniform fluence is delivered to the patient from any given position of the treatment beam to optimize the composite dose distribution
B. Radiation therapy technique in which uniform fluence is delivered to the patient from one to maximum of ten field position of the treatment beam to optimize the composite dose distribution
C. Radiation therapy technique in which beams of radiation used in treatment are shaped to match the tumor
D. Radiation therapy technique in which treatment planning is limited to generating dose distributions in a single or a few planes of the patient's target volume

7. Which of the following is true about IMRT treatment planning?
A. I, II, and III.
B. I and III only.
C. II and IV only.
D. IV only.
E. All are correct.
I. Each beam is divided into large number of beamlets.
II. The treatment planning determines the field's fluence.
III. The treatment planning determines the field weight.
IV. The treatment planning is based on inverse planning.

8. Which of the following are recommended as a check of the mechanical accuracy of a dynamic multileaf collimator (DMLC)?
A. I, II, and III.
B. I and III only.
C. II and IV only.
D. IV only.
E. All are correct.
I. Stability of leaf speed
II. Dose profile across adjacent leaves
III. Leaf acceleration and deceleration
IV. Position accuracy of leaves

9. What is the purpose of IMRT optimization?
A. I, II, and III.
B. I and II.
C. I and III.
D. I only.
E. All are correct.
I. To minimize the dose in normal tissue
II. To maximize the dose in target volume
III. To generate a dose fluence
IV. To reduce the treatment time

10. The prescription for mediastinal lymphoma is 36 Gy, treated in 20 fractions. The physician decided to treat the patient with AP/PA instead of IMRT. The reason could be:
A. AP/PA gives less doses to normal tissue than IMRT.
B. To save time because it might take too long to plan and treat with IMRT.
C. There is no need to use IMRT because the prescription dose is low.
D. AP/PA has better outcome for mediastinal lymphoma.

11. VMAT is superior to standard IMRT at fixed gantry angles because of:
A. I, II, and III.
B. II and IV.
C. II only.
D. II and III.
E. All correct.
I. Better dose homogeneity in the target
II. Short treatment time
III. Easier in achieving dose goals in optimizations
IV. Less intra-fraction motion for the patient

12. The physician needs an SBRT plan with the target in the abdomen. The patient has been treated before. In this case, is VMAT a better choice over standard IMRT?
A. Not necessarily because the main advantage for VMAT is fast delivery of the dose.
B. No. Standard IMRT is better because normal tissue can be avoided by choosing appropriate beam angles by beam's eye view (BEV).
C. Yes. VMAT is generally better over standard IMRT in SBRT because the factional dose of SBRT is huge and VMAT may distribute dose to surrounding normal tissues and reduce the probability of normal tissue complication.
D. Both are really bad options because the patient was treated before.

3.3 IMRT and VMAT (Questions)

13. Does an IMRT plan use physical wedges or EDWs?
A. Yes, to achieve homogeneous dose compensators are always needed.
B. No, an IMRT plan does not care about dose homogeneity.
C. Yes, IMRT has its limitations, so wedges are still needed.
D. No, IMRT can achieve homogeneity with DMLCs.

14. Can an IMRT plan use bolus?
A. Yes, since Dmax always exists for photon beams.
B. No, DMLC can play the role of bolus.
C. No, bolus is only used for electron beams, whereas IMRT is for photons only.
D. It depends. For extremities such as the palm, the backscattering is less; thus, a bolus is helpful, although for most IMRT cases, bolus is not needed.

15. What is a normal request for PTV in terms of prescription in an IMRT plan?
A. 100 % of PTV is covered with 100 % of prescription dose.
B. 100 % of PTV is covered with 95 % of prescription dose.
C. 95 % of PTV is covered with 100 % of prescription dose.
D. 95 % of PTV is covered with 95 % of prescription dose.

Quiz 2 (Level 3)

This quiz could be slightly challenging, especially for CMD candidates, since it requires some in-depth understanding of IMRT, mostly at a graduate level.

1. Gamma Knife and CyberKnife are typically used for stereotactic radiosurgery or radiotherapy; however, the difference between those two modalities is:
A. Gamma Knife is forward planned like 3D-CRT, whereas CyberKnife uses inverse planning like IMRT.
B. Gamma Knife can treat larger lesions.
C. CyberKnife plans are more conformal because there are more beams.
D. Gamma Knife has better homogeneity in dose.

2. Compare standard IMRT to 3D conformal radiotherapy:
A. Standard IMRT is superior in both curing the disease and sparing normal tissue doses than 3D-CRT.
B. Standard IMRT is superior in sparing normal tissue dose but not necessarily better in curing the disease than 3D-CRT.
C. 3D-CRT is superior in curing the disease but worse in sparing normal tissue dose than standard IMRT.
D. 3D-CRT is superior in both curing the disease and sparing normal tissue dose than standard IMRT.

3. What is the goal of IMRT optimization?
A. Find the local minimum of the objective (or cost) function.
B. Find the global minimum of the objective function.
C. Find the local maximum of the objective function.
D. Find the global maximum of the objective function.

4. What technique is used to minimize the objective function in IMRT optimization?
A. Least squares
B. Stimulated annealing.
C. Standard deviation
D. Analytic methods

5. What comes out right after IMRT optimization?
A. IMRT fluence for each field
B. IMRT dose volume histogram
C. IMRT MLC motion file
D. MU numbers

6. Considering the margin from CTV to PTV, which statement below is right?
A. IMRT has smaller margin than 3D-CRT because IMRT uses optimization.
B. The margin is independent to modality (either IMRT or 3D-CRT).
C. IMRT can use IGRT, whereas 3D-CRT cannot; thus, IMRT has smaller PTV margins than 3D-CRT.
D. Those treatment modalities are not comparable.

7. For Gamma Knife, CyberKnife, standard IMRT, and VMAT, if all normalized to body maximum, approximately which one of following is correct for reasonable isodose lines to prescribe to?
A. 60, 70, 95, and 90 %
B. 50, 70, 95, and 90 %
C. 60, 70, 98, and 90 %
D. 50, 60, 95, and 90 %

8. In a VMAT QA using a cylindrical phantom of over 1,300 diodes, the readings of the diodes are all 4 % lower than the plan dose. The reason for this could be:
A. The phantom is placed too close to the gantry.
B. The phantom is placed too far to the gantry.
C. The calibration of the VMAT QA phantom is wrong.
D. The diodes in the phantom are all broken.

9. What is the name of the optimization object of IMRT?
A. IMRT fluence
B. Objective function
C. MLC optimization algorithm
D. Iteration function

10. Mathematically, is the IMRT optimization function analytical?
A. No, that's why we need optimization.
B. Yes, but it takes some time since the calculation is complicated.
C. Yes, but optimization is faster, so it is not used.
D. No, but optimization cannot find the solution either.

3.4 Special Procedures and SRS (Questions)

Quiz 1 (Level 2)

1. Total body irradiation (TBI) with megavoltage photon beams is most commonly used for patients with:
A. Mycosis fungoides
B. Bone marrow transplantation
C. Lung cancer
D. Skin cancer

2. TBI treatments are required to achieve dose uniformity:
A. Within ±10%
B. Within ±5%
C. Within ±2%
D. Within ±20%

3. Tissue lateral effect is defined as:
A. The excessively higher dose to the subcutaneous tissues compared with the midpoint dose when a lower-energy beam is used or a thicker patient is treated with parallel-opposed beams for TBI.
B. The lower dose to the subcutaneous tissues compared with the midpoint dose when a lower-energy beam is used or a thicker patient is treated with parallel-opposed beams for TBI.
C. The excessively higher dose to the subcutaneous tissues compared with the Dmax dose when a higher-energy beam is used or a thicker patient is treated with parallel-opposed beams for TBI.
D. The excessively higher dose to the subcutaneous tissues compared with the midpoint dose when a higher-energy beam is used or a thinner patient is treated with parallel-opposed beams for TBI.

4. Which of the following statements is true about parallel-opposed beams on TBI treatments?
   A. I, II, and III.
   B. I and III only.
   C. II and IV only.
   D. IV only.
   E. All are correct.
   I. The higher the beam energy, the greater the dose uniformity for any thickness patient.
   II. The higher the beam energy, the lower the dose uniformity for any thickness patient.
   III. For patients of thickness greater than 35 cm, energies higher than 6 MV should be used to minimize the tissue lateral effect.
   IV. For patients of thickness less than 35 cm, energies higher than 6 MV should be used to minimize the tissue lateral effect.

5. Which of the following is used to bring the surface dose to at least 90 % of the prescribed TBI dose?
   A. I, II, and III.
   B. I and III only.
   C. II and IV only.
   D. IV only.
   E. All are correct.
   I. Bolus
   II. Wedges
   III. Large spoiler screen
   IV. Blocks

6. Which of the following techniques can be used to treat TBI?
   A. I, II, and III.
   B. I and III only.
   C. II and IV only.
   D. IV only.
   E. All are correct.
   I. Bilateral total body irradiation
   II. AP/PA total body irradiation
   III. Reclined AP/PA total body irradiation
   IV. Oblique total body irradiation

7. Which of the following is used as a reference point on calculation when doing TBI treatment?
   A. Midplane at the level of the chest
   B. Midplane at the level of the waist
   C. Midplane at the level of the umbilicus
   D. Both knees

3.4 Special Procedures and SRS (Questions)

8. Compensator design for TBI is complex because of:
A. I, II, and III.
B. I and III only.
C. II and IV only.
D. IV only.
E. All are correct.
I. Large variation in body thickness
II. Lack of complete body immobilization
III. Internal tissue heterogeneities
IV. Thickness of compensator

9. Stereotactic radiosurgery (SRS) is:
A. A single radiation therapy procedure for treating intracranial lesions
B. A multiple-dose fraction procedure for treating intracranial lesions
C. A single radiation therapy procedure for treating lung lesions
D. A multiple radiation therapy procedure for treating spine lesions

10. Which of the following statements is/are true about stereotactic radiosurgery?
A. I, II, and III.
B. I and III only.
C. II and IV only.
D. IV only.
E. All are correct.
I. It involves three-dimensional imaging to localize the lesion.
II. It has a high degree of conformity.
III. It uses dynamic conformal arcs with mini multileaf collimators (MLCs).
IV. It uses appropriate circular beams to fit the lesion.

11. What is the maximum error accepted in view of the unavoidable uncertainties in target localization when treating stereotactic radiosurgery?
A. ±0.1 mm
B. ±0.2 mm
C. ±1 mm
D. ±3 mm

12. Which of the following types of radiation is used in SRS?
A. I, II, and III.
B. I and III only.
C. II and IV only.
D. IV only.
E. All are correct.
I. Heavy charged particles
II. Cobalt-60
III. Megavoltage x-rays
IV. Electrons

13. Which of the following devices is used in a stereotactic radiosurgery linac treatment for immobilization?
A. Stereotactic aquaplast mask
B. Stereotactic alpha cradle
C. Stereotactic frame
D. Stereotactic bolus

14. Which of the following cone diameters are used for SRS treatments?
A. 1–5 mm cones
B. 5–20 mm cones
C. 5–30 mm cones
D. 20–50 mm cones

15. 15 cm long circular cones are used on SRS linac treatments to?
A. Minimize geometric penumbra
B. Increase the distance (SSD)
C. Maximize the number of noncoplanar arcs
D. Shape the beam's eye aperture

16. Which of the following statements are true about Gamma Knife?
A. I, II, and III.
B. I and III only.
C. II and IV only.
D. IV only.
E. All are correct.
I. Gamma Knife delivers radiation to a target lesion in the brain only.
II. Gamma Knife units are composed of 201 cobalt-60 sources housed in a hemispherical shield.
III. Gamma Knife source-to-focus distance is 40.3 cm.
IV. Gamma Knife central beam is tilted through an angle of 55° with respect to the horizontal plane.

17. Which of the following statements is/are true about Gamma Knife?
A. I, II, and III.
B. I and III only.
C. II and IV only.
D. IV only.
E. All are correct.
I. The central axes of all 201 beams intersect at the focus with a mechanical precision of ±3 mm.
II. The central axes of all 201 beams intersect at the focus with a mechanical precision of ±5 mm.
III. The alignment of helmet channels with the central body channels must have a positioning accuracy of ±0.1 mm.
IV. The alignment of helmet channels with the central body channels must have a positioning accuracy of ±0.3 mm.

3.4 Special Procedures and SRS (Questions)

18. The maximum channel diameter or field size on a Gamma Knife helmet is?
A. 4 mm
B. 8 mm
C. 14 mm
D. 18 mm

19. Which of the following detectors can be used to do QA and dosimetry for stereotactic radiosurgery (SRS)?
A. I, II, and III.
B. I and III only.
C. II and IV only.
D. IV only.
E. All are correct.
I. Ion chambers
II. Film
III. Thermoluminescent dosimeters
IV. Diodes

20. When using film for stereotactic radiosurgery (SRS) dosimetry, care must be taken because?
A. I, II, and III.
B. I and III only.
C. II and IV only.
D. IV only.
I. Films have a size limitation.
II. Films show energy dependence.
III. Films show possible directional dependence.
IV. Films have high statistical uncertainty.

21. Which of the following are the detectors of choice to measure cross-beam profiles and depth-dose distribution for stereotactic radiosurgery (SRS)?
A. I, II, and III.
B. I and III only.
C. II and IV only.
D. IV only.
E. All are correct.
I. Ion chambers
II. Film
III. Thermoluminescent dosimeters
IV. Diodes

22. Some of the major QA for stereotactic radiosurgery (SRS) include:
A. I, II, and III.
B. I and III only.
C. II and IV only.
D. IV only.
E. All are correct.
I. Stereotactic frame accuracy
II. Pedestal or couch mount
III. Frame alignment with gantry and couch eccentricity
IV. Congruence of target point with radiation isocenter

23. Which of the following are advantages of CyberKnife treatments?
A. I, II, and III.
B. I and III only.
C. II and IV only.
D. IV only.
E. All are correct.
I. Frameless treatment
II. Non-isocentric
III. Fractionated treatment
IV. Very complex and conformal treatment

24. Accuray CyberKnife can be used to treat:
A. I, II, and III.
B. I and III only.
C. II and IV only.
D. IV only.
E. All are correct.
I. Intracranial lesions
II. Thoracic-lung tumors
III. Intra-abdmonial-hepatic tumors, pancreatic tumors
IV. Spine-cervical, thoracic, and lumbar lesions

25. CyberKnife's simulation CT scan must:
A. I, II, and III.
B. I and III only.
C. II and IV only.
D. IV only.
E. All are correct.
I. Have a minimum of 10–15 cm above and below the area of interest
II. Slices of 1.0–1.5 mm (1.25 mm)
III. Use contrast if necessary
IV. Gantry tilts at 5°

3.4 Special Procedures and SRS (Questions)

26. CyberKnife's MRI scan must:
A. I, II, and III.
B. I and III only.
C. II and IV only.
D. IV only.
E. All are correct.
I. Use true axial images only
II. Have slices of 1.0–3.0 mm
III. Use contrast if necessary
IV. Have 512×512 acquisitions

27. CyberKnife skull tracking has an accuracy of:
A. 5 mm translation error; 5° rotation error
B. 0.5 mm translation error; 0.5° rotation error
C. 0.5 mm translation error; 10° rotation error
D. 10 mm translation error; 0.5° rotation error

28. How many DRRs are generated as reference images from the CT data set used for planning?
A. 20 pairs of DRRs
B. 33 pairs of DRRs
C. 60 pairs of DRRs
D. 120 pairs of DRRs

29. For soft tissue treatments using fiducial markers, a CT scan must be obtained when?
A. One week after fiducial placement.
B. 24–48 h after fiducial placement.
C. Four weeks after fiducial placement.
D. CT is not required after fiducial placement.

30. How many fixed collimators does CyberKnife have?
A. 5
B. 10
C. 12
D. 15

31. The dynamic collimator on CyberKnife is called?
A. IRIS
B. MLC
C. Jaw
D. EDW

32. What is the typical alpha/beta (α/β) ratio in Gy assumed for spinal cord myelitis?
A. 2.1
B. 2.5
C. 1.6–4.5
D. 10–20

33. Which of the following statements are true about biological effective dose (BED)?
A. I, II, and III.
B. I and III only.
C. II and IV only.
D. IV only.
E. All are correct.
I. BED=$nd_1(1+d_1/\alpha/\beta)$, where n=number of fractions, d_1=dose per fraction, and α/β is the alpha/beta ratio.
II. Given different fractionation schemes, one can sum the BEDs.
III. Given different fractionation schemes, d or n can be solved to get an equivalent regimen.
IV. BED=$nd_1(1+d_1/\alpha/\beta)+nd_2(1+d_2/\alpha/\beta)+nd_3(1+d_3/\alpha/\beta)$ ….

34. Which of the following is the definition of an ablative treatment of radiosurgery?
A. Single large dose
B. Multiple small doses
C. Several large doses
D. Single small dose

35. Which of the following are potential benefits of fractionation in CyberKnife?
A. I, II, and III.
B. I and III only.
C. II and IV only.
D. IV only.
E. All are correct.
I. Exploiting deference in α/β between tumor and normal tissue
II. Better treatment of hypoxic tumors through reoxygenation
III. Exploiting differences in radiation repair between tumor and normal tissue
IV. Manipulating radiosensitivity through cell cycle redistribution

36. How often should the end-to-end QA test be done in CyberKnife?
A. Daily
B. Monthly
C. Bimonthly
D. Four-month intervals

3.4 Special Procedures and SRS (Questions)   259

37. CyberKnife lung tumor is best treated using?
A. Deep inspiration breath hold
B. Deep expiration breath hold
C. Normal breathing
D. Shallow breathing only

38. Some benefits of CyberKnife radiosurgery are?
A. I, II, and III.
B. I and III only.
C. II and IV only.
D. IV only.
E. All are correct.
I. Noninvasive treatment alternative for patients with lung tumors
II. Outpatient procedure usually completed in less than a week
III. Minimized patient-related side effects and toxicity
IV. No need for chemotherapy

39. Which of the following patient can benefit from CyberKnife radiosurgery?
A. I, II, and III.
B. I and III only.
C. II and IV only.
D. IV only.
E. All are correct.
I. Medically inoperative patients
II. Poor/borderline surgical candidates
III. Patients with few other treatment options
IV. All lung tumor patients

40. Some components of CyberKnife is/are?
A. I, II, and III.
B. I and III only.
C. II and IV only.
D. IV only.
E. All are correct.
I. Synchrony camera
II. Ultrasound detector
III. Diagnostic x-ray source
IV. BAT

41. The CyberKnife safety zone is?
A. The distance between the robot position and virtual obstacle
B. The distance between the robot point of radiation and the personnel
C. Where radiation is below tolerance
D. The distance between the robot and the couch

Quiz 2 (Level 3)

1. Some of the benign lesions treated by stereotactic radiosurgery (SRS) are?
A. I, II, and III.
B. I and III only.
C. II and IV only.
D. IV only.
E. All are correct.
I. Meningiomas
II. Acoustic neuromas
III. Arteriovenous malformations (AVMs)
IV. Gliomas

2. Which of the following diseases are best treated with stereotactic irradiation?
A. I, II, and III.
B. I and III only.
C. II and IV only.
D. IV only.
E. All are correct.
I. Functional disorders
II. Chest wall malignancies
III. Metastatic tumors
IV. Whole brain metastases

3. The main components of the Gamma Knife unit are?
A. I, II, and III.
B. I and III only.
C. II and IV only.
D. IV only.
E. All are correct.
I. Radiation unit with an upper hemispherical shield and a central body
II. An operating table and sliding cradle
III. A set of four collimator helmets providing circular beams
IV. A robotic arm that holds the linac

4. A CyberKnife treatment machine uses?
A. I, II, and III.
B. I and III only.
C. II and IV only.
D. IV only.
E. All are correct.
I. A noninvasive image-guided target localization
II. A 6 MV linac mounted on an industrial robotic manipulator
III. A non-isocentric treatment technique
IV. A dual-energy (6 and 18 MV) linac mounted on an industrial robotic manipulator

3.4 Special Procedures and SRS (Questions)

5. CyberKnife offers the following improvements over standard radiosurgical techniques:
A. I, II, and III.
B. I and III only.
C. II and IV only.
D. IV only.
E. All are correct.
I. It allows frameless radiosurgery.
II. It monitors and tracks the patient's position continuously.
III. It allows for frameless radiosurgical dose delivery to extracranial targets such as spine, lung, and prostate.
IV. It allows the patient to move during treatment without affecting the treatment.

6. Which of the following dose is categorized as low-dose TBI?
A. Single fraction or up to six fractions of total dose 1,200 cGy
B. Ten to 15 fractions of 10–15 cGy each
C. Single fraction of 8 Gy delivered to the upper or lower half body
D. Twenty fractions with total dose of 40 Gy.

7. The most notable diseases treated with bone marrow transplantation (BMT) are?
A. I, II, and III.
B. I and III only.
C. II and IV only.
D. IV only.
E. All are correct.
I. Leukemia
II. Malignant lymphoma
III. Aplastic anemia
IV. Lymphoma

8. Which of the following are total body irradiation techniques?
A. I, II, and III.
B. I and III only.
C. II and IV only.
D. IV only.
E. All are correct.
I. Two short SSD parallel opposed beams
II. A dedicated TBI cobalt-60
III. Extended SSD with patient standing
IV. Extended SSD with patient on a stretcher

9. Which of the following devices are used to produce the large and uniform electron fields on total skin electron irradiation (TSEI) treatments?
A. I, II, and III.
B. I and III only.
C. II and IV only.
D. IV only.
E. All are correct.
I. Beam spoilers
II. Blocks
III. Special filters
IV. Wedges

10. Which of the following dosimetric parameters is considered on large total skin electron irradiations (TSEI)?
A. I, II, and III.
B. I and III only.
C. II and IV only.
D. IV only.
E. All are correct.
I. Field flatness at Dmax
II. Electron beam output at dose calibration point
III. PDDs measured at a depth of 15 cm
IV. TMR measured at a depth of 15 cm

11. Which of the following statements are true about intraoperative radiotherapy (IORT)?
A. I, II, and III.
B. I and III only.
C. II and IV only.
D. IV only.
E. All are correct.
I. IORT is a single-fraction special radiotherapeutic technique.
II. IORT delivers a radiation dose of the order of 10–20 Gy.
III. IORT combines surgery and radiotherapy treatments.
IV. Once the IORT is performed, external beam radiotherapy cannot be done in the same area.

12. Which of the following personnel are involved in intraoperative radiotherapy (IORT) treatment?
A. I, II, and III.
B. I and III only.
C. II and IV only.
D. IV only.
E. All are correct.
I. Surgeon
II. Radiation oncologist
III. Medical physicist
IV. Radiation therapist

3.4 Special Procedures and SRS (Questions) 263

13. Which of the following modalities can be used to deliver radiation dose intraoperatively?
A. I, II, and III.
B. I and III only.
C. II and IV only.
D. IV only.
E. All are correct.
I. Orthovoltage x-ray
II. Megavoltage electron beams
III. High-dose rate (HDR) Ir-192 brachytherapy sources
IV. CyberKnife

14. Which of the following statements are true about endocavitary rectal irradiation?
A. I, II, and III.
B. I and III only.
C. II and IV only.
D. IV only.
E. All are correct.
I. Endocavitary rectal irradiation is a sphincter-saving procedure used in the treatment of selected rectal carcinomas with superficial x-rays.
II. There must be a mobile lesion with a maximum diameter of 3 cm.
III. The location of the lesion must be within 10 cm from the anal canal.
IV. No evidence of lymph node or distance metastases can be found.

15. Endorectal treatment technique includes?
A. I, II, and III.
B. I and III only.
C. II and IV only.
D. IV only.
E. All are correct.
I. Short SSD technique of the order of 4 cm
II. Tumor dose of 80 Gy delivered in two or three fractions of 20–30 Gy given 2 weeks apart
III. Long SSD technique of the order of 20 cm
IV. Short SSD technique of the order of 10 cm

16. Which of the following diseases is primarily treated with radiosurgery CyberKnife treatment?
A. I, II, and III.
B. I and III only.
C. II and IV only.
D. IV only.
E. All are correct.
I. Meningiomas
II. Acoustic neuroma
III. Gliomas
IV. Trigeminal neuralgia

17. Stereotactic radiosurgery with CyberKnife treatments requires?
A. I, II, and III.
B. I and III only.
C. II and IV only.
D. IV only.
E. All are correct.
I. High precision
II. Steep dose gradients
III. Reliability
IV. Reproducibility

18. Which of the following problems can be seen on a linac radiosurgery machine?
A. I, II, and III.
B. I and III only.
C. II and IV only.
D. IV only.
E. All are correct.
I. Tolerance errors
II. Focal spot size
III. Inferior treatment planning system
IV. Flattening filter

19. Which of the following planning systems are used in CyberKnife?
A. Eclipse planning system
B. Multiplan planning system
C. Corvus-Nomus planning system
D. ADAC-Pinnacle

20. Which of the following is/are true about CyberKnife?
A. I, II, and III.
B. I and III only.
C. II and IV only.
D. IV only.
E. All are correct.
I. It is made by KUKA.
II. It has six degrees of freedom.
III. It has 0.2 mm repeatability.
IV. Arms allow rotational and translational movements.

21. CyberKnife is:
A. I, II, and III.
B. I and III only.
C. II and IV only.
D. IV only.
E. All are correct.
I. An isocentric treatment
II. A non-isocentric treatment

3.4 Special Procedures and SRS (Questions)   265

III. A noncoplanar treatment
IV. A coplanar treatment

22. Which of the following algorithm is used in CyberKnife?
A. AAA calculation
B. Pencil beam calculation
C. Monte Carlo calculation
D. Acuros

23. Which of the following TG is associated with QA for robotic radiosurgery?
A. TG-142
B. TG-135
C. TG-179
D. TG-51

24. What is the CyberKnife geometric isocenter?
A. Is a reference point in the room which serves as the origin for several coordinate systems used within the CyberKnife application
B. Refers to an isocentric treatment to a target
C. Refers to the isocenter selected on the planning system
D. Refers to the robot cough isocenter

25. The source-to-axis distance (SAD) on a CyberKnife machine is?
A. 150 cm SAD
B. 100 cm SAD
C. 80 cm SAD
D. 50 cm SAD

26. As per TG-135, which of the following QAs must be done daily on a CyberKnife machine?
A. I, II, and III.
B. I and III only.
C. II and IV only.
D. IV only.
E. All are correct.
I. Safety interlocks
II. Accelerator output
III. Accelerator warm-up
IV. Imager alignment

27. The CyberKnife path is defined as?
A. Preassigned points in space where the linac can deliver radiation from multiple beam angles
B. Preassigned points in space where the manipulator is allowed to stop in order to deliver radiation dose
C. A fixed and predetermined workspace where the robotic arm can move
D. The geometric isocenter where the beam is aimed

3.5 Nuclear Medicine Therapy (Questions)

Quiz 1 (Level 3)

1. 60–80 % of patients with a history of colorectal carcinoma, pancreatic carcinoma, breast cancer, and others will develop?
A. Brain metastases
B. Lung metastases
C. Liver metastases
D. Pancreas metastases

2. Which of the following are considered liver-directed treatments?
A. I, II, and III.
B. I and III only.
C. II and IV only.
D. IV only.
E. All are correct.
I. Conformal radiation therapy
II. Hepatic arterial infusion chemotherapy (HAC)
III. Transarterial chemoembolization (TACE)
IV. Radioembolization (RE) using yttrium-90.

3. Hepatic metastases and primary neoplasm are often?
A. Focal and regular in shape
B. Focal and irregular in shape
C. Multifocal and regular in shape
D. Multifocal and irregular in shape

4. A nonsurgical, outpatient therapy that uses microscopic radioactive spheres to deliver high dose of radiation directly to the site of the liver tumors is called?
A. Low-dose radiosurgery therapy (LDR)
B. High-dose radiosurgery therapy (HDR)
C. Selective internal radiation therapy (SIRT)
D. Stereotactic radiation therapy (SRT)

5. The main advantage of selective internal radiation therapy (SIRT) over a traditional method is?
A. Low toxicity
B. No adverse effects
C. Curative treatment
D. Fewer treatments

6. Which of the following radioisotopes are used for selective internal radiation therapy (SIRT)?
A. Iridium-192 (Ir-192)
B. Yttrium-90 (Y-90)
C. Iodine-125 (I-125)
D. Phosphorus-32 (P-32)

3.5 Nuclear Medicine Therapy (Questions)

7. The dose administered for selective internal radiation therapy (SIRT) is?
A. 150–500 Gy
B. 50–150 cGy
C. 50–150 Gy
D. 30 Gy

8. Which of the following studies is/are used on selective internal radiation therapy (SIRT) workup?
A. I, II, and III.
B. I and III only.
C. II and IV only.
D. IV only.
E. All are correct.
I. Computed tomography (CT)
II. Magnetic resonance imaging (MRI)
III. Positron emission tomography
IV. Ultrasound

9. Which organ would be the major concern for normal tissue complication if the patient is treated with Y-90?
A. Gallbladder
B. Lung
C. Stomach
D. Pancreas

10. AAPM Task Group has an important document for Y-90 treatments; which of the following is the right document?
A. TG-143
B. TG-138
C. TG-144
D. TG-101

11. To treat hepatocellular carcinoma (HCC), to which part of the body is the Y-90 microsphere solution injected with the image guidance of angiography?
A. Femoral artery
B. Hepatic artery
C. Splenic artery
D. Pulmonary vein

12. How could therapy with Y-90 selectively treat hepatocellular carcinoma (HCC) alone in the liver without putting a lot of dose to most healthy part of the liver?
A. Hepatocellular carcinoma selectively absorbs Y-90 solution.
B. The uptake of Y-90 in other parts of the liver is negligible.
C. Arteries are chosen that carry blood through the part of the organ which has the disease.
D. Tumor is more sensitive to radiation than healthy normal tissues in the organ.

13. Which of the following isotopes of iodine is used to treat thyroid cancer?
A. I-123
B. I-124
C. I-125
D. I-131

14. What is the standard method for the patient to acquire iodine isotopes to treat thyroid cancer?
A. Injection of solutions with iodine ions
B. Swallow iodine salt tabulates with juice
C. Implant iodine seeds to the thyroid
D. Being exposed to radiation of iodine isotopes

3.6 Isodose Curve Parameters and Isodose Distributions (Answers)

Quiz 1 (Level 2)

1. **B**   A plot of the volume of a given structure receiving a certain dose or higher as a function of dose is the definition of integral DVH; differential DVH is a plot of volume receiving a dose within a specified dose interval (or dose bin) as a function of dose. An isodose chart is a dose distribution in the form of isodose curves or surfaces showing regions of uniform dose, high dose, or low dose, and a beam's eye view is a view of patient from the target, through the beam portal showing patient anatomy within the treatment beam.

2. **A**   Dose volume histogram (DVH) provides quantitative information with regard to how much dose is absorbed in how much volume. It is also a great tool for evaluating a given plan or comparing competing plans. A DVH summarizes the entire dose distribution into a single curve for each anatomic structure of interest; unfortunately, a DVH does not display the area where hot spot is located; it just shows how hot the plan is. In other words, it takes a complex 3-dimensional dose distribution and simplifies it into two dimensions at the cost of losing spatial information.

3. **A**   Isodose charts consist of a family of isodose curves which are usually drawn for equal increments of percent depth dose; they have lines representing equal percentage depth dose for a particular field size and SSD at a specific plane in tissue, but isodose charts do not give you information of the spatial location of the dose distribution.

4. **E**   All of the statements are true. Line A max dose is 9 Gy. The maximum dose can be found by looking at the dose received by 0 % of the volume. As the volume gets closer to 0 %, this represents the hottest voxel in the structure. The V20 Gy refers to the volume of the structure receiving 20 Gy. In this

case, the V20 Gy is about 19 % which is less than 20 %. This could also be written as the D20 % must be less than 20 Gy. This means that 20 % of the volume should receive less than 20 Gy. For line B, the D20 % is about 18 Gy which is again less than 20 Gy. For line C, 30 % of the volume is receiving just about 30 Gy. Finally, the dose received by 95 % of the structure (D95 %) is about 59 Gy which is less than the prescription dose of 60 Gy which is not acceptable.

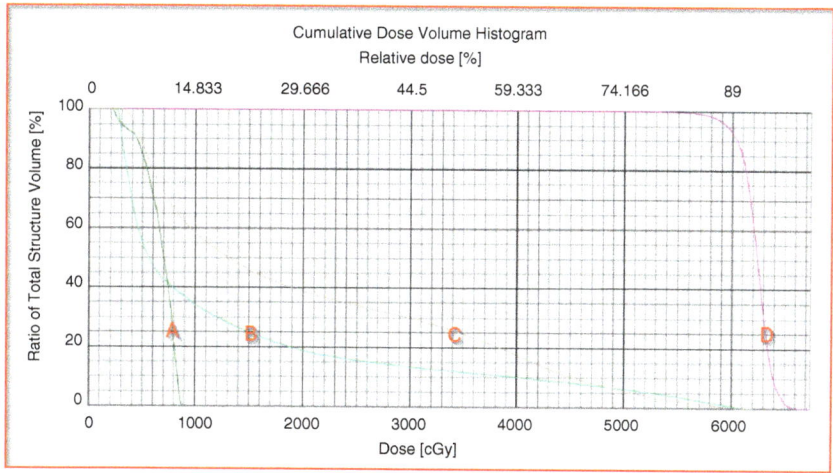

Fig. 3A.1.1 Courtesy of the University of Miami, Sylvester Cancer Center

5.B Based on the following graph, the oral cavity max dose is approximately 65 Gy and about 20 % of the volume received at least 60 Gy.

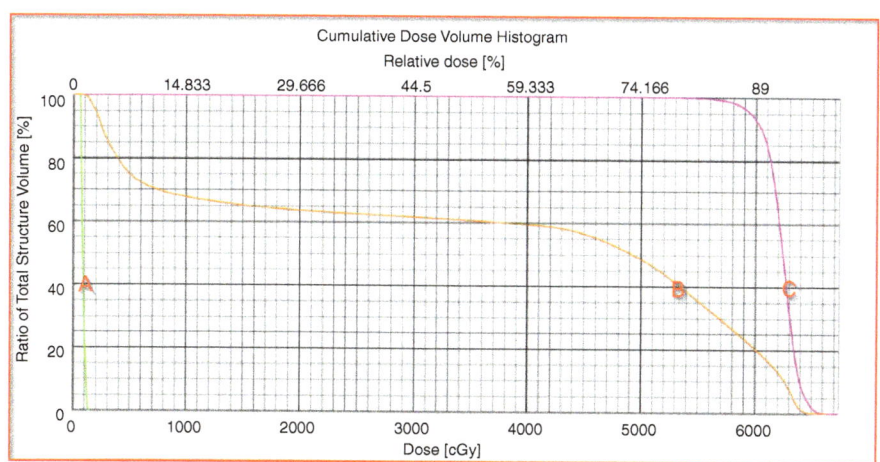

Fig. 3A.1.2 Courtesy of the University of Miami, Sylvester Cancer Center

6. **B** Of the two forms of DVH, the cumulative DVH has been found to be more useful and more commonly used than the differential DVH.

Cumulative DVH – each bin shows the volume of the structure receiving that dose and greater.

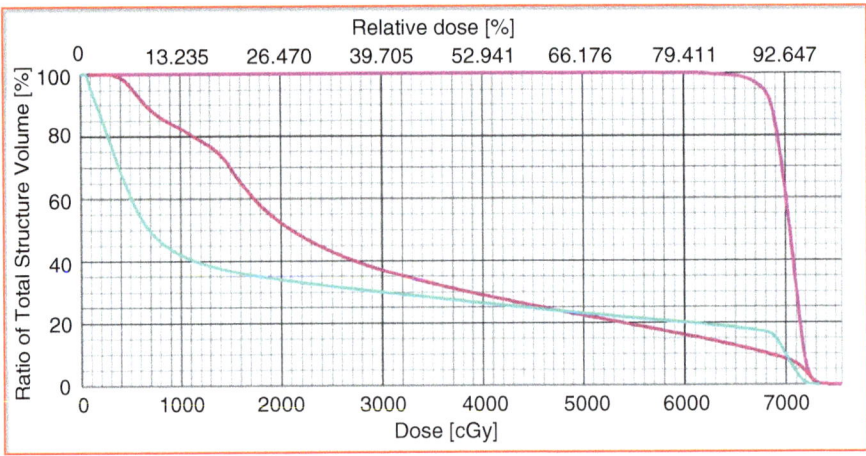

Fig. 3A.1.3 Courtesy of the University of Miami, Sylvester Cancer Center

Differential DVH – each bin represents the volume receiving that dose exactly.

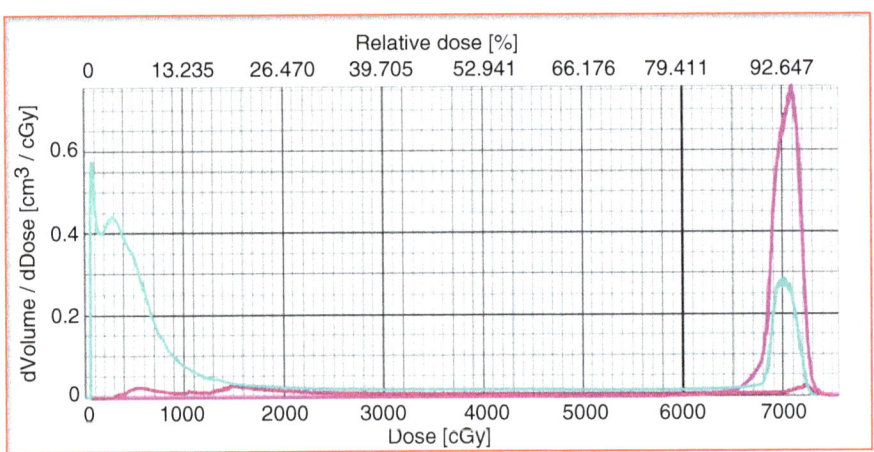

Fig. 3A.1.4 Courtesy of the University of Miami, Sylvester Cancer Center

3.6 Isodose Curve Parameters and Isodose Distributions (Answers)

7. **D** A three-dimensional image set like a CT scan of the patient is needed to create isodose distributions and DVHs since there needs to be a structure and a dose distribution. Electron clinical setups do not require a CT scan or any drawn structures. During a clinical setup, only hand MU calculations are needed. Rule of thumb: no structure contours, no DVH.

8. **E** All of the following may contain a dose volume histogram (DVH) of the PTV and organs at risk (depending what the physician contours). Remember, the only radiation treatments that cannot have DVH are clinical setups where a 3D image set is not acquired.

9. **C** The 50 % isodose line will typically represent the field edge or border.

10. **B** When a composite plan is done, it is essential that the doses contributed by each plan be added together and a composite isodose distribution be displayed. Isodose charts are produced by measuring the dose distribution in a water phantom and a DVH is an essential tool to evaluate a plan, but other parameters must be considered such as isodose distribution in the transverse, coronal, and sagittal view as the DVH loses the spatial information in the dose distribution.

11. **B** In general, 95 % of the PTV must receive 100 % of the prescribed dose and 5 % of the volume should not receive more than 110 % of the prescribed dose. In an ideal world, 100 % of the target would receive 100 % of the prescription dose and 0 % of the target would receive 101 % of the prescription dose, but a dose distribution like this is impossible to deliver, even with protons or heavy ions. Therefore, in a clinical situation, a compromise is made to achieve the best deliverable plan.

12. **A** Isodose curves are lines passing through points of equal dose expressed as a percentage of the dose at a reference point and they represent levels of absorbed dose. To determine the location of a hot spot, a three-dimensional image set and dose distribution with isodose curves are required.

13. **B** The depth dose values of the isodose curves are typically normalized to a certain depth on the central axis or to the global maximum dose point. Isodose lines can be normalized to any point the user wants; these two are usually chosen as they make sense in terms of prescribing the dose and it avoids confusion.

14. **A** The dose at depth is greatest on the central axis of the beam and gradually decreases toward the edges of the beam. Remember that near the field edges, the dose rate decreases rapidly as a function of lateral distance from the beam axis. Isodose curves at a specified depth are important as the penumbra is defined as the lateral distance between two specified isodose curves at a specified depth such as 80 and 20 %.

15. B Horns are high-dose areas near the surface in the periphery of the field created by the flattening filter. As the depth increases, the horns go away because as photons scatter, the central portion of the beam gains scatter contribution from both edges of the beam while the edges of the beam also lose photons to scatter out of the field.

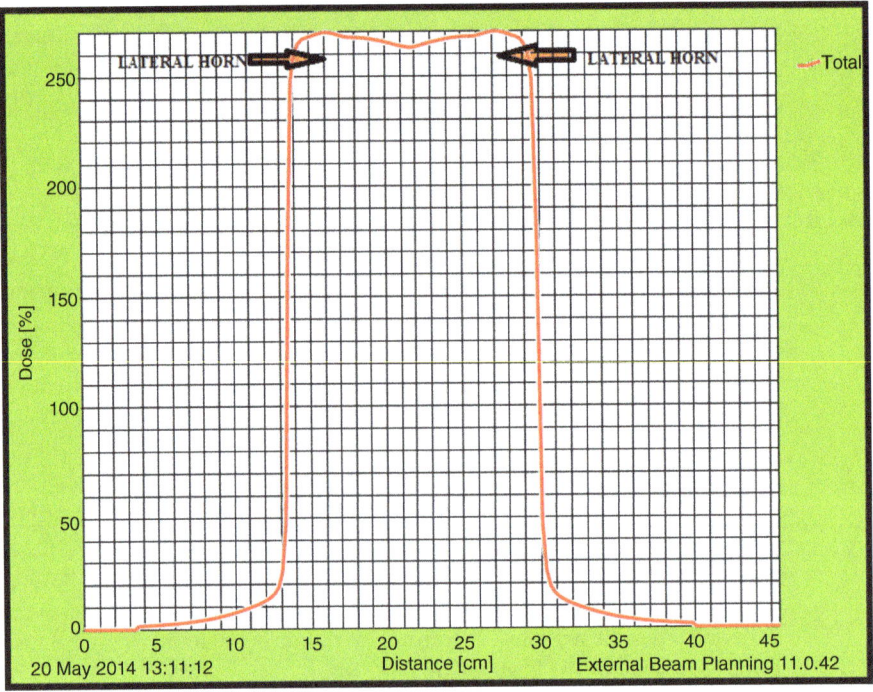

Fig. 3A.1.5 Courtesy of the University of Miami, Sylvester Cancer Center

16. C The field size is defined as the lateral distance between the 50 % isodose lines at a reference depth. The field-defining light is made to coincide with the 50 % isodose lines of the radiation beam projected on a plane perpendicular to the beam axis.

17. D The following graph represents a beam profile which shows the dose variation across the field at a specified depth.

3.6 Isodose Curve Parameters and Isodose Distributions (Answers)

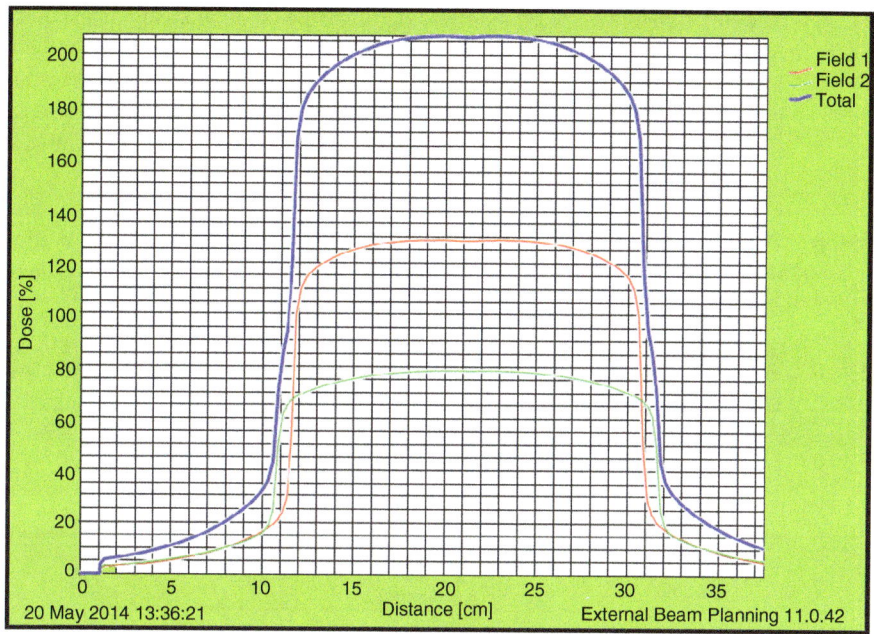

Fig. 3A.1.6 Courtesy of the University of Miami, Sylvester Cancer Center

18. **E** Isodose distributions are affected by beam energy or quality, source size, beam collimator, field size, SSD, and SDD.

19. **E** All statements are correct. Lower-energy beams cause the isodose curves outside the field to bulge out due to the increased side scatter at lower energies. As photon energy increases, scatter tends to be in the forward direction.

20. **B** The flattening filter has the greatest influence in determining the shape of the isodose curves. Without a flattening filter, the isodose curves will be conical in shape, showing markedly increased x-ray intensity along the central axis and a rapid reduction transversely. Modern linear accelerators actually allow treatment with flattening filter-free (FFF) beams. The reason for this is that the flattening filter attenuates the beam which lowers the dose rate, makes the beam harder, and adds contamination to the beam. With the increased use of IMRT and SBRT, the size of fields is becoming smaller, so the peaked dose distribution of an FFF beam is not a problem. Additionally, new planning systems can model the peaked dose distribution therefore treating with an FFF beam is not problematic. Removing the flattening filter allows for an increased dose rate and less beam contamination.

21. C The function of the flattening filter is to make the beam intensity distribution relatively uniform across the field. Trimmers are used to reduce the penumbra of a therapy beam, and a monitor chamber measures and verifies precise amounts of radiation delivered to the patient. Finally, the klystron is a high-power microwave amplifier used to power high-energy linear accelerators.

22. B The most commonly used isodose beam-modifying device is the wedge which causes a progressive decrease in the intensity across the beam, resulting in a tilt of the isodose curves from their normal positions.

23. B Wedges tilt the isodose curves toward the thin end of the wedge and this degree of tilt depends on the slope of the wedge.

24. B Cumulative DVH graph absolute dose

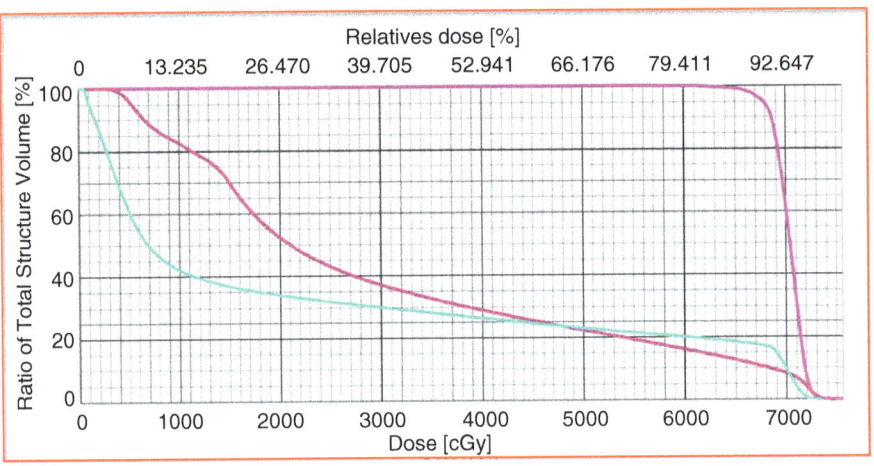

Fig. 3A.1.7 Courtesy of the University of Miami, Sylvester Cancer Center

3.6 Isodose Curve Parameters and Isodose Distributions (Answers)

C. Cumulative DVH graph absolute volume

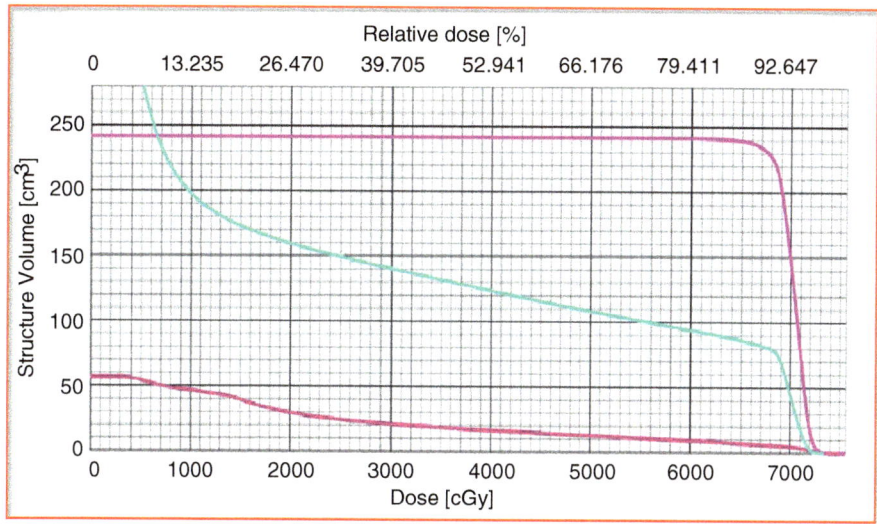

Fig. 3A.1.8 Courtesy of the University of Miami, Sylvester Cancer Center

A. Differential DVH graph absolute dose

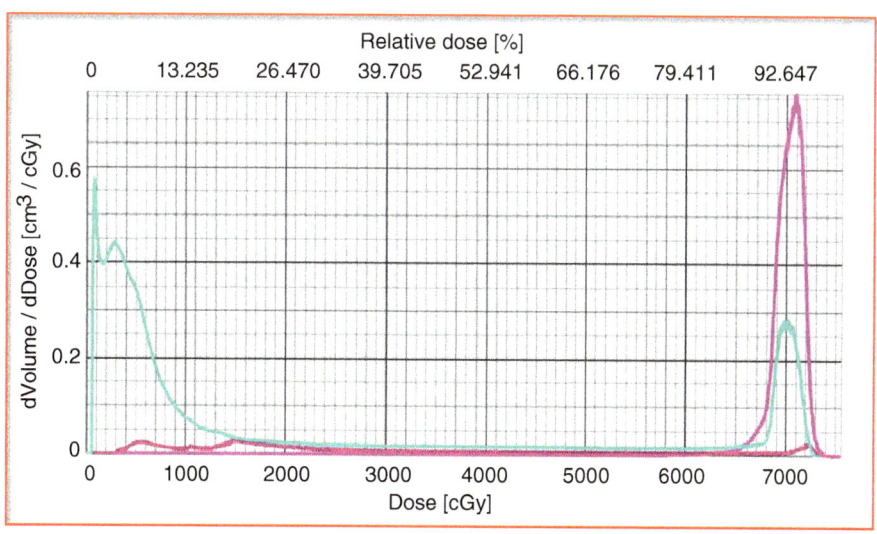

Fig. 3A.1.9 Courtesy of the University of Miami, Sylvester Cancer Center

25. C Cumulative DVH displayed in absolute volume is used to evaluate a particular volume of structures receiving certain dose instead of the relative percentage of that structure receiving that dose.

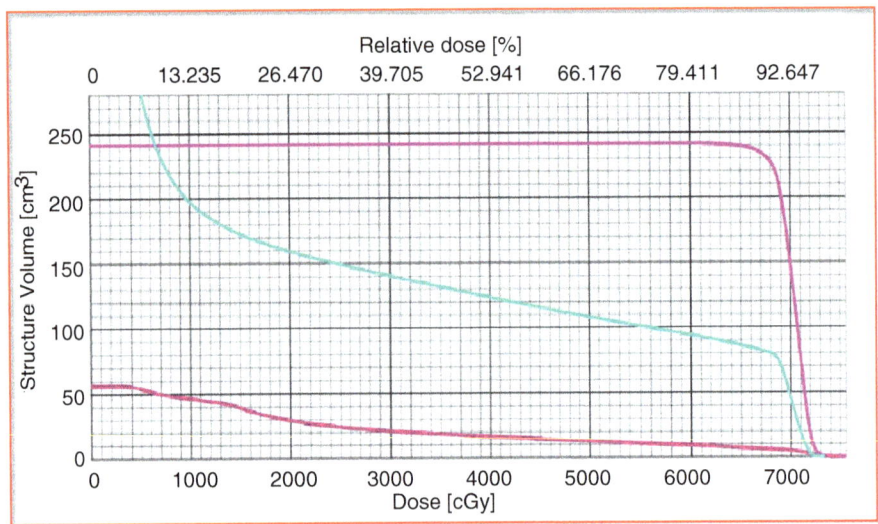

Fig. 3A.1.10 Courtesy of the University of Miami, Sylvester Cancer Center

26. A The advantages of parallel opposed fields are the simplicity and reproducibility of the setup, a more homogeneous dose to the tumor than a single field, and less chances of geometrical miss. The disadvantage of parallel opposed fields is the excessive dose to normal tissues and critical organs above and below the tumor. To reduce the dose to the critical structures, additional fields can be added to increase the dose conformity to the target.

27. E In general, the isodose uniformity distribution depends on patient thickness and beam energy. As the patient thickness increases and the beam energy decreases, the central axis maximum dose near the surface increases relative to the midpoint dose. Also, beam flatness is an important parameter, and by using the appropriate beam weighting, the dose distribution within the irradiated volume can be made more uniform.

28. A NIST = National Institute of Standards and Technology
ADCL = Accredited Dosimetry Calibration Laboratory

3.6 Isodose Curve Parameters and Isodose Distributions (Answers)

NIST or ADCL performs absolute dose measurements with calorimeters, ionization chambers, or Fricke (chemical) dosimeters. Calorimetry is the most basic method for the determination of absorbed dose, but because of technical difficulties, it is not practical in the clinical setting. Integral dose is a measure of the total energy absorbed in the treated volume. If the mass of tissue receives a uniform dose, then the integral dose is simply the product of mass and dose. Remember that integral dose is basically the product of mass and dose, and its unit is the gram-rad or kilogram-gray or simply joule. Relative dose is the ratio of the dose at one point in a phantom to the dose at another point.

29. E Some strategies used to maximize dose to the tumor while minimizing dose to surrounding tissue are using fields of appropriate size, increasing the number of fields, selecting appropriate beam direction, adjusting beam weights, using appropriate beam energy, and using beam modifiers. All of these increase the conformity of the dose distribution.

30. E The isocenter is defined as the point of intersection of the collimator axis and the gantry axis of rotation. An isocentric treatment technique consists of placing the isocenter of the machine at a depth within the patient and directing the beams from different directions meaning that the distance of the source from the isocenter (SAD) remains constant irrespective of the beam direction, but the source-to-skin distance (SSD) may change, depending on the beam direction and shape of the patient contour. With an SSD technique, the SSD is held constant which would mean that the patient might have to be shifted for multiple beam angles. With an isocentric technique, multiple beam angles can be treated without shifting the patient which reduces the possibility of a treatment error.

31. A The source-to-skin distance is equal to source-to-axis distance minus depth ($SSD = SAD - d$).

32. C The lateral distance between two specified isodose curves at specified depth is used to estimate the physical penumbra. The transmission penumbra is the region irradiated by photons which are transmitted through the edge of the collimator block. A beam profile is a graph which represents the dose variation across the field at a specified depth, and tissue lateral effect is the increase of the central axis maximum dose near the surface relative to the midpoint dose as the patient thickness increases and the energy decreases.

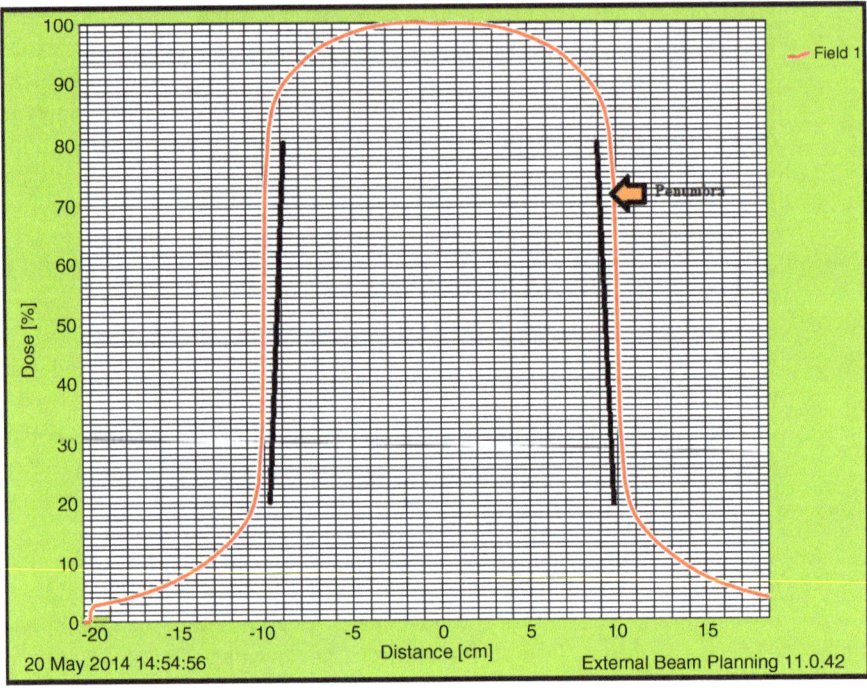

Fig. 3A.1.11 Courtesy of the University of Miami, Sylvester Cancer Center

33. **B** Outside the geometric limits of the beam and the penumbra, the dose variation is the result of side scatter from the field and leakage and scatter from the collimator. Beyond this collimator zone, the dose distribution is governed by the lateral scatter from the medium and leakage from the head of the machine.

34. **A** Isodose charts can be measured by means of an ion chamber, solid-state detector, or film. Of these dosimetry methods, ion chambers are the most reliable method, mainly because of the relatively flat energy response. Calorimetry is the most direct method of determining absorbed dose, but it is not practical to measure a full dose distribution.

35. **B** The ionization chamber used for isodose measurements should be small and be energy independent so that the energy response of the chamber should be as flat as possible. If the volume is too large, then there will be volume averaging in the chamber and the dose distribution will be smoothed out. If the chamber is not energy independent, then as the spectrum changes with depth, the chamber response would also change which is not ideal.

36. **C** A wedge pair is normally used for treating small, superficial tumor volumes. When this technique is used, the high-dose region (hot spot) is moved toward the thin end of the wedge (toe). The hot spot increases with

3.6 Isodose Curve Parameters and Isodose Distributions (Answers)

field size and wedge angle as this effect is related to the differential attenuation of the beam under the thick end relative to the thin end of the wedge. In the case below, the wedge is helping to compensate for the reduced thickness anteriorly.

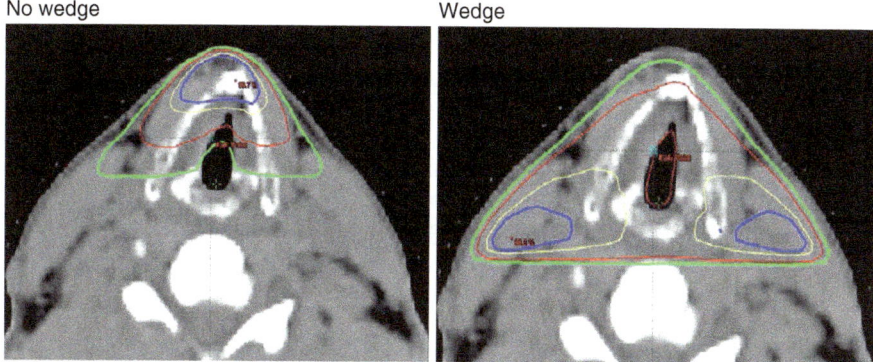

Fig. 3A.1.12 Courtesy of the University of Miami, Sylvester Cancer Center

37. E All of the following techniques can be used to obtain an acceptable uniform dose distribution depending on the clinical situation.

38. E Radiation treatment planning process is based on the pathology, staging, diagnostic exams, and Karnofsky score of the patient.

39. A In 1978, the International Commission on Radiation Units and Measurements (ICRU) Report No. 50 and 62 (24, 25) established a general dose specification system to be adopted universally using a schematic representation of various volumes (GTV, CTV, PTV, treatment volume, irradiated volume). NCRP is a group of experts who evaluate ICRP recommendations in terms of their applicability to the uses of ionizing radiation in the United States as well as develop standards for issues that are unique to the use of radiation in this country. The Atomic Energy Commission (AEC) is a predecessor to the US Nuclear Regulatory Committee (NRC).

40. B The gross tumor volume (GTV) is the extent and location of the visible tumor only. The clinical target volume (CTV) is the tumor(s) if present and any other tissue with presumed tumor or microscopic disease, and the internal target volume (ITV) compensates for internal physiological movements and variation in size, shape, and position of the CTV. Finally, the planning target volume (PTV) includes the CTV (or ITV) with setup margin for patient movement and setup uncertainties.

41. E All statements are correct.

42. B Planning organ at risk (OR) needs adequate protection, and once the planning organ at risk volume is identified, margins may be needed to compensate for its movements, internal, as well as setup to ensure the dose remains below tolerance. Organs at risk (OR) must be evaluated independently so the margin can change depending on the location of the OAR and the distance from the OAR to the PTV. All organs at risk are extremely important, and more care might have to be taken if the OAR is abutting the PTV. In all cases, caution must be taken so that the OAR dose is as low as reasonably achievable (ALARA).

43. A The treatment volume is a margin added to the target volume to allow for limitations of treatment technique and depends on a particular treatment technique used. The treatment volume is larger than the planning target volume, but smaller than the irradiated volume.

44. C The maximum target dose is the highest dose in the target area that covers a minimum of 2 cm^2. A hot spot is an area *outside* the target volume that receives a higher dose than the specified target dose. The mean target dose is the mean of the absorbed dose values at discrete points uniformly distributed in the target area, and the modal target dose is the absolute dose that occurs most frequently within the target area.

45. A The reference point used to record target dose recommended by the ICRU should be selected so that the dose at this point is of clinical relevance and representative of the dose throughout the PTV. It also should be located where the dose can be accurately calculated and be easy to define in a clear and unambiguous way. The point should not lie in the penumbra region or where there is a steep dose gradient as there is a high degree of uncertainty in this location in the dose distribution.

46. C The reference point used to record target dose recommended by the ICRU for parallel opposed, unequally weighted beams should be specified on the central axis placed within the PTV. For rotational arc therapy, the point should be specified at the center of rotation in the principal plane. For parallel opposed, equally weighted beams, the point should be on the central axis midway between the beam entrances, and, finally, for more than two beams, the point should be at the intersection of the central axes of the beams placed within the PTV.

47. A Ionization chambers should be calibrated by an Accredited Dose Calibration Laboratory (ADCL) or the National Institute of Standards and Technology (NIST) if they are to be used to calibrate a linear accelerator or brachytherapy source for patient treatments. Radiochromic film, silicon detectors, and TLDs are used to find the relative dose or the ratio of the dose at one point in a phantom to the dose at another point but are not usually used to measure the absolute dose at a point or calibrate a linac or brachytherapy source.

3.7 Electron Beam Dose Distributions (Answers)

Quiz 1 (Level 2)

1. **E** All of these. Similar to photon beams, when the field size is changed, the dose rate and isodose distribution will change.

2. **D** The depth where there is a rapid dose falloff depends on the incident electron energy. This is why electron energy selection must be considered based on the tumor depth.

3. **C** As a rule of thumb, the electron energy in MeV should be three times the maximum depth of a given tumor; that is, for a 4 cm treatment depth, a 12 MeV electron beam should be used.

4. **C** The most clinically useful energy range for electrons is 6–20 MeV since at these energies the electron can be used to treat superficial tumors (less than 5 cm deep) with a characteristically sharp drop-off in dose beyond the tumor. A downside to high-energy electron beams is the bremsstrahlung tail which is a dose that is deposited beyond the electron dose. It is a result of the bremsstrahlung photons that are created as the electrons are slowed down in the tissue. The higher the electron beam energy, the larger the dose carried deeper by the bremsstrahlung photons, reducing the effectiveness of the electron treatment.

5. **D** Electron treatment can be used for any superficial lesions. For deep-seated tumors, the use of electrons is not recommended. The best treatment for prostate cancer is photon IMRT.

6. **E** Electrons interact with atoms through inelastic collisions with atomic electrons (ionization and excitation), inelastic collisions with nuclei (bremsstrahlung), elastic collisions with atomic electrons, and elastic collisions with nuclei.

7. **A** The rate of electron energy loss depends primarily on electron density of the medium. The rate of energy loss in tissue or water can be approximated as 2 MeV/cm.

8. **C** II and IV only, the rate of energy loss per gram per cm squared (stopping power) is greater for low atomic number materials or low-Z materials; this is because high-Z materials have fewer electrons per gram than low-Z materials and high-Z materials have more tightly bound electrons.

9. **B** Rule of thumb: the energy loss rate of electrons per cm in water is roughly about 2 MeV/cm of water.

10. B The rate of energy loss to bremsstrahlung interactions in an electron beam per cm is proportional to the electron energy and the square of the atomic number (Z^2). Remember that the rest mass of an electron is 0.511 MeV.

11. C II and IV only, the electron scattering power varies approximately as the square of the atomic number (Z^2) and inversely as the square of the kinetic energy.

12. A The practical electron range is defined as the depth of the point where the tangent to the descending linear portion of the curve intersects the extrapolated background. The R_{50} is defined as the depth at which the dose is 50 % of the maximum dose. A point in space that is the same distance from the source for all gantry angles is called the isocenter, and finally, the thickness of the material that reduces the intensity of the beam to half (50 %) its original value is the half-value layer (HVL).

13. A As electron beam energy increases, dose increases, the penumbra at the surface decreases, and the penumbra at depth increases. This bulging of the isodose lines at depth makes it difficult to match electron fields as a hot spot can result where the bulging isodose lines overlap at depth.

14. C The correct energy if a physician asks the dosimetrist that he would like to prescribe an electron treatment at a depth of 3 cm using 90 % depth dose is 12 MeV. Remember:
At 90 % PDD $\approx$ E (MeV)/4.
At 80 % PDD $\approx$ E (MeV)/3.
$R_p \approx$ E (MeV)/2.

15. D The higher the energy, the higher the surface dose or less skin-sparing effect. This is the opposite for photons where a higher energy results in more skin sparing. This is due to the fact that electrons are directly ionizing and photons are indirectly ionizing.

16. B Superficial tumors are best treated with electron beam treatments due to the superficial dose and rapid falloff of dose. Photon beam treatments are best suited for deep tumors as dose can be deposited at depth but still maintain skin sparing. Protons have an advantage over conventional photons due to the Bragg peak and no exit dose. CyberKnife treatments utilize a robotic delivery that can compensate for target motion and are used for SRS and SRT treatments.

17. B The most useful treatment depth or therapeutic range of electrons is given by the 90 % depth dose.

18. C The choice of beam energy is much more critical for electrons than for photons. Because the dose decreases abruptly beyond the 90 % dose level, the

3.7 Electron Beam Dose Distributions (Answers)

treatment depth and the required electron energy must be chosen very carefully. The guiding principle is that when in doubt, use higher electron energy to make sure that the target volume is well within the specified isodose curve.

19. E All the statements are correct; at lower energies, the electrons are scattered more easily and through larger angles, and the ratio of surface dose to maximum dose is less for the lower-energy electrons than for the higher-energy electrons.

20. B Uniformity or flatness of the electron beam is usually specified in a plane perpendicular to the beam axis and at the depth of the 95 % isodose beyond the depth of dose maximum.

21. E All the statements are true.

22. C Acceptable field flatness and symmetry on an electron beam can be obtained by using proper design of beam scatterers. Typically, one or more scattering foils could be used; the first foil widens the beam by multiple scattering, whereas the additional foils make the beam uniform in cross section like a flattening filter. Also, by using proper beam-defining collimators, primary collimation defines the maximum field size and a secondary collimator placed close to the patient defines the treatment field. MLCs are not used for electron treatments and are used on photon beams to shape the field electron cones, and cutouts are used to shape electron fields and should have a minimum distance of 15 cm from the skin surface so that electron contamination or scatter does not affect the patient.

23. B The linear accelerator generates a pencil beam of electrons that exits the vacuum and impinges on the scattering foils spreading the pencil beam into a clinically useful, flat beam. Because of this scattering, the electron beam appears to emanate from a point that is closer than the target where photons originate from. The apparent point where the electron beam appears to originate from is called the virtual point or virtual source. This point is closer to the patient than the photon target (<100 cm).

24. D The tail of the electron depth-dose curve at the point where it becomes straight is due to bremsstrahlung interactions of electrons with the patient. Remember that the target is moved out of the way for electron treatments and that photons undergo photoelectric interactions, not electrons.

25. E All electron broad fields are equivalent because their depth-dose distribution is the same irrespective of field size. Field equivalence is relevant only for small fields in which the lateral scatter equilibrium does not exist and, consequently, the PDD is field size dependent. The size at which this occurs is energy dependent since the scattering distance increases as energy increases.

26. A In an electron treatment, energy should be selected based on depth of target volume, minimum target dose required, and clinically acceptable dose to critical organs. The choice of field size in electron beam therapy should be strictly based on the isodose coverage of the target volume.

27. A Electron beam obliquity tends to increase side scatter at Dmax, decrease the depth of penetration, and shift Dmax toward the surface.

28. D The dose distribution for an electron beam beyond an inhomogeneity can be corrected by using the coefficient of equivalent thickness (CET) method. The CET for a given material is approximately given by its electron density relative to that of water. Remember that some methods of inhomogeneity corrections for photon beams are the TAR and isodose shift methods. The effective SSD method is used when corrections for surface obliquities are needed.

29. A Bolus is often used in electron beam therapy to flatten out an irregular surface, reduce the penetration of the electrons in parts of the field, and increase the surface dose. Remember that the bolus will decrease the depth-dose.

30. E All these can be used as bolus material.

31. B Plates of low atomic number material used on the patient's skin to reduce the energy of an electron beam are known as decelerators. Lucite and polystyrene are both examples of decelerators. Compensators are used when a radiation beam incident on an irregular or sloping surface produces skewing of the isodose curves; wedges are considered compensators.

32. B Large air gaps between the bolus and the surface would result in reduction in dose due to scattering of electrons outside the field.

33. C When an electron field is abutted at the surface with a photon field, a hot spot develops on the side of the photon field, and a cold spot develops on the side of the electron field. This is caused by outscattering of electrons from the electron field into the photon field at depth. We addressed this phenomenon earlier when we were talking about the bulging of the isodose lines at depth in electron beams.

3.7 Electron Beam Dose Distributions (Answers)

Fig. 3A.2.1

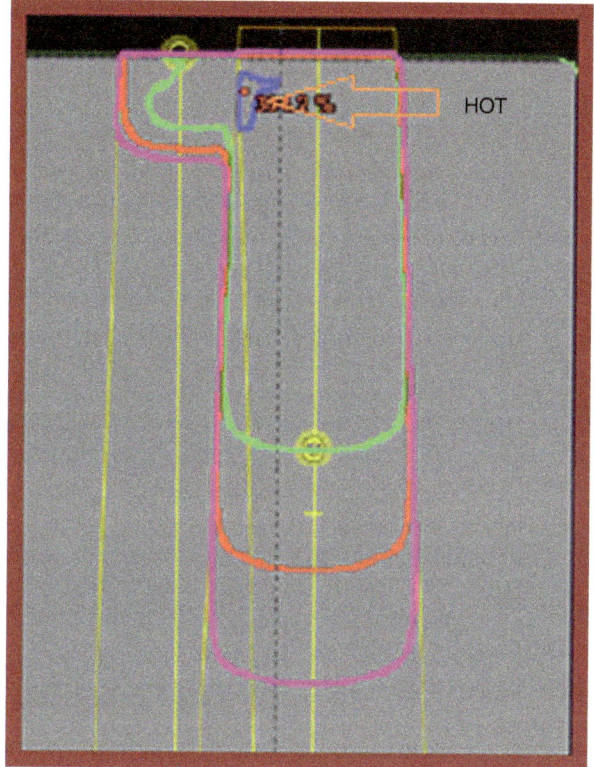

34. **C** Field shaping can be accomplished in electron beam therapy by using lead cutouts. The cutouts are typically placed on the end of the cone to reduce the contamination dose at the patient's surface. Wedges and the MLC are used for photon beams.

35. **A** Adequate cutout transmission on an electron beam treatment is ≤5 % transmission.

36. **B** The required thickness of lead cutouts using electron energies less than 10 MeV in order to keep an acceptable transmission is 5 mm of lead or its equivalent of Cerrobend (20 % greater than lead). For higher energies lead cutouts should have a minimum thickness of lead in mm of electron energy in MeV divided by 2.

37. **C** The required thickness of Cerrobend is approximately 20 % greater than that of pure lead due to the lower density of Cerrobend. The benefit of Cerrobend is its low melting point which makes it easy to form into blocks and cutouts.

38. B As a rule of thumb, the minimum lead thickness required to stop electrons as a function of the most probable electron energy incident on lead in mm is given by electron energy in MeV/2. Another mm of lead may be added as a safety margin.

39. A An internal shield is a piece of high-Z material that is placed behind the treated area, for example, inside the mouth when a buccal mucosa (cheek) is being treated. This shield protects the healthy tissue but allows treatment of the tumor. Lip treatments, buccal mucosa, and eyelid lesions often require internal shielding to protect normal structures beyond the target volume. Stoma lesions are treated using a bolus to increase dose to the skin.

40. C The enhancement in dose at the tissue-lead interface can be quite substantial from 30 to 70% in the range of 1–20 MeV, having a higher value for the lower-energy beams. To dissipate the effect of electron backscatter, a suitable thickness of low atomic number absorber may be placed between the lead shield and the preceding tissue surface. Another consideration when shielding electron is the production of bremsstrahlung photons. Because of this, if a high-Z material is used to block half of an electron field, there might actually be an increase in doe at the edge of the shield due to bremsstrahlung photons. To reduce this effect, cover the shield in wax to reduce the electron energy and reduce the bremsstrahlung photons.

41. A To dissipate the effect of electron backscatter and bremsstrahlung production, a suitable thickness of low atomic number absorber may be placed between the lead shield and the preceding tissue surface. Examples of this include an aluminum sheath around any lead can be used for internal shielding and dental acrylic around any oral shielding. Paraffin wax can also be molded around a lead shield.

42. C The practical range (Rp) must be found first =9 MeV/2 = 4.5 cm, so that the most probable energy can be established. Remember that the Rp is the depth of the point where the tangent to the descending linear portion of the curve intersects the extrapolated background.

The most probable energy at the lead-lower lip interface (2 cm depth) is found by using the following formula:

$$E_z = E_0 \left(1 - z/R_p\right) \text{ where } z \text{ the depth of the interface}$$

$$E_z = 9\,\text{MeV}\left(1 - 2/4.5\right) = 5\,\text{McV}$$

The incident energy at the lead-lower lip interface is 5 MeV. This could also be estimated remembering that electrons lose energy at about 2 MeV/cm in water. Therefore, the lead requires to shield the structures beyond the lip 5 MeV/2 MeV/mm =2.5 mm of lead thickness for shielding. Remember that as a rule of thumb, the minimum thickness of lead required for blocking in millimeters is given by the electron energy in MeV incident on lead divided by 2. Another millimeter of lead may be added as a safety margin. The required thickness of Cerrobend is approximately 20 % greater than that of pure lead.

43. B Electron arc therapy is most suited for treating superficial volumes that follow curved surfaces. The conventional tangential photon beams will irradiate too much to the underlying lung and using multiple abutting electron fields will produce junction problems such as hot and cold spots. The pseudo-arc technique is designed to achieve the results of a continuous arc by using a sufficiently large number of overlapping fields directed isocentrically.

44. C Electron energies in the range of 2–9 MeV have been found useful for treating superficial lesions covering large areas of the body. Superficial lesions like mycosis fungoides which extend to about 1 cm depth can be effectively treated without exceeding bone marrow tolerance.

45. B Pencil beam algorithms (PBA) based on multiple scattering theories are the most common algorithm for electron beam treatment planning. This algorithm models a broad electron beam as many small individual pencil beams and then adjusts the properties of the pencil beam until the distribution closely represents measure dose distribution by convolving various functions accounting for scatter in the collimator, air, patient, etc. The convolution-superimposition algorithm is calculated by modeling the incidence energy fluence as it exits the accelerator head and projects into a patient to compute the total energy release per unit mass (TERMA), which is then three-dimensionally superimposed with an energy deposition kernel. This algorithm is more computationally extensive and handles the dose distribution of scatter photons more accurately than PBA. Monte Carlo algorithms are the most accurate but are very computationally intensive. Some planning systems are beginning to use Monte Carlo for electron dose calculations. Monte Carlo algorithms work by tracking many particles through a medium and recording where the dose is deposited.

46. B As a rule of thumb, if the smallest dimension of the cutout is less than the practical range of the electron (Energy/2), there might not be lateral equilibrium in the field. In these cases, a special measurement might need to be done to determine the cutout factor unless these values have already been tabulated in your department.

3.8 IMRT and VMAT (Answers)

Quiz 1 (Level 2)

1. **D** Rotational therapy is best suited for small, deep-seated tumors, but it can be used for almost any treatment except very superficial tumors where electrons would be better.

2. **E** All are correct.

3. **A** Delivery of IMRT treatments can be accomplished via segmented MLC mode (SMLC) where the MLC moves to one segment; the beam is turned on for the correct number of MU and then turned off so the leaves can move to the next segment. In dynamic MLC mode (DMLC), the leaves are continually moving and the beam never turns on or off. Intensity-modulated arc therapy (IMAT) uses DMLC delivery with gantry rotation. Synchronized MLC mode (SYMLC) does not exist.

4. **B** In dynamic MLC mode (DMLC), the intensity-modulated fields are delivered in a dynamic fashion with the leaves of the MLC moving during the irradiation of the patient. Remember that for segmented MLC mode (SMLC) or step and shoot technique, the beam is only turned on when the MLC leaves are stationary in each of the prescribed subfield position, so there is no MLC motion while the beam is turned on.

5. **C** IMRT stands for intensity-modulated radiation therapy.

6. **A** IMRT refers to radiation therapy technique in which nonuniform fluence is delivered to the patient from any given position of the treatment beam to optimize the composite dose distribution. 3D conformal therapy uses multiple beams shaped like the tumor to deliver a conformal dose. In 2D radiation therapy planning, we are limited to generating dose distributions in a single plane or a few planes of the patient's target volume.

7. **E** The IMRT treatment planning program divides each beam into a large number of beamlets and determines optimum setting of their fluence and weights. The optimization process involves inverse planning in which beamlet weights or intensities are adjusted to satisfy predefined dose distribution criteria for the composite plan rather than the planner defines the beam shape and beam weight as in 3D conformal forward treatment planning.

8. **E** There are five tests as a check of the mechanical accuracy of DMLC which are fundamental to the accurate delivery of IMRT; (1) stability of leaf speed because if the leaf speeds are not stable, the intensity profiles uniformity can be affected; (2) dose profile across adjacent leaves to check any

irregularity in the expected dose profile pattern in the direction perpendicular to the path of leaf motion; (3) leaf acceleration and deceleration, leaves are instructed to move at different speeds from one segment of the field to another; discontinuities in planned intensity profiles could possibly occur as a result of acceleration or deceleration of leaves due to inertia; (4) positional accuracy of leaves, if any of the leaves were to under-travel or over-travel, there would be a hot spot or cold spot; and (5) routine mechanical check to evaluate positioning error of a leaf. All these are checked by medical physicists on a monthly basis.

9. A   The purpose of IMRT optimization is to minimize the dose in normal tissue, maximize the dose in target volume, and generate a dose fluence which is generated at the end of optimization. IMRT treatments usually take longer than 3D conformal treatments because more MUs are needed due to the smaller beamlets.

IMRT optimization is done by minimizing an objective function. The objective function is created when the planner enters the specific dose constraints. The computer then attempts to generate a plan that meets all of these constraints. A simple way to optimize is to subtract the computer-generated objective function from the planner's objective function. If the computer has met the planner's constraints, the result will be zero as the computer and planner's plans should be identical. That is why optimization involves minimization of the objective function.

10. C   The purpose of IMRT is to reduce dose in normal tissue. If the prescription dose is too low, there is no need to use IMRT because the dose in normal tissue is already within tolerance, e.g., $TD_{5/5}$. Also, it does take more time to plan and deliver an IMRT plan as QA and other parameters must be checked.

11. B   VMAT takes less time in dose delivery; thus, the patient in general moves less during the treatment. VMAT does not necessarily provide a better plan but it is usually delivered in a much shorter time.

12. C   One of the advantages of VMAT is that in SBRT cases the dose in normal tissue could be more evenly distributed although a larger volume of tissue is irradiated to this low dose.

13. D   Wedges are not used in IMRT. The intensity modulation is created by using the MLC.

14. A   To treat superficial lesions, bolus is normally needed because MV beams spare the surface.

15. C   The normal request of an IMRT plan is that 95 % of PTV is covered with 100 % of prescription dose.

Quiz 2 (Level 3)

This quiz could be slightly challenging, especially for CMD candidates, since it requires some in-depth understanding of IMRT, mostly at a graduate level.

1. **A**   Gamma Knife planning is done by adding "shots" of radiation. The Gamma Knife contains many cobalt-60 sources that focus on a single isocenter with several collimators of different diameters that determine the shot size. Multiple shots can be added to create a conformal dose distribution. CyberKnife is a linear accelerator on a robotic arm with various diameter circular collimators. Planning is done inversely like IMRT where the planner inputs constraints to create an objective function to be minimized.

2. **B**   There is no evidence that IMRT is better in local control of disease than 3D-CRT. Due to the higher degree of beam modulation, the dose distribution can be more conformal than 3D-CRT. In addition, one of the main reasons for the invention of IMRT was to reduce normal tissue complications.

3. **B**   As discussed in an earlier question, optimization is done by minimizing the objective function, meaning the plan generated by the computer is as close as possible to the plan wanted by the planner. As these are complex functions, minimization is not a simple process. One reason is that there is a global minimum (lowest possible value) but there are also local minimum values where the function has a low point, but this is not the best possible value. Some optimization algorithms can get trapped in local minimums meaning that there is a better plan that could be generated but the algorithm is not able to generate it.

4. **B**   Stimulated annealing is typically used to minimize the objective function. Think about the objective function as a slope that has hills going up and down. At some point, there is a global minimum that is the ideal solution, but there are also local minimum points on the function. A quick way to find the minimum is to just follow the function down the slope. This is called a "gradient optimization" and it is very quick, but it tends to trap the optimization in local minimum points. Simulated annealing lets the algorithm "climb" up some of the hills and potentially finds the global minimum value. A downside is that simulated annealing is more computationally intensive.

5. **A**   The IMRT fluence is the direct result of the optimization process. Using this fluence, the MLC motion can be calculated.

6. **B**   A PTV margin is used to account for setup uncertainties and motion during treatment. Therefore, the margin will be dependent on how well the setup

can be done and how much the tumor and OARs experience motion during treatment. Since 3D-CRT can use the same image guidance as IMRT, the margin is independent of modality.

7. **B** Gamma Knife and CyberKnife are used for treating stereotactic radiosurgery (single fraction) or stereotactic radiotherapy (2–5 fractions). Stereotactic means that a special 3D coordinate system is used to accurately position the patient. For Gamma Knife, the patient has a frame that is attached to the skull with screws. This provides much more accuracy in terms of positioning than something like a thermoplastic mask. Also, both Gamma Knife and CyberKnife utilize very small field sizes meaning the dose can be delivered very conformably. Because of this, the isodose lines chosen to prescribe dose to are much lower than in linac treatments. Prescribing to a low isodose line means that the plan becomes much hotter. For example, if the prescription is 10 Gy, prescribing to the 90 % IDL results in an 11.1 Gy maximum dose, but prescribing to the 50 % IDL results in a 20 Gy maximum dose. With stereotactic treatments, this is fine because with the high conformity, the hot spot falls inside the tumor which actually improves the chance of destroying the tumor. CyberKnife is not quite as conformal as Gamma Knife and the prescription isodose line is usually around 70 %, but the same principle still applies.

8. **C** Since all diodes are off by the same percentage, it could be a dose calibration problem. If this were to happen in a clinic, the cause of the deviation must be investigated before this plan is approved for treatment.

9. **B** The name of the optimization object of IMRT is the objective (or cost) function.

10. **A** Analytical means the mathematical expression can be found by directly solving the equations using variables and mathematical expression.
The cost function for IMRT optimization is complex and has no analytical solution.

3.9 Special Procedures and SRS (Answers)

Quiz 1 (Level 2)

1. **B** TBI with megavoltage photon beams is most commonly used as part of the conditioning regimen for bone marrow transplantation. Its role is to destroy the recipient's bone marrow and tumor cells and to immunosuppress the patient sufficiently to avoid rejection of the donor bone marrow transplant. The dose is typically around 12 Gy, delivered in 2 Gy fractions, BID (twice daily). The fractions are at least 6 h apart.

2. A   TBI treatments should achieve dose uniformity along the body axis to within ±10 %, although extremities and some noncritical structures may exceed this specification.

3. A   The term tissue lateral effect has been used to describe the situation in which an excessively higher dose is delivered to the subcutaneous tissues compared with the midpoint dose when a lower-energy beam is used or a thicker patient is treated with parallel-opposed beams for TBI.

4. B   If the maximum thickness of the patient parallel to the beam central axis is less than 35 cm and SSD is 300 cm, a 6 MV beam can be used without increasing the peripheral dose to greater than 110 % of the midline dose. If the thickness is greater, then a higher energy should be used. A downside of using beams with an energy >10 MV is the generation of secondary particles like neutrons that add contamination to the beam.

5. B   Most TBI protocols do not require skin sparing. Instead, a bolus or a beam spoiler is specified to bring the surface dose to at least 90 % of the prescribed TBI dose. A large spoiler screen of 1–2 cm thick acrylic is sufficient to meet these requirements.

6. A   Bilateral total body irradiation is a technique involving left and right lateral opposing fields with the patient seated on a couch in a semi-fetal position, arms positioned laterally covering the lungs. To achieve dose uniformity within approximately ±10 % along the sagittal axis of the body, compensators are designed for head and neck, lungs, and legs. This is due to the varying anatomical thickness of the different regions of the body when treating laterally. For the AP/PA total body irradiation, the patient is irradiated anteroposteriorly by parallel-opposed fields while positioned in a standing upright position. The AP/PA technique can also be adopted for treating small children in the reclined position. The children will be treated in the supine and posterior positions while lying down on a low-height couch, with the couch top only a few inches off the floor

7. C   Midplane at the level of the umbilicus is used as the reference point when doing TBI treatments.

8. A   All are correct. Compensator design for TBI is complex because of large variations in body thickness (especially when treating laterally), lack of complete body immobilization, and internal tissue heterogeneities.

9. A   Stereotactic radiosurgery (SRS) is a single-fraction radiation therapy procedure for treating intracranial lesions using a combination of a stereotactic apparatus and narrow multiple beams delivered through noncoplanar isocentric arcs (or a modality such as CyberKnife or Gamma Knife).

3.9 Special Procedures and SRS (Answers)

Stereotactic radiotherapy (SRT) is the same procedure but using 2–5 dose fractions.

10. E Stereotactic radiosurgery involves three-dimensional imaging to localize the lesion and it has a high degree of conformity. Typically, circular collimators are used, but it is possible to use mini-MLCs and dynamic conformal arcs.

11. C The best achievable mechanical accuracy in terms of isocenter displacement from the defined center of target image is 0.2 mm ± 0.1 mm, although a maximum error of ±1 mm is commonly accepted in view of the unavoidable uncertainties in target localization.

12. E Currently, there are three types of radiation used in SRS and SRT: heavy charged particles, cobalt-60 (Gamma Knife), and megavoltage x-rays (CyberKnife or linac).

13. C Pedestal-mounted frames and couch-mounted frames are the devices used in stereotactic radiosurgery treatments. It must be attached to the patient's skull as well as to the couch or pedestal to provide a rigidly fixed frame of coordinates for relating the center of the imaged target to the isocenter of the treatment. This provides the high degree of accuracy necessary for the delivery.

14. C Depending on the modality, typical cone sizes range from 4 to 30 mm in diameter. For the Gamma Knife 5C, the collimator diameters are 4, 8, 14, and 18 mm (the new Gamma Knife Perfexion only has collimators of 16, 8, and 4 mm). For linac- and CyberKnife-based treatments, the cones are 15 cm long made of a high-Z material. CyberKnife cones range from 5 mm up to 60 mm although the larger cones are not typically used for SRS. A few cones of larger diameter may also be available for treating larger lesions with SRT.

15. A The geometric penumbra is inversely proportional to source-to-diaphragm distance. The 15 cm long cone is designed to bring the collimator diaphragm closer to the surface in order to maintain the penumbra as small as possible.

16. E All are correct. The most recent Gamma Knife model called the Perfexion has the ability to treat upper cervical spine lesions and is also going to include CBCT image guidance in the near future. Also, the Perfexion only uses 192 sources.

17. B The central axes of all 201 beams intersect at the focus with a mechanical precision of ±3 mm, and the alignment of helmet channels with the central body channels must have a positioning accuracy of ±0.1 mm. The new Perfexion model does not use helmets to collimate the beams, rather the sources move on moveable sectors.

18. D Each Gamma Knife helmet is characterized by its channel diameter that produces a circular field opening of 4, 8, 14, or 18 mm at the focus point. Selected channels can be blocked with 6 cm thick tungsten alloy plugs to shield the eyes or to optimize the dose distribution. Again, the Perfexion model has made some changes and eliminated the use of helmets.

19. E Several types of detector systems can be used in SRS dosimetry: ion chambers, film, thermoluminescent dosimeters, and diodes.

20. C An ion chamber is the most accurate and the least energy-dependent system but usually has a size limitation which can be a problem for the small field sizes with SRS. Film has the best spatial resolution but shows energy dependence and a high statistical uncertainty (±3 %). Thermoluminescent dosimeters show little energy dependence and can have a small size in the form of chips but suffer from the same degree of statistical uncertainty as the film and diodes have small size but show energy dependence as well as possible directional dependence. Therefore, the choice of detector for SRS dosimetry depends on the quantity to be measured and the measurement conditions.

21. C Diodes and film are the detectors of choice when measuring cross-beam profiles and depth-dose distribution on SRS treatments because of their small size and there is little change in the photon energy spectrum across small fields, so energy dependence is not an issue.

22. E Some of the major QAs for SRS include stereotactic frame accuracy including phantom-based accuracy, CT/MRI/angiographic localizer accuracy, pedestal or couch mount accuracy, imaging data transfer, treatment plan parameters, target position, monitor unit (time) calculation, frame alignment with gantry and couch eccentricity, congruence of target point with radiation isocenter, collimator settings, cone diameters, couch position accuracy, patient immobilization and safety locks, and treatment console programming of beam energy, monitor units, and arc angles.

23. E When compared to linac stereotactic radiosurgery or Gamma Knife, CyberKnife treatments are frameless, non-isocentric, and can fractionated if needed. The precision is on the order of 0.47 ± 0.17 mm.

24. E Accuracy CyberKnife can be used to treat intracranial lesions as well as full body targeting. The CyberKnife has a respiratory tracking system that

3.9 Special Procedures and SRS (Answers)

can move the robotic arm to compensate for the breathing pattern when treating lung or abdominal lesions.

25. A CyberKnife's simulation CT scan must be done so that the scans have a minimum of 10–15 cm above and below the area of interest, the FOV must include the entire circumference of the patient, slices of 1.0–1.5 mm must be used, and contrast must be used if necessary. Additional slices are required because the non-isocentric delivery can bring beams in from multiple off-axis directions.

26. E CyberKnife's MRI scan must use true axial images only, slices must be in the range of 1.0–3.0 mm, and contrast may be used if necessary. Three hundred slices is the maximum number of slices allowed.

27. B CyberKnife skull tracking has an accuracy of 0.5 mm translation error and 0.5° rotation error.

28. A 33 pairs of DRRs are generated as reference images from the CT data set used for planning.

29. A Because fiducial migration will degrade the accuracy of fiducial-based targeting, the time between the simulation CT study and treatment should be minimized. Typically, simulation CT is acquired 1 week after soft tissue fiducial placement and within 24–48 h if the fiducials are placed on the bone so that migration can be evaluated.

30. C Twelve (12) fixed collimators can be used on CyberKnife treatment. They will be selected when planning is performed and it depends on the size of the tumor in treatment. The 12 collimators' diameters are 5.0, 7.5, 10, 12.5, 15, 20, 25, 30, 35, 40, 50, and 60 mm.

31. A The IRIS variable aperture collimator is the name of the dynamic collimator used in CyberKnife. This dynamic collimator can create the same field sizes as the fixed cones, but time can be saved as there is no need to switch cones during treatment. A limitation is that the IRIS should not be used to treat with a 5 mm aperture due to the uncertainty in the mechanical reproducibility at the very small size. The MLC is used on the linac where the leaves shape the field.

32. B The alpha/beta (α/β) ratio is a radiation biology parameter that is used to calculate how a tissue will respond to a radiation dose. The α/β ratio in Gy for spinal cord myelitis is 2.5 Gy. For the optic nerve/chiasm, α/β is 2.1 Gy. For lung toxicity, the α/β is 1.6–4.5 Gy, and for skin desquamation, α/β is between 10 and 20 Gy.

33. E All statements are true about biological effective dose (BED). $BED = nd_1(1 + d_1/\alpha/\beta)$, where n = number of fractions, d_1 = dose per fraction, and α/β is the alpha/beta ratio. Given different fractionation schemes, one can sum the BEDs, and given different fractionation schemes, d or n can be solved to get an equivalent regimen. Finally, $BED = nd_1(1 + d_1/\alpha/\beta) + nd_2(1 + d_2/\alpha/\beta) + nd_3(1 + d_3/\alpha/\beta)...$ The BED is used in SRS and SRT because most of the data for radiotherapy treatments are based off 2 Gy fractionation schemes. As the dose is increased and the number of fractions reduced, an equivalent dose needs to be determined to provide similar tumor control and normal tissue complications.

34. A An ablative treatment dose from radiosurgery is a single large dose. For conventional radiotherapy, multiple small doses are delivered. For stereotactic radiotherapy, several large doses are given.

35. E Potential benefits of fractionation in CyberKnife include any of the benefits that are seen during normal radiotherapy treatments. The benefits of fractionation are due to the 4 Rs of radiobiology: repair, repopulation, reassortment, and reoxygenation. Basically, fractionation exploits the difference in α/β between tumor and normal tissue. Repair is the ability of the healthy cells to repair sublethal damage before the next dose of radiation. Repopulation refers to the healthy cells being able to divide and increase their numbers before the next treatment. Reassortment refers to the redistribution of the tumor cells into more sensitive phases of the cell cycle as some cells will stay at more resistant phases when they receive a dose of radiation. Finally, reoxygenation refers to the cells in the center of the tumor receiving blood supply again. This is because in a tumor, the center is usually necrotic (or dead) as there is no blood flow or oxygen. When one fraction is delivered, the outer cells of the tumor are destroyed allowing blood to flow into the center of the tumor. Oxygen enhances the effects of radiation, so the center of the tumor becomes more radiosensitive for the next fraction.

36. D The end-to-end QA test in CyberKnife should be done every 4 months, one modality each month (skull, fiducials, synchrony respiratory tracking, X-sight). Since it is very time-consuming to perform E2E tests for all tracking modalities and path combinations every month, it is recommended that one intracranial and one extracranial be performed at least monthly. The E2E test phantom consists of a ball in a cube in which a pair of orthogonal radiochromic films can be placed. When a beam is delivered, the ball attenuates the radiation and then the film can be processed and the ball should be perfectly in the center of the radiation aperture. CyberKnife daily QA includes system warm-up, output constancy, and a BB test (single fiducial). Bimonthly QA includes full-scatter output, linac energy and symmetry checks, and isopost image center check. Yearly QA includes acquiring

3.9 Special Procedures and SRS (Answers) 297

PDDs, profiles, and output factors. All QA for CyberKnife can be found in AAPM TG-135.

37. C CyberKnife lung treatments use the synchrony system to predict the respiratory motion and move the robotic arm to compensate for the motion. Therefore, the patient must breathe normally.

38. A CyberKnife radiosurgery is a noninvasive treatment alternative for patients with lung tumors. It is also an outpatient procedure that is usually completed in less than a week. There are minimal patient-related side effects and toxicity due to the sparing of healthy tissue. Some patients must have chemotherapy to treat any metastasis.

39. A Not all lung patients can benefit from CyberKnife because their breathing pattern might be irregular or the tumor might be too large.

40. B Some components of CyberKnife are a diagnostic x-ray source for positioning based on bony anatomy or fiducial markers, a 6 MV linear accelerator, a synchrony camera system for respiratory motion tracking, image detectors, and a robotic couch.

41. A The CyberKnife safety zone is the distance between the robot position and virtual obstacle. ESTOP triggers when proximity detection program (PDP) distance is <5 cm which avoids any collision to the patient. There are two safety zones: one zone is called the fixed zone because it is fixed with respect to the robot and includes system components that do not move, such as imaging system components, floor, walls, and ceiling, and the second is the patient safety zone which is relative to the patient couch.

Quiz 2 (Level 3)

1. A Stereotactic radiosurgery was originally developed for benign lesions such as arteriovenous malformations (AVMs), meningiomas, and acoustic neuroma. Today, SRS is also the treatment of choice of malignant tumors such as gliomas and some brain metastases; also it is used to treat functional disorders such as trigeminal neuralgia and movement disorders.

2. B Stereotactic irradiation is suitable for treatment of functional disorders, vascular lesions, primary benign and malignant tumors, and metastatic tumors.

3. A The main components of the Gamma Knife unit are the radiation unit with an upper hemispherical shield and a central body, an operating table and sliding cradle, and a set of four collimator helmets providing circular beams. A robotic arm that holds the linac is used in CyberKnife machine.

4. A   A CyberKnife treatment machine uses a noninvasive image-guided target localization, a 6 MV linac mounted on an industrial robotic manipulator, and a non-isocentric treatment technique.

5. A   CyberKnife treatment allows frameless radiosurgery; it also monitors and tracks the patient's position continuously, and it allows for frameless radiosurgical dose delivery to extracranial targets such as spine, lung, and prostate. If the patient moves during treatment outside the limits, the machine automatically stops.

6. B   Low-dose TBI typically delivers a dose in 10–15 fractions of 10–15 cGy each; high-dose TBI delivers a single fraction or up to six fractions of 200 cGy each in 3 days for a total dose of 1,200 cGy. Half-body irradiation delivers a dose of 8 Gy to the upper or lower half body in a single session and, finally, total nodal irradiation with a typical nodal dose of 40 Gy delivered in 20 fractions.

7. A   The most notable diseases treated with bone marrow transplantation (BMT) are some leukemias such as acute non-lymphoblastic, acute lymphoblastic, and chronic myelogenous, malignant lymphoma, and aplastic anemia.

8. E   All are correct.

9. B   Both beam spoilers and special filters are used on TSEI to produce a large and uniform electron fields in the patient treatment plane. The use of beam spoilers will degrade the electron beam energy striking the patient, and special filters improve the electron beam flatness through electron beam scattering.

10. A   The basic dosimetry parameters of the large TSEI electron field are field flatness at Dmax, electron beam output at dose calibration point, and PDDs measured to a depth of 15 cm. Remember that TMR is used for SAD setups with photons.

11. A   IORT is a special radiotherapeutic technique that delivers a dose on the order of 10–20 Gy in a single session following the surgical resection of the tumor. Following the surgery, the patient is transported to the linac (or treatment device) before the surgical opening is closed so the dose can be delivered directly to the tumor bed to ensure that if any tumor was not able to be resected, it is still destroyed. Typically, electrons are used. The initial treatment attempts to shrink the tumor and can be followed by chemotherapy and external beam radiotherapy modalities.

3.9 Special Procedures and SRS (Answers)

12. E All are involved in the IORT treatment. The team consists of a surgeon, radiation oncologist, medical physicist, anesthesiologist, nurse, and pathologist and radiation therapist.

13. A Orthovoltage x-rays, megavoltage electron beams, and high-dose rate (HDR) Ir-192 brachytherapy sources are modalities used to deliver radiation dose intraoperatively.

14. E Endocavitary rectal irradiation is a sphincter-saving procedure used in the treatment of selected rectal carcinomas with superficial x-rays. In order to be performed, there must be a mobile lesion with a maximum diameter of 3 cm, the location of the lesion must be within 10 cm from the anal canal, and no evidence of lymph node or distance metastases can be found. Also there has to be a biopsy proven a well- or moderately well-differentiated rectal adenocarcinoma.

15. A The two techniques used for endorectal treatments are short SSD with the SSD on the order of 4 cm where the x-ray tube is inserted into the proctoscopic cone and an SSD treatment with the SSD of the order of 20 cm with the x-ray tube coupled to the cone externally. The tumor dose for endorectal treatments is around 80 Gy delivered in two or three fractions of 20–30 Gy given 2 weeks apart.

16. E Meningiomas, pituitary adenomas, acoustic neuromas, metastatic tumors, gliomas, arteriovenous malformations, and trigeminal nerve disease are primary diseases treated with radiosurgery using CyberKnife.

17. E Stereotactic radiosurgery CyberKnife treatments require high precision, steep dose gradients, reliability, and reproducibility.

18. E All of them are problems involving linac radiosurgery due to the required precision and tight margins used in these procedures. As linacs have many moving parts, each has to have a much tighter tolerance than the final tolerance as each error compounds with other errors. The focal spot size on a linac is larger than for Gamma Knife, and if the flattening filter is required, the highest dose rate is limited. Also, the treatment planning systems are not optimized for SRS treatments.

19. B The planning system used in CyberKnife is called Multiplan. This system provides a comprehensive set of tools available for high-precision radiosurgery treatment planning. Eclipse, Corvus, and ADAC planning system simplify modern radiation therapy planning for all kinds of treatment such as forward planning (3D conformal therapy), intensity-modulated radiation therapy (IMRT), ARC treatment planning, and brachytherapy.

20. E All are true.

21. A CyberKnife has great flexibility to deliver both isocentric and non-isocentric treatments. It also delivers a noncoplanar treatment where the robotic mobility allows for the ability to deliver hundreds of uniquely angled beams. Linacs are limited to clockwise/counterclockwise rotation making a noncoplanar beam delivery very difficult, except if the couch is rotated.

22. C CyberKnife planning system supports Monte Carlo dose calculation for both fixed collimators and the IRIS. Monte Carlo is widely accepted as the most accurate method for calculating radiation dose, especially stereotactic radiosurgery. Acuros is Varian's next-generation radiotherapy dose calculation software, and it uses a deterministic method to solve the Boltzmann transport equation.

23. B Task Group-135 is the one that involves QA for robotic radiosurgery including CyberKnife. The TG-142 report is for the QA of medical accelerators, the TG-179 report includes QA for image-guided radiation therapy utilizing CT-based technologies, and TG-51 is associated with absolute dose calibration for linac.

24. A The CyberKnife geometric isocenter is a reference point in the room which serves as the origin for several coordinate systems used within the CyberKnife application, not to be confused with treatment isocenter which refers to an isocentric treatment to a target located at a distance from the geometric isocenter. Remember that most CyberKnife treatments are non-isocentric.

25. C CyberKnife SAD is 800 mm or 80 cm. Linac SADs used to be 80 cm but most of them are now 100 cm SAD.

26. A As per TG-135 daily CyberKnife, QA includes safety interlocks, accelerator warm-up (6,000 MU must be delivered if the chamber is open and 3,000 MU if it is closed), accelerator output, detection of incorrect or missing secondary collimator, a visual check of beam laser and a standard floor mark, and the AQA test.

27. C The robotic manipulator is programmed to move in a fixed and predetermined workspace which accounts for the positions of objects in the treatment suite including the treatment couch, imaging sources and detectors, the floor, and the ceiling and eliminates collision hazards by creating suitable paths. Additionally, the workspace is comprised of preassigned points in space, termed nodes where the manipulator is allowed to stop in order to deliver radiation dose. At each node, the linac can deliver radiation from multiple beam angels; the paths are composed of a series of nodes where the linac delivers radiation from 12 different positions per node. During treatment delivery, the manipulator will move from node to node.

3.10 Nuclear Medicine Therapy (Answers)

Quiz 1 (Level 3)

1. **C** 60–80 % of patients with a history of colorectal carcinoma, pancreatic carcinoma, breast cancer, and others will develop liver metastases.

2. **E** All are correct; there has been a significant progress in hepatobiliary surgery, but other innovative liver-directed treatments have been developed, such as conformal radiation therapy, hepatic arterial infusion chemotherapy (HAC), transarterial chemoembolization (TACE), radiofrequency ablation (RFA), and radioembolization (RE) using yttrium-90 (Y-90) microspheres.

3. **D** Hepatic metastases and primary neoplasms are often multifocal and irregular in shape as well as potentially replacing large parts of the liver volume. Only a small population of patients is considered optimal candidates for conformal or stereotactic radiation therapy.

4. **C** Selective internal radiation therapy (SIRT) is a nonsurgical, outpatient therapy that uses microscopic radioactive spheres, called SIR-Spheres (or TheraSpheres), to deliver high dose of radiation directly to the site of the liver tumors. TheraSpheres are used to treat primary hepatocellular carcinoma and SIR-Spheres are used to treat metastatic disease. Low-dose rate (LDR) brachytherapy is an inpatient procedure which involves implanting radiation sources directly into or near the tumor that emit radiation at a rate of up to $2 \text{ Gy} \cdot \text{h}^{-1}$. High-dose rate (HDR) brachytherapy is when the rate of dose delivery exceeds $12 \text{ Gy} \cdot \text{h}^{-1}$. Stereotactic radiation therapy (SRT) is an outpatient procedure that uses external beam high dose of radiation focused on the tumor, minimizing damage to the surrounding structures. SRT can be done on a linac or CyberKnife.

5. **A** The main advantage of selective internal radiation therapy (SIRT) over traditional methods is low toxicity due to minimal dose to tissues outside the region of angioplasty. SIRT is a non-curative treatment, but it has been associated with improved survival, reduction in tumor marker, and regression in the number and size of lesions.

6. **B** All the radioisotopes mentioned are possible isotopes for intraluminal brachytherapy, but due to specific characteristics, Y-90, a pure β emitter, produced by neutron bombardment of yttrium-89 in a reactor (limited tissue penetration of mean, 2.5 mm; max, 11 mm; and short half-life of 64 h (2.67 days)), is the radioisotope used for selective internal radiation therapy (SIRT) treatments.

7. C   SIRT can provide extremely high local tumor doses ranging from 50 to 150 Gy, in contrast to the traditional whole-liver external beam radiation where radiation doses have to be limited to 30 Gy to prevent serious hepatic dysfunction. Additionally, the SIRT procedure causes the spheres to block the vasculature to the tumor causing it to die. This is called embolization.

8. A   Selective internal radiation therapy (SIRT) workup includes contrast computed tomography (CT) and gadolinium-enhanced magnetic resonance imaging (MRI) of the liver, portal vein patency, and extent of extrahepatic disease. Also for tumors with a high glucose metabolism rate, whole-body ^{18}F-fluorodeoxyglucose positron emission tomography/computed tomography (FDG-PET/CT) is used. There are additional nuclear medicine scans acquired to determine the lung shunt fraction (amount of blood that flows from the liver to the lung) and the ratio of tumor to normal liver uptake. These are important because it allows the toxicity to the lung and normal liver to be calculated. Sometimes, the procedure must be canceled if too much dose will end up in the lung or normal liver.

9. B   Lung dose is the major concern, due to the blood flow. This is calculated with the lung shunt fraction determined with the nuclear medicine scan.

10. C   AAPM TG-144

11. A   Injection through femoral artery with guidance of angiography is the prevalent method.

12. C   Hepatocellular carcinoma (HCC) is typically located in the small lobe of the liver where the hepatic artery provides blood flow while the majority of the blood supply to the rest of the liver comes from the hepatic vein. Therefore, during the injection, by using embolization to block other veins and by using the hepatic artery, the dose can be directed to the tumor and spare the healthy liver.

13. D   I-123 is used for single-photon computed tomography (SPECT) imaging. SPECT imaging is a nuclear medicine procedure where one or more gamma cameras are rotated around a patient who has been injected with a photon-emitting radionuclide. Using a collimator (e.g., pinhole or parallel hole) a 3D image of the radionuclide location in the patient can be reconstructed. I-124 is used for positron emission tomography (PET) imaging. PET is a nuclear medicine procedure where a positron emitter is injected into the patient. When the positron annihilates with an electron, two 511 keV photons are produced that travel in opposite directions. The PET scanner consists of a ring of detectors around the patient, so when the two photons are detected, a line can be drawn between the

3.10 Nuclear Medicine Therapy (Answers)

two detectors and in the end a 3D image can be reconstructed of the radionuclide in the patient. I-125 has a longer half-life than the other isotopes of iodine and is used for LDR brachytherapy procedures like prostate seed implants or eye plaques. I-131 has a lifetime of 8 days and is ideal to treat thyroid cancer due to the proclivity of the thyroid to uptake iodine.

14. B Typically, the iodine is administered orally.

Patient Immobilization

Contents

4.1 Patient Positioning and Treatment Devices (Questions) 306
4.2 Image-Guided Radiotherapy (Questions) 308
4.3 Margins Accounting for Positioning (Questions) 312
4.4 Patient Positioning and Treatment Devices (Answers) 314
4.5 Image-Guided Radiotherapy (Answers) 316
4.6 Margins Accounted for Positioning (Answers) 318

Patient immobilization and positioning is very important in radiotherapy (RT). There are 2 aspects to immobilizing and positioning a patient that we must be concerned about: intra-treatment (during the actual delivery) motion and immobilization and inter-treatment (reproducibility from one fraction to the next) motion and immobilization. To ensure that the patient is positioned and immobilized properly for every fraction, immobilization devices and imaging techniques are used.

The purpose of intra-treatment immobilization is to ensure that the patient is not moving during dose delivery and remains in the same position as simulation. An exception to this is when gating is used because the delivery is controlled by patient respiration so motion is expected. In a standard treatment plan, a margin to account for patient motion is added to the clinical target volume (CTV) to ensure that the CTV is always covered in treatment. The added margin is called the planned target volume (PTV). The PTV margin is determined based on the uncertainty in the patient positioning, the amount of motion the target experiences, and the proximity of critical structures. Without an immobilization device, e.g., a mask for head/neck treatments, the PTV margin would have to be very large to ensure that the CTV does not move outside of the PTV and receives the appropriate dose. Another way of reducing the uncertainty in patient setup is to use image guidance like orthogonal x-rays or cone beam CT (CBCT).

© Springer International Publishing Switzerland 2015
W. Amestoy, *Review of Medical Dosimetry: A Study Guide*,
DOI 10.1007/978-3-319-13626-4_4

The purpose of inter-treatment immobilization is to ensure the reproducibility of every fraction of treatment. The role of the PTV is also to ensure CTV coverage during every fraction, and using an immobilization device or image guidance can help reproduce the patient's position daily so that the CTV is covered by the prescription dose.

It is important to mention the procedures of post-planning simulation (so-called second simulation). After a plan is calculated and approved on the simulation CT, a patient will often undergo a second simulation and have external marks placed such as tattoos or BBs, to localize the treatment isocenter prior to treatment, as well as be able to reproduce the patient's position at every fraction. This can be done in a simulator using fluoroscopy to visualize the patient's anatomy and treatment area, or nowadays, most linear accelerators have KV imaging capabilities allowing for the second simulation to be done on the linac. In the case of image-guided radiotherapy (IGRT), target localization is also confirmed visually with imaging prior to each fraction. The choice to use image guidance is based on the complexity of the treatment and the proximity of OARs. An IMRT plan with steep dose gradients requires more accurate positioning to ensure the dose is being delivered to the correct area.

4.1 Patient Positioning and Treatment Devices (Questions)

Quiz 1 (Level 2)

1. Which of the following devices is/are used for patient positioning reproducibility?
A. I, II, and III
B. I and III only
C. II and IV only
D. IV only
E. All are correct
I. Total body cast
II. Triangle pillow under knees
III. Headrest
IV. Arm support

2. Daily patient-treatment setup positions include:
A. I, II, and III
B. I and III only
C. II and IV only
D. IV only
E. All are correct
I. Supine
II. Prone
III. Head and thorax slightly upright
IV. Trendelenburg

4.1 Patient Positioning and Treatment Devices (Questions)

3. Which of the following treatments can benefit from using an Alpha Cradle mold for patient immobilization?
A. RT of head and neck and nasopharynx
B. RT of lower leg sarcoma
C. RT of chest wall
D. RT of whole brain

4. Which of the following treatment devices is used to move the small bowel away from the treatment field?
A. Alpha Cradle
B. Aquaplast mask
C. Belly board
D. Bite block

5. Patient's positioning and the immobilization device used depend on:
A. I, II, and III
B. I and III only
C. II and IV only
D. IV only
E. All are correct
I. Patient's medical condition
II. CT scanner bore dimension
III. Location of the disease
IV. Patient's preference

6. Which of the following devices is/are used for immobilization of head and neck radiation treatments?
A. I, II, and III
B. I and III only
C. II and IV only
D. IV only
E. All are correct
I. Aquaplast mask
II. Shoulder straps
III. Headrest
IV. Bite block

7. Which of the following devices is/are used for immobilization of thorax radiation treatment?
A. I, II, and III
B. I and III only
C. II and IV only
D. IV only
E. All are correct

I. Vac-Lok bag
II. Alpha Cradle
III. Wing board
IV. Prone pillow

8. Which of the following devices is used for immobilization CNS patients?
A. Sandbags
B. Belly board
C. Wing board
D. Duncan face mask

9. The belly board's main advantage is:
A. Minimize lung dose
B. Reduce pelvic tilt
C. Reproducibility
D. Minimize small bowel dose

10. What is the Calypso® 4D localization system used for?
A. Intra-fractional prostate motion tracking
B. Inter-fractional prostate motion tracking
C. Intra-fractional prostate motion monitoring
D. Inter-fractional prostate motion monitoring

11. Which of the following are components of Calypso® 4D systems?
A. I, II, III, and IV
B. II, III, and IV
C. I, III, and IV
D. All of them
I. 4D electromagnetic array
II. Implanted electromagnetic transponders
III. 4D console inside treatment room
IV. 4D tracking system
V. Infrared cameras and optic targets

4.2 Image-Guided Radiotherapy (Questions)

Quiz 1 (Level 2)

1. Image-guided radiotherapy (IGRT) refers to:
A. A RT delivery technique where an image is acquired just before or during delivery of a fraction to improve the accuracy of target localization for delivery and avoidance of organs at risk

B. View of patient through the beam portal image showing patient anatomy within treatment beam
C. A combined radiation therapy technique in which a single beam is irradiated both with an electron and a photon beam
D. An x-ray film taken on the treatment machine with the patient in treatment position and with the beam settings as used for treatment

2. Some IGRT systems include:
A. I, II, and III
B. I and III only
C. II and IV only
D. IV only
E. All are correct
I. Cone beam computed tomography (CBCT)
II. Megavoltage computed tomography (MVCT)
III. Portal imaging
IV. Online imaging with paired orthogonal planar images

3. Which of the following IGRT systems enable visualization of the exact tumor location by integrating a CT imaging system with a linac and involve acquiring multiple planar images?
A. BAT
B. BrainLab
C. Paired orthogonal planar imagers
D. CBCT

4. The advantage of megavoltage beams for CBCT is:
A. The beams come from the linac beamline and thus no additional equipment is required to produce the cone beam.
B. It produces better soft tissue contrast.
C. It is lower energy.
D. It can produce radiographic and fluoroscopic images.

5. A CT-on-rails system is comprised of:
A. A detector panel already present for use in electronic portal imaging opposite to the linac head
B. A conventional x-ray tube mounted on a retractable arm at 90° to the high-energy treatment beam and a flat panel x-ray detector mounted on a retractable arm opposite the x-ray tube
C. A linac and a CT unit on rails approach at opposite ends of a standard radiotherapy treatment table
D. A 2D or 3D ultrasound imaging system integrated with an isocentric medical linac

6. TomoTherapy systems include:
A. I, II, and III
B. I and III only
C. II and IV only
D. IV only
E. All are correct
I. IMRT treatment capability using a 6 MV linear accelerator
II. A CT-type gantry ring that rotates around the patient
III. A couch that advances the patient through the gantry bore
IV. IMRT treatment using dual energy (6 and 18 MV)

7. TomoTherapy IGRT consists of:
A. I, II, and III
B. I and III only
C. II and IV only
D. IV only
E. All are correct
I. An MVCT scan of patient anatomy at any time before, during, or after treatment
II. MVCT image data acquired with a xenon ionization chamber array
III. MVCT guidance to adjust patient's position at every fraction
IV. An MVCT that can be taken after radiation delivery with patient still in the treatment position to evaluate the true dose distribution delivered to the patient

8. BAT stands for:
A. Brain acquisition and targeting system
B. B-mode acquisition and targeting system
C. Best algorithm treatment system
D. B-section alteration tolerance

9. The BAT system consists of:
A. A detector panel already present for use in electronic portal imaging opposite to the linac head
B. A conventional x-ray tube mounted on a retractable arm at 90° to the high-energy treatment beam and a flat panel x-ray detector mounted on a retractable arm opposite the x-ray tube
C. A linac and a CT unit on rails approaching at opposite ends of a standard radiotherapy treatment table
D. A cart-based ultrasound unit positioned next to a linac treatment table to image the target volume prior to each fraction of a patient's treatment

10. The BAT system is most commonly used for:
A. Prostate localization
B. Liver metastasis localization
C. Brain boost localization
D. Pancreas localization

4.2 Image-Guided Radiotherapy (Questions)

11. ExacTrac consists of:
A. A cart-based ultrasound unit positioned next to a linac treatment table to image the target volume prior to each fraction of a patient's radiotherapy
B. A reflective marker array attached to an ultrasound probe using infrared tracking system relative to reflective markers attached to patient
C. A set of paired orthogonal x-ray tubes and detectors to determine the location of the lesion in the room coordinate system
D. A special accessory added to a linac to compensate automatically and instantly for the effects of respiratory movement

12. CyberKnife IGRT is based on:
A. A pair of orthogonal x-ray images to determine the location of the lesion in the target relative to the room's coordinate system
B. A cart-based ultrasound unit positioned next to a linac treatment table to image the target volume prior to each fraction of a patient's radiotherapy
C. A reflective marker array attached to an ultrasound probe using infrared tracking system relative to reflective markers attached to patient
D. A conventional x-ray tube mounted on a retractable arm at 90° to the high-energy treatment beam and a flat panel x-ray detector mounted on a retractable arm opposite the x-ray tube

13. CyberKnife IGRT uses:
A. I, II, and III
B. I and III only
C. II and IV only
D. IV only
E. All are correct
I. A pair of orthogonal x-ray images to determine the location of the lesion in the target relative to the room's coordinate system
II. A set of digitally reconstructed radiographs (DRR) from a CT scan acquired prior to treatment
III. A mechanism to communicate the actual target position to the robotic arm, which then adjusts the linac's beam to maintain alignment with the target
IV. Online tracking of target motion

14. Adaptive radiotherapy:
A. Modifies dose distribution for subsequent treatment fractions of a course of radiotherapy
B. Modifies patient position for subsequent treatment fractions of a course of radiotherapy
C. Alternates CBCT and orthogonal x-ray images for subsequent treatment fractions of a course of radiotherapy
D. Alternates CBCT and ultrasound images for subsequent treatment fractions of a course of radiotherapy

15. Adaptive radiotherapy is useful to account for:
A. I and II
B. I and III only
C. II and IV only
D. IV only
E. All are correct
I. Tumor shrinkage
II. Patient loss of weight
III. Increased hypoxia due to fractionated treatments
IV. Patient movement

4.3 Margins Accounting for Positioning (Questions)

Quiz 1 (Level 2)

1. Compared to standard IMRT treatments, stereotactic radiosurgery (SRS) and stereotactic body radiotherapy (SBRT) treatments have:
A. The same margins but fewer fractions
B. Tighter margins but similar fractions
C. The same margins and similar fractions
D. Tighter margins and fewer fractions

2. Comparing hypo-fractionation RT and SBRT, they are:
A. Essentially the same, just being called by different names
B. Similar, both have tighter margins to account for motion or setup uncertainty but except that SBRT must have less than 5 fractions
C. Similar, but SBRT has 5 fractions or less and usually utilizes much smaller margins when accounting for motion or setup uncertainty
D. Very different both in margin size and in number of fractions

3. In the past, most of the radiotherapy treatments were
A. SBRT
B. Hypo-fractionated
C. Hyper-fractionation with large margins accounting for motion or setup uncertainty
D. Hyper-fractionation with small margins accounting for motion or setup uncertainty

4. A patient threw away his immobilization mask before being treated to the neck with a boost plan, what should the therapists do? Assume the linear accelerator has KV imaging capabilities.
A. Make a new mask for the patient at linear accelerator couch, and treat with the original boost plan.
B. Redo a CT with a new mask, and ask the dosimetrist to replan the boost using the new CT.

4.3 Margins Accounting for Positioning (Questions)   313

C. Forget about the mask since it was already lost. Ask the dosimetrist to do a simple plan like bilateral or AP/PA fields for the same dose.
D. Treat the patient without the mask.

5. Historically, why did hyper-fractionation become main stream after CT was used for planning?
A. The margins used to account for motion and setup uncertainty were not small, thus hypo-fractionation treatments with large margins would cause severe normal tissue complications.
B. Hyper-fractionation treatments have better treatment outcome over hypo-fractionation treatments because more dose can be delivered in each treatment.
C. The devices used for immobilization enabled the reproducibility of treatments, allowing physicians to prescribe more fractions.
D. The application of image-guided radiotherapy (IGRT) ensured the reproducibility of fractional treatments and directly led to the popularity of hyper-fractionations.

6. Single-fraction SRS normally has zero or 1 mm margin on the CTV, whereas a standard hyper-fractionated treatment normally has more than a 5 mm margin on the CTV. In addition, SRS gives a much larger dose than standard fractionation. Why is this the case for SRS?
A. I and III are correct.
B. III is correct.
C. II and III are correct.
D. All of them are correct.
I. The idea of radiosurgery is to completely ablate the target with radiation. To avoid healthy tissue from being obliterated and causing complications, only a very small margin is allowed.
II. Since single fractional treatment is used, there is no need to worry about setup uncertainty, thus the margin for that is unnecessary.
III. Small margins allow minimal normal tissue complications as the irradiated volume decreases. Therefore, much larger doses can be given avoiding normal tissue complications.

7. What is the difference between 3D-CRT hyper-fractionation strategy and IMRT hyper-fractionation strategy?
A. Both are efforts to minimize normal tissue complications, and IMRT does a better job.
B. Both are efforts to enhance better treatment outcomes, and IMRT does a better job.
C. IMRT does a better job in both minimizing normal tissue complications and treatment outcomes.
D. Both are efforts to enhance treatment outcomes and to minimize normal tissue complications and IMRT does a better job in both of them.

8. Recently, hypo-fractionation has gradually gained popularity, although this strategy had vanished for decades and the reason for this is:
   A. Actually it is still controversial since hypo-fractionation caused a lot of normal tissue complications (NTC) in the early time of radiotherapy.
   B. With the advent of image-guided radiotherapy (IGRT), much smaller margins can be used, significantly reducing NTC.
   C. After treating patients with radiotherapy for a century, people have a much better understanding on NTCs, thus hypo-fractionation is no longer dangerous.
   D. Gamma Knife has showed that a high fractional dose is fine as long as the target is precisely located, causing hypo-fractionation to be picked up again.

9. Adaptive radiotherapy is another hot topic in radiation therapy. It consists of replanning on a daily basis or when needed to account for changes in patient anatomy or daily motion variations. Will this method help to reduce setup uncertainty?
   A. Not really, since it focuses on replanning due to the target's change with time.
   B. Sure, replanning reduces the setup uncertainty because the new plan follows the change of target.
   C. Actually it depends on whether the target changes with time or not.
   D. It is too early to judge this since it is too new.

4.4 Patient Positioning and Treatment Devices (Answers)

Quiz 1 (Level 2)

1. **E** All of these are used for patient positioning reproducibility. Total or whole body casts have been used in Europe for many years to reproduce and immobilize the patient's position during treatment; the drawback is the time and effort invested in the construction and it may not be suitable for all patients such as obese patients or children. The triangle pillow under the knees is used to relax the back and arm support is used for arm stability. The headrest is one of the most commonly used devices.

2. **A** Some daily treatment setup positions include supine where the patient is positioned lying on his/her back, prone where the patient is lying on his/her stomach, and head and thorax slightly upright, used specially on patients that have difficulty breathing. Trendelenburg is not a treatment setup position used in RT, it is a position used in surgical procedures where the body is laid flat on the back with the feet higher than the head by 15 to 30°.

3. **B** RT lower leg sarcoma. An Alpha Cradle mold consists of a strong plastic bag filled with a set of chemicals which solidify and conform to the patient's treatment area. An Alpha Cradle is very useful in immobilization of extremities, but it can also be used for abdominal and pelvic treatments if additional immobilization and accuracy is required.

4. **C** The belly board can be used in rectum or abdomen treatment sites where the patient is placed in a prone position lying on the belly board which causes the small bowel to be displaced anterior and cephalic by gravity and pressure. Another method is to maintain a full bladder, thereby displacing the small bowel away from the pelvis. In the past, the small bowel could be surgically moved cephalic by placing a Vicryl mesh sling within the abdomen to hold the small bowel in place. The mesh would dissolve within a few weeks, allowing the bowel to return to its normal position.

5. **A** Patient's positioning and device used depend on the patient's medical condition since the patient must lie still during the whole treatment process. The CT scanner bore dimension is of concern since not all CT scanners can fit larger patients or certain devices like breast boards. The setup and device used depend primarily on the location of the disease and the proximity to critical structures as this determines if there are steep dose gradients in the plan.

6. **E** The most common setup uses an Aquaplast mask, shoulder straps, and a headrest. The Aquaplast mask is heated so that it can conform to the patient's head and neck and hardens as it cools. The shoulder straps help move the shoulders inferiorly if the lymph nodes in the lower neck need to be treated. Bite blocks and tongue blades are immobilization devices used for head and neck radiation treatments with tumors near the oral cavity and are used to provide more reproducible jaw position or, in the case of a bite block, can be attached to an external frame to provide additional immobilization.

7. **A** The Vac-Lok bag, Alpha Cradle, wing board, headrest, and breast board are the most commonly used devices for immobilization of thorax radiation treatment. The prone pillow is used for abdomen and pelvic radiation treatments.

8. **D** The Duncan face mask is used for immobilization of CNS patients. The patient is positioned prone using an elevation headrest so that the chin is hyperextended, and so the upper PA spine field exit dose does not affect the mandible. The Duncan face mask holds the head in a reproducible position.

9. **D** Belly boards are used for patients having rectum or other pelvic treatments. The patient is set up prone on the board and the patient's belly will fall into the opening in the board, moving the small bowel away from the treatment volume and minimizing the dose.

10. **C** The Calypso® system consists of radiofrequency (RF)-emitting "beacons" that are implanted in the patient's prostate and an external radiofrequency detector panel. The panel detects the location of the beacons in real time so intra-fraction motion can be tracked, and if the motion is too large, the beam can be stopped. Calypso® cannot modify the beam to track the target, but it can notify the user if the target has moved out of limits.

   CyberKnife is capable of motion tracking because the beam position can be adjusted by the robotic arm to account for organ motion in real time.

11. **D** The 4D electromagnetic array is a flat plate on which there are optical targets. The optical targets are tracked by the infrared cameras in the treatment room so the position of the array is known relative to the treatment isocenter. The implanted electromagnetic transponders are 3 "beacons" implanted into the patient's prostate. They transmit an RF signal and the array can convert this signal into a 3D location in the patient. Using these components together, the system can notify the user if the implanted beacons are outside of the limits.

4.5   Image-Guided Radiotherapy (Answers)

Quiz 1 (Level 2)

1. **A** Image-guided radiotherapy (IGRT) refers to an RT delivery technique where an image is acquired just before or during delivery of a fraction to improve accuracy target localization for delivery and avoidance of organs at risk. Examples of IGRT used today are CBCT, ultrasound, MV portal imaging, etc. A view of the patient from the target, through the beam portal showing patient anatomy within treatment beam, is called a portal image, and this can be compared to the beam's eye view and DRR generated in the planning system to verify patient position.

2. **E** IGRT systems include cone beam computed tomography (CBCT), megavoltage computed tomography (MVCT), portal imaging, and online imaging with paired orthogonal planar images.

3. **D** CBCT imaging enables visualization of the exact tumor localization just prior to treatment on a linac. This technique integrates a CT imaging system with a linac and involves acquiring multiple planar images

4.5 Image-Guided Radiotherapy (Answers)

(called projections) produced by a kilovoltage or megavoltage cone beam rotating a full 360°. The projections can be reconstructed into a 3D image.

4. A The only advantage of megavoltage beams for CBCT is that the beams come from the linac beamline and thus no additional equipment is required to produce the cone beam. Kilovoltage beams produce better soft tissue contrast due to the photoelectric effect and are thus deemed more useful.

5. C A CT-on-rails system is comprised of a linac and a CT unit on rails approaching at opposite ends of a standard radiotherapy treatment table. An advantage of this is that a diagnostic quality CT can be acquired at each fraction. This helps with positioning and also could detect changes in the tumor size. CBCT has much lower soft tissue contrast than a standard CT due to increased scatter. A megavoltage CBCT system is comprised of a detector panel already present for use in electronic portal imaging opposite to the linac head. A kV CBCT system is comprised of a conventional x-ray tube mounted on a retractable arm at 90° to the high-energy treatment beam and a flat panel x-ray detector mounted on a retractable arm opposite the x-ray tube. A BAT system is comprised of a 2D or 3D ultrasound imaging system integrated with an isocentric medical linac.

6. A A TomoTherapy system consists of a 6 MV linear accelerator that rotates around the patient in a CT-type gantry ring. The couch advances the patient through the gantry bore so that the radiation dose is delivered in a helical geometry around the target volume. A binary MLC (leaf position is either open or closed) is used to deliver IMRT treatments.

7. E TomoTherapy IGRT consists of an MVCT scan of patient anatomy at any time before, during, or after treatment as the CT is acquired using the treatment beam. The MVCT image data is acquired with a set of xenon ionization chambers. MVCT guidance can be used to adjust the patient's position at every fraction and an MVCT can be taken after radiation delivery with patient still in the treatment position to evaluate the true dose distribution delivered to the patient.

8. B BAT stands for B-mode acquisition and targeting system. B-mode is a type of ultrasound acquisition technique. An advantage to using ultrasound for IGRT is that no extra ionizing radiation is delivered to the patient.

9. D A BAT system consists of a cart-based ultrasound unit positioned next to a linac treatment table to image the target volume prior to each fraction of a patient's treatment. The advantage is that no ionizing radiation is used but disadvantages include difficulty in reading the ultrasound image, difficulties in acquiring a quality image, and the inability to image past tissue-air interfaces or bone-tissue interfaces.

10. A   The BAT system has found its widest application in pelvic radiotherapy, particularly for prostate cancer. The prostate is imaged transabdominally (or transperitoneal) with an ultrasound probe on a daily basis.

11. C   BrainLab's ExacTrac consists of a set of paired orthogonal x-ray tubes and detectors to determine the location of the lesion in the room coordinate system.

12. A   CyberKnife IGRT is based on a pair of orthogonal x-ray images (similar to BrainLab's ExacTrac) to determine the location of the target relative to the room's coordinate system and communicates these coordinates to the robotic arm, which then adjusts the linac's beam to maintain alignment with the target.

13. E   CyberKnife IGRT uses a pair of orthogonal x-ray images to determine the location of the target relative to the room's coordinate system. These images are compared to a set of digitally reconstructed radiographs (DRRs) obtained from the planning CT. This comparison provides a mechanism to communicate the actual target position to the robotic arm which then adjusts the linac's beam to maintain alignment with the target. Online tracking of target motion is also available.

14. A   Adaptive radiotherapy adapts the treatment plan to account for motion or changes in patient anatomy during the course of treatment. The adaptation could be on a daily basis or as needed. There are many issues with adaptive radiotherapy such as the time it takes to modify the plan, the need for a physician to reapprove an adapted plan, and the QA required on the adapted plan. These issues are being investigated by many groups, and hopefully in the near future, true adaptive radiotherapy will be possible.

15. A   Adaptive radiotherapy adjusts the dose distribution for subsequent treatment fractions of a course of radiotherapy to compensate for inaccuracies in dose delivery that cannot be corrected for by simply adjusting the patient's positioning. It is very useful to correct for tumor shrinkage and patient weight loss.

4.6   Margins Accounted for Positioning (Answers)

Quiz 1 (Level 2)

1. D   SRS and SBRT normally have minimal margins to account for motion and setup uncertainty and are delivered in less than 5 fractions. The reason for the tighter margins is that the lesions are usually found in the brain which does not have any motion. Also, the immobilization is typically better for these cases such as a headframe. All these factors allow for reduced margins which in turn lead to a smaller treated volume and lower normal tissue complications.

4.6 Margins Accounted for Positioning (Answers) 319

2. C Conventional radiotherapy is usually defined by delivery of daily doses of 2 Gy or less, five times a week for several weeks. The term hypo-fractionation can be used to describe any course of radiation with fractional doses greater than 2 Gy and delivered in fewer fractions than a conventional course of treatment. Any RT course that fits any of these criteria may be considered hypo-fractionated such as the Canadian breast hypo-fractionation protocol delivering 267 cGy per fractions for 16 fractions. SBRT is delivered in 5 fractions or less, with each dose delivering very high doses of radiation, greater than 4 Gy/fraction. To do this, the setup accuracy for SBRT must be much tighter than conventional treatments because missing on one fraction would result in a huge underdose. Typically IGRT is done every fraction and sometimes even two or three times per fraction. Because of this, SBRT can typically have smaller margins, although this is not always true. Again, margin size is dependent on the setup accuracy along with proximity to OARs and the motion in that region.

3. B In the past, most treatments were hypo-fractionated, meaning patients were treated in a small number of fractions. However, the only imaging techniques available were radiographic films so the margins could not be tightened. SBRT did not exist at the time as it was impossible to ensure the positioning accuracy that is required for SBRT. Hyper-fractionation was not usually performed, mainly because hypo-fractionation was more convenient and the radiation-induced normal tissue complications were not well understood.

4. B Answer D is definitely incorrect. A mask is necessary for the purpose of immobilization and daily reproducibility. Answer C is not right either, because the doses for organs at risk (OARs) cannot be guaranteed as planned. Answer A is incorrect, because the position of the patient could be quite different from the planned position, introducing uncertainty in dose delivery. Although kV images will allow you to position the patient as in the original CT based on comparison to the DRRs, this position can't be guaranteed and possibly reproduced; therefore a new CT and plan is the appropriate choice.

Answer B is correct. Unfortunately, the patient has to be re-simulated (CT), and a new mask is created for the new CT. A new boost plan should be done on the new CT. The original CT may also be registered to the new CT to evaluate the total prescribed dose (from original plan and new boost plan) and that the involved organs are within the dose tolerance.

Immobilization devices are very important in RT; thus losing them usually requires repeating everything.

5. A Normal tissue complications used to be a major concern in RT. Since imaging modalities were not quite developed, a large margin to account for motion and setup uncertainty was always needed to ensure adequate coverage of the disease volume.

Answer B is incorrect, Hypo-fractionated treatments usually involve relatively larger fractional dose.

Answer C is incorrect. The number of fractionations is still limited by the tolerance of normal tissues.

Answer D is incorrect, mature IGRT techniques were not developed at the time when hyper-fractionation started to become popular.

6. **A** Stereotactic radiosurgery (SRS) means you can accurately localize the target with a fixed coordinate system using something like a fixed headframe. Because of the increased immobilization, the margins can be reduced to 1 mm or less which reduces the treatment volume.

7. **A** Hyper-fractionation is done in an effort to avoid normal tissue complications (NTCs) by taking advantage of the radiobiology of tumors and normal tissues. By hyper-fractionating, the normal tissues have more time to recover. In the past, most of the treatments were hypo-fractionated and caused a lot of NTCs. Later it was found that smaller fractional doses and more fractions may significantly reduce NTCs, leading to the use of hyper-fractionated treatments.

   Hyper-fractionated IMRT has even better results in minimizing NTCs than 3D-CRT because it allows better normal tissue sparing by modulating the dose to avoid OARs and target the tumor. The downside to hyper-fractionation is that it is very inconvenient for the patient and the cost of care is increased. The current fractionation schemes aim to balance the NTCs and the costs of the treatment. As more research is done on hypo-fractionation and as image guidance and positioning accuracy increases, hypo-fractionation is starting to gain popularity again (plus there is a reduction in cost which is very important in modern healthcare).

8. **B** IGRT is extremely helpful in precisely locating the target, thus the margin used to account for setup uncertainty can be minimized. This reduces the amount of normal tissues being irradiated for treatment, allowing for increase in fractional doses and reduction in number of fractions. Another benefit of hypo-fractionation is convenience for the patient and reduced cost of care. In current healthcare environments, anything that can cut cost and still be effective is desirable.

9. **A** The primary goal of adaptive radiotherapy is to account for the change in the target throughout multiple fractions of a treatment course. To minimize the setup uncertainty, IGRT (CBCT, kV planar image, MV port film, etc.) is needed which is already the standard of care for most cases where adaptive therapy would be beneficial.

Brachytherapy 5

Contents

5.1	General Concepts on Brachytherapy (Questions)	322
5.2	Radioactive Source Characteristics (Questions)	326
5.3	Implant Methods (Questions)	335
5.4	Temporary Implant Procedures (Questions)	340
5.5	Permanent Implant Procedures (Questions)	348
5.6	Dose Delivery (Questions)	351
5.7	Brachytherapy Dose Calculations (Questions)	354
5.8	ICRU and AAPM TG Reports on Brachytherapy (Questions)	364
5.9	General Concepts on Brachytherapy (Answers)	368
5.10	Radioactive Source Characteristics (Answers)	370
5.11	Implant Methods (Answers)	377
5.12	Temporary Implant Procedures (Answers)	380
5.13	Permanent Implant Procedures (Answers)	384
5.14	Dose Delivery (Answers)	386
5.15	Brachytherapy Dose Calculations (Answers)	388
5.16	ICRU and AAPM TG Reports on Brachytherapy (Answers)	403

In some institutions, dosimetrists are responsible for high-dose brachytherapy (HDR) planning followed by a physics check and signature. Dose delivery procedures for HDR, however, are always handled by certified medical physicists because special training is required.

There is no significant difference in dosimetry between low-dose rate (LDR) and HDR brachytherapy planning, but there are biological differences in terms of the dose delivery.

5.1 General Concepts on Brachytherapy (Questions)

Quiz-1 (Level 2)

1. Which of the following statements are true about brachytherapy?
A. I, II, and III
B. I and III only
C. II and IV only
D. IV only
E. All are correct
I. Sources may be left in place for a limited period of time to irradiate the tissues.
II. Brachytherapy delivers fractionated doses of 120–400 cGy multiple times separated by many hours or days.
III. Brachytherapy uses sealed sources of ionizing radiation placed within the patient.
IV. Brachytherapy is an external beam radiation therapy.

2. Methods used in brachytherapy are:
A. I, II, and III
B. I and III only
C. II and IV only
D. IV only
E. All are correct
I. Interstitial
II. Intracavitary
III. Surface application
IV. Intravascular

3. A procedure where a radioactive source is implanted and then left for several days before being removed describes:
A. HDR brachytherapy
B. LDR brachytherapy
C. Permanent brachytherapy
D. Local brachytherapy

4. Which of the following is/are the advantages of the remote afterloading technique in HDR brachytherapy?
A. I, II, and III
B. I and III only
C. II and IV only
D. IV only
E. All are correct

5.1 General Concepts on Brachytherapy (Questions)

I. Reducing unnecessary exposure to personnel.
II. Plan in advance.
III. Prepare needed apparatus in advance.
IV. Facilitate optimal loading of an implant after the apparatus is inserted but before the radioactivity is actually loaded.

5. Packing material (gauze, etc.) is commonly used along with intracavitary applicators like a vaginal cylinder. What is the function of the packing in these implants?
A. I, II, and III
B. I and III only
C. II and IV only
D. IV only
E. All are correct
I. Keep the applicator sterilized in the body
II. Hold the applicator firmly in position
III. Avoidbody fluids in contact with the applicator
IV. Pushe normal tissues away from the source, reducing the dose to healthy tissue

6. Which of the following is the best approach to reduce personnel exposure during a brachytherapy treatment?
A. Hot implant technique
B. Using dummy wires while treatment
C. Remote afterloading technique
D. Manual afterloading technique

7. In 2D brachytherapy planning, to aid dose calculations and precise localization of the sources, which of the following is/are correct?
A. I, II, and III
B. I and III only
C. II and IV only
D. IV only
E. All are correct
I. At least two radiographs are necessary.
II. Orthogonal films are taken at right angles (90°).
III. Magnification factors are carefully determined for each film.
IV. Two posterior oblique films at 120° are required.

8. Modern remote afterloading units consist of:
A. I, II, and III
B. I and III only
C. II and IV only
D. IV only
E. All are correct

I. Lead-shielded storage area for radioactive source
II. Several channels for source transport
III. A remote loading and unloading system
IV. A variety of applicators that are inserted into the patient

9. Which of the following are examples of applicator types with which remote afterloading systems can be used?
A. I, II, and III
B. I and III only
C. II and IV only
D. IV only
E. All are correct
I. Interstitial brachytherapy
II. Skin applicators
III. Gynecologic intracavitary brachytherapy applicator
IV. Endobronchial catheters

10. The film magnification factor used in brachytherapy is given by:
A. SFD/SAD
B. SFD×SAD
C. 0.693/HVL
D. $F=[(SSD_2+d_m)/(SSD_1+d_m)\times(SSD_1+d)/(SSD_2+d)]^2$

11. In 2D brachytherapy planning, three-dimensional reconstruction of the source geometry is usually accomplished by using:
A. Isodose curves
B. Tandem and ovoid method
C. Manchester system
D. Orthogonal imaging or the stereo-shift method

12. When planning an HDR treatment using a remote afterloader unit, the desired isodose distributions can be obtained by:
A. Programming dwell position and dwell time of the source
B. Using MLC to control dwell position and time
C. Using compensators to control source position
D. Programming how far the source travels

13. Disadvantages of remote afterloader units include:
A. I, II, and III
B. I and III only
C. II and IV only
D. IV only
E. All are correct
I. Quality assurance requirements are significantly greater.
II. The units are expensive and require a substantial capital expenditure.
III. Additional costs must be considered for room shielding.
IV. Increase exposure to medical personnel.

5.1 General Concepts on Brachytherapy (Questions)

14. Which of the following are advantages of remote afterloading units?
A. I, II, and III
B. I and III only
C. II and IV only
D. IV only
E. All are correct
I. Provide the capability of optimizing dose distributions beyond what is possible with manual afterloading.
II. Treatment techniques can be made more consistent and reproducible.
III. HDR remote afterloading permits treatment on an outpatient basis.
IV. HDR remote afterloading is suited for treating large patient populations.

15. According to the ICRU, the dose rate criteria at the dose specification point(s) for an LDR brachytherapy treatment is:
A. 0.4–2 Gy/h
B. 2–12 Gy/h
C. >12 Gy/h
D. >1,200 cGy/h

16. The advantage(s) of using HDR systems over LDR systems is/are:
A. I, II, and III
B. I and III only
C. II and IV only
D. IV only
E. All are correct
I. Optimization of dose distribution
II. Outpatient treatments
III. Elimination of staff radiation exposure
IV. Minimum QA

17. Disadvantages of HDR systems include:
A. I, II, and III
B. I and III only
C. II and IV only
D. IV only
E. All are correct
I. Uncertainty in biological effectiveness
II. Potential for accidental high exposures and serious errors
III. Increased staff commitment
IV. Inpatient treatment

18. What are the differences between LDR and HDR system?
A. LDR uses multiple sources together with inactive spacers to achieve typical treatment dose rates of about 0.4–2 Gy/h. HDR uses a single source, with a typical activity of 10–20 Ci.
B. LDR uses a single source with a typical activity of 0.4–2 Gy/h. HDR uses multiple sources together with inactive spacers to achieve typical treatment dose rates of about 10–20 Ci.

C. LDR uses multiple sources together with inactive spacers to achieve typical treatment dose rates of about 0.4–12 Gy/h; HDR uses a single source with a typical activity of 0.4–2 Gy/h.
D. LDR uses a single source with a typical activity of 0.4–12 cGy/h. HDR uses multiple sources together with inactive spacers to achieve typical treatment dose rates of about 0.4–2 cGy/h.

19. Which of the following are essential components of remote afterloading system?
A. I, II, and III
B. I and III only
C. II and IV only
D. IV only
E. All are correct
I. Safe to house the radioactive source
II. A local or remote operating console
III. A source control and drive mechanism
IV. Source transfer guide tubes and treatment applicators

5.2 Radioactive Source Characteristics (Questions)

Quiz-1 (Level 2)

1. Which of the following radioisotopes is most commonly used in remote afterloader units?
A. ^{137}Cs
B. ^{60}Co
C. ^{192}Ir
D. ^{226}Ra

2. Which of the following particles emitted in the radium decay series is of importance for clinical use?
A. Alpha particles
B. Beta particles
C. Electrons
D. Gamma rays

3. Match the following radionuclides with their corresponding half-life:

A.	^{226}Ra	I.	(30.0 years)
B.	^{222}Rn	II.	(73.8 days)
C.	^{60}Co	III.	(3.83 days)
D.	^{137}Cs	IV.	(59.4 days)
E.	^{192}Ir	V.	(1,600 years)
F.	^{198}Au	VI.	(17 days)

5.2 Radioactive Source Characteristics (Questions)

G.	^{125}I	VII.	(2.7 days)
H.	^{103}Pd	VIII.	(5.26 years)
E.	^{90}Sr	IX.	(14.0 days)
F.	^{90}Y	X.	(64 h)
G.	^{32}P	XI.	(28 years)

4. Match the following radionuclides with their corresponding exposure rate constant Γ (Rcm^2/mg-h):

A.	^{226}Ra	I.	(13.07)
B.	^{222}Rn	II.	(4.69)
C.	^{60}Co	III.	(10.15)
D.	^{137}Cs	IV.	(2.38)
E.	^{192}Ir	V.	(1.48)
F.	^{198}Au	VI.	(8.25)
G.	^{125}I	VII.	(1.45)
H.	^{103}Pd	VIII.	(3.28)

5. Match the following radionuclides with their corresponding effective photon energy (MeV):

A.	^{226}Ra	I.	(1.25)
B.	^{222}Rn	II.	(0.42)
C.	^{60}Co	III.	(0.37)
D.	^{137}Cs	IV.	(0.83 avg)
E.	^{192}Ir	V.	(0.02)
F.	^{198}Au	VI.	(0.028)
G.	^{125}I	VII.	(0.83 avg)
H.	^{103}Pd	VIII.	(0.66)

6. Match the following radionuclides with their corresponding decay rate:

A.	^{226}Ra	I.	(4 % daily)
B.	^{222}Rn	II.	(18 % daily)
C.	^{60}Co	III.	(1 % yearly)
D.	^{137}Cs	IV.	(2.3 % yearly)
E.	^{192}Ir	V.	(1 % monthly)
F.	^{198}Au	VI.	(25 % daily)
G.	^{125}I	VII.	(1 % daily)
H.	^{103}Pd	VIII.	(>1 % yearly)

7. What do ^{131}I, ^{32}P, ^{90}Y, and ^{90}Sr have in common?
A. They all emit gamma rays.
B. They all emit β^-.
C. They all emit β^+.
D. They all have a very long $T_{1/2}$.

8. Radium-226 (^{226}Ra) has been replaced by other radioactive nuclides because:
A. I, II, and III
B. I and III only
C. II and IV only
D. IV only
E. All are correct
I. Any leakage from a ^{226}Ra source can result in deposition of a high radiation dose in bone.
II. ^{226}Ra high average gamma ray energy can result in high exposures to medical personnel.
III. Radon gas leakage represents a significant hazard if source is broken.
IV. ^{226}Ra has a very short $T_{1/2}$ which makes the radionuclide impractical for brachytherapy treatments.

9. Which of the following statements are true about ^{226}Ra?
A. I, II, and III
B. I and III only
C. II and IV only
D. IV only
E. All are correct
I. ^{226}Ra is a decay product of ^{238}U and decays to stable form of lead, ^{206}Pb.
II. Radium $T_{1/2}$ is 1,622 years.
III. ^{226}Ra emits alpha particles, beta particles, and gamma rays.
IV. ^{226}Ra sources are manufactured as needles or tubes in a variety of lengths and activities.

10. What is the active length of a radium source?
A. The distance between the actual ends of the source
B. Milligrams of radium content
C. The distance between the ends of the radioactive material
D. Transverse thickness of the capsule wall, usually expressed in terms of millimeters of platinum

11. How does one obtain the uniformity of activity distribution of a radioactive source?
A. Taking orthogonal images (90°) apart of the source in the simulation room
B. Placing the source on an unexposed x-ray film for a time long enough to obtain reasonable darkening of the film
C. Doing a leak test to determine how much uniform activity the source has
D. Using a well-type ion chamber

5.2 Radioactive Source Characteristics (Questions)

12. Historically, what was characteristic of an Indian club radium needle?
A. The amount of radium activity was uniformly spread throughout the active length.
B. The amount of radium activity was uniform, but with higher activity at one end of the needle.
C. The amount of radium activity was uniform, but with higher activity at both ends of the needle.
D. Are usually furnished in multiples of 5 mg of radium filtered by 1 mm platinum.

13. Which is the exposure rate constant of radium (^{226}Ra)?
A. 3.27 R-cm^2/mg-h
B. 8.25 R-cm^2/mg-h
C. 13.07 R-cm^2/mg-h
D. 8.25 R-cm^2/mg-h

14. The activity of radioactive nuclide-emitting photons is related to the exposure rate by:
A. The exposure rate constant (Γ)
B. The source construction
C. The physical length of the source
D. The half-life ($T_{1/2}$)

15. The exposure rate constant of radium (^{226}Ra) is measured:
A. At a distance of 1 cm from a 1 mCi point source filtered by 0.5 mm platinum
B. At a distance of 1 cm from a 1 mg point source filtered by 0.5 mm platinum
C. At a distance of 1 mm from a 1 mCi point source filtered by 0.5 mm platinum
D. At a distance of 1 cm from a 1 mg point source filtered by 0.5 mm lead

16. Brachytherapy treatment sources are chosen based on:
A. I, II, and III
B. I and III only
C. II and IV only
D. IV only
E. All are correct
I. The half-life ($T_{1/2}$) of the source
II. The photon energy (MeV) of the source
III. The activity of the source
IV. The half-value layer of the source

17. Advantages of cesium-137 (^{137}Cs) over radium include:
A. I, II, and III
B. I and III only
C. II and IV only
D. IV only
E. All are correct

I. ^{137}Cs requires less shielding than radium (^{226}Ra).
II. ^{137}Cs has a longer $T_{1/2}$ than radium (^{226}Ra).
III. ^{137}Cs is less hazardous in the microsphere form than radium (^{226}Ra).
IV. ^{137}Cs can be used clinically for 1,000 years without replacement.

18. Match the following radionuclides with their form used. Answers can be used more than once:

A.	^{226}Ra	I.	Wire
B.	^{103}Pd	II.	Needles
C.	^{60}Co	III.	Powder
D.	^{137}Cs	IV.	Seeds
E.	^{192}Ir	V.	Grains
F.	^{198}Au	VI.	Tubes
G.	^{125}I		

19. Which of the following radionuclides emit gamma (γ) rays for radiotherapy?
A. I, II, and III
B. I and III only
C. II and IV only
D. IV only
E. All are correct
I. Radium-226 (^{226}Ra)
II. Cobalt-60 (^{60}Co)
III. Cesium-137 (^{137}Cs)
IV. Gold-198 (^{198}Au)

20. The main advantage of cobalt-60 (^{60}Co) is:
A. It is an inexpensive source.
B. It has a very long $T_{1/2}$.
C. ^{60}Co inventory system is simple.
D. It has a high specific activity.

21. ^{60}Co can be used to replace which of the following sources on an intracavitary application?
A. Radium-226 (^{226}Ra)
B. Gold-198 (^{198}Au)
C. Iodine-125 (^{125}I)
D. Palladium-103 (^{103}Pd)

22. Which of the following statements are true about iridium-192 (^{192}Ir)?
A. I, II, and III
B. I and III only
C. II and IV only
D. IV only
E. All are correct

5.2 Radioactive Source Characteristics (Questions)

I. ^{192}Ir is composed of 30 % alloy Ir and 70 % Pt.
II. Because of the low energy, these sources require less shielding for personnel protection.
III. The half-life is relatively short requiring frequent source replacement.
IV. The source can be used in nonpermanent implants similar to radium and cesium.

23. Gold-198 is used for:
A. Intracavitary implant
B. Surface molds implants
C. Temporal implant
D. Permanent implant

24. Which are the advantages of iodine-125 (^{125}I) when used for permanent implants over radon and gold-198 (^{198}Au)?
A. I, II, and III
B. I and III only
C. II and IV only
D. IV only
E. All are correct
I. Its encapsulation in titanium
II. Its longer half-life ($T_{1/2}$)
III. Its simple dosimetry
IV. Its low photon energy

25. The anisotropic dose distribution around iodine-125 (^{125}I) sources creates:
A. Hot spots near the source ends
B. Cold spots near the source ends
C. A change on its exposure rate constant
D. Cold spots at the center of the source

26. The advantage of palladium-103 (^{103}Pd) over iodine-125 (^{125}I) for permanent implants is:
A. There are not any advantages; both are the same.
B. ^{103}Pd is not encapsulated.
C. ^{103}Pd can deliver a much faster dose rate.
D. ^{103}Pd photon fluence distribution around the source is *not* anisotropic.

27. The source strength for any radionuclide may be specified in terms of:
A. Millicurie (mCi)
B. Kilovoltage potential (kVp)
C. Sievert (Sv)
D. rem

28. The exposure rate of a radionuclide at any particular point is:
A. Proportional to the product of its mass and its exposure rate constant
B. Proportional to the product of its activity and its exposure rate constant
C. Proportional to its milligram of radium equivalent
D. Proportional to the air kerma strength

29. The National Council on Radiation Protection and Measurements (NCRP) recommends that the strength of any γ-emitter should be specified directly in terms of:
A. Exposure rate in air at a specified distance such as 1 m
B. Exposure rate in tissue at a specified distance such as 1 m
C. Exposure rate in tissue at Dmax
D. Exposure rate in air at Dmax

30. Historically, brachytherapy sources are specified in terms of the equivalent mass of radium because:
A. It is an accurate measurement.
B. This is the only method used for source specification.
C. Some users accustomed to radium sources continue to use mg-Ra eq.
D. The best way to specify brachytherapy sources is in terms of mg-Ra eq.

31. Apparent activity is defined as:
A. The product of air kerma rate in free space and the square of the distance of the calibration point from the source center along the perpendicular bisector
B. The activity of a bare point source of the same nuclide that produces the same exposure rate at 1 m as the source to be specified
C. The thickness of material necessary to reduce the number of photons in a beam or intensity to 50 % of its initial value
D. The activity of a source that produces different exposure rate at 1 m as the source to be specified

32. 1 mg-Ra eq is equal to:
A. 8.25×10^{-4} mR/h at 1 m
B. 8.25×10^{-4} R/h at 1 m
C. 8.25×10^{-2} R/h at 1 m
D. 8.25×10 R/h at 1 m

33. The rapid falloff of radium-226 (^{226}Ra), cobalt-60 (Co^{60}), and cesium-137 (^{137}Cs) at a distance of about 5 cm in tissue is due to:
A. Inverse square law
B. Tissue attenuation
C. Double encapsulation of the isotopes
D. Apparent activity

34. A dosimeter used to calibrate brachytherapy source is:
A. Thimble ionization chamber
B. Extrapolation chamber
C. Parallel-plate chamber
D. Well-type ion chamber

5.2 Radioactive Source Characteristics (Questions)

35. The dose rate constant of a radionuclide depends on:
A. I, II, and III
B. I and III only
C. II and IV only
D. IV only
E. All are correct
I. The type of source
II. Its construction
III. Its encapsulation
IV. Its physical length

36. Which of the following is true about radium sources?
A. Because the half-life for radioactive decay is much longer for radium-226 than for any of its daughter products, radium achieves secular equilibrium with its daughters.
B. Because the half-life for radioactive decay is not much longer for radium-226 than for any of its daughter products, radium achieves transient equilibrium with its daughters.
C. Because the half-life for radioactive decay is much longer for radium-226 than for any of its daughter products, radium achieves transient equilibrium with its daughters.
D. Because the half-life for radioactive decay is not much longer for radium-226 than for any of its daughter products, radium achieves secular equilibrium with its daughters.

37. According to the AAPM and ICRU, the strength of a brachytherapy source must be specified in terms of:
A. Air kerma rate $K_{air}(d_{ref})$
B. Activity
C. Number of disintegrations per unit time
D. Exposure rate produced at a given distance from the source

38. Air kerma strength is defined as:
A. The sum of the products of the reference air kerma rate and the duration of the application of each source.
B. The product of air kerma rate in "free space" and the square of the distance of the calibration point from the source center along the perpendicular bisector
C. The activity of a bare point source of the same nuclide that produces the same exposure rate at 1 m as the source to be specified
D. Kinetic energy released in matter, measured in gray or rad

39. The SI unit of the reference air kerma rate is:
A. Gy/s
B. cGy/Ci
C. Curie (Ci)
D. Becquerel (Bq)

40. Brachytherapy source encapsulation:
   A. I, II, and III
   B. I and III only
   C. II and IV only
   D. IV only
   E. All are correct
   I. Contains the radioactivity
   II. Provides source rigidity
   III. Absorbs any (α) alpha and, for photon-emitting sources, (β) beta radiation produced through the source decay
   IV. Allows for handling of the source without any complications.

41. The useful radiation fluence from a brachytherapy source generally consists of:
   A. I, II, and III
   B. I and III only
   C. II and IV only
   D. IV only
   E. All are correct
   I. Gamma (γ) rays
   II. Characteristic x-rays
   III. Bremsstrahlung radiation
   IV. Alpha (α) rays

42. The choice of an appropriate photon-emitting radionuclide for a specific brachytherapy treatment depends on:
   A. I, II, and III
   B. I and III only
   C. II and IV only
   D. IV only
   E. All are correct
   I. Photon energies and penetration
   II. Half-life and half-value layer (HVL)
   III. Specific activity and source strength
   IV. Encapsulation

43. Some brachytherapy sources are doubly encapsulated in order to provide adequate shielding against:
   A. I, II, and III
   B. I and III only
   C. II and IV only
   D. IV only
   E. All are correct
   I. Beta (β) particles
   II. Alpha (α) particles
   III. Leakage of radioactive material
   IV. Gamma (γ) rays

44. Some of the radioactive isotopes used in liquid form include:
A. I, II, and III
B. I and III only
C. II and IV only
D. IV only
E. All are correct
I. ^{131}I
II. ^{32}P
III. ^{198}Au
IV. ^{90}Y

5.3 Implant Methods (Questions)

Quiz-1 (Level 2)

1. The Paterson-Parker or Manchester system of implant dosimetry:
A. Uses uniform strength sources implanted in parallel lines or in an array
B. Uses uniform strength sources to achieve a nonuniform dose distribution, higher in the central region of treatment
C. Uses nonuniform strength sources to archive uniform dose distribution (within ±10 %) to a plane or volume
D. Uses uniform strength sources spaced 1 cm apart

2. Some methods used to provide optimal brachytherapy dose distributions in the irradiated volume are:
A. I, II, and III
B. I and III only
C. II and IV only
D. IV only
E. All are correct
I. The Paterson-Parker system
II. The Memorial system
III. The Paris system
IV. The MLC system

3. The implant types used in the Manchester system are:
A. I, II, and III
B. I and III only
C. II and IV only
D. IV only
E. All are correct
I. Planar implant
II. Circular implant
III. Volume implant
IV. Triangular implant

4. In the case of planar implants for the Paterson-Parker or Manchester system:
A. I, II, and III
B. I and III only
C. II and IV only
D. IV only
E. All are correct
I. The prescribed dose is 10 % higher than the minimum dose.
II. The prescribed dose is 10 % lower than the minimum dose.
III. The maximum dose should not exceed 110 % of the prescribed dose.
IV. The maximum dose should exceed 110 % of the prescribed dose.

5. In the case of planar implants with the Paterson-Parker or Manchester system, if the size of the implant is 50 cm^2, what fraction of radium is used in the periphery and what fraction is used in the center?
A. 1/3 in the center, 2/3 in the periphery.
B. 2/3 in the center, 1/3 in the periphery.
C. The distribution is even throughout the area.
D. ½ in the center, ½ in the periphery.

6. Which of the following statements are true about planar implants with the Paterson-Parker or Manchester system?
A. I, II, and III
B. I and III only
C. II and IV only
D. IV only
E. All are correct
I. The spacing of the needles should not exceed 1 cm from each other or from the crossing ends.
II. If the ends cannot be crossed, reduce the activity by 10 % from the area for each uncrossed end.
III. One needle should touch the end of the next around the periphery, while in the central area, they should be spread out uniformly.
IV. The needles should lie parallel to each other within the plane.

7. If it is impossible to cross both ends on a single-plane Paterson-Parker or Manchester system implant, then:
A. I, II, and III
B. I and III only
C. II and IV only
D. IV only
E. All are correct
I. The treatment area should be considered as 90 % of the length of the implant.
II. The treatment area should be considered as 80 % of the length of the implant.
III. Use of Indian club needles eliminates the need for crossing needles at both ends.
IV. Use of dumbbell needles eliminates the need for crossing needles at both ends.

5.3 Implant Methods (Questions)

8. A volume implant is required if the lesion is:
A. Less than 2.5 cm thick.
B. More than 2.5 cm thick.
C. Less than 2 cm thick.
D. It could be perform at any lesion thickness.

9. Which of the following are types of volume implants used in the Paterson-Parker or Manchester system?
A. I, II, and III
B. I and III only
C. II and IV only
D. IV only
E. All are correct
I. Cylinder volume shape
II. Sphere volume shape
III. Cuboid volume shape
IV. Octagon volume shape

10. Which of the following statements are true about the distribution of sources in a volume implant using the Paterson-Parker or Manchester system?
A. I, II, and III
B. I and III only
C. II and IV only
D. IV only
E. All are correct
I. The amount of radium is divided into eight parts for all the volume types.
II. The cylinder is composed of a belt (four parts), a core (two parts), and each end (one part).
III. The sphere is made up of a shell (six parts) and a core (two parts).
IV. The cuboid consists of each side (one part), each end (one part), and a core (two parts).

11. Which of the following statements are true about volume implants used in Paterson-Parker or Manchester system?
A. I, II, and III
B. I and III only
C. II and IV only
D. IV only
E. All are correct
I. The needles should be spaced as uniformly as possible, not more than 1 cm apart.
II. The prescribed dose is stated 10 % higher than the minimum dose within the implanted volume.
III. There should be at least eight needles in the belt and four in the core.
IV. If the ends of the volume implant are uncrossed, 7.5 % is deducted from the volume for uncrossed end.

12. In the case of an implant using the Quimby system:
A. I, II, and III
B. I and III only
C. II and IV only
D. IV only
E. All are correct
I. For the planar implant, the stated dose is the maximum dose in the plane of treatment.
II. For the planar implant, the stated dose is the minimum dose in the plane of treatment.
III. For the volume implant, the stated dose is the minimum dose within the implant volume.
IV. For the volume implant, the stated dose is the maximum dose within the implant volume.

13. Which of the following is an extension of the Quimby system?
A. The Paris system
B. The Paterson-Parker system
C. The Memorial system
D. The Manchester system

14. The Paris system:
A. I, II, and III
B. I and III only
C. II and IV only
D. IV only
E. All are correct
I. Uses sources of uniform linear activity.
II. The line source spacing must be constant, but the space is selected according to implant dimensions.
III. Uses sources implanted in parallel lines.
IV. Crossing needles are not used.

15. What is the minimum and maximum source separation according to implant dimensions allowed using the Paris system?
A. Minimum of 1 cm, maximum of 2 cm
B. Minimum of 8 mm, maximum of 2 cm
C. Minimum of 8 mm, maximum of 1.5 cm
D. Minimum of 1 cm, maximum of 15 mm

16. The reference isodose in the Paris system is fixed at:
A. 85 % of the basal dose
B. 50 % of the basal dose
C. 95 % of the prescribed dose
D. 95 % of the volume to receive 100 % of the dose

5.3 Implant Methods (Questions)

17. The basal dose is defined as:
A. The average of the maximum dose between sources
B. The average of the minimum dose between sources
C. The maximum dose in the plane of treatment
D. The total dose contribution from each point

18. Mach the following types of brachytherapy implants with its corresponding description.
A. Intracavitary
B. Interstitial
C. Surface (mold)
D. Intraluminal
E. Intraoperative
F. Intravascular
G. Temporal
H. Permanent
I. Dose is delivered over the lifetime of the source until completely decayed.
II. A single source is placed into small or large arteries.
III. Sources are placed into body cavities close to the tumor volume.
IV. Dose is delivered over a short period of time, and the sources are removed after the prescribed dose has been reached.
V. Sources are placed over the tissue to be treated.
VI. Sources are implanted surgically within the tumor volume.
VII. Sources are implanted into the target tissue during surgery.
VIII. Sources are placed in a lumen.

19. The brachytherapy hot loading method is defined as:
A. The applicator is placed first into the target position and the radioactive sources are loaded later, either by hand or by a machine.
B. The applicator is preloaded and contains radioactive sources at the time of placement into the patient.
C. The applicator is hot, so it cannot be inserted directly into the patient.
D. The applicator contains hot sources, so it cannot be inserted directly into the patient.

20. Match the following applicators with its corresponding definition.
A. Fletcher-Suit
B. Vaginal cylinder
C. Rectal applicator
D. Intraluminal catheter
E. Nasopharyngeal applicator
F. Interstitial implant

I. Used for treatments of prostate gland, gyn malignancies, breast, and some head and neck tumors. Hollow needles are implanted into the tumor, and the source is introduced into the needle.
II. Used for treatment of endobronchial carcinoma. Suitable diameter catheters of various lengths.
III. Used for treatment of nasopharyngeal tumors with HDR. The applicator set includes tracheal tube, catheter, and a nasopharyngeal connector.
IV. Used for treatment of gynecological malignancies of the uterus, cervix, and pelvic side walls. Consists of rigid intrauterine tandems with curvatures of 15°, 30°, and 45° and a pair of ovoids.
V. Used for treatment of vaginal wall. Consists of acrylic cylinders having a variety of diameters and an axially drilled hole to accommodate a catheter.
VI. Used for treatment of superficial tumors of the rectum. Consists of acrylic cylinders of different diameters. Selected shielding is incorporated to spare normal tissue.

5.4 Temporary Implant Procedures (Questions)

Tandem and ovoids (LDR, HDR), vaginal cylinder (HDR), and eye plaque (LDR)

Quiz-1 (Level 2)

1. Which of the following are considered surface applicators?
A. I, II, and III
B. I and III only
C. II and IV only
D. IV only
E. All are correct
I. Sr-90 applicator
II. COMS eye plaque
III. Molds applicator
IV. Tandem and ovoid

2. A Sr-90 applicator is used to treat:
A. Choroidal melanoma
B. Pterygium
C. Ocular melanoma
D. Skin lesions

3. Sr-90 is a:
A. Gamma (γ) emitter
B. Alpha emitter
C. Beta-minus emitter
D. Neutron emitter

5.4 Temporary Implant Procedures (Questions)

4. The sources typically used for COMS eye plaques are:
A. I, II, and III
B. I and III only
C. II and IV only
D. IV only
E. All are correct
I. Radium-226 (^{226}Ra)
II. Iodine-125 (^{125}I)
III. Gold-198 (^{198}Au)
IV. Palladium-103 (^{103}Pd)

5. For a volume implant using the Manchester system, the radioactive material is distributed on the belt, the core, and the ends. Which part of the implant is the belt?
A. The inner needles
B. The crossing needles
C. The periphery
D. The uncrossing end

6. What does the acronym COMS stand for?
A. Cornea obstruction melanoma study
B. Choroidal ocular melanoma study
C. Concave obstructive melanoma study
D. Custom ocular mold study

7. The two major parts of a COMS eye plaque are:
A. Gold backing and Silastic seed insert
B. Tungsten backing and Silastic seed insert
C. Lead backing and silicone
D. Wax backing and plaster of Paris

8. Surface molds can be used to treat:
A. I, II, and III
B. I and III only
C. II and IV only
D. IV only
E. All are correct
I. Superficial skin lesions
II. Lesions of the oral and nasal cavity
III. Lesions of the hard palate
IV. Lesions to the prostate

9. In interstitial therapy, the radioactive sources are fabricated in the form of:
A. I, II, and III
B. I and III only
C. II and IV only
D. IV only
E. All are correct

I. Needles
II. Wires
III. Seeds
IV. Grains

10. Which of the following sources are used in a temporal interstitial implant?
A. I, II, and III
B. I and III only
C. II and IV only
D. IV only
E. All are correct
I. Radium needles
II. Gold (^{198}Au) seeds
III. Iridium wires or seeds
IV. Iodine-125 (^{125}I) seeds

11. Intracavitary therapy is mostly used for cancers of the:
A. I, II, and III
B. I and III only
C. II and IV only
D. IV only
E. All are correct
I. Vagina
II. Cervix
III. Uterine body
IV. Bladder

12. The most common method of intracavitary brachytherapy is:
A. COMS eye plaque applicator
B. Needles using the Paris system
C. Fletcher tandem and ovoid applicator
D. Henschke applicator

13. Which of the following systems of dose specification for cervix treatment is the most extensively used?
A. Milligram-Hours
B. The Manchester system
C. The International Commission on Radiation Units and Measurements System
D. The Quimby system

14. The Milligram-Hours system is not used because:
A. I, II, and III
B. I and III only
C. II and IV only
D. IV only
E. All are correct

5.4 Temporary Implant Procedures (Questions) 343

I. It lacks information on source arrangement.
II. It lacks information for the position of the tandem relative to the ovoids.
III. It lacks information of packing for the applicators.
IV. It lacks information of tumor size and patient anatomy.

15. The Manchester system used for treatment of the cervix is characterized by dose to?
A. I, II, and III
B. I and III only
C. II and IV only
D. IV only
E. All are correct
I. Point A and B
II. Rectum point
III. Bladder point
IV. Bowel point

16. The duration of the implant for a brachytherapy treatment of the cervix using the Manchester system is based on:
A. Dose rate calculated at point B
B. Dose rate calculated at the bladder point
C. Dose rate calculated at the rectum point
D. Dose rate calculated at point A

17. The point of prescription for a brachytherapy treatment of the cervix using the Manchester system is:
A. Point A
B. Point B
C. Bladder point
D. Rectum point

18. On a brachytherapy treatment of the cervix, point A is defined as:
A. 2 cm superior to the lateral vaginal fornix and 2 cm lateral to the cervical canal
B. 2 cm superior to the external cervical os and 2 cm lateral to the cervical canal
C. 2 cm superior to the internal cervical os and 2 cm lateral to the cervical canal
D. 2 cm inferior to the lateral vaginal fornix and 2 cm lateral to the cervical canal

19. On a brachytherapy treatment of the cervix, point B is defined as:
A. 2 cm superior to the external cervical os or head of the ovoids and 5 cm lateral to point A if the uterus is tipped
B. 3 cm superior to the external cervical os or head of the ovoids and 2 cm lateral to point A if the uterus is not tipped
C. 2 cm superior to the external cervical os or head of the ovoids and 3 cm lateral to point A if the uterus is not tipped
D. 5 cm superior to the external cervical os or head of the ovoids and 4 cm lateral to point A if the uterus is tipped

20. On a brachytherapy treatment of the cervix, point A represents:
A. The location where the uterine vessels cross the ureter
B. The location of the obturator nodes
C. The location of the bladder
D. The location of the rectum

21. Limitations to using point A as a prescription point on a brachytherapy treatment of the cervix include:
A. I, II, and III
B. I and III only
C. II and IV only
D. IV only
E. All are correct
I. It relates to the position of the sources and not to a specific anatomic structure.
II. Dose to point A is very sensitive to the position of the ovoid sources relative to the tandem sources.
III. Depending on the size of the cervix, it may lie inside the tumor or outside.
IV. Dose prescription at point A could risk underdosage of large cervical cancers or overdosage of small ones.

22. Recently, for an intracavitary treatment, the ICRU has recommended a system of dose specification that relates the dose distribution to:
A. Point A
B. Point B
C. Target volume
D. Bladder and rectum points

23. Tandem and ovoid applicators are used for:
A. Cervical cancer patients after a hysterectomy has been performed
B. Cervical cancer patients when no hysterectomy has been performed
C. Any patient who has cervical cancer
D. Bladder and rectum cancer patients when surgery cannot be achieved

24. On a brachytherapy treatment of the cervix, the bladder point is located radiographically:
A. I, II, and III
B. I and III only
C. II and IV only
D. IV only
E. All are correct
I. At the center of the balloon on the frontal radiograph
II. 3 cm lateral from the center of the balloon on the frontal radiograph
III. On the lateral radiograph, on a line drawn anteroposteriorly through the center of the balloon, at the posterior surface
IV. On the lateral radiograph, on a line drawn anteroposteriorly through 3 cm lateral from the center of the balloon, at the anterior surface on the lateral radiograph

5.4 Temporary Implant Procedures (Questions) 345

25. On a brachytherapy treatment of the cervix, the rectal point is located radiographically:
A. I, II, and III
B. I and III only
C. II and IV only
D. IV only
E. All are correct
I. 3 cm lateral from the ovoid sources on the frontal radiograph.
II. At the midpoint of the ovoid sources on the frontal radiograph
III. On the lateral radiograph, on a line drawn 3 cm lateral from the ovoid sources, 5 cm in front the posterior vaginal wall
IV. On the lateral radiograph, on a line drawn from the middle of the ovoid sources, 5 mm behind the posterior vaginal wall

26. On a brachytherapy treatment of the cervix, which of the following points corresponds to the para-aortic and iliac nodes?
A. Point A
B. Point B
C. Lymphatic trapezoid of Fletcher
D. Pelvic wall points

27. Which of the following organs are at risk during a brachytherapy treatment of the cervix?
A. I, II, and III
B. I and III only
C. II and IV only
D. IV only
E. All are correct
I. Rectum
II. Seminal vesicles
III. Bladder
IV. Prostate

28. The anterior rectal wall and the sigmoid colon dose can be minimized by:
A. I, II, and III
B. I and III only
C. II and IV only
D. IV only
I. Using a rectal retractor
II. Using packing
III. Using a tandem with appropriate degree of angulation
IV. Minimizing the treatment time

29. The Radiation Therapy Oncology Group or RTOG states that the bladder and rectum doses should be limited to:
A. 10 % or less than point A
B. 5 % or less than point A
C. 80 % or less than point A
D. Equal to that of point A

30. Which of the following statements are true about the position of the tandem and ovoids?
A. I, II, and III
B. I and III only
C. II and IV only
D. IV only
E. All are correct
I. The tandem is inserted through the cervical os into the body of the uterus or uterine canal.
II. Ovoids are inserted into the vagina.
III. The cervical clamp is fitted to the tandem and rests at the location of the cervix.
IV. The cervical clamp prevents the tandem from penetrating deeper into the uterus.

31. Which of the following statements are true about ovoid position?
A. I, II, and III
B. I and III only
C. II and IV only
D. IV only
E. All are correct
I. Ovoids rest snugly against the vaginal fornices.
II. Ovoids are clamped to the tandem to hold them as a single unit.
III. Ovoids use plastic cylinders like cup to ensure the vaginal mucosa does not come in direct contact with the ovoids.
IV. Ovoid cups should be as large as possible to keep vaginal surface dose down.

32. For a brachytherapy treatment of the cervix:
A. The longest tandem length as well as the largest set of ovoids that fit the patient's anatomy should always be used.
B. The longest tandem length but the smallest set of ovoids should always be used.
C. The smallest tandem length as well as the smallest set of ovoids should always be used.
D. The tandem length and the size of the ovoids are not important on a brachytherapy treatment of the cervix.

5.4 Temporary Implant Procedures (Questions)

33. Where is the prescription point for a vaginal cylinder high-dose brachytherapy normally located?
A. Vaginal surface
B. 5 mm posterior to the vaginal surface
C. 5 mm superior to the vaginal surface
D. Anywhere in the pelvis

34. In a standard HDR applicator, how far can the radioactive source go?
A. To the tip end of the catheter
B. Normally 1–2 mm from the tip end of the catheter
C. Normally 4–5 mm from the tip end of the catheter
D. Normally 8–10 mm from the tip end of the catheter

35. Recently, in GYN HDR, the field has moved away from the ICU points and is now using 3D planning and DVHs. Rather than looking at the point max dose, what volume is typically looked at as the OAR constraint?
A. 5 cc of the given structure
B. 4 cc of the given structure
C. 3 cc of the given structure
D. 2 cc of the given structure

36. Which of the following applicators is used for endometrial cancer in the case where a hysterectomy has been performed?
A. I, II, and III
B. I and III only
C. II and IV only
D. IV only
E. All are correct
I. Cylinder
II. Tandem and ovoids
III. Burnett applicator
IV. Catheters

37. The methods of dose optimization for an endometrial cancer using a cylinder are:
A. I, II, and III
B. I and III only
C. II and IV only
D. IV only
E. All are correct
I. Prescribing to point A
II. Prescribing to the surface and dome of the cylinder
III. Prescribing to point B
IV. Prescribing to 5 mm from the surface of the cylinder

38. According to ICRU report #38, what is the difference when determining the dose to rectum using a tandem and ovoid versus using a vaginal cylinder?
A. There is no difference.
B. On the lateral film, the rectal point is 5 mm posterior to the vaginal wall for both applicators, but on the anterior film, the rectal point is located at the lower end of the intrauterine source for the tandem and ovoid and in the middle of the intrauterine source for the cylinder.
C. On the lateral film, the rectal point is 5 mm posterior to the vaginal wall but is 5 mm anterior for the cylinder. On the anterior film, the rectal point is located at the lower end of the intrauterine source for both applicators.
D. On the lateral film, the rectal point is 5 mm anterior to the vaginal wall for both applicators. On the anterior film, the rectal point is located in the middle of the intrauterine source for both applicators.

39. As recommended by the ICRU, the lymphatic trapezoid points correspond to:
A. I, II, and III
B. I and III only
C. II and IV only
D. IV only
E. All are correct
I. Para-aortic lymph nodes
II. Common iliac lymph nodes
III. External iliac lymph nodes
IV. Pelvic wall point

5.5 Permanent Implant Procedures (Questions)

Quiz-1 (Level 2)

1. Which of the following are factors that must be known when doing a permanent prostate seed implant?
A. I, II, and III
B. I and III only
C. II and IV only
D. IV only
E. All are correct
I. Choice of radionuclide
II. Planning technique
III. Source delivery technique
IV. Total prescribed dose

5.5 Permanent Implant Procedures (Questions)

2. Which of the following radionuclides are used for permanent radioactive seed implants?
A. I, II, and III
B. I and III only
C. II and IV only
D. IV only
E. All are correct
I. Palladium (^{103}Pd)
II. Iridium (^{192}Ir)
III. Iodine (^{125}I)
IV. Radium (^{226}Ra)

3. Which of the following permanent radioactive seed implants is used to treat fast-growing high-grade tumors?
A. Iodine (^{125}I)
B. Gold (^{198}Au)
C. Palladium (^{103}Pd)
D. Iridium (^{192}Ir)

4. The surgical approaches to perform seed implantation of the prostate are:
A. I, II, and III
B. I and III only
C. II and IV only
D. IV only
E. All are correct
I. Retropubic
II. Ultrasound guided
III. Transperineal
IV. Retroperitoneal

5. Which of the following image guidance technique is used during seed implantation of the prostate?
A. I, II, and III
B. I and III only
C. II and IV only
D. IV only
E. All are correct
I. MRI
II. Ultrasound
III. PET
IV. Fluoroscopy

6. Which of the following statements is true about post-implant dosimetry?
A. Post-implant dosimetry is usually performed 1 week post-implantation using MRI images.
B. Post-implant dosimetry is usually performed 1 month post-implantation using CT images.
C. Post-implant dosimetry is usually performed 1 month post-implantation using MRI images.
D. Post-implant dosimetry is usually not necessary unless patient has side effects due to the surgery.

7. The position adopted by the patient for a transperineal prostate seed implant is:
A. Supine
B. Prone
C. Decubitus
D. Dorsal lithotomy

8. In the case of a large prostate gland or significant pubic arch interference on a permanent prostate implant procedure:
A. The patient may need hormonal therapy for a few months.
B. The patient is positioned on Trendelenburg as much as possible.
C. The patient implant must be done retropubically.
D. Patient cannot have a permanent prostate implant done.

9. A preplanned permanent prostate pre-implant includes:
A. I, II, and III
B. I and III only
C. II and IV only
D. IV only
E. All are correct
I. Number of needles to be used
II. Number of seeds in each needle
III. Template coordinates
IV. Size of the needles to be used

10. Which of the following organs should be contoured on a permanent prostate pre-implant treatment plan?
A. I, II, and III
B. I and III only
C. II and IV only
D. IV only
E. All are correct
I. Prostate
II. Urethra
III. Rectum
IV. Bladder

5.6 Dose Delivery (Questions)

11. The major problems with permanent seed implants are:
A. I, II, and III
B. I and III only
C. II and IV only
D. IV only
E. All are correct
I. Disagreement between the pre-implant and post-implant dose distributions
II. Patient recovery
III. Source anisotropy
IV. Radiation safety

12. What is the purpose of doing a cystoscopy after a permanent prostate implant procedure?
A. Make sure that all the seeds are in correct position
B. Look for any seeds that may have been accidentally implanted into the bladder
C. Look for any seeds that may have been accidentally implanted into the rectum
D. In vivo count of all the implanted seeds in the prostate

13. The average life of a radionuclide is:
A. The sum of the lifetimes of all the individual atoms divided by the total number of atoms present originally
B. The number of disintegrations per second of a radioactive source
C. The thickness of a given material needed to reduce the intensity of a photon beam to 50 % of its initial value
D. The time necessary for a radioactive material to decay to 50 % of its original activity

5.6 Dose Delivery (Questions)

Applicators, source calibration, and dwell position accuracy

Quiz-1 (Level 2)

1. What devices are used to calibrate HDR source strength?
A. Rule, radiochromical film, or any feasible films
B. A calibrated G-M counter
C. Well-type ion chamber and electrometer
D. Farmer-type ion chamber and electrometer

2. What is the "sweet spot"?
A. The center of the well chamber
B. The position in the well chamber having the maximum reading of charge
C. The position in the well chamber having the maximum reading of current
D. 3 cm in the catheter to the top of the well chamber

3. The correct applicator for a lung intralumen implant is a:
A. Tandem and ovoids
B. Cylinder
C. Heyman capsules
D. Catheter

4. Which of the following statements are true?
A. I, II, and III only
B. I and III only
C. II and IV only
D. IV only
E. All are correct
I. For intracavitary applications, radium and cesium are equally effective as far as the therapeutic effects are concerned.
II. For interstitial implants, iridium-192 is the best available source although iodine-125 offers some advantages for particular techniques.
III. For intracavitary applications, cesium has replaced radium mainly for radiation protection considerations relating to storing and handling the sources.
IV. Afterloading procedures are the current standard of practice in brachytherapy.

5. Which of the following checks are recommended for intracavitary sources and manual afterloading source identification?
A. I, II, and III only
B. I and III only
C. II and IV only
D. IV only
E. All are correct
I. Source physical length
II. Source diameter
III. Source serial number
IV. Source color coding

6. Which of the following statements is/are true?
A. I, II, and III only
B. I and III only
C. II and IV only
D. IV only
E. All are correct
I. Active length and source distribution activity can be checked using an autoradiograph.
II. The source symmetry may be ascertained by leaving it on a film for an appropriate length of time.
III. All sources should be checked for source uniformity and symmetry.
IV. The iso-optical density curve is obtained by autoradiograph of one random source from each group of designated strength.

5.6 Dose Delivery (Questions)

7. If a disagreement between the vendor and the user source calibration is within ±5 %:
A. The user calibration should be used.
B. The vendor calibration should be used.
C. The source would require recalibration by the vendor.
D. The source would require recalibration by the user.

8. Intracavitary applicator's internal positioning may be examined by:
A. Orthogonal radiographs.
B. Visual inspection.
C. No internal structure exam is required.
D. CT scan.

9. Source position accuracy can be checked by:
A. I, II, and III only
B. I and III only
C. III and IV only
D. IV only
E. All are correct
I. The dummy sources in CT scan
II. Radiographs of dummy sources in the applicators
III. Visual inspection
IV. Autoradiography

10. The position of dummy sources and radioactive sources should correspond:
A. Within ±1 mm
B. Within ±3 mm
C. Within ±5 mm
D. Within ±1 cm

11. What is the smallest step size for a typical HDR source?
A. 5 mm
B. 3 mm
C. 2.5 mm
D. 2 mm
E. 1.5 mm

12. In an endobronchial HDR case, the treatment site is 11 cm long. What is the most appropriate step size to be chosen if a Nucletron remote afterloading unit is used?
A. 10 mm
B. 5 mm
C. 2.5 mm
D. 2 mm

5.7 Brachytherapy Dose Calculations (Questions)

Quiz-1 (Level 2)

1. Which of the following equations is used to calculate exposure rate of a radio-nuclide at any distance?
   A. $D_0 \times t_{avg}$
   B. # of mCi of radionuclide $\times \Gamma$ of radionuclide/Γ Ra
   C. $\Gamma \times A/d^2$
   D. $X \times t$

2. You have a 10 mCi source of ^{137}Cs. How many Becquerel is this?
   A. 301,550,000 Bq
   B. 8.15 Bq
   C. 300,000,000 Bq
   D. 603,100,000 Bq

3. The exposure rate at 1 cm of any 15 mg-Ra eq source is:
   A. 8.25 R/h
   B. 123.75 R/h
   C. 8.25 mR/h
   D. 123.75 mR/h

4. If the exposure rate at 3 cm from a source of ^{137}Cs is 3.62 R/h, what would be the exposure rate at 7 cm from the source?
   A. 0.66 R/h
   B. 19.71 R/h
   C. 1.55 R/h
   D. 0.051 R/h

5. How many mg-Ra eq are contained in 0.53 mCi of ^{192}Ir?
   A. 0.0212 mg-Ra eq
   B. 13.25 mg-Ra eq
   C. 0.301 mg-Ra eq
   D. 0.0373 mg-Ra eq

6. If the exposure rate at 3 cm from a 10 mCi source of ^{137}Cs is said to be 3.62 R/h, what would be the exposure rate at 7 cm from the source using an additional 25 % filtration?
   A. 0.499 R/h
   B. 0.665 R/h
   C. 1.164 R/h
   D. 0.1662 R/h

5.7 Brachytherapy Dose Calculations (Questions)

7. Calculate the mg-Ra eq from a Ra-226 source which has a dose rate of 3.20 R/h at 5 cm.
   A. 0.103 mg-Ra eq
   B. 9.697 mg-Ra eq
   C. 80 mg-Ra eq
   D. 1.939 mg-Ra eq

8. What is the strength of iridiun-192 (^{192}Ir) in mg-Ra eq if its exposure rate is 0.495 mR/h at 1 m?
   A. 0.408 mg-Ra eq
   B. 0.603 mg-Ra eq
   C. 1.666 mg-Ra eq
   D. 0.330 mg-Ra eq

9. Using the Manchester system and the table below (mg-h to deliver 1,000 cGy to each depth), calculate the number of mg-Ra eq to deliver a dose of 2,000 cGy in 40 h to 1.5 cm depth for a 4.44 cm² single-plane implant that is crossed on one end only.

Table 5.7.1

Area cm²	0.5 cm	1.0 cm	1.5 cm	2.0 cm
0	30	119	268	476
2	97	213	375	598
4	141	278	462	698
6	177	333	536	782
8	206	384	599	855

   A. 2,000 mg
   B. 10.23 mg
   C. 23.10 mg
   D. 462 mg

10. What is the amount of radioactive material on the periphery and center of the treatment volume using Manchester planar distribution rules if 20 mg-h is used on an area less than 25 cm²?
    A. Periphery 6.66 mg, center 13.33 mg
    B. Periphery 13.33, center 6.66 mg
    C. Periphery 10 mg, center 10 mg
    D. Periphery 15 mg, center 5 mg

11. What is the amount of radioactive material on the belt, core, and each end for a cylinder implant using the Manchester volume implant system if both ends are crossed and 20 mg-h is delivered?
    A. Belt 10 mg-h, core 5 mg-h, and each end 5 mg-h
    B. Belt 5 mg-h, core 10 mg-h, and each end 2.5 mg-h
    C. Belt 10 mg-h, core 5 mg-h, and each end 2.5 mg-h
    D. Belt 10 mg-h, core 10 mg-h, and each end 5 mg-h

12. What is the amount of radioactive material in the belt, core, and each end using a cylinder implant with the Manchester volume implant system if one end is uncrossed and if 20 mg-h is delivered?
    A. Belt 11.43 mg-h, core 5.7 mg-h, and the crossing end 2.9 mg-h
    B. Belt 11.43 mg-h, core 5.7 mg-h, and each end 2.9 mg-h
    C. Belt 5.7 mg-h, core 11.43 mg-h, and the crossing end 2.9 mg-h
    D. Belt 2.9 mg-h, core 11.43 mg-h, and the crossing end 5.7 mg-h

13. What is the amount of radioactive material in the belt, core, and each end using a SPHERE implant with the Manchester volume implant system if 20 mg-h is delivered?
    A. Belt 5 mg-h, core 10 mg-h, and each end 0 mg-h
    B. Belt 5 mg-h, core 10 mg-h, and each end 5 mg-h
    C. Belt 10 mg-h, core 10 mg-h, and each end 0 mg-h
    D. Belt 15 mg-h, core 5 mg-h, and each end 0 mg-h

14. Which of the following formulas is used to calculate basal dose using the Paris system?
    A. $D_{total} = D_0 \times t_{avg}$
    B. $BD = BD_1 \times BD_2 \times BD_3/3$
    C. $BD = BD_1 - BD_2 - BD_3/3$
    D. $BD = BD_1 + BD_2 + BD_3/3$

15. In a typical survey meter, what would the reading in mR/hr be if the meter needle were pointing to 5.5 and the multiplication factor were positioned to the ×10 scale?
    A. 15.5 mR/h
    B. 55 mR/h
    C. 4.5 mR/h
    D. 1.8 mR/h

16. For permanent implants, the total dose to a point may be found from the initial dose rate by:
    A. $D_{total} = D_0/t_{avg}$
    B. $D_{total} = D_0 - t_{avg}$
    C. $D_{total} = D_0 \times t_{avg}$
    D. $D_{total} = D_0 \times t_{avg}[1 - e^{t/t_{avg}}]$

17. Calculate the total dose to a point for a permanent implant using ^{198}Au if the initial dose rate is 5 Gy per day.
    A. 19.45 Gy
    B. 2.66 Gy
    C. 17.14 Gy
    D. 9.35 Gy

5.7 Brachytherapy Dose Calculations (Questions)

18. The physician wants to deliver a total dose of 150 Gy for a permanent implant using ^{125}I. What is the correct initial dose rate of the source used?
A. 0.57 Gy/day
B. 1.75 Gy/day
C. 1.75 Gy/h
D. 0.57 Gy/h

19. An ^{125}I source implant was performed on a patient on June 15, 2014, with the intention to deliver 70 Gy to the tumor. Due to emergency, the sources were removed on September 1, 2014. Calculate the dose delivered to the tumor:
A. 89 cGy
B. 5,987 cGy
C. 4,187 cGy
D. 7,210 cGy

20. What is the total dose to a point for a permanent implant using ^{198}Au if the initial dose rate is 15 cGy per hour?
A. 93.31 cGy
B. 673.6 cGy
C. 0.160 cGy
D. 1,399 cGy

21. For temporary implants, the total dose to a point may be found from the initial dose rate by:
A. $D_{total} = D_0/t_{avg}$
B. $D_{total} = D_0/[1 - e^{t/t_{avg}}] \times t_{avg}$
C. $D_{total} = D_0 \times t_{avg}$
D. $D_{total} = D_0 \times t_{avg}[1 - e^{t/t_{avg}}]$

22. How long must a temporary ^{192}Ir implant be left in place to deliver 2,000 cGy if the initial dose rate is 0.7 Gy/h?
A. 25 h
B. 10 h
C. 50 h
D. 24 h

23. The formula to find t_{avg} used in the equation of permanent and temporary implant is:
A. $t_{avg} = 1.44/t_{1/2}$
B. $t_{avg} = 1.44 \times t_{1/2}$
C. $t_{avg} = 0.693/t_{1/2}$
D. $t_{avg} = 0.693/\lambda$

24. Calculate the t_{avg} of ^{60}Co.
A. 0.273 days
B. 7.57 days
C. 7.57 years
D. 0.312 years

25. 0.75 mCi of ^{192}Ir is needed in your department, but the order must be placed in number of mg-Ra eq. What is the correct amount order?
A. 1.34 mg-Ra eq
B. 134 mg-Ra eq
C. 0.42 mg-Ra eq
D. 50.83 mg-Ra eq

26. 0.60 mCi of radium equivalent is needed in your department, but the order must be placed in mCi of ^{137}Cs. What is the correct amount order?
A. 23 mCi of ^{137}Cs
B. 0.23 mCi of ^{137}Cs
C. 15.9 mCi of ^{137}Cs
D. 1.59 mCi of ^{137}Cs

27. A ^{198}Au source has been calibrated and its exposure rate is 0.350 mR/h at 1 m. What is the strength of this source in terms of effective mg-Ra eq?
A. 0.042 mg-Ra eq
B. 2.357 mg-Ra eq
C. 0.424 mg-Ra eq
D. 23.57 mg-Ra eq

28. Calculate the mCi of ^{103}Pd used if a physical length of 30 cm ^{103}Pd titanium tube contains two graphite pallets plated with an active length of 20 cm at 0.85 mg-Ra eq/cm.
A. 85.4 mCi of ^{103}Pd
B. 178 mCi of ^{103}Pd
C. 4.73 mCi of ^{103}Pd
D. 0.15 mCi of ^{103}Pd

29. How many mCi of ^{131}I are present in a 1-mg-Ra eq ^{131}I?
A. 3.587 mCi of ^{131}I
B. 0.279 mCi of ^{131}I
C. 356.9 mCi of ^{131}I
D. 18.97 mCi of ^{131}I

30. 12 mg-Ra eq is equal to how many mCi of ^{137}Cs, ^{198}Au, and ^{125}I?
A. 4.742 mCi of ^{137}Cs, 3.462 mCi of ^{198}Au, 2.124 mCi of ^{125}I
B. 30.36 mCi of ^{137}Cs, 41.59 mCi of ^{198}Au, 67.81 mCi of ^{125}I
C. 67.81 mCi of ^{137}Cs, 30.36 mCi of ^{198}Au, 41.59 mCi of ^{125}I
D. 2.124 mCi of ^{137}Cs, 3.462 mCi of ^{198}Au, 4.742 mCi of ^{125}I

5.7 Brachytherapy Dose Calculations (Questions)

31. Calculate how many mg-Ra eq of ^{137}Cs, ^{198}Au, and ^{125}I are present in 12 mCi.
A. 2.124 mg-Ra eq of ^{137}Cs, 3.462 mg-Ra eq of ^{198}Au, 4.742 mg-Ra eq of ^{125}I
B. 30.36 mg-Ra eq of ^{137}Cs, 41.59 mg-Ra eq of ^{198}Au, 67.81 mg-Ra eq of ^{125}I
C. 4.74 mg-Ra eq of ^{137}Cs, 3.46 mg-Ra eq of ^{198}Au, 2.12 mg-Ra eq of ^{125}I
D. 67.81 mg-Ra eq of ^{137}Cs, 30.36 mg-Ra eq of ^{198}Au, 41.59 mg-Ra eq of ^{125}I

32. A physician wants a treatment done using 30 mCi-min of ^{125}I, but the documents must be filled out in mg-Ra eq-h. How many mg-Ra eq-h should be documented?
A. 318.54 mg-Ra eq-min
B. 10,171 mg-Ra eq-h
C. 5.309 mg-Ra eq-h
D. 318.54 mg-Ra eq-h

33. A vaginal treatment was performed using a cylinder loaded with two ^{137}Cs sources with activities of 100 and 120 mCi. What is the total number of mg-Ra eq?
A. 86.90 mg-Ra eq
B. 39.50 mg-Ra eq
C. 47.40 mg-Ra eq
D. 556.6 mg-Ra eq

34. The exposure rate constant of radium is said to be 8.25 R cm^2/mg-h because:
A. The exposure rate at 1 cm from a 1-mg point source of radium-226 unfiltered is 8.25 R cm^2/mg-h.
B. The exposure rate at 10 cm from a 1-mg point source of radium-226 unfiltered is 8.25 R cm^2/mg-h.
C. The exposure rate at 1 cm from a 1-mg point source of radium-226 filtered by 0.5 mm of platinum (Pt) is 8.25 R cm^2/mg-h.
D. The exposure rate at 10 cm from a 1-mg point source of radium-226 filtered by 0.5 mm of platinum (Pt) is 8.25 R cm^2/mg-h.

35. The exposure rate of any radionuclide at any distance and at any length of time can be calculated by:
A. $X = \lambda \times A/r^2 \times t$
B. $X = r^2 \times A/\Gamma \times t$
C. $X = \Gamma \times A/r^2 \times t$
D. $X = 1.44 \times t_{1/2}$

36. What would be the weekly exposure to an accountant who is sitting 2 m from 15 mCi of ^{137}Cs?
A. 0.049 mCi
B. 0.049 mrem
C. 0.049 R
D. 49 Ci

37. Calculate the exposure rate (R/h) at 2 m from 250 mg-Ra eq of ^{198}Au.
    A. 1.250 R/h
    B. 0.006 R/h
    C. 2.975 R/h
    D. 0.051 R/h

38. Which of the following formulas is used to calculate activity of a radionuclide after a specific time?
    A. $A = A_0 e^{-\lambda t}$
    B. $A = t \times A_0 e^{-\lambda/T_{1/2}}$
    C. $A = t \times e^{-\lambda/A}$
    D. $A = A_0 e^{\lambda t}$

39. A ^{103}Pd has arrived to your department with an initial activity of 15 mCi. Calculate the activity of this source after 15 days.
    A. 27.64 mCi
    B. 81.38 mCi
    C. 8.138 mCi
    D. 216.01 mCi

40. A physician wants to deliver a total dose of 70 Gy using ^{103}Pd sources. Calculate the delivered dose 5 days after the implant:
    A. 12.95 Gy
    B. 1.295 Gy
    C. 57.09 Gy
    D. 15.82 Gy

41. A package of ^{137}Cs sources was received in your department on January 1, 2010. Each source had an initial activity of 80 mCi. What will be the activity of each source on July 2, 2012?
    A. 84.76 mCi
    B. 75.52 mCi
    C. 8.476 mCi
    D. 7.552 mCi

42. Calculate the activity of ^{192}Ir having an original activity of 12.5 Ci and the source is 3 months old.
    A. 5.250 Ci
    B. 12.15 Ci
    C. 2.934 Ci
    D. 9.395 Ci

43. What is the approximate activity of a ^{137}Cs source after 180 months?
    A. 70 %
    B. 12.5 %
    C. 50 %
    D. 25 %

5.7 Brachytherapy Dose Calculations (Questions)

44. A permanent implant was scheduled to be done using a group of ^{125}I seeds on January 1, but due to patient health issues, the implant was done 2 weeks later using the same seeds. To maintain the same prescription dose, approximately how many more seeds will have to be implanted?
A. 15 %
B. 85 %
C. 17 %
D. 2 %

45. If a procedure is scheduled at specific time in the future, which of the following formulas is used to calculate initial activity of a radionuclide?
A. $A_0 = A_t e^{-\lambda/T_{1/2}} \times t$
B. $A_0 = t \times A_t e^{-\lambda/T_{1/2}}$
C. $A_0 = t \times e^{-\lambda/A}$
D. $A_0 = A_t \times e^{\lambda t}$

46. What will be the ^{198}Au source activity at the time of order if at the implant 5 days later the activity is 10 mCi?
A. 2.77 mCi
B. 6.88 mCi
C. 9.04 mCi
D. 36.14 mCi

47. A temporary implant of ^{192}Ir has been scheduled for Monday, the 1st of the month at 8:00 am. The physician wants to deliver 15 Gy and the initial dose rate of the ^{192}Ir source is 0.6 Gy/h. When does the source have to be removed so that the patient receives the correct dose?
A. Wednesday, 3rd at 8:00 am
B. Monday, 1st at 10:00 pm
C. Tuesday, 2nd at 9:00 am
D. Thursday, 4rd at 10:00 am

48. How many Bq should you order if 100 mCi of ^{198}Au is needed?
A. 3.7×10^9 Bq
B. 3.7×10^7 Bq
C. 37,000,000 Bq
D. 3.7×10^5 Bq

49. One Ci is equal to:
A. 3.7×10^4 Bq
B. 3.7×10^7 Bq
C. 3.7×10^{10} Bq
D. 3.7×10^1 Bq

50. The R to rad (or cGy) conversion factor in air is:
A. 8.25 Rcm²/mg-h
B. 0.876 cGy/R
C. 0.693
D. 0.511 MeV

51. What is the equation used to find the air kerma strength of 1 mCi of ¹⁰³Pd?
A. 1.48×0.693
B. 1.44×17 days
C. 1.48×0.876
D. 0.696/17 days

52. How much is 1 mg-Ra eq in terms of air kerma strength in cGy?
A. 9.418 cGy/h
B. 0.106 cGy/h
C. 7.227 cGy/h
D. 7.374 cGy/h

53. What is the air kerma strength in microgray (μGy/h) at 2 m if it has been calculated that at 1 cm from the source, the air kerma strength is 7.227 cGy/h?
A. 361.35 μGy/h
B. 0.0002 μGy/h
C. 0.0361 μGy/h
D. 1.8067 μGy/h

54. What would be the total reference air kerma if 90 mCi of ¹⁹²Ir was planned to be left on the patient's skin for 72 h?
A. 26,622 μGy at 1 cm
B. 26,622 μGy at 1 m
C. 4.108 μGyh⁻¹m²
D. 369.72 μGy/hr at 1 m

55. Which of the following answers is correct if a physicist asks you to calculate the fraction of decay per year of ¹³⁷Cs so that a new order can be placed?
A. 2.2 %/year
B. 0.22 %/year
C. 97 %/year
D. 33.3 %/year

56. ¹⁹²Ir source was placed in the new HDR machine. An evaluation of the source must be done monthly, so the physicist asks you to calculate the fraction of decay of ¹⁹²Ir per month. Which of the following answers is correct?
A. 0.9 %/month
B. 24.4 %/month
C. 13.23 %/month
D. 0.755 %/month

5.7 Brachytherapy Dose Calculations (Questions)

57. An incident occurred at your department where a therapist worked for 2 h at 5 m from a ^{125}I source whose exposure rate at 2 m is known to be 200 mR/h. What was the exposure received by the therapist?
A. 2,500 mR
B. 160 mR
C. 64 mR
D. 32 mR

58. The formula to calculate HVL is composed of?
A. I, II, and III
B. I and III only
C. II and IV only
D. IV only
E. All are correct
I. Half-life ($T_{1/2}$)
II. Linear attenuation coefficient (μ)
III. Exposure rate constant (Γ)
IV. Natural log of 2 (0.693)

59. Calculate the HVL if the linear attenuation coefficient is 0.050 cm^{-1}.
A. 0.035 cm
B. 13.86 cm
C. 0.072 cm
D. 0.0743 cm

60. If the thickness of a material needed to reduce the intensity to one-half of its original value is 15 m, what will be the linear attenuation coefficient?
A. 21.64 m^{-1}
B. 10.39 m^{-1}
C. 15.69 m^{-1}
D. 0.046 m^{-1}

61. A part-time accountant will be working for 10 h/week in an area next to an HDR room. Her desk will be 4.6 m from the ^{192}Ir source. The RSO measured a dose rate of 200 mrem/h at 5 ft from the source. Calculate how many HVLs are needed to reduce the dose to the accountant to less than 100 mrem per year.
A. 10 HVL
B. 7 HVL
C. 1 TVL
D. 5 HVL

62. Calculate the dose to point P from sources A, B, and C using the following table (cGy/mg-Ra eq-h) and diagram:
A. 7.83 cGy/h
B. 40.30 cGy/h
C. 18.75 cGy/h
D. 17.30 cGy/h

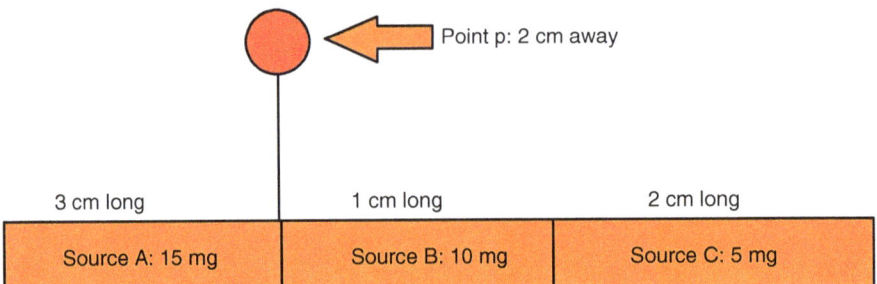

Fig. 5.7.1

Table 5.7.2

Distance along the source, cm						
Distance away cm	0	1.0	1.5	2.0	2.5	3
1.0	6.69	4.11	2.48	1.54	0.99	0.68
2.0	1.89	1.56	1.25	0.97	0.74	0.57
3.0	0.86	0.77	0.70	0.60	0.51	0.42
4.0	0.49	0.46	0.43	0.39	0.35	0.31
5.0	0.31	0.30	0.29	0.27	0.25	0.22

5.8 ICRU and AAPM TG Reports on Brachytherapy (Questions)

Quiz-1 (Level 2)

1. ICRU 58 was written to:
A. Generate a guideline about the dose specification and reporting for interstitial brachytherapy
B. Generate a guideline about fundamental quantities and units for ionization radiation
C. Generate a guideline about prescribing, recording, and reporting dose for photon beam therapy
D. Generate a guideline about the dose and volume specification for reporting intracavitary therapy in gynecology

2. Per ICRU 58, the total time of implantation on a temporary implant depends on:
A. I, II, and III
B. I and III only
C. II and IV only
D. IV only
E. All are correct
I. Number of sources used
II. Strengths and type of the source
III. Pattern of distribution of sources
IV. Organs at risk

5.8 ICRU and AAPM TG Reports on Brachytherapy (Questions) 365

3. Which of the following is true about volume and planes as defined in ICRU 58?
A. I, II, and III
B. I and III only
C. II and IV only
D. IV only
E. All are correct
I. The clinical treatment volume on an interstitial implant is defined as the palpable extent of the malignant growth.
II. The dose value at the treatment volume encompassed by a specific isodose surface is the minimum target volume.
III. GTV is not of concerned on interstitial brachytherapy treatment.
IV. For interstitial brachytherapy, the PTV is, in general, identical to the CTV.

4. What is the minimum target dose (MTD) as specified by ICRU 58?
A. I, II, and III
B. I and III only
C. II and IV only
D. IV only
E. All are correct
I. Is specified at the periphery of the CTV
II. Is specified as the minimum doses between sources, in the central plane
III. Most be equal of approximately 90 % of the prescribed dose in the Manchester system for interstitial therapy
IV. The volume of tissue receiving 150 % of the mean central dose

5. As per ICRU 58, dose uniformity is measured using:
A. I, II, and III
B. I and III only
C. II and IV only
D. IV only
E. All are correct
I. The volume within the CTV encompassed by the isodose line corresponding to 90 % of the prescribed dose
II. Individual minimum doses used to calculate the mean central dose in the central plane
III. The ratio of the maximum target dose to minimum target dose
IV. The ratio of minimum target dose to the mean central dose

6. As per ICRU 58, the time and dose rate for temporary implants can be calculated by:
A. Time = prescribed dose × initial dose rate
B. Time = prescribed dose/initial dose rate
C. Time = prescribed dose + initial dose rate
D. Time = prescribed dose − initial dose rate

7. As per ICRU 58, which of the following parameters must be recorded and reported on temporary interstitial brachytherapy?
A. I, II, and III
B. I and III only
C. II and IV only
D. IV only
E. All are correct
I. Detailed description of volumes (GTV, CTV…)
II. Description of the radioisotope and filtration used
III. Description of the pattern of source distribution
IV. Description of the technique used

8. In compliance with the NRC regulations, the leakage radiation levels outside the HDR unit:
A. Should not exceed 1 R/h at a distance of 10 mm with the source in the shielded position
B. Should not exceed 10 mR/h at a distance of 5 cm with the source in the shielded position
C. Should not exceed 1 mR/h at a distance of 10 cm with the source in the shielded position
D. Should not exceed 10 mR/h at a distance of 10 mm with the source in the shielded position

9. Which of the AAPM TG reports refers to brachytherapy source dose calculation?
A. TG-51
B. TG-43
C. TG-21
D. TG-40

10. Which of the following is the comprehensive AAPM TG report for permanent prostate seed implant brachytherapy?
A. TG-43
B. TG-40
C. TG-64
D. TG-128

11. Which of the following AAPM TG reports provides the dosimetry guidelines for COMS eye plaque with ^{125}I or ^{103}Pd to treat intraocular tumors?
A. TG-64
B. TG-128
C. TG-129
D. TG-151

5.8 ICRU and AAPM TG Reports on Brachytherapy (Questions)

12. In terms of HDR brachytherapy QA, what are the four major components that must be checked periodically?
A. Temporal accuracy, dosimetric accuracy, positional accuracy, and safety
B. Temporal accuracy, HDR source length, positional accuracy, and safety
C. Afterloader location, HDR source length, positional accuracy, and applicator length
D. Temporal accuracy, dosimetric accuracy, positional accuracy, and applicator length

13. What is the formalism typically used for brachytherapy dose calculations?
A. Pencil beam
B. TG-43
C. Monte Carlo
D. Superposition

14. In TG-43, source strength is specified in terms of what?
A. mg-Ra eq
B. mCi
C. cGy
D. Air kerma (U)

15. When the dose rate constant is multiplied by the source strength in TG-43, the result is:
A. Activity (mCi)
B. Activity (Bq)
C. Dose rate (cGy/h)
D. Dose (cGy)

16. The inverse square effect is taken into account in the TG-43 formalism by which component?
A. Source strength
B. Anisotropy factor
C. Geometry factor
D. Radial dose function

17. The radial dose function corrects for the fact that in tissue, the inverse square law can break down due to scatter and attenuation. Which radionuclide would this affect the most?
A. Co-60
B. Cs-137
C. Ir-192
D. I-125

18. The anisotropy function corrects for what effect in the TG-43 formalism?
A. Angular dependence of the dose distribution
B. Inverse square law
C. Source strength
D. Length of the source

5.9 General Concepts on Brachytherapy (Answers)

Quiz-1 (Level 2)

1. **B** I and III only are correct. Brachytherapy uses sealed sources of ionizing radiation placed within the patient, in or close to the diseased tissues. Also, sources may be left in place for a limited period of time to irradiate the tissues. Teletherapy is considered external beam therapy, and doses are typically fractionated over a period of time and usually range from 1.2 Gy per fraction to 4 Gy per fraction (unless SRS or SRT).

2. **E** All of these are used for brachytherapy. The benefit of brachytherapy is that a high radiation dose is delivered locally to the tumor with rapid dose falloff in the surrounding normal tissue. Interstitial brachytherapy is delivered by placing needles or catheters directly into the tumor and placing the source in these catheters. Intracavitary brachytherapy involves placing an applicator into a body cavity such as the vagina. Surface applicators can be used to treat skin cancer, and intravascular brachytherapy delivers the dose through catheters in the blood vessels (this method is not very common).

3. **B** A typical LDR implant lasts for several days while an HDR procedure only takes a few minutes. Some LDR implants are permanent, meaning the sources are implanted and never removed. Prostate seed implants are permanent implants.

4. **E** All of them are correct. Remote afterloading refers to HDR brachytherapy delivery where the source is housed in a shielded container which is then connected to the applicator or catheter that has been implanted in the patient. Once the applicator is connected, all personnel can leave the room, and the afterloader will send the source out through the applicator to deliver the dose to the patient. This reduces the dose to the personnel caring for the patient. It also allows applicator insertion without having radioactivity present.

5. **C** The use of packing material helps stabilize the applicator, and it can also push critical structures such as the rectum away from the applicator. Remember that due to the inverse square law, the dose in brachytherapy falls off very quickly so moving the OARs slightly can make a large impact on the dosimetry and reduce toxicity.

5.9 General Concepts on Brachytherapy (Answers)

6. C The best approach to reduce personnel exposure during a brachytherapy treatment is by using the remote afterloading technique because all the personnel stay outside the room when the source is loaded and unloaded into the patient. A hot implant technique is basically the opposite technique where the physician physically loads hot sources into the applicator. Dummy wire is used during simulation so the location of the catheters can be determined. The manual afterloading technique is similar to the hot implant except the time near the source can be reduced as the applicator has already been implanted so the source just needs to be inserted.

7. A In 2D brachytherapy planning, a simulation CT is not obtained. In order to aid dose calculations and precise localization of the sources, at least two radiographs are necessary and these films must be orthogonal, taken at right angles (90°). Additionally, magnification factors are carefully determined for each film.

8. E Modern remote afterloading units consist of a lead-shielded storage area for the radioactive source and a remote system for delivering the source through multiple catheters (depending on the applicator and site).

9. E All are correct.

10. A The film magnification factor used in brachytherapy is given by SFD/SAD, where the SFD is the source-to-film distance and SAD is source-to-axis distance. Remember that magnification is the image size/object size.

11. D Three-dimensional reconstruction of the source geometry is usually accomplished by using orthogonal imaging taken at right angles with the central axes of the x-ray beams meeting approximately in the middle of the implant. The stereo-shift method can also be used by taking two radiographs of the same view but the patient or the x-ray tube is shifted a certain distance between the two exposures. The Manchester system is a method of determining the activity needed for a brachytherapy implant.

12. A To modulate the dose for an HDR treatment using a remote afterloading unit, two parameters can be changed. The first parameter is the location of the dwell position. A dwell position is a location where the radioactive source sits. The second parameter is the length of the dwell time. The longer the source remains at the dwell position, the more doses are delivered. The activity of the source can be calculated using the calibrated activity and radioactive decay. MLCs and compensators are used for external beam treatment units.

13. A Only I, II, and III are the disadvantages of remote afterloading units. The major advantage of the remote afterloading unit is the elimination or reduction of exposure to medical personnel.

14. E All are advantages. Traditional LDR implants are limited in terms of dose optimization because the number of sources implanted is limited and the activity for that source is fixed. With HDR, even though there is only one source, that source can be programmed to dwell in many different locations simulating multiple sources and the dwell time can be changed simulating multiple source activities. Furthermore, the patient typically does not have to spend the night in the hospital as most procedures are outpatient.

15. A According to the ICRU, the dose rate at the dose specification point(s) for an LDR brachytherapy treatment is 0.4–2 Gy/h. Medium dose rate (MDR) is 2–12 Gy/h and HDR is >12 Gy/h or >1,200 cGy/h. Be careful with the units 12 Gy = 1,200 cGy.

   We suggest the readers to memorize this number: LDR means dose rate <2 Gy/h.

16. A All are advantages except that HDR units require additional QA due to the extra functionality.

17. A Disadvantages of HDR systems include uncertainty in biological effectiveness, potential for accidental high exposures and serious errors, and increased staff commitment. Remember that one advantage of HDR is that treatment is usually done as an outpatient procedure.

18. A LDR uses multiple sources together with inactive spacers to achieve typical treatment dose rates of about 0.4–2 Gy/h vs. HDR systems which use a single source with a typical activity of 10–20 Ci. Remember to be careful with the units Gy vs. cGy, Ci vs. cGy/h, etc. Also, remember the dose rates: LDR, 0.4–2 Gy/h; MDR, 2–12 Gy/h; HDR, >12.0 Gy/h.

19. E All of these are essential components of remote afterloading system.

5.10 Radioactive Source Characteristics (Answers)

Quiz-1 (Level 2)

1. C ^{192}Ir is the most commonly used radioisotope in remote afterloaders although ^{137}Cs or ^{60}Co sources are used in some units. ^{226}Ra is not used anymore due to its disadvantages over artificial radioisotopes.

2. D Radium decays to stable forms of lead; in the process, it emits alphas, beta particles, and gamma rays. Alpha and beta particles have limited clinical use because of their short range. To use them, they must be tagged to a molecule that can be injected and preferentially uptake into the tumor. Gamma rays penetrate deeply into tissues and have more uses.

5.10 Radioactive Source Characteristics (Answers)

3. Half-life of each important radionuclide must be well known by the student; remember that half-life is the time necessary for a particular radioactive material to decay to 50 % of its original activity; the unit of half-life is time.

A.	V	^{226}Ra	(1,600 years)
B.	III	^{222}Rn	(3.83 days)
C.	VIII	^{60}Co	(5.26 years)
D.	I	^{137}Cs	(30.0 years)
E.	II	^{192}Ir	(73.8 days)
F.	VII	^{198}Au	(2.7 days)
G.	IIV	^{125}I	(59.4 days)
H.	VI	^{103}Pd	(17 days)
E.	XI	^{90}Sr	(28 years)
F.	X	^{90}Y	(64 h)
G.	IX	^{32}P	(14.0 days)

4. Radionuclides with their corresponding exposure rate constant Γ (Rcm²/mg-h)

A.	VI	^{226}Ra	(8.25)
B.	III	^{222}Rn	(10.15)
C.	I	^{60}Co	(13.07)
D.	VIII	^{137}Cs	(3.28)
E.	II	^{192}Ir	(4.69)
F.	IV	^{198}Au	(2.38)
G.	VII	^{125}I	(1.45)
H.	V	^{103}Pd	(1.48)

5. Radionuclides with their corresponding effective photon energy (avg-MeV)

A.	VII	^{226}Ra	(0.83 avg)
B.	IV	^{222}Rn	(0.83 avg)
C.	I	^{60}Co	(1.25)
D.	VIII	^{137}Cs	(0.66)
E.	III	^{192}Ir	(0.37)
F.	II	^{198}Au	(0.42)
G.	VI	^{125}I	(0.028)
H.	V	^{103}Pd	(0.02)

6. The decay rate or constant is a statistical phenomenon where one can predict in a large collection of atoms the proportion that will disintegrate in a given time. The differential equation is $\lambda = 0.693/T_{1/2}$ or $N = N_0\,e^{-\lambda t}$ where λ is a constant of proportionality called the decay constant $\ln(2) = 0.693$.

A.	^{226}Ra	VIII.	(>1 % yearly)
B.	^{222}Rn	II.	(18 % daily)
C.	^{60}Co	V.	(1 % monthly)
D.	^{137}Cs	IV.	(2.3 % yearly)
E.	^{192}Ir	III.	(1 % yearly)
F.	^{198}Au	VI.	(25 % daily)
G.	^{125}I	VII.	(1 % daily)
H.	^{103}Pd	I.	(4 % daily)

7. **B** ^{131}I, ^{32}P, ^{90}Y, and ^{90}Sr all emit β⁻ particles. ^{131}I and ^{90}Y also release γ-rays. All these radioisotopes have a relatively short $T_{1/2}$.

8. **A** Only I, II, and III are correct. Radium-226 behaves like calcium (same column in the periodic table); therefore, any leakage from ^{226}Ra can result in deposition of high radiation dose in the bone. Its high average gamma ray energy can result in high exposures to medical personnel, and radon gas leakage represents a significant hazard if the source is broken. Remember that ^{226}Ra has a very long $T_{1/2}$ of 1,622 years.

9. **E** All the statements are true about ^{226}Ra.

10. **C** The active length of a radium source is the distance between the ends of the radioactive material in the source. The physical length is the measured distance between the actual ends of the source. The activity or strength of source can be expressed in milligrams of radium content, air kerma strength, or Curies. Finally, the source filtration is the transverse thickness of the capsule wall, usually expressed in terms of millimeters of platinum.

11. **B** The uniformity of activity distribution of a source can be obtained by placing the source on an unexposed x-ray film for a time long enough to obtain reasonable darkening of the film. The leak test does not determine how much activity the source has, but rather if the source is leaking and a well-type ion chamber is used for routine calibration of brachytherapy sources and determination of the source activity.

12. **B** An Indian club radium needle used higher activity at one end of the needle with the rest of the needles having uniform activity. A uniform activity needle had radium activity uniformly spread throughout the active length, and a dumbbell needle had higher activity at both ends of the needle.

5.10 Radioactive Source Characteristics (Answers)

13. D The exposure rate constant of radium (^{226}Ra) is 8.25 R-cm^2/mg-h. Answer B is wrong because the source strength of radium is specified in milligrams instead of mCi. 3.27 R-cm^2/mg-h is the exposure rate constant of ^{137}Cs, and 13.07 R-cm^2/mg-h is the exposure rate constant of ^{60}Co. All the energies, $T_{1/2}$, and exposure rate constants of each individual radioisotope must be known.

14. A The activity of a radioactive nuclide-emitting photons is related to the exposure rate by the exposure rate constant (Γ).

15. B The International Commission on Radiation Units and Measurements (ICRU) has recommended that the exposure rate constant (Γ) of radium (^{226}Ra) is measured at a distance of 1 cm from a 1 mg point source filtered by 0.5 mm platinum.

16. A Brachytherapy treatment sources are chosen based on their half-life which determines the dose rate, their energy which determines the penetration and dose distribution, and the activity which determines the dose.

17. B Advantages of cesium-137 (^{137}Cs) over radium are that ^{137}Cs requires less shielding than radium (^{226}Ra) and ^{137}Cs is less hazardous in the microsphere from that of radium (^{226}Ra). Remember that ^{137}Cs's $T_{1/2}$ is 30 years and radium's (^{226}Ra) $T_{1/2}$ is 1,600 years.

18. Radionuclides come in different forms:

A.	II, VI	^{226}Ra	Needles or tubes
B.	VI, IV	^{103}Pd	Seeds or tubes
C.	I	^{60}Co	Wire
D.	II, III, VI	^{137}Cs	Powdered solution encapsulated in needles and tubes
E.	I, VI	^{192}Ir	Wire or seeds
F.	VI, V	^{198}Au	Seeds or grains
G.	VI	^{125}I	Seeds

19. E All of the radionuclides emit gamma rays (γ) for radiotherapy.

Radium-226 (^{226}Ra) emits gamma rays (γ) for therapy with energies ranging from 0.184 to 2.45 MeV with an average energy of 0.83 MeV; filtration provided by the source case absorbs all alpha (α) and most of the beta (β) particles emitted.

Palladium-103 (^{103}Pd) is another important radionuclide that decays by electron capture with the emission of characteristic x-rays in the range of 20–23 keV (average energy 20.9 keV) and Auger electrons.

Cobalt-60 (^{60}Co) is a gamma (γ)-emitting radioisotope with energies of 1.17 and 1.33 MeV.

Cesium-137 (^{137}Cs) is a gamma (γ)-emitting radioisotope of energy 0.662 MeV; it also emits beta (β) particles, and low-energy characteristic x-rays are absorbed and not used in therapy.

Iridium-192 (^{192}Ir) is a gamma (γ)-emitting radioisotope with an average energy of 0.38 MeV.

Gold-198 (^{198}Au) is a gamma (γ)-emitting radioisotope with an average energy of 0.412 MeV.

Iodine-125 (^{125}I) is a gamma (γ)-emitting radioisotope with energy of 35.5 keV. Characteristic x-rays in the range of 27–35 keV are also produced due to the electron capture and internal conversion processes.

20. D The main advantage of cobalt-60 (^{60}Co) is its high specific activity, which allows fabrication of small sources required for some special applicators. Remember that specific activity is activity per unit mass. ^{60}Co is considered to be an expensive source, even more expensive than ^{137}Cs. ^{60}Co has a relatively short half-life of 5.26 years which means the source has to be replaced every 5 years or so. Finally, due to its short half-life and frequent replacement, the inventory is complex.

21. A Cobalt-60 (^{60}Co) can be used to replace radium-226 (^{226}Ra) on an intracavitary application. Gold-198 (^{198}Au) is used for interstitial implants, and iodine-125 (^{125}I) and palladium-103 (^{103}Pd) are commonly used for permanent prostate seed implants.

22. E All of the statements are correct about iridium-192 (^{192}Ir); it is composed of 30 % Ir and 70 % Pt, and because of the low energy, these sources require less shielding for personnel protection. The short half-life of 73.8 days is a disadvantage because the source must be replaced quarterly. The source can be used in nonpermanent implants similar to radium and cesium.

23. D Gold-198 can be used for permanent implants where the sources are left permanently in the implanted tissue.

24. C The advantages of iodine-125 when used for permanent implants over radon and gold-198 (^{198}Au) are its longer half-life of 59.4 days which is convenient for storage and its low photon energy which requires less shielding. Its encapsulation in titanium serves to absorb liberated electrons and x-ray with energies less than 5 keV. Due to the encapsulation and source geometry, its dosimetry can be much more complex than the conventional interstitial sources.

5.10 Radioactive Source Characteristics (Answers) 375

25. B Because of the presence of titanium end welds, the dose distribution around iodine-125 (^{125}I) is highly anisotropic (not uniform), which creates cold spots near the source ends due to extra attenuation.

26. C Palladium-103 (^{103}Pd) provides a biologic advantage over iodine-125 (^{125}I) for permanent implants because the dose is delivered at a much faster rate due to the shorter half-life. Palladium-103 (^{103}Pd) is encapsulated in a laser-welded titanium tube, and the ^{103}Pd photon fluence distribution around the source is anisotropic due to self-absorption by the source pallets, the welds, and the lead x-ray marker.

27. A The source strength for any radionuclide may be specified in terms of millicurie (mCi). The unit of dose equivalent is rem, while in the SI system, it is the sievert (Sv). The National Council on Radiation Protection and Measurements (NCRP) recommends that the strength of any gamma (γ) emitter should be specified directly in terms of exposure rate in air at a specified distance such as 1 m.

28. B The exposure rate of a radionuclide at any particular point is proportional to the product of its activity and its exposure rate constant.

29. A The National Council on Radiation Protection and Measurements (NCRP) recommends that the strength of any γ-emitter should be specified directly in terms of exposure rate in air at a specified distance such as 1 m

30. C Historically, brachytherapy sources are specified in terms of the equivalent mass of radium because some users, especially the physicians who are accustomed to radium sources, continue to use mg-Ra eq. The best way to specify brachytherapy sources strength is in terms of exposure rate or air kerma rate at a distance of 1 m. This is the current method to document source strength.

31. B Apparent activity is defined as the activity of a bare point source of the same nuclide that produces the same exposure rate at 1 m as the source to be specified. The product of air kerma rate in free space and the square of the distance of the calibration point from the source center along the perpendicular bisector is the definition of air kerma strength, and the thickness of the material necessary to reduce the number of photons in a beam or intensity to 50 % of its initial value is the definition of HVL.

32. B 1 mg-Ra eq is equal to 8.25×10^{-4} R/h at 1 m.

33. A One advantage of brachytherapy is that the dose falls off very quickly in tissue due to the inverse square law.

34. D A well-type ion chamber is used to determine the activity of brachytherapy sources. The advantage of the well-type chamber is that the active volume almost completely surrounds the source to ensure all particles are collected.

35. A The dose rate constant of a radionuclide depends on the type of source, its construction, and its encapsulation. The physical length is the distance between the actual ends of the source and does not affect dose rate.

36. A Because the half-life for radioactive decay is much longer for radium-226 than for any of its daughter products, radium achieves a secular equilibrium with its daughters. Remember that if the half-life of the parent IS SLIGHTLY LONGER than that of the daughter, then the type of equilibrium established is called the transient equilibrium. On the other hand, if the half-life of the parent IS MUCH LONGER than that of the daughter, then it can give rise to what is known as the secular equilibrium. Therefore, the remaining answers are incorrect because the half-life for ^{226}Ra is much longer than for any of its daughter products.

37. A According to the AAPM and ICRU, the strength of a brachytherapy source must be specified in terms of air kerma rate $K_{air}(d_{ref})$. In the past, there were many accepted ways to document source strength including activity, mg-Ra eq, and exposure rate produced at a given distance from the source.

38. B Air kerma strength is defined as the product of air kerma rate in "free space" and the square of the distance of the calibration point from the source center along the perpendicular bisector. The total reference air kerma is defined as the sum of the products of the reference air kerma rate and the duration of the application of each source, the activity of a bare point source of the same nuclide that produces the same exposure rate at 1 m as the source to be specified is the apparent activity of a radionuclide, and finally, kinetic energy released in matter, measured in gray or rad, is the definition of kerma.

39. A The SI unit of the reference air kerma rate is Gy/s (which can be converted into cGy/h). The curie (Ci) and Becquerel (Bq) are both units of activity.

40. A I, II, and III are correct. Brachytherapy sources must always be handled with care even with the encapsulation. One never wants to pick up a source with their fingers.

41. A The useful radiation fluence from a brachytherapy source generally consists of gamma (γ) rays which form the most important component of the emitted radiation. Characteristic x-rays emitted incidentally through electron capture or internal conversion that occurs in the source and Bremsstrahlung radiation which originates in the source capsule are pres-

ent but not a major component of the source activity as these tend to be very low energy.

42. **E** All are correct.

43. **A** Some brachytherapy sources are doubly encapsulated in order to provide adequate shielding against beta (β) particles, alpha (α) particles, and leakage of radioactive material as all of these components require minimal shielding. The gamma (γ) ray emission is the most useful radiation component from a brachytherapy source although low-energy Bremsstrahlung photons and characteristic x-rays will be absorbed in the encapsulation but these photons do not significantly contribute to the patient dose, either.

44. **E** All are correct. Radionuclides in liquid form are better suited for ingestion or injection. ^{131}I in doses of ≥100 mCi is given orally in the treatment of thyroid malignancies, and ^{32}P and ^{90}Y are injected into cystic craniopharyngiomas. At the same time, one must be very careful with liquid radionuclides because a spill can be hard to contain and decontaminate.

5.11 Implant Methods (Answers)

Quiz-1 (Level 2)

1. **C** The Paterson-Parker or Manchester system of implant dosimetry uses non-uniform strength sources to archive a uniform dose distribution (within ±10 %) to a plane or volume. This method achieves a uniform dose distribution but it can be difficult to acquire sources with different activities. The Paris system uses uniform strength sources implanted in parallel lines or in an array, and the Quimby system uses uniform strength sources to achieve a nonuniform dose distribution. If uniform strength sources are implanted, the dose in the central region will be higher and lower in the periphery. Finally, the Memorial system uses uniform strength sources spaced 1 cm apart.

2. **A** The MLC system is not a system of implant dosimetry.

3. **B** Planar implants consist of one or two planes of interest and volume implants consist of more than two planes (cuboid, sphere, or cylinder).

4. **B** Only I and III are correct. In the case of planar implants with the Manchester system, the prescribed dose is 10 % higher than the minimum dose and the maximum dose should not exceed 110 % of the prescribed dose to satisfy the uniformity criterion.

5. D In the case of planar implants with the Paterson-Parker or Manchester system, the ratio between the amount of radium used in the periphery and the center is as follows:

area (cm^2) 0–25 = 1/3 in the center, 2/3 in the periphery; area (cm^2) 25–100 = ½ in the center, ½ in the periphery;

area (cm^2) over 100 = 2/3 in the center, 1/3 in the periphery.

6. E All statements are true.

7. C If it is impossible to cross both ends on a single-plane Paterson-Parker system implant, the treatment area should be considered as 80 % of the length of the implant. The treatment area should be considered as 90 % of the length of the implant when only one end is crossed, that is, for each uncrossed end, the treatment area should be taken as 10 % less than the nominal area. The use of Indian club needles eliminates the need for a crossing needle at one end of the implant and dumbbell needles have greater activity at both ends and do not require crossing at either end.

8. B A volume implant is required if the lesion is more than 2.5 cm thick.

9. A Due to the dimension and shape of different tumors, some are better implanted using three-dimensional shapes such as cylinders, spheres, and cuboids.

10. E All statements are correct about the distribution of sources on volume implants used for a Paterson-Parker or Manchester system implant.

11. E All statements are correct about volume implants. Remember that in a planar implant, if the ends cannot be crossed, the treatment area is reduced by 10 % from the area for each uncrossed end.

12. B In the case of an implant using the Quimby system, for the planar implant, the prescribed dose is the maximum dose in the plane of treatment, and for the volume implant, the prescribed dose is the minimum dose within the implant volume.

13. C The Memorial system is an extension of the Quimby system and is characterized by complete dose distributions around lattices of point sources of uniform strength spaced 1 cm apart. Remember that the Paterson-Parker system and the Manchester system are the same systems and use nonuniform sources to achieve a uniform dose. The Quimby (Memorial) system uses uniform sources but accepts a nonuniform dose distribution.

14. E All are correct about the Paris system.

5.11 Implant Methods (Answers)

15. C Using the Paris system, sources could be spaced at a minimum of 8 mm and a maximum of 15 mm intervals, depending on implant dimension.

16. A The reference isodose in the Paris system is fixed at 85 % of the basal dose.

17. B The basal dose is defined as the average of the minimum dose between sources. The maximum dose in the plane of treatment is defined as the stated dose.

18. Match the brachytherapy implants with its corresponding description:
A. III. Intracavitary (Sources are placed into body cavities close to the tumor volume.)
B. VI. Interstitial (Sources are implanted surgically within the tumor volume.)
C. V. Surface (mold) (Sources are placed over the tissue to be treated.)
D. VIII. Intraluminal (Sources are placed in a lumen.)
E. VII. Intraoperative (Sources are implanted into the target tissue during surgery.)
F. II. Intravascular (A single source is placed into small or large arteries.)
G. IV. Temporal (Dose is delivered over a short period of time and the sources are removed after the prescribed dose has been reached.)
H. I. Permanent (Dose is delivered over the lifetime of the source until completely decayed.)

19. B The brachytherapy hot loading method is when the applicator is preloaded and contains radioactive sources at the time of placement into the patient. An afterloading method is when the applicator is first placed into the treatment position and the radioactive sources are loaded later, either by hand (manual afterloading) or by a machine (remote afterloading).

20. Applicators with its corresponding definition
A. IV. Fletcher-Suit: Used for treatment of gynecological malignancies of the uterus, cervix, and pelvic side walls. Consists of rigid intrauterine tandems with curvatures of 15°, 30°, and 45° and a pair of ovoids (or a ring).
B. V. Vaginal cylinder: Used for treatment of vaginal wall. Consists of acrylic cylinders having a variety of diameters and an axially drilled hole to accommodate a central catheter.
C. VI. Rectal applicator: Used for the treatment of superficial tumors of the rectum. Consists of acrylic cylinders of different diameters. Selected shielding is incorporated to spare normal tissue.
D. II. Intraluminal catheter: Used for treatment of endobronchial carcinoma. Different diameter catheters of various lengths.
E. III. Nasopharyngeal applicator: Used for treatment of nasopharyngeal tumors with HDR. The applicator set includes tracheal tube, catheter, and a nasopharyngeal connector.
F. I. Interstitial implants: Used for treatments of prostate gland, gyn malignancies, breast, and some head and neck tumors. Hollow needles are implanted into the tumor and the source is introduced into the needle.

5.12 Temporary Implant Procedures (Answers)

Tandem and ovoids (LDR, HDR), vaginal cylinder (HDR), and eye plaque (LDR)

Quiz-1 (Level 2)

1. **A** A tandem and ovoid is used in intracavitary therapy such as the treatment of uterine cancer.

2. **B** Sr-90 applicator is used to treat pterygium which is a non-cancerous growth that covers the white of the eye. Choroidal melanomas and ocular melanoma are treated using COMS eye plaques and skin lesions are treated with surface molds.

3. **C** Sr-90 is a ß-emitter with energy of 2.2 MeV. This isotope is chosen because it does not penetrate very deep. This energy covers the tumor which is very superficial, but the lens can be spared. Remember that a ß-particle is an electron which loses energy at around 2 MeV/cm in tissue.

4. **C** The sources typically used for COMS eye plaques are iodine-125 (^{125}I) and palladium-103 (^{103}Pd). Radium-226 (^{226}Ra) was used in the past for temporal interstitial implants, and gold-198 (^{198}Au) is used for permanent interstitial implants.

5. **C** For a volume implant in the Manchester system, the radioactive material is distributed on the belt, which is the periphery of implant; the core, which is the inner needles of the implant; and the end, which is the location where the needles cross.

6. **B** Choroidal ocular melanoma study

7. **A** The two major parts of a COMS eye plaque are the gold backing which serves the purpose of attenuating radiation that is not directed towards the target and also helps to scatter some of the photons back towards the tumor and the Silastic seed insert composed of a soft silicon rubber which carries the seeds. These are precast slots in the insert that hold the seeds in a symmetrical, pre-calculated array.

8. **A** Surface molds can be used to treat superficial skin lesions such as those in the oral and nasal cavity and hard palate. Prostate lesions are deep-seated tumors and cannot be treated with surface molds.

9. **A** In interstitial therapy, the radioactive sources are fabricated in the form of needles, wires, and seeds, depending on the application.

5.12 Temporary Implant Procedures (Answers)

10. B Sources used in a temporal interstitial implant are radium needles, iridium wires, or iridium seeds. Gold (^{198}Au) seeds and iodine-125 (^{125}I) seeds are typically used in a permanent interstitial implant.

11. A Intracavitary therapy is mostly used for cancers of the vagina, cervix, and uterine body. There are no body cavities near the bladder.

12. C The most common method of intracavitary brachytherapy is the Fletcher tandem and ovoid applicator. The Henschke applicator is similar to the Fletcher system, and the COMS eye plaque applicator is used as a surface applicator to treat choroidal melanomas and ocular melanomas. Needles are used for interstitial implants.

13. B The most extensively used systems of dose specification for cervix treatment is the Manchester system. The Milligram-Hours system is one of the oldest systems but is fraught with large uncertainties in the dose distribution from patient to patient. The ICRU system is used also but not as frequently as the Manchester system. Remember that the Quimby system is used for interstitial implantation characterized by a uniform distribution of sources of equal linear activity resulting in a nonuniform dose distribution, higher in the central region of treatment.

14. E All answers are true.

15. A The Manchester system used for the treatment of the cervix is characterized by dose to four points: point A, point B, a bladder point, and a rectum point. Point A is located 2 cm superior to the external cervical os and 2 cm lateral to the cervical canal. As the tandem is in the cervical canal, these points move with the tandem and represent the intersection of the uterine arteries and ureters. Point B represents the obturator lymph nodes and is located 2 cm superior and 5 cm lateral to the patient's midline. These points are fixed in space regardless of the tandem orientation. The rectal point is 5 mm posterior to the posterior vaginal wall. The bladder point is defined using the posterior surface of the Foley balloon.

16. D The duration of the implant on a brachytherapy treatment of the cervix using the Manchester system is based on the dose rate calculated at point A, although the dose at the other points is taken into consideration in evaluating the treatment plan.

17. A Point A is the point of prescription on a brachytherapy treatment of the cervix using the Manchester system.

18. B On a brachytherapy treatment of the cervix, point A is defined as 2 cm superior to the external cervical os and 2 cm lateral to the cervical canal. Originally, point A was defined as 2 cm superior to the lateral vaginal fornix and 2 cm lateral to the cervical canal. Remember that this point moves with the tandem as the tandem is inside the cervical canal.

19. **C** On a brachytherapy treatment of the cervix, point B is defined as 2 cm superior to the external cervical os or the head of the ovoids and 3 cm lateral to point A if the uterus is not tipped. Remember that point B remains fixed at 5 cm lateral to the midline of the body. Thus, point A and point B might not lie along the same line if the uterus is tilted with respect to the patient's midline.

Fig. 5A.4.1

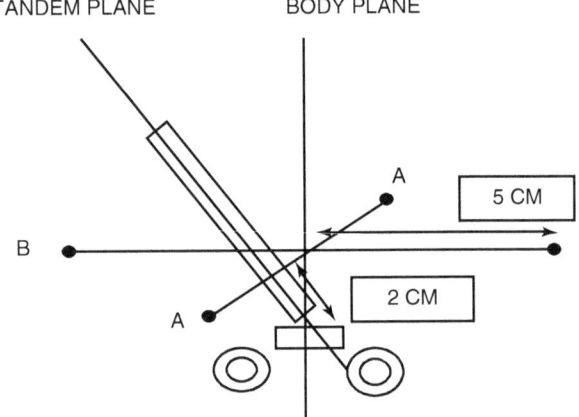

20. **A** On a brachytherapy treatment of the cervix, point A represents the location where the uterine arteries cross the ureters. The tolerance of these structures is the main limiting factor in the irradiation of the uterine cervix. Point B represents the location of the obturator nodes.

21. **E** All statements are limitations to prescribing to point A on a brachytherapy treatment of the cervix.

22. **C** Due to the limitation imposed by prescribing to a single point, for an intracavitary treatment, the ICRU has recently recommended a system of dose specification that relates the dose distribution to the target volume and not to a specific point. This is also related to the use of CT scans for planning rather than orthogonal films. Now, the locations of the tumor and OARs can be defined and the dose can be calculated more accurately.

23. **B** Tandem and ovoid applicators together are used for cervical cancer patients when no hysterectomy has been performed. In a case where the patient has had hysterectomy done, the ovoids can be used to boost the cervix. Sometimes, a tandem can be used alone if there is no room for the ovoids although this is not ideal.

5.12 Temporary Implant Procedures (Answers)

24. B On a brachytherapy treatment of the cervix, the bladder point is located at the center of the balloon on the frontal radiograph and on a line drawn anteroposterioly through the center of the balloon, at the posterior surface of the balloon on the lateral radiograph.

25. C On a brachytherapy treatment of the cervix, the rectal point is located radiographically at the midpoint of the ovoid sources on the frontal radiograph and, on the lateral radiograph, on a line drawn from the middle of the ovoid sources, 5 mm behind the posterior vaginal wall.

26. C On a brachytherapy treatment of the cervix, lymphatic trapezoid of Fletcher corresponds to the para-aortic and iliac nodes. Remember that point A represents the location where the uterine vessels cross the ureter and point B represents the location of the obturator nodes. The pelvic wall points are located at the intersection of a horizontal tangent to superior aspect of the acetabulum and a vertical line touching the medial aspect of the acetabulum. On the lateral view, these points are marked as the highest middistance points of the right and left acetabulum. Many of these points are required because external beam treatments are used to boost the dose to the lymph nodes because the brachytherapy applicator cannot push the dose out that far. Tracking these points allows for a composite dose to be calculated from the brachytherapy and external beam treatments.

27. B The rectum and the bladder are organs at risk on a brachytherapy treatment of the cervix. The prostate and seminal vesicles belong to male anatomy.

28. A The anterior rectal wall and the sigmoid colon dose can be minimized by using a rectal retractor as well as packing material which at the same time will hold the tandem and ovoids in place. Also, the tandem can be straight or have some degree of angulation. The angle the tandem draws the uterus into a central position in the pelvis away from the sigmoid colon and the anterior rectal wall.

29. C The maximum dose to the bladder and rectum should be as far as possible, less than the dose to point A and, preferably, 80 % or less than point A.

30. E All the statements are correct.

31. E All the statements are correct about ovoid applicator.

32. A On a brachytherapy treatment of the cervix, the longest tandem length as well as the largest set of ovoids that fit the patient's anatomy should always be used. As the tissue is pushed further from the source, the dose distribution becomes more uniform.

33. A The most common prescription is to vaginal surface although sometimes a depth of 5 mm is chosen.

34. C The source cannot reach the tip end seen from the CT or film; normally, the deepest point it can reach is about 4–5 mm from the tip end of the catheter. The reason for this is that the source is designed to retract if it encounters any resistance in the catheter. This is to prevent a source becoming stuck inside the patient. Therefore, if the source was allowed to travel to the very end of the catheter, there is a chance it could hit the end of the catheter and retract. The source moves very quickly and there are mechanical limitations on how accurately the source can stop, usually <1 mm, but this could be enough to collide with the end of the catheter.

35. D The typical volume is 2 cc. Some physicians still like to look at the point max or the 1 cc volume.

36. B Endometrial cancer where a hysterectomy has been performed is done using a cylinder, also called a Burnett applicator.

37. C The most common method of dose optimization for an endometrial cancer using a cylinder is to optimize the dose to the surface and dome of the cylinder. Prescribing and optimizing to 5 mm from the surface of the cylinder is also done.

38. B On the lateral film, the rectal point is 5 mm posterior to the vaginal wall for both applicators, but on the anterior film, the rectal point is located at the LOWER end of the intrauterine source for the tandem and ovoid and in the MIDDLE of the intrauterine source for the cylinder.

39. A The ICRU recommends placing reference points at certain locations in the pelvis to monitor the dose. They are the lymphatic trapezoid which includes the para-aortic lymph nodes and the common and external iliac lymph nodes, and the second reference point is the pelvic wall point.

5.13 Permanent Implant Procedures (Answers)

Quiz-1 (Level 2)

1. E All are correct; depending on the desired radiobiological effect, different radionuclides can be chosen with different energies and half-lives. Some seed implants are preplanned meaning the plan is generated using images taken before the procedure and others are planned intraoperatively meaning the plan is generated on images acquired real time. The sources can be delivered manually on a seed-by-seed basis or using stranded seeds that are preloaded into needles. The manual technique allows for more freedom but can take extra time. The total prescribed dose will vary based on the radionuclide used and if the therapy is monotherapy (seed implant only) or a boost treated in conjunction with external beam therapy.

5.13 Permanent Implant Procedures (Answers)

2. B Permanent radioactive seed implants include palladium-103 (^{103}Pd) and iodine-125 (^{125}I). Gold-198 (^{198}Au) was used in the past, but the unnecessary radiation exposure hazard prevented the use of it from gaining wide acceptance. Iridium and radium are typically used as a temporary implant.

3. C Palladium-103 (^{103}Pd), which has a shorter half-life (17 days) than iodine-125 (^{125}I) (60 days), delivers a higher initial dose rate and hence has been found useful in treating fast-growing high-grade tumors.

4. A The primary options for early prostate stage disease (T1c, Gleason <7, and PSA from 10 to 15 ng/ml) confined to the prostate and immediately surrounding area are surgery, external beam irradiation, seed implantation, and observation. Of those options, ultrasound-guide permanent seed implantation is a popular choice due to higher radiation dose to the prostate and surrounding tissue and lower dose to adjacent organs such as rectum and bladder due to the rapid dose falloff. Observation is also gaining popularity as this reduces the cost of care for the patient, and the data is still being collected for long-term outcomes for observation vs. seed implant. I-125 (energy of 28 keV, $T_{1/2}$ 60 days) or Pd-103 (energy of 21 keV, $T_{1/2}$ 17 days) can be used to deliver doses of around 145 Gy for I-125 and 125 Gy for Pd-103. The difference in dose is related to the higher rate of decay for Pd-103. Retropubic (needles inserted through the abdomen) seed implantation can be done, but the contraindications include poor seed distribution, complications, and poor long-term clinical control. The transperineal (needles inserted through the perineum) approach using ultrasound guidance is preferred due to quick recovery, minimal blood loss, and the ability to deliver complex seed distributions.

5. C Fluoroscopy and ultrasound are the two modalities typically used to perform seed implantation of the prostate. The benefit of ultrasound is that no ionizing radiation is delivered to the patient or to the personnel in the room. Because of this, transperineal needle insertion with transrectal (probe in the rectum) ultrasound guidance has become the technique of choice because it is carried out as an outpatient 1-day procedure. CT and MRI can be used to do preplanning and to determine the size of the prostate prior to the implant.

6. B Post-implant dosimetry is usually performed 1 month post-implant to allow for reduction in edema and any migration of seeds. Using CT images, the location of the seeds is determined and dose calculations are performed and compared with pre-implant dose distributions. MRI is not used because the metal in the seeds creates artifacts in the image. Post-implant dosimetry can be done on the day of the procedure, but the prostate is usually swollen so the dosimetry is not as accurate.

7. D The position adopted by the patient for a transperineal prostate seed implantation is the dorsal lithotomic position. The patient is supine with their legs held up in stirrups. The transrectal ultrasound probe is securely anchored to the table to obtain transverse and sagittal images of the prostate gland.

8. A In the case of a large gland and significant pubic arch interference on a permanent prostate implant procedure, the patient may need hormonal therapy for a few months to shrink the gland to allow for an adequate implant. The hormone therapy can help shrink the gland to a more manageable size.

9. A If a treatment plan is generated prior to the procedure, the plan must include the number of needles to be used and the number of seeds in each needle and the template coordinate for each needle.

10. A On a permanent prostate pre-implant treatment plan, the prostate, urethra, and rectum need to be contoured for planning purposes. Usually the bladder wall can be seen but most of the bladder cannot be visualized.

11. B The major problems with permanent seed implants are the disagreement between the pre-implant and post-implant dose distributions. Hot and cold spots can develop as a result of source movement with time and gland shrinkage after surgery. Also, source anisotropy can cause cold spots of greater than 50 % (reduction in dose) at the ends of the implant.

12. B The purpose of doing a cystoscopy after a permanent prostate implant procedure is to look for any seeds that may have been accidentally implanted into the bladder. A cystoscopy is a test that allows doctors to look at the inside of the bladder and the urethra using a thin, lighted instrument called a cystoscope. Any seeds that might have ended up in the bladder can be removed.

13. A The average lifetime of a radionuclide is the sum of the lifetimes of all the individual atoms divided by the total number of atoms present originally, not to be confused with the half-life which is the time necessary for a radioactive material to decay to 50 % of its original activity. Activity is the number of disintegrations per second of a radioactive source, and HVL is the thickness of a given material needed to reduce the intensity of a photon beam to 50 % of its initial value.

5.14 Dose Delivery (Answers)

Applicators, source calibration, and dwelling position accuracy

Quiz-1 (Level 2)

1. C Well ion chambers and electrometers are used together to measure HDR source strength. The "current" mode of electrometer must be used meaning that the current (nA) generated in the chamber by the source is measured in

5.14 Dose Delivery (Answers)

real time rather than integrating the total charge (nC) collected for a period of time which is done in linac QA.

2. C The sweet spot is defined as the position in the well chamber having the maximum current. When calibrating an HDR source, the source should dwell at this position. The well chamber has a calibration factor from an ADCL that relates the current to an activity.

3. D The correct applicator on a lung implant is the catheter that is inserted into the bronchus. Tandem and ovoids, cylinders, and Heyman capsules are used for gynecologic brachytherapy treatments.

4. E All statements are correct.

5. E All are correct. Source dimensions may be checked by physical measurement or by radiography, and the serial number and color coding can be checked by visual inspection. For HDR brachytherapy, a source certificate is provided following each source exchange and the source never leaves the afterloader until a new source is needed.

6. E All are correct. An autoradiograph is generated by placing a source on a film which causes the film to darken and the dose distribution can be visualized. Additionally, a normal radiograph can be taken of the source so the physical dimension of the source can be seen along with the dose.

7. A If the disagreement between the vendor and the user calibration is within ±5 %, the user calibration should be used although using one or the other would not cause any significant changes in dosimetry. Differences larger than ±5 % are not acceptable and would require recalibration by the vendor and issuance of a new calibration certificate.

8. A Before 3D planning, applicator positioning was verified by orthogonal radiographs. Now, the position can be verified by CT, scout images, or orthogonal radiographs, depending on the equipment in the department.

9. C Source position accuracy is one of the main QA components of HDR brachytherapy. This can be verified through visual inspection using the in-room camera and a source ruler. The source ruler is a device that can be attached to the afterloader and has a transparent channel with a ruler. The actual position of the source can be seen and compared to the value on the ruler. Another method is to take an autoradiograph of the applicator with the source programmed at several dwell positions. Next, the marker cable is introduced into the applicator and a radiograph is taken. The position of the source should overlay the position on the marker cable. This also checks the integrity of the marker cable which is critical because this is how the catheter and applicator is digitized during treatment planning from the CT scan.

10. A   The position of dummy sources and radioactive sources should correspond within ±1 mm.

11. C   The smallest step size is 2.5 mm for the Nucletron HDR system. This allows for more dose modulation in the plan. The number of dwell positions is limited, so if a long treatment length is required, step sizes of 5 mm or 1 cm might be required.

12. B   The correct answer is B. Most remote afterloading units have an upper limit of dwell positions. In the Nucletron remote afterloading unit, the maximal positions allowed is 40. If using the normal 2.5 mm step size, the system might reach its limit. Of course, 1 cm step size is an option, but fewer dwelling positions will reduce the conformity of dose distribution.

5.15 Brachytherapy Dose Calculations (Answers)

Quiz-1 (Level 2)

1. C   To calculate exposure rate of a radionuclide at any distance: $X = \Gamma \times A/d^2$, where X = exposure, exposure rate constant (Γ), activity (A), and distance (d^2). Total dose to a point for a permanent implant = initial dose rate of the implant (D_0) × average life of the radionuclide used (t_{avg}). To convert the # of mCi of radionuclide to mg-Ra eq: # of mCi of radionuclide × exposure rate constant (Γ) of radionuclide/exposure rate constant (Γ) of radium. Finally, to calculate the exposure rate from the point source: exposure rate (X) × time (t).

2. C   Be organized:
   $A = 10$ mCi
   1 mCi $= 3.7 \times 10^7$ Bq
   10 mCi $= 3.7 \times 10^8$ Bq
   $A = 300{,}000{,}000$ Bq

3. B   Remember that the exposure rate constant of radium is 8.25 R cm²/mg-h (or 8.25 R cm²/mg-Ra eq-h) because the exposure rate at 1 cm from a 1-mg point source of radium-226 filtered by 0.5 mm of platinum (Pt) is 8.25 R/h. Therefore, the exposure rate at 1 cm of a 15 mg-Ra eq source is 123.75 R/h.
   8.25R/h × 15 mg-Ra eq = 123.75 R/h at 1 cm
   Exposure rate formula:
   $X = \Gamma \times A/d^2$
   $X = 8.25$ R cm²/mg-Ra eq-h × 15 mg-Ra eq/(1 cm)²
   $X = 123.75$ R/h
   Remember, to convert between mg-Ra eq and mCi, you need to know the ratio of the radionuclide exposure rate constant to the exposure rate constant for Ra-226. In this case, the ratio is 1 since the 8.25/8.25 = 1. This is why the exposure rate constant for Ra-226 can have mg-Ra eq or mCi in the denominator.

5.15 Brachytherapy Dose Calculations (Answers)

4. A If the exposure rate at some other distance from the source is needed, then all that has to be done is to use the inverse square law:
3.62 R/h × (3/7 cm)² = 0.66 R/h. Remember that since the distance has increased, the exposure rate must go down.

5. C ^{192}Ir activity = 0.53 mCi
Γ of ^{192}Ir = 4.69 R cm²/mg-h
Γ of ^{226}Ra = 8.25 R cm²/mg-h
A conversion must be done from mCi to mg-Ra eq. The correct formula is the ratio of the exposure rate constant of Ir-192 to Ra-226:
Mg-Ra eq = Γ ^{192}Ir/Γ ^{226}Ra × # of mCi ^{192}Ir
Mg-Ra eq = 4.69/8.25 × 0.53 mCi
Mg-Ra eq = 0.0121 mg-Ra eq

6. A If the exposure rate at some other distance from the source is needed, then the inverse square law can be used. In this case, the source has been filtrated by an additional 25 %, so a factor of 0.75 must be included as well:
3.62 R/h × 0.75 (3/7 cm)² = 0.499 R/h

7. B Collect the data:
mg-Ra eq = ?
Γ mg-Ra eq = 8.25 R cm²/mg-Ra eq-h
Distance = 5 cm
Dose rate = 3.20 R/h at 5 cm
First, use the inverse square law as the exposure rate constant is defined at 1 cm:
3.20 × (5/1)² = 80 R/h at 1 cm
Convert to mg-Ra eq using the known exposure rate constant at 1 cm.
80 R/h / 8.25 R/mg-Ra eq-h = 9.697 mg-Ra eq

8. B The strength of any radionuclide in mg-Ra eq can be calculated by the ratio of the radionuclide exposure rate constant divided by that of Ra-226. This question requires a few steps.
First, notice the units of the exposure rate. Now let's convert this into R/h:
0.495 mR/h × 1 R/1,000 mR = 0.000495 R/h
This is the exposure rate at 1 m; we need to be at 1 cm so use the inverse square law:
0.000495 R/h × (100 cm/1 m)² = 4.95 R/h at 1 cm
Now we can use the exposure rate constant for Ir-192 to determine how many mCi of Ir-192 we have here:
Γ Ir-192 = 4.69 R cm²/mg-h
mCi of Ir-192 at 1 cm = (4.95 R/h)/(4.69 R cm²/mg-h) = 1.06 mCi
mg-Ra eq = (exposure rate constant of radionuclide/exposure rate constant of radium) × # mCi radionuclide
mg-Ra eq = (4.69/8.25) × 1.06 mCi
mg-Ra eq Ir-192 = 0.603 mg-Ra eq

9. C The number of mg-Ra eq to deliver a dose of 2,000 cGy in 40 h to 1.5 cm for a 4.44 cm² single-plane implant that is crossed on one end only is 23.10 mg.
Be organized;
Dose = 2,000 cGy
Time = 40 h
Area = 4.44 cm²
Table = 1.5 cm for a 4 cm² single plane = ?
Crossed on one end only = 10 % reduction
First, find the corrected area. Since the planar implant is crossed on one end only, a 10 % reduction on the treatment area needs to be done:
4.44 cm² × 0.9 = 4.0 cm²
Second, calculate the number of mg/h:
From the table, a 4 cm² area at a depth of 1.5 cm requires 462 mg-h to deliver.
1,000 cGy:
(462 mg-h/1,000 cGy) × 2,000 cGy = 924 mg-h needed
A total of 924 mg-h is needed to deliver 2,000 cGy to a distance of 1.5 cm.
Finally, find out the total mg needed for a 40 h implant:
924 mg-h/40 h = 23.10 mg

Table 5A.7.1

Area cm²	0.5 cm	1.0 cm	1.5 cm	2.0 cm
0	30	119	268	476
2	97	213	375	598
4	141	278	462	698
6	177	333	536	782
8	206	384	599	855

10. B The amount of radioactive material on the periphery is 13.33 mg and in the center is 6.66 mg if Manchester planar distribution rules are used for an area less than 25 cm².
Remember the distribution rules for a planar implant:
Area (cm²) 0–25 = fraction in the center 1/3, faction in the periphery 2/3
Area (cm²) 25–100 = fraction in the center 1/2, faction in the periphery 1/2
Area (cm²) over 100 = fraction in the center 2/3, faction in the periphery 1/3
So, periphery = 2/3 × 20 mg = 13.33 mg
Center = 1/3 × 20 mg = 6.66 mg

11. C Remember the distribution rule for a cylinder using a Manchester volume implant:
If both ends are crossed, there would be a total of 8 parts.
Cylinder:
4 parts go to the belt or ½ of the total activity.
2 parts go to the core or ¼ of the total activity.
1 part goes to each end or 1/8 of the total activity.

5.15 Brachytherapy Dose Calculations (Answers)

The activity is 20 mg-h.
So,
Belt = 1/2 × 20 mg = 10 mg-h total
Core = 1/4 × 20 mg = 5 mg-h total
Each end = 1/8 × 20 mg = 2.5 mg-h per end (×2 ends = 5 mg-h total)
Remember that the activity is 20 mg-h so be careful; first, all the answers must add up to 20 mg-h.

12. A If one end is uncrossed, then only seven (7) parts will be distributed. Remember the distribution rule for a cylinder on a Manchester volume implant:
If one end is uncrossing, there would be a total of 7 parts.
Cylinder:
4 parts go to the belt or 4/7 of the total activity.
2 parts go to the core or 2/7 of the total activity.
1 part goes to one end or 1/7 of the total activity.
The activity is 20 mg-h.
So,
Belt = 4/7 × 20 mg-h = 11.43 mg-h
Core = 2/7 × 20 mg-h = 5.7 mg-h
One end = 1/7 × 20 mg-h = 2.9 mg-h
Remember that the activity is 20 mg/h, so be careful; first, all the answers must add up to 20 mg/h.

13. D Remember that on a sphere implant, no crossing is needed. The distribution rule for a sphere on a Manchester volume implant:
Sphere:
6 parts go to the belt or 3/4 of the activity.
2 parts go to the core or 1/4 of the activity.
Crossing ends = 0
The activity is 20 mg-h.
So,
Belt = 3/4 × 20 mg-h = 15 mg-h
Core = 1/4 × 20 mg-h = 5 mg-h
Crossing ends = 0 mg-h

14. D The basal dose rate (BD) gives a measurement of dose rate in the center of the treatment volume, and it is an average of the individual base dose rate, in this case $BD = BD_1 + BD_2 + BD_3/3$.

15. B In a typical survey meter, if the meter needle were pointing to 5.5 and the multiplication factor were positioned to the ×10 scale, the reading will be 55 mR/h.

16. C For permanent implants, the total dose to a point may be found from the initial dose rate by the equation $D_{total} = D_0 \times t_{avg}$, where D_0 is the initial dose rate and t_{avg} is the average life of the radionuclide in question. $D_{total}=D_0 \times t_{avg}[1-e^{t/t_{avg}}]$ is the formula used to find out total dose on a temporary implants where t is the implant time. $T_{avg}=1.44 \times T_{1/2}$.

17. A For permanent implants, the total dose to a point may be found from the initial dose rate by the equation:
$D_{total}=D_0 \times t_{avg}$ $t_{avg}=1.44 \times T_{1/2}$ ^{198}Au
$D_{total}=?$ $t_{avg}=1.44 \times 2.7$ days
$D_0=5$ Gy/day $t_{avg}=3.89$ days
$t_{avg}=3.89$ days
$D_{total}=D_0 \times t_{avg}$
$D_{total}=5$ Gy $\times 3.89$
$D_{total}=19.45$ Gy

18. B For permanent implants, the total dose to a point may be found from the initial dose rate by the equation:
$D_{total}=D_0 \times t_{avg}$ $t_{avg}=1.44 \times T_{1/2}$ ^{125}I
$D_{total}=150$ Gy $t_{avg}=1.44 \times 59.4$ days
$D_0=?$ $t_{avg}=85.54$ days
$t_{avg}=85.54$ days
$D_{total}=D_0 \times t_{avg}$
150 Gy $= D_0 \times 85.54$ days
$D_0=1.75$ Gy/day

19. C Be organized and collect all the data available.
June 15, 2014, to September 1, 2014 = 78 days
Total dose = 70 Gy $t_{avg}=1.44 \times T_{1/2}$ ^{125}I
$^{125}I T_{1/2}=59.4$ days $t_{avg}=1.44 \times 59.4$ days
$t_{avg}=85.54$ days $t_{avg}=85.54$ days
$t=78$ days
Temporary implant dose formula:
$D_{total}=D_0 \times t_{avg}(1-e^{-t/t_{avg}})$
We need to find D_0, the initial dose rate that was implanted. We can use the planned dose to calculate this:
$D_0=D_{total}/t_{avg}=70$ Gy/85.54 days $=0.82$ Gy/day
Therefore:
$D_{total}=0.82$ Gy/day $\times 85.54$ days $(1-e^{-78/85.54})$
$D_{total}=70.14(1-0.4018)$
$Dc=70.14(0.5982)$
$Dc=42$ Gy

20. D For permanent implants, the total dose to a point may be found from the initial dose rate by the equation:
$D_{total}=D_0 \times t_{avg}$ $t_{avg}=1.44 \times T_{1/2}$ ^{198}Au
$D_{total}=?$ $t_{avg}=1.44 \times 64.8$ h
$D_0=15$ cGy/h $t_{avg}=93.31$ h
$D_{total}=D_0 \times t_{avg}$

5.15 Brachytherapy Dose Calculations (Answers)

$D_{total} = 15$ cGy/h $\times 93.31$ h
$D_{total} = 1{,}399$ cGy

21. D For temporary implants, the total dose to a point may be found from the initial dose rate by $D_{total} = D_0 \times t_{avg}[1 - e^{-t/t_{avg}}]$.

22. A The total time a temporary Ir-192 implant must be left in place if the total dose delivered is 2,000 cGy and the initial dose rate is 0.7 Gy/h is 25.335 h.
Be organized;
$D_{total} = 2{,}000$ cGy or 20 Gy
$D_0 = 0.7$ Gy/h
$t_{avg} = 2{,}550$ h
$T_{1/2}\ ^{192}I = 73.8$ days
$t_{avg} = 1.44 \times T_{1/2}\ ^{192}I$
$t_{avg} = 1.44 \times 73.8$ days
$t_{avg} = 106.27$ days
$D_{total} = D_0 \times t_{avg}[1 - e^{-t/t_{avg}}]$
20 Gy $= 0.7$ Gy $\times 2{,}550$ h $[1 - e^{-t/2{,}250\ h}]$
20 Gy $= 1{,}785$ Gy/h $[1 - e^{-t/2{,}250\ h}]$
$1 - e^{-t/2{,}250\ h} = 20$ Gy/1,785 Gy/h
$1 - e^{-t/2{,}250\ h} = 0.0112$ h
$e^{-t/2{,}250\ h} = 1 - 0.0112$ h
$e^{-t/2{,}250\ h} = 0.9888$ h
Solve for t
Ln $(e^{-t/2{,}250\ h}) = $ ln (0.9888)
$-t/2{,}250$ h $= -0.01126$ h
$-t = -0.01126 \times 2{,}250$ h
$-t = -25.335$ h
$t = -25.335$ h/-1
$t = 25.335$ h

23. B The formula to find t_{avg} used in the equation of permanent and temporary implant is $t_{avg} = 1.44 \times t_{1/2}$, where 1.44 is a constant and $t_{1/2}$ is the time necessary for a radioactive material to decay to 50 % of its original activity.

24. C The $t_{1/2}$ of ^{60}Co is 5.26 years, and the formula to find t_{avg} is:
$t_{avg} = 1.44 \times t_{1/2}$
$t_{avg} = 1.44 \times 5.26$ years
$t_{avg} = 7.57$ years

25. C Be organized and know the formula.
The question is simple, it is asking to covert 0.75 mCi of ^{192}Ir to mg of radium equivalent (mg-Ra eq).
Γ radium $= 8.25$ R cm²/mg-h
$\Gamma\ ^{192}$Ir $= 4.62$ R cm²/mg-h
mCi of ^{192}Ir $= 0.75$
Formula:
mg-Ra eq $= \Gamma\ ^{192}$Ir/Γ radium $\times$ # of mCi of ^{192}Ir
mg-Ra eq $= 4.62/8.25 \times 0.75$ mCi
0.75 mCi of ^{192}Ir $= 0.42$ mg-Ra eq

26. D Be organized and know the formula.
The question is simple, it is asking to covert 0.60 mCi of Ra eq to mCi of ^{137}Cs.
Γ radium = 8.25 R cm²/mg-h
Γ ^{137}Cs = 3.1 R cm²/mg-h
mCi of Ra eq = 0.60
Formula:
mCi of ^{137}Cs = Γ radium/Γ ^{137}Cs × mCi of Ra eq
mCi of ^{137}Cs = 8.25/3.1 × 0.60 mg-Ra eq
0.60 mCi of Ra eq = 1.59 mCi of ^{137}Cs

27. C Whenever a question involves conversion from exposure to mg-Ra eq, use the conversion formula based on the exposure rate constant:
Mg-Ra eq = Γ ^{198}Au/Γ radium × # of mCi of ^{198}Au
Now, be organized and analyze the question.
Γ radium = 8.25 R.cm²/h = 0.825 mR/h
Γ ^{198}Au = 2.35 R cm²/mg-h = 0.235 mR m²/mg-h
Exposure rate of ^{198}Au = 0.350 mR/h at 1 m
mCi ^{137}Cs = (0.350 mR/h)/(0.235 mR m²/mg-h) = 1.49 mCi
Formula:
mg-Ra eq = Γ ^{198}Au/Γ radium × # of mCi of ^{198}Au
mg-Ra eq = (2.35/8.25) × 1.49 mCi
mg-Ra eq = 0.424 mg-Ra eq

28. B First, analyze the question and collect the data. Remember that the physical length is the distance between the actual ends of the source, but the active length is the distance between the ends of the radioactive material. This is important and we will use this later. Also, the question asked to answer in mCi, but the activity is given in mg-Ra eq/cm.
Γ ^{103}Pd = 1.48 R cm²/mg-h
Γ ^{226}Ra = 8.25 R cm²/mg-h
mCi of ^{103}Pd = ?
Active length = 20 cm
Multiply the ACTIVE length by the activity per length, not the physical length.
Activity = 0.85 mg-Ra eq/cm × 20 cm = 17 mg-Ra eq total
# mCi of ^{103}Pd = 17 (8.25/1.48)
# mCi of ^{103}Pd = 178 mCi

29. A # mCi of ^{131}I = ?
1 mg-Ra eq of ^{131}I
Γ ^{226}Ra = 8.25 R/mg-h at 1 cm
Γ ^{131}I = 2.3 R/mg-h at 1 cm
Conversion from mg-Ra eq to mCi of ^{131}I
mCi of ^{131}I = 1 mg-Ra eq of ^{131}I × (8.25/2.3)
mCi of ^{131}I = 3.587 mCi
Be aware that the exposure rate at 1 cm from a 1-mg point source of radium-226 filtered by 0.5 mm of platinum (Pt) is 8.25 R/h. The question

5.15 Brachytherapy Dose Calculations (Answers)

affirms that ^{226}Ra has been filter by 0.5 mm of Pt. If the ^{226}Ra is filtered by a different thickness, the % difference must be added to the equation.

30. B Be organized and collect all the data:
$\Gamma\ ^{226}$Ra = 8.25 R cm^2/mg-h
$\Gamma\ ^{137}$Cs = 3.26 R cm^2/mg-h
$\Gamma\ ^{198}$Au = 2.38 R cm^2/mg-h
$\Gamma\ ^{125}$I = 1.46 R cm^2/mg-h
Activity = 12 mg-Ra eq
Conversion from mg-Ra eq to mCi
mCi radionuclide = $\Gamma\ ^{226}$Ra/Γ radionuclide × activity in mg-Ra eq
mCi ^{137}Cs = $\Gamma\ ^{226}$Ra/$\Gamma\ ^{137}$Cs × activity
mCi ^{137}Cs = 8.25/3.26 × 12 mg-Ra eq
mCi ^{137}Cs = 30.36 mCi
mCi ^{198}Au = $\Gamma\ ^{226}$Ra/$\Gamma\ ^{198}$Au × activity
mCi ^{198}Au = 8.25/2.38 × 12 mg-Ra eq
mCi ^{198}Au = 41.59 mCi
mCi ^{125}I = $\Gamma\ ^{226}$Ra/$\Gamma\ ^{125}$I × activity
mCi ^{125}I = 8.25/1.46 × 12 mg-Ra eq
mCi ^{125}I = 67.81 mCi

31. C Be organized and collect all the data:
$\Gamma\ ^{226}$Ra = 8.25 R cm^2/mg-h
$\Gamma\ ^{137}$Cs = 3.26 R cm^2/mg-h
$\Gamma\ ^{198}$Au = 2.38 R cm^2/mg-h
$\Gamma\ ^{125}$I = 1.46 R cm^2/mg-h
Activity = 12 mCi
Conversion from mCi to mg-Ra eq
mg-Ra eq radionuclide = Γ radionuclide/$\Gamma\ ^{226}$Ra × activity in mCi
mg-Ra eq ^{137}Cs = $\Gamma\ ^{137}$Cs/$\Gamma\ ^{226}$Ra × activity
mg-Ra eq ^{137}Cs = 3.26/8.25 × 12 mCi
mg-Ra eq ^{137}Cs = 4.74
mg-Ra eq ^{198}Au = $\Gamma\ ^{198}$Au/$\Gamma\ ^{226}$Ra × activity
mg-Ra eq ^{198}Au = 2.38/8.25 × 12 mCi
mg-Ra eq ^{198}Au = 3.46
mg-Ra eq ^{125}I = $\Gamma\ ^{125}$I/$\Gamma\ ^{226}$Ra × activity
mg-Ra eq ^{125}I = 1.46/8.25 × 12 mCi
mg-Ra eq ^{125}I = 2.12

32. D Be organized and collect all the data:
$\Gamma\ ^{226}$Ra = 8.25 R cm^2/mg-h
$\Gamma\ ^{125}$I = 1.46 R cm^2/mg-h
Activity ^{125}I = 30 mCi-min = 1,800 mg-h
Conversion from mCi to mg-Ra eq
mg-Ra eq radionuclide = Γ radionuclide/$\Gamma\ ^{226}$Ra × activity in mCi
mg-Ra eq radionuclide = 1.46/8.25 × 1,800
mg-Ra eq radionuclide = 318.54 mg-Ra eq-h

33. A Be organized and collect all the data:
Γ ^{226}Ra = 8.25 R cm²/mg-h
Γ ^{137}Cs = 3.26 R cm²/mg-h
Activity ^{137}Cs = 100 mCi, and 120 mCi
Conversion from mCi to mg-Ra eq
\# mg-Ra eq ^{137}Cs = Γ ^{137}Cs/Γ ^{226}Ra × activity in mCi
\# mg-Ra eq ^{137}Cs = 3.26/8.25 × 100 = 39.5
\# mg-Ra eq ^{137}Cs = 3.26/8.25 × 120 = 47.4
39.5 + 47.4 = 86.90 total \# mg-Ra eq

34. C The exposure rate constant of radium is said to be 8.25 R cm²/mg-h because the exposure rate at 1 cm from a 1-mg point source of radium-226 filtered by 0.5 mm of platinum (Pt) is 8.25 R cm²/mg-h.

35. C The exposure rate of any radionuclide at any distance and at any length of time can be calculated by the equation $X = Γ × A/r^2 × t$, where X represents exposure, r is the distance, A is the activity in mCi, and t is the exposure time.

36. C Be organized and know the formula.
Γ (^{137}Cs) = 3.27 (R × cm²)/(mCi × h)
A = 15 mCi
t = 40 h = weekly
d = 2 m = 200 cm
Formula:
$X = Γ × A/r^2 × t$
X = 3.27 (R × cm²)/(mCi × h) × 15 mCi/200 cm² × 40 h
X = 0.049 R or 49 mrem

37. D Be organized and know the formula.
Γ (^{198}Au) = 2.38 R cm²/mg-h
Convert to mCi using the ratio of exposure rate constants:
mCi ^{198}Au = Γ ^{226}Ra/Γ ^{198}Au × mg-Ra eq = (8.25/2.38) × 250 mg-Ra eq
A = 866.6 mCi
D = 2 m = 200 cm
Formula:
$X = Γ × A/r^2 × t$
X = 2.38 R cm²/mg-h × 866.6 mCi × (1/200 cm)²
X = 0.051 R.cm²/h.mg

38. A The formulas used to calculate the activity of a radionuclide AFTER a specific time is $A = A_0 e^{-λt}$, where A is activity, A_0 is initial activity, e is the exponential, lambda (λ) is the probability per unit time of decay (λ = ln(2)/$T_{1/2}$), the – sign indicates that there is a decay on the radioactive nuclide, and t is the time from time zero. Be careful because in answer D, lambda is positive.

5.15 Brachytherapy Dose Calculations (Answers)

39. C The formulas used to calculate activity of a radionuclide AFTER a specific time are:
$A = A_0 e^{-\lambda t}$ $A = A_0 e^{(-\lambda t)}$
Be organized: $A = 15$ mCi $\times e^{(-0.041 \times 15)}$
$A = ?$ $A = 15$ mCi $\times 0.542$
$A_0 = 15$ mCi $A = 8.138$ mCi
$\lambda = 0.693/T_{1/2} = 0.041$ day^{-1}
$T_{1/2}$ ^{103}Pd $= 17$ days
$t = 15$ days

40. A The question is asking for the future dose of a ^{103}Pd source Therefore the formula to be used is the same as the one used to calculate the activity of a radionuclide *after* a specific time: $A = D_{total} = D_0 \times t_{avg}[1 - e^{-t/tavg}]$
Be organized:
Total dose $= 70$ Gy
$T_{1/2}$ ^{103}Pd $= 17$ days
$t = 5$ days
Dose after 5 days $= ?$
Total dose after t days $= D_0 \times t_{avg}[1 - e^{-t/tavg}]$
First, we need to calculate the initial dose rate, D_0:
Remember the total dose for a permanent implant $= D_0 \times t_{avg}$
70 Gy $= D_0 \times 1.44 \times 17$ days
$D_0 = 2.86$ Gy/day
Dose after 5 days $= D_0 \times t_{avg}[1 - e^{-t/tavg}]$
Dose after 5 days $= 2.86$ Gy/day $\times 1.44 \times 17$ days $[1 - e^{-5/(1.44 \times 17)}]$
Dose after 5 days $= 70.01 \times [1 - 0.815]$
Dose after 15 days $= 12.95$ Gy

41. B The formula used to calculate the activity of a radionuclide AFTER a specific time is:
$A = A_0 e^{-\lambda \times t}$ $\lambda = \ln(2)/T_{1/2}$ $T_{1/2}$ ^{137}Cs $= 30$ years $A = 80$ mCi
$e^{(-(0.693/30 \text{ years}) \times 2.5 \text{ years})}$
$t = 2$ years and 6 months or 2.5 years $A = 80$ mCi $\times 0.944$
$A_0 = 80$ mCi $A = 75.52$ mCi

42. A Collect all the data:
Activity of ^{192}Ir at 3 months $= ?$
Original activity $(A_0) = 12.5$ Ci
$t = 3$ months old $= 93$ days
$\lambda = \ln(2)/T_{1/2}$
$T_{1/2}$ of ^{192}I $= 74.3$ days
Formula of activity in the future:
$A = A_0 (e^{-\lambda t})$
Remember that both the half-life and t must have the same unit (days, years, etc.)

$A = 12.5$ Ci $(e^{-(0.693/74.3 \text{ days}) \times 93 \text{ days}})$
$A = 12.5$ Ci $\times 0.420$
$A = 5.250$ Ci

43. C Collect the data:
Original activity of ^{137}Cs $= 100$ %
Activity of ^{137}Cs in 180 months $= 15$ years $= ?$
$T_{1/2}$ ^{137}Cs $= 30$ years
$\lambda = \ln(2)/T_{1/2} = 0.0231$ year^{-1}
$100 =$ original activity
Formula of activity in the future (remember they have consistent units):
$A = A_0 e^{-\lambda \times t} = 100 \times e^{-0.0231 \times 15 \text{ years}}$ $A = 70.7$ %
The activity of ^{137}Cs in 180 months is 70 % of the original activity.
Another way of to look at this is:
180 months $= 1/2$ of a half-life of ^{137}Cs
$(½)^2 = 0.25 = ¼$ has decayed so around 75 % still remains.

44. A Collect the data:
Original activity of ^{125}I $= 1.0$
Activity of ^{125}I in 14 days $= ?$
$T_{1/2}$ ^{125}I $= 59.4$ days
$\lambda = \ln(2)/T_{1/2} = 0.0117$ day^{-1}
Formula of activity in the future:
$A = A_0 e^{-\lambda \times t} = 1 \times e^{-0.0117 \text{ day}^{-1} \times 14 \text{ days}}$ $A = 0.85$
The activity of ^{125}I in 14 days is 85 % of the initial.
This means that the seeds have decayed by 15 %, so approximately 15 % more seeds will have to be used to account for this decay.

45. D If a procedure is scheduled at a specific time in the future and the initial activity needs to be known, the formula is $A_0 = A_t e^{\lambda t}$.

46. D This question does not even need to be calculated as the activity must be larger than the required activity. Just select D as the answer. Anyway, the formula used to calculate the activity of a radionuclide AFTER specific time is $A = A_0 e^{-\lambda t}$, where the sign – in front of λ indicates decay of the source over time. One way to calculate activity in the past is by changing the – sign to +.
$A = A_0 e^{+\lambda t}$ $\lambda = \ln(2)/T_{1/2} = 0.257$ day^{-1}
Be organized: $A_0 = 10$ mCi $\times (e^{+0.257 \times 5 \text{ days}})$
$A = 10$ mCi $A_0 = 10$ mCi $\times 3.614$
$A_0 = ?$ $A_0 = 36.14$ mCi
$T_{1/2}$ ^{198}Au $= 2.7$ days
$t = 5$ days

47. C As we can see, the formula to be used is the formula to calculate temporary implants, but we need to solve for t which is the time needed for the source to be removed.
$D_{\text{total}} = 15$ Gy $t_{\text{avg}} = 1.44 \times T_{1/2}$ ^{192}I

5.15 Brachytherapy Dose Calculations (Answers)

$D_0 = 0.6$ Gy/h $\quad t_{avg} = 1.44 \times 73.8$ days
$\qquad\qquad\qquad t_{avg} = 106.27$ days
$t = ?\qquad\qquad t_{avg} = 2{,}550$ h
Formula:
$D_{total} = D_0 \times t_{avg}[1 - e^{-t/t_{avg}}]$
15 Gy $= 0.6$ Gy/h $\times 2{,}550$ h $[1 - e^{-t/2{,}550}]$
15 Gy $= 1{,}530$ Gy $[1 - e^{-t/2{,}550}]$
15 Gy $= 1{,}530$ Gy $[1 - e^{-t/2{,}550}]$
$1 - e^{-t/2{,}550} = 15$ Gy$/1{,}530$ Gy
$1 - e^{-t/2{,}550} = 0.0098$
Solve for t:
$1 - e^{-t/2{,}550} = 0.0098$
$e^{-t/2{,}550} = 1 - 0.0098$
$e^{-t/2{,}550} = 0.9902$
Ln $(e^{-t/2{,}550}) = \ln (0.9902)$
$-t/2{,}550 = -0.0098$
$-t = 2{,}550 \times -0.0098$
$-t = -25$
$t = -25/-1$
$t = 25$ h
One day is 24 h, so the source should be removed on Tuesday at 9:00 am.

48. A 1 mCi $= 3.7 \times 10^{7\,Bq}$, so 100 mCi $= 3.7 \times 10^9$ Bq.

49. C 1 Ci $= 3.7 \times 10^{10}$.
1 mCi $= (10^{-3}) = 3.7 \times 10^7$ Bq
1 µCi $= (10^{-6}) = 3.7 \times 10^4$ Bq
1 nCi $= (10^{-9}) = 3.7 \times 10^{10}$ Bq
1 pCi $= (10^{-12}) = 3.7 \times 10^1$ Bq

50. B The Γ for ^{226}Ra is 8.25 R cm^2/mg-h; the value of natural logarithm of 2, ln(2), used in radioactivity is 0.693; and the mass of an electron at rest is 0.511 MeV.

51. C To find out the air kerma strength, first you need to find the exposure rate and then use the rad (cGy) to R conversion factor. Remember that the exposure rate constant of ^{103}Pd is 1.48 R cm^2/mg-h. Take this value and multiply by the activity which is 1 mCi to get 1.48 R/h at 1 cm. Multiply this by 0.876 cGy/R to get the answer; 1.44×17 days is the average life equation, $t_{avg} = 1.44 \times t_{1/2}$; and 0.696/17 days is the radioactive decay formula $\lambda = 0.693/T_{1/2}$.

52. C 1 mg-Ra eq in terms of air kerma strength is 7.227 cGy/h.
The rad (cGy) to R or air kerma value is 0.876 cGy/R.
Γ ^{226}Ra is 8.25 R cm^2/mg-h.
$8.25 \times 0.876 = 7.227$ cGy/h.

53. D As always, analyze the question and collect data:
Air kerma strength at 1 cm = 7.227 cGy/h
7.227 cGy/h × 1 Gy/100 cGy × 1,000,000 µGy/1 Gy = 72,270 µGy at 1 cm
Air kerma strength at 200 cm = ?
Inverse square law:
$(1 \text{ cm}/200 \text{ cm})^2 \times 72{,}270$ µGy/h = 1.8067 µGy/h

54. B Collect the data:
^{192}Ir activity = 90 mCi
Γ ^{192}Ir = 4.69 R cm²/mC h
Air kerma value is 0.876 cGy/R
Duration (time) = 72 h
Total reference air kerma = ?
First, convert mCi Γ ^{192}Ir to air kerma strength:
Γ ^{192}Ir × activity × air kerma value
4.69 R cm²/mg-h × 90 mCi × 0.876 cGy/R = 369.7 cGy/h at 1 cm
Convert to microgray
369.7 cGy/h at 1 cm × 10,000 µGy/cGy = 3,697,596 µGy/h at 1 cm
Γ ^{192}Ir is in 1 cm but air kerma is defined at 1 m, so use the inverse square law:
3,697,596 µGy/h × (1 cm/100 cm)² = 396.75 µGy h⁻¹ at 1 m
Finally, to find total reference air kerma at 1 m, multiply 369.72 µGy/h by 72 h.
369.72 µGy/h at 1 m × 72 h = 26,622 µGy at 1 m
Total reference air kerma at 1 m = 26,622 µGy at 1 m

55. A Collect the data:
Fraction of decay per year of ^{137}Cs = ?
^{137}Cs $T_{1/2}$ = 30 years
Initial activity (A_0) = 1
Time (t) = 1 year
$\lambda = \ln(2)/T_{1/2} = 0.0231$ year⁻¹
Decay formula:
$A = A_0 e^{-\lambda t} = 1 \times e^{-0.0231 \text{ year}-1 \times 1 \text{ year}}$
$A = 0.977$
Therefore, 97.7 % of the Cs is still left after 1 year and 2.2 % has decayed away.

56. B Collect the data:
Fraction of decay per year of ^{192}Ir = ?
^{192}Ir $T_{1/2}$ = 74.2 days
Initial activity (A_0) = 1
Time (t) = 1 month = 30 days
$\lambda = \ln(2)/T_{1/2} = 0.0093$ day⁻¹
Decay formula:
$A = A_0 e^{-\lambda t} = 1 \times e^{-0.093 \text{ day}-1 \times 30 \text{ days}}$
$A = 0.756$

5.15 Brachytherapy Dose Calculations (Answers)

Therefore, 75.6 % of the Ir is still left after 1 month and 24.4 % has decayed away.

57. C The exposure received by the therapist is 64 mR in 2 h.
Collect the data:
Exposure rate at 2 m = 200 mR/h
Exposure rate at 5 m = ?
Time spent in place = 2 h
First, use the inverse square law:
200 mR/h × (2/5 m)² = 32 mR/h at 5 m
32 mR/h × 2 h = 64 mR in 2 h

58. C The formula to calculate HVL is composed of the linear attenuation coefficient (μ) for the absorber placed in the beam and the natural log of 2 (0.693), so the formula is HVL = 0.693/μ.

59. B Collect the information and write down the formula.
HVL = ?
μ = 0.050 cm^{-1}
Natural log of 2 = 0.693
Formula:
HVL = 0.693/μ
HVL = 0.693/0.050 cm^{-1}
HVL = 13.86 cm

60. D Collect the information and write down the formula.
HVL = 15 m
μ = ?
Natural log of 2 = 0.693
Formula:
HVL = 0.693/μ
15 = 0.693/μ
μ = 0.693/15 m
μ = 0.046 m^{-1}

61. B Unit conversion, time, distance, and shielding are all variables in this problem. It makes no difference which one is handled first.
Collect the information:
Dose rate at 4.6 m = ?
Dose rate at 5 ft = 200 mrem/h
Working hours = 10 h/week
HVL to reduce dose to less than 100 mrem/year = ?
First, convert meter to feet.
If 1 m = 3.28 ft, then 4.6 m = 15 ft.
Next, use the inverse square law:

200 mrem/h × (5/15 ft)² = 22.22 mrem/h at 4.6 m or 15 ft
22.22 mrem × 10 h/week = 222.22 mrem/week
Now, calculate the # of HVLs to reduce 222.22 mrem/week to less than 100 mrem per year.
If 222.22 mrem were to be received in a week, then 11,111 mrem will be received in a year, since the working year has 50 weeks.
11,111 mrem/year_____5,555.5 mrem/year (1 HVL)
5,555.5 mrem/year_____2,777.7 mrem/year (2 HVL)
2,777.7 mrem/year_____1,388.8 mrem/year (3 HVL)
1,388.8 mrem/year_____694.4 mrem/year (4 HVL)
694.4 mrem/year_____347.2 mrem/year (5 HVL)
347.2 mrem/year_____173.6 mrem/year (6 HVL)
173.6 mrem/year_____86.8 mrem/year (7 HVL)
Alternatively, you could solve for n in the following equation:
Shielded dose = unshielded dose × $(0.5)^n$
100 mrem = 11,111 mrem × $(0.5)^n$
$0.009 = (0.5)^n$
$Log(0.009) = Log((0.5)^n)$
$-2.04 = n × Log(0.5) = n × -0.3$
$n = 6.8$ HVL (are exactly needed to get to 100 mrem)
The above estimation showed that 7 HVLs reduced the dose to 86.6 which makes sense.

62. B Dose to point P = 40.30 cGy/h

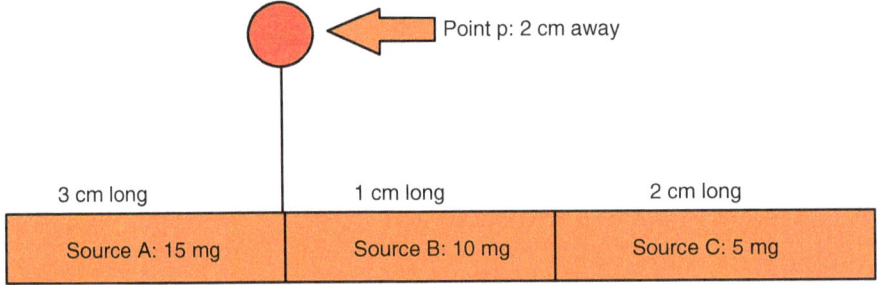

Fig. 5A.7.1

Collect all the data.
The dose from each source is measured from the center of the source to the point; therefore:
Source A (2 cm away and 1.5 cm along) = 1.25 cGy/mg-Ra eq-h
Source A = 1.25 cGy/mg-Ra eq-h × 15 mg-Ra eq = 18.75 cGy/h
Source B (2 cm away and 0.5 cm along) = 1.73 cGy/mg-Ra eq-h
Since 0.5 cm along is not on the table, the values for 0 cm and 1 cm along are taken and divided by two.

1.89 + 1.56 = 3.45/2 = 1.73 cGy/mg-Ra eq
Source B = 1.73 cGy/mg-Ra eq × 10 mg-Ra eq = 17.30 cGy/h
Source C (2 cm away and 2 cm along) = 0.97 cGy/mg-Ra eq-h
Source C = 0.97 cGy/mg-Ra eq-h × 5 mg-Ra eq = 4.85 cGy/h
Finally, add all the result from each source.
Point P dose = 18.75 + 17.30 + 4.25 cGy/h
Point P dose = 40.30 cGy/h

5.16 ICRU and AAPM TG Reports on Brachytherapy (Answers)

Quiz-1 (Level 2)

1. **A** ICRU 58 was developed in 1997, and it was written to generate a guideline about the dose specification and reporting for interstitial brachytherapy. ICRU 60 was written to generate a guideline about fundamental quantities and units for ionizing radiation. ICRU 50 contains guidelines about prescribing, recording, and reporting doses in photon beam therapy, and ICRU 38 was written as a guideline about the dose and volume specification for reporting intracavitary therapy in gynecology.

2. **A** As per ICRU 58, the total time of implantation on a temporary implant depends on the number of sources used, the strength and type of the source used, and the pattern of distribution of the sources. The location of the OARs usually does not affect the total time of implantation.

3. **C** As per ICRU 58 report, the gross tumor volumes (GTV) are the palpable or visible extent of the malignant growth while the clinical tumor volume (CTV) contains the GTV and/or subclinical microscopic malignant disease. The planning target volume (PTV) is the volume receiving the prescribed irradiation and for interstitial brachytherapy. The PTV is, in general, identical to the CTV, and finally, the treatment volume (TV) is the volume of tissue encompassed by an isodose surface specified by the radiation oncologist and the dose value at this isodose line is the minimum target dose.

4. **B** The minimum target dose (MTD) as specified by ICRU 58 is specified at the periphery of the CTV and must be equal to approximately 90 % of the prescribed dose in the Manchester system for interstitial therapy. The mean central dose (MCD) is the minimum doses between sources, in the central plane, and a high-dose volume is the volume of tissue receiving 150 % of the mean central dose.

5. **C** As per ICRU 58, dose uniformity is measured using individual minimum doses used to calculate the mean central dose in the central plane and the ratio of minimum target dose to the mean central dose.

6. B As per ICRU 58, temporary implant time and dose is:
Time = prescribed dose/initial dose rate

7. E As per ICRU 58, all should be reported. For more information, review the tables used in ICRU 58 of the levels of priority for reporting on different interstitial implant techniques.

8. C In compliance with the NRC regulations, the leakage radiation levels outside the HDR unit cannot exceed 1 mR/h at a distance of 10 cm from the nearest accessible surface surrounding the safe with the source in the shielded position.

9. B AAPM TG-43 is the essential report for brachytherapy dose calculations.

10. C AAPM TG-64 is the essential report for permanent prostate seed implant brachytherapy. The procedure of prostate seed implant is rather complicated as discussed in TG-64, including planning techniques with ultrasound imaging, source types, implant procedures, post-implant dosimetry, etc.

AAPM TG-128 is only for the QA of ultrasound system used in the procedure of prostate seed implant.

11. C AAPM TG-129 is for eye plaque dosimetry using ^{125}I or ^{103}Pd.

12. A There are four main components to HDR brachytherapy. The first is temporal accuracy which refers to the accuracy of the dwell time. This can be checked with a stopwatch. Temporal accuracy should be within 1 s. The second is dosimetric accuracy. This refers to the proper decay of the radioactive source. This can be checked by having an independent chart showing the daily decay. The third component is the positional accuracy. This refers to the accuracy of the position of the source. This can be checked using autoradiographs or the source ruler. The accuracy should be <1 mm. The final component is the safety equipment which consists of door and afterloader interlocks, Prime Alert radiation monitors, the audio/visual system, and emergency kit to name a few.

13. B The most common dose calculation formalism is TG-43. Other algorithms are beginning to gain momentum such as Monte Carlo and collapsed cone convolution, but they are just beginning to be implemented clinically.
TG-43 is what is known as a modular dose formalism meaning that the various components of the dose distribution are broken down into simpler parts. In TG-43, these components are the source strength, the gamma ray dose constant, the geometry function, the radial dose function, and the anisotropy function. These components have been tabulated for the various commercial sources using measurement and Monte Carlo simulations. The

5.16 ICRU and AAPM TG Reports on Brachytherapy (Answers)

benefit of this method is that it is very quick and provides sufficient clinical accuracy. A limitation is that it assumes that the entire calculation volume is water, so heterogeneities are not accounted for. Modern methods account for heterogeneities but require much more computing time.

14. **D** In TG-43, source strength is specified in terms of air kerma, or U. The units are cGy cm^2/h. This quantity must be measured for each source that is used in the clinic. The other choices besides cGy have been used in the past to specify source strength.

15. **C** In TG-43, the dose rate constant is unique to each commercially available brachytherapy source and has been calculated using a combination of measurement and simulation. The units are cGy/h-U, meaning that when this value is multiplied by the source strength, the resulting value is the dose rate at 1 cm in units of cGy/h.

16. **C** In TG-43, the inverse square effect is taken into account by the geometry function. For a simple point source, this function is simple $1/r^2$. It becomes more complex for a line source approximation. Refer to TG-43 for more information on this topic.

17. **D** As the energy of the source increases, the inverse square law tends to hold true. The effects of scatter and attenuation in tissue affect the inverse square law more for low-energy sources. Therefore, I-125 with an average energy of around 28 keV would have the most pronounced effect.

18. **A** The anisotropy function corrects for the fact that the dose distribution around a line source is not constant due to self-attenuation at the ends of the source. This factor is not used if a point source approximation is used.

Radiobiology

Contents

6.1	Cellular Biology (Questions)	408
6.2	Cell Death Due to Irradiation (Questions)	410
6.3	Normal Tissue Complication (NTC) (Questions)	412
6.4	Cell Survival Curves and Models (Questions)	422
6.5	BED and Fractionations (Questions)	425
6.6	Oxygen Enhancement and Hyperthermia Treatments (Questions)	427
6.7	Summary (Questions)	430
6.8	Cellular Biology (Answers)	432
6.9	Cell Death Due to Irradiations (Answers)	433
6.10	Normal Tissue Complication (NTC) (Answers)	435
6.11	Cell Survival Curves and Models (Answers)	442
6.12	BED and Fractionations (Answers)	444
6.13	Oxygen Enhancement and Hyperthermia Treatments (Answers)	446
6.14	Summary (Answers)	447

Radiobiology is the study of how ionizing radiation affects living cells. This is extremely important in radiation therapy as the decision to use a particular treatment strategy is closely related to radiobiology.

The purpose of radiotherapy is to kill the cancer cells using ionizing radiation while minimizing normal tissue complications. The theoretical basis to accomplish this goal stems from how normal tissue and tumor tissue respond to radiation. Readers are expected to understand cell survival curves, cell cycles, and the mechanism of cell death by radiation and other factors related to cell death such as hypoxia.

6.1 Cellular Biology (Questions)

Quiz-1 (Level 2)

1. The main constituent(s) of a cell is/are:
A. I, II, and III
B. I and III only
C. II and IV only
D. IV only
E. All are correct
I. Cytoplasm
II. Parenchyma
III. Nucleus
IV. Stroma

2. Human cells are:
A. I, II, and III
B. I and III only
C. II and IV only
D. IV only
E. All are correct
I. Eukaryotic cells
II. Somatic cells
III. Germ cells
IV. Prokaryotic cells

3. Which of the following is the definition of a mature cell?
A. Cells which exist to self-perpetuate and produce cells for a differentiated cell population
B. Cells which are fully differentiated and do not exhibit mitotic activity
C. Cells which are in movement to another population
D. Cells that divide and reproduce abnormally with uncontrolled growth

4. Which of the following cells are classified as mature cells?
A. Mucosa lining of the intestine
B. Reticulocyte that is differentiating to become erythrocyte
C. Epidermis
D. Nervous tissue

5. A group of cells that together perform one or more functions is referred as:
A. Organ
B. Organism
C. Tissue
D. Organ system

6.1 Cellular Biology (Questions)

6. The cell cycle is composed of:
A. I, II, and III
B. I and III only
C. II and IV only
D. IV only
E. All are correct
I. G1 or gap 1
II. S or synthesis
III. G2 or gap 2
IV. M or mitoses

7. In which part of the cell cycle do chromosomes separate and cell division takes place?
A. Gap 1
B. Synthesis
C. Gap 2
D. Mitoses

8. The cell cycle in mammalian cells takes approximately:
A. 5 days
B. 10 days
C. 10–20 h.
D. 2 days

9. Cells are most radiosensitive in:
A. I, II, and III
B. I and III only
C. II and IV only
D. IV only
E. All are correct
I. M phase
II. S phase
III. G2 phase
IV. G1 phase

10. Cells are most radioresistant in:
A. I, II, and III
B. I and III only
C. II and IV only
D. IV only
E. All are correct
I. M phase
II. G1 phase
III. G2 phase
IV. S phase

11. The biological effects of radiation result mainly from:
A. Damage to the cytoplasm
B. Damage to the DNA
C. Damage to the ribosome
D. Damage to the nucleus

12. When directly ionizing radiation is absorbed in biological material, the damage to the cell may occur by:
A. I, II, and III
B. I and III only
C. II and IV only
D. IV only
E. All are correct
I. Double ionization
II. Direct action
III. Single ionization
IV. Indirect action

13. Which of the following actions produce free radicals within the cell, damaging the critical target within?
A. Double ionization
B. Direct action
C. Single ionization
D. Indirect action

6.2 Cell Death Due to Irradiation (Questions)

Quiz-1 (Level 2)

1. The dominant action in the interaction of high linear energy transfer (LET) particles with a biological material is:
A. Double ionization
B. Direct action
C. Single ionization
D. Indirect action

2. Select the proper order involving biological damage produced by indirect action:
A. High electron interaction; photon produced; photon produces free radicals in water; free radicals produce changes in DNA; biological effects occur.
B. Primary photon interaction; high-energy electron produced; electron produces free radicals in water; free radicals produce changes in DNA; biological effects occur.

6.2 Cell Death Due to Irradiation (Questions)

C. Primary photon interaction; produces free radicals in water; free radicals produce changes in DNA; biological effects occur.
D. Free radical interaction; photon produced; photon produces a change in DNA; biological effects occur.

3. Irradiation of a cell will result in which of the following outcomes?
A. I, II, and III
B. I and III only
C. II and IV only
D. IV only
E. All are correct
I. No effect
II. Division delay
III. Apoptosis
IV. Reproductive failure

4. Irradiation of a cell can result in apoptosis which means:
A. The cell dies when attempting the first or subsequent mitosis.
B. There is a delayed form of reproductive failure as a result of induced genomic instability.
C. The cell dies before it can divide or afterward by fragmentation into smaller bodies, which are taken up by neighboring cells.
D. The cell is delayed from going through division.

5. Match the following irradiation cell outcomes with its corresponding definition.
A. Apoptosis
B. Division delay
C. Reproductive failure
D. Genomic instability
E. Mutation
F. Transformation
G. Bystander effects
H. Adaptive response
I. The cell dies when attempting the first or subsequent mitosis.
II. Programmed death of a cell following irradiation to prevent mutation or genomic instability.
III. Delayed form of reproductive failure as a result of induced genomic instability.
IV. The cell is delayed from going through mitosis.
V. The cell survives but the mutation leads to a transformed phenotype and possibly carcinogenesis.
VI. The irradiated cell is stimulated to react and become more resistant to subsequent irradiation.
VII. The cell survives but reproduced incorrectly.
VIII. An irradiated cell can send signals to neighboring unirradiated cells and induce biological effects.

6. At what dose level will a double-strand break occur in DNA?
A. 1 Gy
B. 2 Gy
C. 5 Gy
D. 10 Gy
E. No dose threshold

7. Which of the following types of radiation can be stopped by a human body?
A. Neutrons
B. Gamma rays
C. Beta particles
D. Alpha particles

8. Which of the following is considered electromagnetic radiation?
A. Neutrons
B. Gamma rays
C. Beta particles
D. Alpha particles

6.3 Normal Tissue Complication (NTC) (Questions)

Quiz-1 (Level 2)

1. Ionizing radiation has been proven to cause:
A. I, II, and III
B. I and III only
C. II and IV only
D. IV only
E. All are correct
I. Leukemia
II. Thyroid cancer
III. Breast cancer
IV. Bone cancer

2. In addition to carcinogenesis, late effects of radiation include:
A. I, II, and III
B. I and III only
C. II and IV only
D. IV only
E. All are correct
I. Fibrosis
II. Generic damage
III. Life span shortening
IV. Hair loss

6.3 Normal Tissue Complication (NTC) (Questions)

3. Which of the following radiation damage categories is irreversible and irreparable and leads to cell death?
A. Sublethal damage
B. Lethal damage
C. Potentially lethal damage
D. Somatic effect

4. What are somatic effects?
A. Harm that exposed individuals suffer during their lifetime
B. Radiation-induced mutations to an individual's genes and DNA that can contribute to the birth of defective descendants
C. An effect where the probability of occurrence increases with increasing dose but the severity in the affected individual does not depend on the dose
D. An effect that increases in severity with increasing dose, usually above a threshold dose

5. Which of the following is true about stochastic effect?
A. I, II, and III
B. I and III only
C. II and IV only
D. IV only
E. All are correct
I. There is no threshold dose.
II. There is a threshold dose.
III. Probability increases with increasing dose.
IV. Increase in severity with increasing dose.

6. Which of the following are considered acute effects?
A. I, II, and III
B. I and III only
C. II and IV only
D. IV only
E. All are correct
I. Inflammation
II. Edema
III. Hemorrhage
IV. Ulceration

7. Which of the following syndromes is caused when the dose to the total body in a single fraction is 50 Gy?
A. Bone marrow syndrome
B. Central nervous system syndrome
C. Gastrointestinal syndrome
D. Organ system syndrome

8. What is the proper order of fetal stages of development from conception to birth?
A. Organogenesis, preimplantation, growth stage
B. Growth stage, organogenesis, preimplantation
C. Organogenesis, preimplantation, growth stage
D. Preimplantation, organogenesis, growth stage

9. How long does organogenesis last?
A. From day 1 to day 10
B. From day 11 to day 42
C. From day 43 to birth
D. From birth to 1 year old

10. The effects produced on the fetus due to radiation depend on:
A. I, II, and III
B. I and III only
C. II and IV only
D. IV only
E. All are correct
I. Mother's health
II. Dose delivered
III. Fetus gender
IV. Stage of development at the time of exposure

11. The principal effects of radiation on a fetus are:
A. I, II, and III
B. I and III only
C. II and IV only
D. IV only
E. All are correct
I. Neonatal death
II. Malformations
III. Growth retardation
IV. Congenital defects and cancer induction

12. An abortion to avoid the possibility of radiation-induced congenital abnormalities should be considered:
A. If fetal total dose exceeded 10 Gy
B. If fetal total dose exceeded 10 cGy
C. If fetus is exposed to any radiation
D. If fetus is exposed only during the growth stage

13. What is the aim of radiotherapy?
A. Deliver enough radiation to the tumor to destroy it.
B. Deliver enough radiation to the tumor to destroy it without irradiating normal tissue to a dose that will lead to serious complications.

6.3 Normal Tissue Complication (NTC) (Questions)

C. Deliver enough radiation to the tumor and surrounding normal tissue to a dose that will lead to serious complications.
D. Deliver some dose to the tumor so that the surrounding normal tissue does not have serious complications.

14. Which of the following statements are true?
A. Normal cells are less sensitive to single doses of radiation than tumor cells.
B. Tumor cells are less sensitive to single doses of radiation than normal cells.
C. Both malignant cells and normal cells exhibit similar characteristics.
D. Tumor cells are less sensitive to late reactions than early reactions.

15. Which of the following statements are true?
A. For the same radiation dose, radiation delivered at a lower dose rate may produce more cell killing than radiation delivered at a higher dose rate.
B. For the same radiation dose, radiation delivered at a lower dose rate may produce less cell killing than radiation delivered at a higher dose rate.
C. Dose rate is not an important factor on cell killing when same radiation dose is delivered.
D. Fractionation of radiation treatment so that it is given over a period of weeks rather than in a single session results in a worst therapeutic ratio.

16. The four Rs of radiobiology include:
A. Radiosensitivity, reconstruction, redistribution, and reoxygenation
B. Radiosensitivity, repair, repopulation, and reoxygenation
C. Radioresistant, repopulation, redistribution, and reoxygenation
D. Repair, repopulation, redistribution, and reoxygenation

17. Which of the following are true about the four Rs of radiotherapy?
A. I, II, and III
B. I and III only
C. II and IV only
D. IV only
E. All are correct
I. Cells repopulate while receiving fractionated doses of radiation.
II. Redistribution in proliferating cell populations throughout the cell cycle phases increases the cell kill from a fractionated treatment relative to a single session treatment.
III. Reoxygenation of hypoxic cells occurs during a fractionated course of treatment, making them more radiosensitive to subsequent doses of radiation.
IV. Cells can repair from radiation damage.

18. Radioprotectors are:
A. Chemical agents that enhance cell response to radiation
B. Chemical agents that reduce cell response to radiation
C. Multileaf collimators used on a linac to block radiation
D. Systemic antineoplastic drugs used to kill or destroy cancer cells

19. Radioprotectors:
A. I, II, and III
B. I and III only
C. II and IV only
D. IV only
E. All are correct
I. Reduce the biological effect of radiation.
II. Protect normal tissues.
III. Must be present during radiation to take effect, usually within 30 min.
IV. Amifostine is considered a radioprotector.

20. Normal tissue tolerance dose (NTTD) is most dependent on:
A. I, II, and III
B. I and III only
C. II and IV only
D. IV only
E. All are correct
I. The number of fractions
II. Overall duration between the first and last fraction
III. The size of fractions
IV. The total dose

21. The response of a tissue or organ to radiation depends on:
A. I, II, and III
B. I and III only
C. II and IV only
D. IV only
E. All are correct
I. The sensitivity of the individual cells
II. The kinetics of the tissue as a whole of which the cells are a part
III. The way the cells are organized in that tissue
IV. Time of the day the cells are irradiated

22. $TD_{5/5}$ refers to:
A. The minimum tolerance dose that causes a 5 % complication rate within 5 years of radiation completion
B. The maximum tolerance dose that causes a 5 % complication rate within 5 years of radiation completion
C. The total dose that causes 5 % of the population to die within 5 years of radiation completion
D. The time delay that takes 5 % of the cell population to duplicate in 5 years

6.3 Normal Tissue Complication (NTC) (Questions)

23. Match the following tissues and organ sensitivities with their corresponding $TD_{5/5}$:
A. Liver (acute and chronic hepatitis)
B. Stomach (perforation, ulcer, and hemorrhage)
C. Brain (infarction, necrosis)
D. Kidney (acute and chronic nephrosclerosis)
I. $TD_{5/5}$ 45 Gy
II. $TD_{5/5}$ 30 Gy
III. $TD_{5/5}$ 50 Gy
IV. $TD_{5/5}$ 50 Gy

24. Match the following tissues and organ sensitivities with their corresponding $TD_{50/5}$:
A. Bladder (contracture) III
B. Lens (cataract) I
C. Lung (acute and chronic pneumonitis) IV
D. Rectum (ulcer, stenosis, fistula) II
I. $TD_{50/5}$ 18 Gy
II. $TD_{50/5}$ 80 Gy
III. $TD_{50/5}$ 80 Gy
IV. $TD_{50/5}$ 24.5 Gy

25. Match the following tissues and organ sensitivities with the corresponding injury if the $TD_{5/5}$ or $TD_{50/5}$ is exceeded:
A. Ovaries ($TD_{5/5}$ 2–3 Gy; $TD_{50/5}$ 6–12 Gy)
B. Ureters ($TD_{5/5}$ 70 Gy; $TD_{50/5}$ 100 Gy)
C. Oral cavity and pharynx ($TD_{5/5}$ 60 Gy; $TD_{50/5}$ 75 Gy)
D. Whole intestine ($TD_{5/5}$ 40 Gy; $TD_{50/5}$ 55 Gy)
I. Stricture
II. Obstruction, perforation, fistula
III. Sterilization
IV. Ulceration, mucositis

26. Bergonie and Tribondeau defined radiosensitivity as:
A. I, II, and III
B. I and III only
C. II and IV only
D. IV only
E. All are correct
I. Mitotic activity
II. Level of differentiation
III. Directly proportional to a cell's reproductive activity and inversely proportional to a cell's degree of differentiation
IV. Directly proportional to a cell's degree of differentiation and inversely proportional to a cell's reproductive activity

27. Bergonie and Tribondeau state that the most radiosensitive cells are:
A. I, II, and III
B. I and III only
C. II and IV only
D. IV only
E. All are correct
I. Cells that have a high division rate
II. Cells that are nonspecialized
III. Cells that have a high metabolic rate
IV. Cells that are well nourished

28. Bergonie and Tribondeau state that:
A. I, II, and III
B. I and III only
C. II and IV only
D. IV only
E. All are correct
I. Undifferentiated cells or immature cells that divide and replace other cells are radiosensitive.
II. Undifferentiated cells or immature cells that divide and replace other cells are radioresistant.
III. Differentiated cells or mature cells that do not divide are radioresistant.
IV. Differentiated cells or mature cells that do not divide are radiosensitive.

29. Match the cell type with its radiosensitivity.
A. Vegetative intermitotic cells (VIM)
B. Differentiating intermitotic cells (DIM)
C. Reverting postmitotic cells (RPM)
D. Fixed postmitotic cells (FPM)
I. Radiosensitive cell
II. Extremely radiosensitive cell
III. Radioresistant cell
IV. Highly radioresistant cell

30. Which of the following organs are composed of RPM or FPM cells making them radioresistant?
A. I, II, and III
B. I and III only
C. II and IV only
D. IV only
E. All are correct
I. Liver
II. Muscle
III. Nerves
IV. Bone marrow

6.3 Normal Tissue Complication (NTC) (Questions)

31. Which of the following are characteristics of DNA?
A. I, II, and III
B. I and III only
C. II and IV only
D. IV only
E. All are correct
I. DNA is a large molecule with double helix structure consisting of two strands.
II. The two strands are held together by hydrogen bonds between bases.
III. The backbone of individual strands is composed of sugar and phosphate groups.
IV. DNA is the principal target for the biological effects of radiation, including cell killing, carcinogenesis, and mutation.

32. The four bases attached to the backbone of DNA are composed of:
A. I, II, and III
B. I and III only
C. II and IV only
D. IV only
E. All are correct
I. Pyrimidines (thymine and cytosine)
II. Pyrimidines (adenine and guanine)
III. Purines (adenine and guanine)
IV. Purines (thymine and cytosine)

33. The correct pair of the bases on opposite strands is:
A. Adenine pairs with guanine, and thymine pairs with cytosine.
B. Adenine pairs with cytosine, and guanine pairs with thymine.
C. Adenine pairs with cytosine, and guanine pairs with adenine.
D. Adenine pairs with thymine, and guanine pairs with cytosine.

34. The phases of mitosis are:
A. I, II, and III
B. I and III only
C. II and IV only
D. IV only
E. All are correct
I. Prophase
II. Metaphase
III. Anaphase
IV. Telophase

35. Match the phase of mitosis with its correct description.
A. Prophase
B. Metaphase
C. Anaphase
D. Telophase

I. Movement of chromosomes on spindle to the opposite poles of the cell.
II. Thickening of the chromatin as the chromosomes condense into light coils. The chromosomes reach maximal condensation and the nuclear membrane disappears.
III. Chromosomes begin to uncoil and the nuclear membrane reappears.
IV. Chromosomes move to the center of the cell, spindles form, and centromeres divide.

36. Prodromal radiation syndrome is defined as:
A. Signs and symptoms that occur in the first 48 h following irradiation of the central nervous system.
B. A dose of ionizing radiation sufficient to cause death.
C. It is the time between an injury occurring and the effects of the injury expressing themselves as disease.
D. Biological changes and symptoms, including death, that occur within weeks after a high-intensity total-body irradiation.

37. How long does it take for hematopoietic syndrome death to occur?
A. 24 to 48 h after exposure.
B. In a matter of days (usually between 3 and 10 days).
C. Several weeks to 2 months after exposure.
D. All syndromes are associated with 3 weeks death after exposure to radiation.

38. Which of the following radiation syndromes is associated with extensive bloody diarrhea and destruction of the GI mucosa?
A. Hematopoietic syndrome
B. Acute radiation syndrome
C. Cerebrovascular syndrome
D. Gastrointestinal syndrome

39. Mean lethal dose (D_{50}) is:
A. Lethal dose that causes mortality in 50 % of the exposed population or group in 30 days
B. Lethal dose that causes mortality in 50 % of the exposed population or group within a specific period of time
C. Lethal dose that causes death in 50 % of the exposed population or group in 60 days
D. Dose received by 50 % of the exposed population or group within a specific period of time

40. Which is the correct order of tissues from radiosensitive to radioresistant?
A. Testes, ovaries, lens, lung, liver, brain
B. Lung, testes, liver, ovaries, lens, brain
C. Testes, brain, ovaries, liver, lens, lung
D. Ovaries, brain, lung, lens, testes, liver

6.3 Normal Tissue Complication (NTC) (Questions)

41. The forms of electromagnetic radiation are:
A. I, II, and III
B. I and III only
C. II and IV only
D. IV only
E. All are correct
I. Alpha (α) particles
II. Gamma (γ) particles
III. Electrons
IV. X-rays

42. Radio waves, microwaves, infrared radiation, visible light, ultraviolet light, x-rays, and gamma (γ) particles all have the same what?
A. I, II, and III
B. I and III only
C. II and IV only
D. IV only
E. All are correct
I. Wavelengths (λ)
II. Frequency (ν)
III. Origin
IV. Velocity (c)

43. Which of the following statements is/are true?
A. I, II, and III
B. I and III only
C. II and IV only
D. IV only
E. All are correct
I. The longer the wavelength, the shorter the frequency.
II. The longer the wavelength, the smaller the energy.
III. The shorter the wavelength, the larger the biological effect.
IV. Radio waves have a longer wavelength than visible light.

44. Which of the following statements are true?
A. I, II, and III
B. I and III only
C. II and IV only
D. IV only
E. All are correct
I. If a cell has a single-strand DNA break, the cell will either die, mutate, or undergo carcinogenesis because it cannot be repaired.
II. If a cell has a double-strand DNA break directly opposite to one another on the DNA molecule, the cell either dies, mutates, or undergoes carcinogenesis because it cannot be repaired.

III. If a cell has a double-strand DNA break but well separated along the molecule, the cell either dies, mutates, or undergoes carcinogenesis because it cannot be repaired.
IV. If a cell has a single-strand DNA break, the cell rapidly repairs itself using the opposite strand as a template.

6.4 Cell Survival Curves and Models (Questions)

Quiz-1 (Level 2)

1. What does a cell survival curve describe?
A. The relationship between the surviving fraction of cells and the absorbed dose
B. A plot of a biological effect observed against absorbed dose
C. A plot of volume of a given structure receiving a certain dose or higher as a function of dose
D. A plot of volume receiving a dose within a specified dose interval as a function of dose

2. What is a cell survival curve in the multi-target model composed of?
A. I, II, and III
B. I and III only
C. II and IV only
D. IV only
E. All are correct
I. Extrapolation number
II. Initial slope
III. Quasithreshold dose
IV. Practical range

3. Advantages of conventional fractionation in radiotherapy include:
A. I, II, and III
B. I and III only
C. II and IV only
D. IV only
E. All are correct
I. Spares normal tissues through repair of sublethal damage between dose fractions and repopulation of cells
II. Increases tumor damage through reoxygenation and redistribution of tumor cells
III. Spares late reactions
IV. Regeneration of early-responding tissues and tumor reoxygenation

6.4 Cell Survival Curves and Models (Questions)

4. More than one fraction per day with a smaller dose per fraction (<1.8 Gy) is the definition of:
A. Standard fractionation
B. Accelerated fractionation
C. Hyperfractionation
D. CHART

5. Which of the following statements are true?
A. I, II, and III
B. I and III only
C. II and IV only
D. IV only
E. All are correct
I. Differentiated cells do not proliferate.
II. Nerve and muscle cells are considered differentiated cells.
III. Stem and intestinal epithelium cells are considered proliferating cells.
IV. Secretory cells are considered proliferating cells.

6. The n symbol in the cell survival curve (multi-target model) represents:
A. Extrapolation number
B. Dose
C. Quasithreshold dose
D. Practical range

7. The quasithreshold dose (D_0) in the cell survival curve:
A. I, II, and III
B. I and III only
C. II and IV only
D. IV only
E. All are correct
I. Is a measure of the width of the shoulder region of the curve
II. Is the dose at which survival curve becomes exponential
III. Measures a cell's ability to accumulate and repair sublethal damage
IV. Is defined as the dose at which the straight portion of the survival curve, extrapolated backward, cuts the dose axis drawn through a survival fraction of unity

8. The D_0 in the cell survival curve (multi-target model) represents:
A. I, II, and III
B. I and III only
C. II and IV only
D. IV only
E. All are correct
I. 37 % cell survival
II. 50 % cell survival
III. Cell radiosensitivity
IV. Cell's ability to accumulate sublethal damage

9. Match the following letters with its corresponding survival curve parameters?
A. Extrapolation number
B. D_0
C. Quasithreshold dose

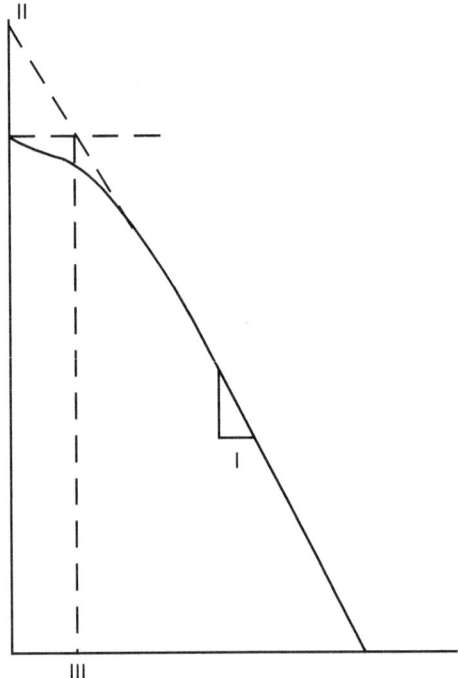

Fig. 6.4.1

10. Which of the following is the correct formula used to represent the three parameters of the survival curve?
A. $SF = 1 - (1 - e^{-D/D_0})^n$
B. $N(D) = N_0 \times e^{-D/D_0}$
C. $N(D) = N_0 [1 - (1 - e^{-D/D_0})^n]$
D. $\mathrm{Log}_e n = D_Q/D_0$

11. Which of the following is the model of choice to describe survival curves?
A. Cell survival curve
B. Linear–quadratic model
C. Dose–volume histogram
D. Linear model

6.5 BED and Fractionations (Questions)

Quiz-1 (Level 2)

1. Which of the following is used in radiobiology to calculate the dose required to kill a cell population?
   A. D_5
   B. $T_{1/2}$
   C. D_{10}
   D. LET

2. The formula used to calculate the D_{10} is:
   A. $D_{10} = \log(2) \times D_0$
   B. $D_{10} = 2.3 \times D_0$
   C. $D_{10} = 0.693 \times D_0$
   D. $D_{10} = \log(10)/D_0$

3. What will be the total dose required to kill 90 % of the tumor population if the D_0 is 5 Gy?
   A. 11.5 Gy
   B. 3.46 Gy
   C. 11.5 Gy
   D. 34.65 Gy

4. Radiation-induced damage to mammalian cells includes:
   A. I, II, and III
   B. I and III only
   C. II and IV only
   D. IV only
   E. All are correct
   I. Sublethal damage
   II. Lethal damage
   III. Potentially lethal damage
   IV. Reversible lethal damage

5. Which of the following statements are true?
   A. I, II, and III
   B. I and III only
   C. II and IV only
   D. IV only
   E. All are correct

I. The α/β ratio is about 3 Gy for early-responding tissues.
II. The α/β ratio is about 10 Gy for late-responding tissues.
III. The α/β ratio is the dose at which linear and quadratic components of cell killing are equal.
IV. The α/β ratio is about 100 Gy for late-responding tissues.

6. Which of the following are true about hyperfractionation?
A. I, II, and III
B. I and III only
C. II and IV only
D. IV only
E. All are correct
I. The aim of hyperfractionation is to further separate early and late effects.
II. Early reactions may be increased slightly.
III. Late effects are greatly reduced.
IV. Tumor control is slightly improved.

7. Which of the following statements are true?
A. I, II, and III
B. I and III only
C. II and IV only
D. IV only
E. All are correct
I. If fewer and larger dose fractions are given, late reactions are more severe.
II. For early effects, α/β is large.
III. For late effects, α/β is small.
IV. Late-effect tissues are more sensitive to changes in fractionation patterns than are early-responding tissues.

8. Which of the following is correct about α/β values?
A. They estimate the sensitivity of the tumor or normal tissue to fractionation.
B. They estimate the sensitivity of the tumor or normal tissue to LET.
C. They describe the process by which a radioactive element moves toward stability.
D. Determined by adding the dose equivalents to various organs using weighting factors.

9. The intent of an accelerated treatment strategy is:
A. To reduce repopulation in rapidly proliferating tumors
B. To farther separate early and late effects
C. To deliver low dose per fraction to minimize late effects and a very short overall time to minimize tumor proliferation
D. To have good local tumor control owing to short overall time

10. The time interval between multiple daily fractions should be:
A. Less than 4 h.
B. Longer than 4 h.
C. Less than 6 h.
D. Longer than 6 h.

11. Which of the following equations is used to calculate the quantity by which different fractionation regimens are intercompared or the biologically effective dose (E/α)?
A. $1 - (1 - e^{-D/D_0})^n$
B. $nd \times (1 + [d/\alpha/\beta])$
C. $2.3 \times D_0$
D. D_Q/D_0

12. A physician is undecided whether to treat a patient using conventional treatment or hyperfractionation. A conventional treatment will be delivered in 30 fractions of 1.8 Gy given one fraction per day, 5 days per week, for an overall treatment time of 6 weeks. The hyperfractionation treatment will use 70 fractions of 1.2 Gy given twice daily, 6 h apart, and 5 days per week, for an overall treatment time of 6 weeks and 3 days. Calculate the biological effect dose for early and late effects for each case if α/β is assumed to be 3 Gy for late-responding tissues and 10 Gy for early-responding tissues.
A. Conventional: early effects 63.72 Gy_{10}, late effects 86.4 Gy_3
   Hyperfractionation: early effects 121 Gy_3, late effects 96.8 Gy_{10}
B. Conventional: early effects 86.4 Gy_3, late effects 63.72 Gy_{10}
   Hyperfractionation: early effects 121 Gy_3, late effects 96.8 Gy_{10}
C. Conventional: early effects 63.72 Gy_{10}, late effects 86.4 Gy_3
   Hyperfractionation: early effects 96.8 Gy_{10}, late effects 121 Gy_3
D. Conventional: early effects 96.8 Gy_{10}, late effects 121 Gy_3
   Hyperfractionation: early effects 63.72 Gy_{10}, late effects 86.4 Gy_3

6.6 Oxygen Enhancement and Hyperthermia Treatments (Questions)

Quiz-1 (Level 2)

1. Which of the following statements are true?
A. I, II, and III
B. I and III only
C. II and IV only
D. IV only
E. All are correct
I. The presence or absence of molecular oxygen within a cell influences the biological effect of ionizing radiation.

II. The larger the cell oxygenation above anoxia, the larger is the biological effect of ionizing radiation.
III. The biological effect due to presence or absence of molecular oxygen within a cell is much more pronounced for low LET.
IV. The oxygen enhancement ratio increases as the LET increases.

2. Oxygen enhancement ratio (OER) is defined as:
A. The relationship between the surviving fraction of cells and the absorbed dose
B. The processes by which cells that are hypoxic become oxygenated after irradiation, through the killing and removal of toxic radiosensitive cells from the tumor
C. The ratio of doses without and with oxygen (hypoxic versus well-oxygenated cells) to produce the same biological effect
D. The ratio of dose to produce an effect with radioprotector to dose to produce the same effect without radioprotector

3. What is the oxygen enhancement ratio (OER) if in order to produce the same biological effect cells under hypoxic condition, one needs to deliver a dose of 150 cGy, versus 70 cGy under oxygenated condition?
A. 10,500
B. 220
C. 2.14
D. 0.46

4. Match the radiation type with its corresponding OER.
A. X-rays and γ-rays
B. Neutrons
C. High-LET radiations (α particle)
I. 1.5 OER
II. 1 OER
III. 2–3.5 OER

5. Which of the following is true?
A. I, II, and III
B. I and III only
C. II and IV only
D. IV only
E. All are correct
I. Oxygen is an effective radioprotector.
II. Oxygen is an effective radiosensitizer.
III. Hypoxic cells are radiosensitive.
IV. Hypoxic cells are radioresistant.

6.6 Oxygen Enhancement and Hyperthermia Treatments (Questions)

6. What type of cell exists in the center of tumors?
A. Oxygenated cells.
B. Hypoxic cells.
C. Neutral cells.
D. A cell becomes well oxygenated when duplicated.

7. Hydroxyurea is a powerful chemotherapy agent used to:
A. Block radiation damage repair
B. Slow the normal cycle of the cell
C. Kill cells resistant to radiotherapy
D. Coordinate cells in a phase of the cycle that is more sensitive to radiation (M and G2)

8. Which of the following are correct about hyperthermia?
A. I, II, and III
B. I and III only
C. II and IV only
D. IV only
E. All are correct
I. It inhibits the repair to radiation damage.
II. It increases blood flow to normal tissues.
III. It damages tumor cell blood vessels.
IV. It burns tumor cells.

9. Which of the following are the disadvantages of hyperthermia?
A. I, II, and III
B. I and III only
C. II and IV only
D. IV only
E. All are correct
I. Thermotolerance.
II. Difficult to keep an area at constant temperature.
III. Distribution of the heat.
IV. Not all body tissues respond the same way to heat.

10. Which of the following is true about hyperthermia treatment?
A. I, II, and III
B. I and III only
C. II and IV only
D. IV only
E. All are correct
I. Hyperthermia uses heat to kill cancer cells.
II. Microwaves, radio waves, and ultrasound waves can be used to heat the treatment area.
III. Hyperthermia doses are expressed in cumulative equivalent minutes at 43 °C.
IV. Thermotolerance is a problem when using fractionation hyperthermia treatments.

11. Which of the following techniques are used in hyperthermia treatments?
A. I, II, and III
B. I and III only
C. II and IV only
D. IV only
E. All are correct
I. Microwaves
II. Radio waves
III. Ultrasound waves
IV. Electricity

6.7 Summary (Questions)

Quiz-1 (Level 3)

1. Gene mutation occurs in self-repairing of DNA after irradiation. Which of the following repair processes might cause gene mutation?
A. Single-strand break (SSB) of DNA only
B. Double-strand break (DSB) of DNA only
C. Both SSB and DSB
D. Fragment repairing

2. Which of the following strategies is prevalent in current radiotherapy?
A. Hyperfractionated IMRT
B. Hypofractionated IMRT
C. Both hyperfractionated IMRT and hypofractionated IMRT
D. 3D-CRT

3. At the time when radiotherapy was implemented in the late nineteenth century, treatments were:
A. All hypofractionated.
B. All hyperfractionated.
C. Some were hyperfractionated and some were hypofractionated.
D. Neither hyperfractionated nor hypofractionated.

4. In the past half century, the major effort of radiotherapy was to:
A. Increase the chance to kill the diseases.
B. Reduce normal tissue complications.
C. Extend patients' lives.
D. Develop more advanced imaging technologies.
E. All of the above.

6.7 Summary (Questions)

5. A physician wants to implement a new hypofractionated strategy to replace the original hyperfractionated IMRT strategy for the patient. The new fractional dose is three times more than the original one. What should he/she do to compute the new fractionation?
A. Of course BED, that is exactly for this.
B. Nothing, BED cannot be applied in this case.
C. Use a modified linear-quadratic model, which BED is based on.
D. The physician should not do so.

6. There is sometimes a "late effect" of normal tissue complications (NTCs) occurring several months after irradiation. What is the reason for this effect?
A. Unfortunately this late effect has not been well understood.
B. It takes a while for radiobiological effects to occur.
C. Cells mutated and thus cannot carry on biological functions.
D. Radiation-induced apoptosis suddenly occurred after a few weeks of irradiations.

7. What is the major function of ribosomes in cells?
A. Duplicate DNA.
B. Duplicate RNA.
C. Synthesize proteins.
D. Provide energy to cells.
E. Collect garbage in cells.

8. An adult receives an x-ray radiograph for the chest. This amount of exposure is equivalent to how many days of normal background exposure?
A. 6 months
B. 1 month
C. 1 week
D. 3 days
E. 1 year

9. Why is it possible in stereotactic radiosurgery (SRS) to deliver a tremendously large dose but with limited normal tissue complications (NTCs)?
A. At huge dose level, NTCs are negligible.
B. SRS only has 1–3 fractions; thus NTCs are not important.
C. The margin for treatment uncertainty is very small.
D. SRS does have NTCs, just like other external beam radiotherapy.

10. Studies showed SBRT has a better outcome over hyperfractionated IMRT. A patient who will be treated for 80 Gy in 2 Gy fractions now will be treated with SBRT in 5 fractions. What is the fractional dose?
A. 8.5 Gy.
B. 11.5 Gy.
C. It depends on the cancer type. The corresponding α/β values are needed for BED calculation.
D. The physician may estimate the dose from the RTOG trials for similar studies. Current research is looking at the BED method based on the LQ model.

6.8 Cellular Biology (Answers)

Quiz-1 (Level 2)

1. **B** The two main constituents of a cell are the cytoplasm, which supports all metabolic functions within the cell, and the nucleus, which contains the genetic information (DNA). Tissues and organs are composed of parenchyma, which contains characteristic cells of that tissue or organ, and stroma which consists of connective tissue and vasculature.

2. **A** Human cells are eukaryotic cells which contain membrane-bound compartments with a nucleus. They are either somatic cells which divide through mitosis producing two cells, each carrying a chromosome complement identical to that of the original cell, or germ cells which divide through meiosis. Prokaryotic cells are single-cell organisms that are the earliest and most primitive form of life on earth. Bacteria are examples of prokaryotes.

3. **B** Mature cells are classified as cells which are fully differentiated and do not exhibit mitotic activity. Stem cells are cells which exist to self-perpetuate and produce cells for a differentiated cell population. Transit progenitor cells are cells which are in movement to another population, and cancer cell are cells that divide and reproduce abnormally with uncontrolled growth.

4. **D** Nervous tissue and muscle cells are classified as mature cells. Mucosa linings of the intestine and epidermis are stem cells, and a reticulocyte that is differentiating to become an erythrocyte is an example of a transit cell.

5. **C** A group of cells that together perform one or more functions is referred to as tissue. A group of tissues that together perform one or more functions is called an organ, and a group of organs that perform one or more function is a system of organs or an organism.

6. **E** The cell cycle is an order of events in which a cell grows and divides. The cycle is composed of gap 1, synthesis, gap 2, and finally mitoses (G1-S-G2-M). The length of time spent in each part is different for each cell type.

7. **D** Mitosis is the stage in the cell cycle where chromosomes separate and cell division occurs. DNA replication occurs during synthesis, and the gap phases prepare the cell for mitosis or synthesis.

8. **C** The cell cycle in mammalian cells takes approximately 10–20 h. S phase is usually 6–8 h. M phase is less than an hour, G2 phase takes around 2–4 h, and G1 is approximately 8 h. G1 demonstrates the most variation in length from cell to cell.

6.9 Cell Death Due to Irradiations (Answers)

9. B Cells are most radiosensitive in the M and G2 phases. These are the phases where the cell is actively dividing or preparing to divide. Radiation damage at this point is usually fatal to the cell.

10. D Cells are most radioresistant in S phase. This is thought to be related to the ability of the cell to repair DNA damage once replication is complete.

11. B The biological effects of radiation result mainly from damage to the DNA, which is the most critical target within the cell. The DNA contains all genetic information that allows the cell to proliferate. If the DNA is damaged, the cell usually dies while trying to divide or mutates, potentially into a malignant cancer. There are also other sites in the cell that, when damaged, may lead to cell death as well.

12. C When directly ionizing radiation is absorbed in biological material, the damage to the cell may occur by direct or indirect action. Direct action refers to excitation and damage of the atoms inside the DNA by the incoming radiation, whereas indirect action refers to DNA damage inflicted by free radicals (molecules with an unpaired electron formed by the incoming radiation) which are extremely reactive.

13. B In indirect action, the radiation interacts with other molecules (usually H_2O) and atoms within the cell to produce free radicals, which damage the DNA within the cell. In direct action, the radiation interacts directly with the critical target in the cell.

6.9 Cell Death Due to Irradiations (Answers)

Quiz-1 (Level 2)

1. B Direct action is the dominant process in the interaction of high-LET particles. High LET means that the particle is depositing a lot of energy over a short distance (densely ionizing). High-LET particles are energetic neutrons, protons, and heavy charged particles. About two thirds of the biological damage from low-LET radiations like x-rays or electrons is due to indirect action.

2. B The correct sequence in producing biological damage by the indirect action is first there is a primary photon interaction (photoelectric effect, Compton effect, or pair production) which produces high-energy electrons. These electrons in turn produce free radicals in water which cause damage in DNA. The damage in DNA might result in a biological effect.

3. **E** Irradiation of a cell can result in nine possible outcomes: no effect, division delay, apoptosis, reproductive failure, genomic instability, mutation, transformation, bystander effects, or adaptive responses. These will be addressed in the following questions.

4. **C** Irradiation of a cell can result in apoptosis which means the cell dies before it can divide. Apoptosis is an important cellular process because it prevents a cell from dividing if it is damaged. The cell realizes it is damaged and undergoes a programmed death rather than risk a mutation. Apoptosis does not always occur when a cell is damaged. Division delay is a process by which the cell pauses before going through mitosis. It is another means of preventing mutation. The delay gives the cell time to repair the damage before dividing during mitosis. If the cell cannot repair itself or does not undergo apoptosis, reproductive failure might occur if the cell attempts mitosis but it is damaged beyond repair. If the cell loses any genetic information through DNA damage, this is referred to as genomic instability.

5. Match the term with its corresponding definition.
   - **A.** II. Apoptosis: Programmed death of a cell following irradiation to prevent mutation or genomic instability.
   - **B.** IV. Division delay: The cell is delayed from going through division to allow for repair of damage.
   - **C.** I. Reproductive failure: The cell dies when attempting the first or subsequent mitosis.
   - **D.** III. Genomic instability: Delayed form of reproductive failure as a result of induced genomic instability.
   - **E.** VII. Mutation: The cell survives but reproduced incorrectly.
   - **F.** V. Transformation: The cell survives but the mutation leads to a transformed phenotype and possibly carcinogenesis.
   - **G.** VIII. Bystander effect: An irradiated cell can send signals to neighboring unirradiated cells and induce biological effects.
   - **H.** VI. Adaptive responses: The irradiated cell is stimulated to react and become more resistant to subsequent irradiation.

6. **E** There is no threshold dose for a double-strand break to occur. Double-strand breaks are more common with high-LET radiation or very high dose rates that create many direct and indirect actions in close proximity to each other.

7. **D** Alpha particles only have a range of a few millimeters in tissue due to their relatively large size and mass. Remember that an alpha particle is a helium molecule. Beta particles, or electrons, have a range of several centimeters in tissue as their mass is much smaller than an alpha particle. Gamma rays are indirectly ionizing and experience exponential attenuation rather than the continuous slowing down of charged particles. Therefore, gamma rays have the highest penetration power.

8. B Electromagnetic radiation is classified by wavelength into radio, microwave, infrared, visible light, ultraviolet light, x-ray, and gamma rays. All of these exhibit both wave- and particle-like behaviors as they travel through space. By definition, photons have neither a charge nor mass.

6.10 Normal Tissue Complication (NTC) (Answers)

Quiz-1 (Level 2)

1. E All are correct. Ionizing radiation has been proven to cause leukemia, and it had been implicated in the development of many other cancers in tissues such as the bone, lung, skin, thyroid, and breast.

2. A In addition to carcinogenesis, late effects of radiation include delayed tissue reactions such as fibrosis, life span shortening, genetic damage, and potential effects to the fetus. Hair loss is an early effect of radiation, not a late effect.

3. B When lethal damage is produced in mammalian cells, the damage is irreversible and irreparable and leads to cell death. If sublethal damage occurs, cells can be repaired in hours unless additional sublethal damage is added that eventually leads to lethal damage. Potentially lethal damage can be manipulated by repair when cells are allowed to remain in a nondividing state. Somatic effects are not considered radiation damage to mammalian cells but an effect of radiation on the human population.

4. A Somatic effects are effects that are a result of DNA damage from radiation exposure. Examples of possible effects are carcinogenesis, sterility, opacification of the eye lens, and life shortening. Radiation-induced mutations to an individual's DNA that can contribute to the birth of defective descendants are genetic or hereditary effects. Two other types of effects are deterministic and stochastic radiation effects. A stochastic effect is an effect in which the probability of occurrence increases with increasing dose but the severity in affected individuals does not depend on the dose. Cancer is an example of a stochastic effect as an individual can develop cancer with an exposure of any dose although the probability of developing cancer increases with increasing dose. Additionally, cancer is bad if it is one cell or one million cells. On the other hand, a deterministic effect is one that increases in severity with increasing dose, usually above a threshold dose. An example is a cataract which only develops above a dose of around 10 Gy and the severity increases as the dose increases. This means that a cataract from 20 Gy will be more severe than a cataract from 10 Gy.

5. B Stochastic effects are ones in which the probability of occurrence increases with increasing dose but the severity in the affected individuals does not depend on the dose. There is no threshold dose for the effects that are truly stochastic, and it is assumed that there is always some small probability of the event occurring even at very small doses. For example, cancer from 1 Gy is just as bad a cancer from 100 Gy.

6. A Acute effects manifest themselves soon after exposure to radiation and are characterized by inflammation, edema, desquamation of epithelia and hemopoietic tissue, and hemorrhage. Late effects are delayed and are characterized by fibrosis, atrophy, ulceration, stenosis, or obstruction of the intestine (to name a few).

7. C Acute total-body exposure can cause different syndromes depending on the actual total-body dose above 1 Gy.

1 Gy < dose < 10 Gy: Bone marrow (hematopoietic) syndrome. The quickly dividing red and white blood cells are destroyed. Death can result from infection weeks after the exposure. If the individual is provided hospital care, survival probability is improved. There is a window between 8 and 10 Gy where a bone marrow transplant might help the individual to recover.

10 Gy < dose < 100 Gy: Gastrointestinal syndrome. No human has ever survived a total-body dose of more than 10 Gy. This dose destroys the cells in the lining of the intestines. The individual experiences vomiting, bloody diarrhea, and death within several days.

Dose > 100 Gy: Central nervous system syndrome. At doses this high, death will result within a day or two. It is thought that death results from blood leaking from damaged capillaries in the brain but there have been very few exposures to this dose level.

8. D The proper order of fetal stages of development from conception to birth is preimplantation, organogenesis, and growth stage. If there is an exposure in this period of development, the possible effects will be very different and the threshold for the effects is different.

9. B Fetus stages of development from conception to birth:

Preimplantation (day 1 to day 10). Any exposure during this period usually results in death as there are very few cells and they are dividing quickly.

Organogenesis (day 11 to day 42). Exposure during this period can lead to temporary growth retardation or anatomic malformations.

Growth stage (day 43 to birth). Exposure during this period can lead to mental retardation and small head circumference. The severity is proportional to the exposure. There are also studies that link exposure during this period to latent cancer although these studies have controversial findings.

10. C The effects produced on the fetus due to radiation depend on the dose delivered and the stage of development at the time of exposure.

11. E All are correct. The principal effects of radiation on a fetus are neonatal death, malformations, growth retardation, congenital defects, and cancer induction. Again, the probability of these occurrences depends on the delivered dose and the stage of the fetal development.

12. B An abortion to avoid the possibility of radiation-induced congenital abnormalities should be considered only if fetal total dose exceeded 10 cGy. Even then, this is a decision that must be discussed between the parents and the doctors.

13. B The aim of radiotherapy is to deliver enough radiation to the tumor to destroy it without irradiating normal tissue to a dose that will lead to serious complications (morbidity).

14. D When talking about early and late reactions, one is referring to the α/β ratio, or the dose on a cell survival curve where the linear and quadratic components of cell killing are equal. For early-responding tissues such as tumor cells, the α/β ratio is high, usually accepted to be about 10 Gy. For late-responding tissues like normal tissue, the α/β ratio is much lower, accepted to be about 3 Gy. Late-responding tissues benefit from fractionating the dose because they have much better repair mechanisms than early-responding tissues. By taking advantages of differences in the α/β ratio, multi-fraction treatments spare late-responding tissues while killing early-responding tissues.

15. B For the same radiation dose, radiation delivered at a lower dose rate may produce less cell killing than radiation delivered at a higher dose rate because sublethal damage repair occurs during the protracted exposure. As the dose rate is reduced, the slope of the survival curve becomes shallower and the shoulder (initial region of the cell survival curve that is flatter) tends to disappear. Fractionating radiation treatments over a period of weeks rather than in a single session results in a better therapeutic ratio; however, to achieve the desired level of biological damage, the total dose in a fractionated treatment must be much larger than that in a single treatment.

16. D The four Rs of radiotherapy include repair, repopulation, redistribution, and reoxygenation.
    Repair – repair of sublethal damage in the cell.
    Repopulation – time to allow for the cell to divide and proliferate.
    Redistribution – the cell cycle has phases where the cell is radiosensitive and other times where it is radioresistant. In addition, there might be blocks that prevent the cell from progressing into a radiosensitive phase due to

previous irradiation. Redistribution refers to the cells distributing throughout all phases of the cell cycle over time.

Reoxygenation – when the oxygen content is high, radiation damage to DNA can become permanent if oxygen is present to bond with the damaged area. Reoxygenation refers to oxygen entering a region of a tumor that was previously hypoxic or necrotic. The presence of oxygen makes the cells more radiosensitive.

17. E   All statements are correct.

18. B   Radioprotectors are chemical agents that reduce cell response to radiation. A common radioprotector are sulfhydryl compounds, or compounds with sulfur and hydrogen. They work by helping to remove free radicals that would otherwise damage DNA, and they can also donate hydrogen atoms to help with sublethal DNA repair. Radiosensitizer are chemical agents that enhance cell response to radiation. Chemo therapy uses systemic antineoplastic drugs to kill or destroy cancer cells.

19. E   All are correct. Radioprotectors must be present during the irradiation, so they must be given within 30 min of the exposure.

20. B   Normal tissue tolerance dose (NTTD) is most dependent on the number and size of fractions than the overall duration between the first and last fraction. This is because normal tissues are late-responding tissues with a low α/β ratio. A low α/β ratio means the tissue has a larger shoulder and benefits from receiving many small doses rather than a single large dose to allow the repair mechanisms to function.

21. A   The response of a tissue or organ to radiation depends on the sensitivity of the individual cells because highly differentiated (or mature) cells performing specialized functions are very resistant to radiation because they do not undergo further mitosis. The structure of a tissue or organ is very important as well because if one part of a tissue is dependent on another part, it will be more sensitive to radiation because killing one section would cause damage to another even if that section was not irradiated. If each part in a tissue can function independently, it will be much more radioresistant as a whole. A serial tissue is one where one section is dependent on another section (spinal cord), and a parallel tissue is one where each section functions independently (liver).

22. A $TD_{5/5}$ refers to the minimum tolerance dose that causes a 5 % complication rate within 5 years of radiation completion. Another term, the $TD_{50/5}$, refers to the minimum tolerance dose that causes a 50 % complication rate within 5 years of radiation completion.

6.10 Normal Tissue Complication (NTC) (Answers)

23. **A.** II. TD$_{5/5}$ 30 Gy: Liver (acute and chronic hepatitis)
B. III. TD$_{5/5}$ 50 Gy: Stomach (perforation, ulcer, hemorrhage)
C. I. TD$_{5/5}$ 45 Gy: Brain (infarction, necrosis)
D. IV. TD$_{5/5}$ 50 Gy: Kidney (acute and chronic nephrosclerosis)

24. **A.** III. TD50/5 80 Gy: Bladder (contracture)
B. I. TD$_{50/5}$ 18 Gy: Lens (cataract)
C. IV. TD$_{50/5}$ 24.5 Gy: Lung (acute and chronic pneumonitis)
D. II. TD$_{50/5}$ 80 Gy: Rectum (ulcer, stenosis, fistula)

25. **A.** III. TD$_{5/5}$ 2–3 Gy; TD$_{50/5}$ 6–12 Gy: Ovaries (sterilization)
B. I. Stricture TD$_{5/5}$ 70 Gy; TD$_{50/5}$ 100 Gy: Ureters
C. IV. TD$_{5/5}$ 60 Gy; TD$_{50/5}$ 75 Gy: Oral cavity and pharynx (ulceration, mucositis)
D. TD$_{5/5}$ 40 Gy; TD$_{50/5}$ 55 Gy: Whole Intestine (obstruction, perforation, fistula)

26. **A** The law of Bergonie and Tribondeau states that the radiosensitivity of a cell is directly proportional to its reproductive activity and inversely proportional to its degree of differentiation. Therefore, radiosensitivity is dependent on both mitotic activity and level of differentiation.

27. **E** All are correct. As a cell becomes more differentiated and specialized, it tends to undergo less mitosis and becomes less active and therefore is more radioresistant.

28. **B** Bergonie and Tribondeau state that undifferentiated cells or immature cells that divide and replace other cells are radiosensitive while differentiated cells or mature cells that do not divide as they specialize in performing specific functions are radioresistant.

29. Cell type with its radiosensitivity:
A. II. Extremely radiosensitive cell: vegetative intermitotic cells (VIM)
B. I. Radiosensitive cell: differentiating intermitotic cells (DIM)
C. III. Radioresistant cell: reverting postmitotic cells (RPM)
D. IV. Highly radioresistant cell: fixed postmitotic cells (FPM)

30. **A** The liver, muscle, and nerves are composed of RPM or FPM cells making them radioresistant. Bone marrow contains VIM cells making it highly radiosensitive.

31. **E** All are correct. Deoxyribonucleic acid (DNA) is a double helix with two strands composed of phosphate and sugar groups that are held together by hydrogen bonds like rungs on a ladder.

32. B The four bases attached to the backbone of DNA are pyrimidines (thymine and cytosine) and purines (adenine and guanine). Thymine always pairs with adenine (A-T), and cytosine always pairs with guanine (G-C). The specific order of these base pairs defines the human genetic code. The benefit of this pairing means that if only one of the strands is broken (single-strand break), the DNA can be repaired because the opposite base is known. More serious damage is a double-strand break because this is much more difficult for the cell to repair.

33. D The pairing is *always* A-T and G-C.

34. E Mitosis is divided into four phases: prophase, metaphase, anaphase, and telophase. The following question addresses each phase.

35. A. II. Prophase: Thickening of the chromatin as the chromosomes condense into light coils. The chromosomes reach maximal condensation and the nuclear membrane disappears.
    B. IV. Metaphase: Chromosomes move to the center of the cell, the spindle forms, and centromeres divide.
    C. I. Anaphase: Movement of chromosomes on the spindle to the opposite poles of the cell.
    D. III. Telophase: Chromosomes begin to uncoil and the nuclear membrane reappears.

36. A Prodromal radiation syndrome is defined as signs and symptoms that occur in the first 48 h following irradiation of the central nervous system. A dose of ionizing radiation sufficient to cause death is called a lethal dose, and the latency period is the time between an injury occurring and the effects of the injury expressing themselves as disease.

37. C Hematopoietic syndrome (2.5–10 Gy exposure) death occurs several weeks to two months after exposure, if at all. Remember, this syndrome is due to the depletion of the quickly dividing blood cells, and if death is to occur, it usually is a result of an infection. With proper medical care and perhaps a bone marrow transplant (8–10 Gy exposure), death might be avoided. No one has ever survived a total-body exposure >10 Gy. Above 100 Gy, the cerebrovascular syndrome results in death within 24–48 h after exposure, and with total-body exposures of >10 Gy, the gastrointestinal syndrome results in death usually between 3 and 10 days.

38. D The gastrointestinal syndrome is associated with extensive bloody diarrhea and destruction of the GI mucosa, nausea, vomiting and loss of appetite, dehydration, weight loss, emaciation, complete exhaustion, and finally

death. The cerebrovascular syndrome is associated with neurologic and cardiovascular breakdown, severe nausea and vomiting within minutes, disorientation and loss of coordination, respiratory distress, diarrhea, convulsive seizures, coma, and finally death. The hematopoietic syndrome is associated with lack of circulating blood elements, nausea and vomiting, a latent period, fatigue, petechial hemorrhages in the skin, and ulceration of the mouth.

39. B Mean lethal dose (D_{50}) is the lethal dose that causes mortality in 50 % of the exposed population or group within a specific period of time. The accepted dose for the D_{50} is between 3 and 4 Gy without medical attention. The D_{50} can be raised if medical attention is provided to prevent infection or a bone marrow transplant is completed for a dose between 8 and 10 Gy. The $D_{50/30}$ is the lethal dose that causes mortality in 50 % of the exposed population or group in 30 days, and the $D_{50/60}$ is the lethal dose that causes death in 50 % of the exposed population or group in 60 days.

40. A The correct order of tissues from radiosensitive to radioresistant is testes ($TD_{5/5}$, 1 Gy; $TD_{50/5}$, 2 Gy), ovaries ($TD_{5/5}$, 2–3 Gy; $TD_{50/5}$, 6–12 Gy), lens ($TD_{5/5}$, 10 Gy; $TD_{50/5}$, 18 Gy), lung ($TD_{5/5}$, 17.5 Gy; $TD_{50/5}$, 24.5 Gy), liver ($TD_{5/5}$, 30 Gy; $TD_{50/5}$, 40 Gy), and brain ($TD_{5/5}$, 45 Gy; $TD_{50/5}$, 60 Gy).

41. C X-rays and gamma (γ) particles are forms of electromagnetic radiation. They do not differ in nature or in properties but only in how they are produced. X-rays are produced outside the nucleus (extra-nuclearly) and gamma (γ) particles originate in the nucleus. Other examples of electromagnetic radiation are radio waves, microwaves, visible light, and ultraviolet light. Other types of ionizing radiation that occur in nature are electrons, neutrons, negative π-mesons, and heavy charged ions.

42. D Radio waves, microwaves, infrared radiation, visible light, ultraviolet light, x-rays, and gamma (γ) particles are all forms of electromagnetic radiation having the same velocity (c = the speed of light). Each of these has a range of wavelengths and frequencies that are related by $c = \lambda \nu$.

43. E All statements are correct.

44. C If a cell is irradiated and has a double-strand DNA break opposite to one another, usually the cell dies, mutates, or undergoes carcinogenesis because it cannot repair. If a DNA double-strand break takes place but is well separated, the cell usually can repair rapidly because each break is handled individually using the opposite strand as a template. The same is usually true if a single-strand DNA break occurs.

6.11 Cell Survival Curves and Models (Answers)

Quiz-1 (Level 2)

1. **A** The cell survival curve describes the relationship between the surviving fraction of cells (the fraction of irradiated cells that maintain their reproductive integrity) and the absorbed dose. A dose response curve is a plot of a biological effect against absorbed dose.

2. **A** The cell survival curve following the multi-target model is composed of the extrapolation number which measured the width of the shoulder, the initial and final slopes, and the quasithreshold dose which is another method of measuring the width of the shoulder. The practical range is the maximum depth of penetration by electrons.

3. **E** All are correct.

4. **C** Hyperfractionation uses more than one fraction per day with a smaller dose per fraction (<1.8 Gy). Standard fractionation is based on five daily treatments per week and a total treatment time of several weeks. Accelerated fractionation reduces the overall treatment time by half while the same total dose is delivered, and CHART (continuous hyperfractionated accelerated radiation therapy) was an experimental program that used three fractions per day for 12 continuous days.

5. **A** I, II, and III are correct. Nerve, muscle, and secretory cells are considered differentiated and do not proliferate. On the other hand, stem and intestinal epithelium cells are considered proliferating cells.

6. **A** The n symbol in the cell survival curve represents extrapolation number (n) which is a measure of the width of the shoulder.

7. **E** All are correct.

8. **B** D_0 represents a cell survival of 37 %, or it is the dose required to reduce the fraction of surviving cells to 37 %. It also represents the cell's radiosensitivity. Remember that the cell's ability to accumulate sublethal damage is defined by the quasithreshold dose (D_0).

9. Multi-target model:
    A. II. Extrapolation number (n)
    B. I. Dose (D_0)
    C. III. Quasithreshold dose (D_Q)

6.11 Cell Survival Curves and Models (Answers)

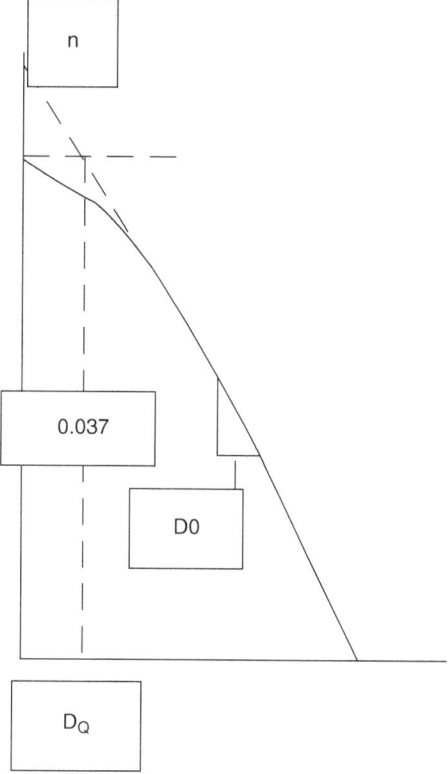

Fig. 6A.4.1

10. D The correct formula used to represent the three parameters of the survival curve is $\log_e n = D_Q/D_0$. The survival fraction is calculated by $SF = 1 - (1 - e^{-D/D_0})^n$. If a single-target model is assumed, single-hit target survival is found by
$N(D) = N_0 \times e^{-D/D_0}$, where N represents the initial number of cells. If a multi-target model is assumed, single-hit survival can be found by
$N(D) = N_0 [1 - (1 - e^{-D/D_0})^n]$ where N represents the number of targets.

11. B Linear-quadratic model is the model of choice to describe survival curves. It assumes that a cell can be killed by a single lethal event (proportional to the dose) or accumulation of sublethal events (proportional to the square of the dose). This is the model used to determine α/β ratios.

6.12 BED and Fractionations (Answers)

Quiz-1 (Level 2)

1. **C** To kill a cell population, at least 90 % of the cells need to be destroyed. This is referred to as the D_{10}, or a 10 % surviving fractions.

2. **B** D_0 is the dose required to reduce the surviving fraction to 37 %.

3. **C** The total dose required to kill 90 % of the tumor population is 11.5 Gy.
   $D_{10} = ?$
   $D_0 = 5$ Gy
   $D_{10} = 2.3 \times 5$
   $D_{10} = 11.5$ Gy

4. **A** Lethal damage is irreversible and irreparable and leads to cell death. Sublethal damage under normal circumstances can be repaired in hours unless additional sublethal damage is added. Potentially lethal damage can be modified by postirradiation environmental conditions.

5. **A** The ratio α/β is the dose at which linear and quadratic components of cell killing are equal and is another measure of the shoulder of the cell survival curve in the linear-quadratic model.

6. **E** All the statements are correct. A downside to hyperfractionation is that it is not convenient for patients and it is also expensive as each treatment costs money.

7. **E** All statements are true. If fewer and larger dose fractions are given, late reactions are more severe, and for early effects, α/β is large (8–10) and for late effects, α/β is small (2–4). Finally, late-effect tissues are more sensitive to changes in fractionation patterns than are early-responding tissues.

8. **A** They estimate the sensitivity of the tumor or normal tissue to fractionation.
   The decay process of radioactive materials describes how a radioactive element moves toward stability, and the effective dose equivalent is determined by adding the dose equivalents to various organs using weighting factors.

9. **A** The intent of an accelerated treatment strategy is to reduce repopulation in rapidly proliferating tumors. Hyperfractionated treatments are based on

separating early and late effects, and continuous hyperfractionated accelerated radiation (CHART) is designed to deliver low dose per fraction to minimize late effects with a very short overall treatment time to minimize tumor proliferation.

10. D The time interval between multiple daily fractions should be longer than 6 h because the repair of sublethal damage in late-responding tissues is slow. RTOG studies indicate that the incidence of late effects is worse for interfraction intervals less than 4 h compared with interfraction intervals longer than 6 h.

11. B The equation used to calculate the quantity by which different fractionation regimens are intercompared is $E/\alpha = nd \times (1+[d/\alpha/\beta])$, where the $\underline{n}$ = number of fractions, d = dose per fraction, and α/β = alpha/beta ratio. $SF = 1 - (1 - e^{-D/D_0})^n$ is the formula to calculate the survival fraction, $D_{10} = 2.3 \times D_0$ is the formula used to calculate the dose required to kill 90 % of the population, and $Log_e n = D_Q/D_0$ is the formula used to represent the three parameters of the survival curve in the multi-target model.

12. C The biological effect dose for a conventional treatment: early effects = 63.72 Gy_{10} and late effects = 86.4 Gy_3. For the hyperfractionated treatment: early effects = 96.8 Gy_{10} and late effects = 121 Gy_3.

Collect the Data:
α/β = 3 Gy for late-responding tissues and 10 Gy for early-responding tissues
Conventional
Total dose (nd) = 54 Gy
$E/\alpha = nd \times (1+[d/\alpha/\beta])$
$E/\alpha = 54 \times (1+[1.8/10])$ Early responding
$E/\alpha = 63.72$ Gy_{10}
$E/\alpha = 54 \times (1+[1.8/3])$ Late responding
$E/\alpha = 86.4$ Gy_3
Hyperfractionation
Total dose (nd) = 84 Gy
$E/\alpha = nd \times (1+[d/\alpha/\beta])$
$E/\alpha = 86.4 \times (1+[1.2/10])$ Early responding
$E/\alpha = 96.8$ Gy_{10}
$E/\alpha = 86.4 \times (1+[1.2/3])$ Late responding
$E/\alpha = 121$ Gy_3

6.13 Oxygen Enhancement and Hyperthermia Treatments (Answers)

Quiz-1 (Level 2)

1. **A** The oxygen enhancement ratio DECREASES as the LET increases.

2. **C** Oxygen enhancement ratio (OER) is defined as the ratio of doses without and with oxygen (hypoxic versus well-oxygenated cells) to produce the same biological effect. The process by which cells that are hypoxic become oxygenated after irradiation, through the killing and removal of toxic radiosensitive cells from the tumor, is called reoxygenation. The relationship between the surviving fraction of cells and the absorbed dose is the definition of the cell survival curves. The ratio of dose to produce an effect with radioprotector to dose to produce the same effect without radioprotector is the dose-modifying factor (DMF).

3. **C** OER = dose under hypoxic condition / under oxygenated condition
   OER = 150/70
   OER = 2.14

4. **A.** III. X-rays and γ-rays (2–3.5 OER)
   B. I. Neutrons (1.5 OER)
   C. II. High-LET radiations (α particle) (1 OER)

5. **C** Oxygen is an effective radiosensitizer and hypoxic cells are radioresistant.

6. **B** The center of tumors cells is consider to be hypoxic and necrotic as there is no vasculature to carry oxygen to the core of the tumor. The exterior of the tumor is considered to be oxygenated and more radiosensitive. During fractionated treatments, the more radiosensitive exterior of the tumor is destroyed allowing for the vasculature to reoxygenate the hypoxic core of the tumor.

7. **D** Hydroxyurea is a powerful chemotherapy agent used to coordinate cells in a phase of the cycle that is more sensitive to radiation (M and G2). Methotrexate is used to block radiation damage repair, fludarabine slows the normal cycle of the cell, and cis-platinum kills cells resistant to radiotherapy.

8. **A** Hyperthermia is a method used to kill tumor cells by heating them up with focused ultrasound or electromagnetic waves. It inhibits the repair to radiation damage, increases blood flow to normal tissues, and damages tumor cell blood vessels.

9. **E** Disadvantages of hyperthermia include thermotolerance or resistance of the cell to a second or third heating, difficulty to keep an area at a constant temperature, difficulty achieving distribution of the heat, and differences in the way that different body tissues respond to heat. Also, monitoring the temperature at the site being treated is difficult.

10. **E** All are correct.

11. **A** Hyperthermia uses microwaves, radio waves, or ultrasound waves to heat the treatment area to kill cancer cells. This can be done internally on the patient using a thin needle or probe into the tumor or externally using a machine that produces high-energy waves to aim the tumor near the surface.

6.14 Summary (Answers)

Quiz-1 (Level 3)

1. **B** When a cell attempts to repair a double-strand break, it is possible that incorrect strands could be connected. This might cause gene mutations because different segments of DNA may be attached.

2. **A** Hyperfractionated treatment is still the standard of care in radiation therapy where the daily doses are between 1.5 and 3 Gy. There is a recent trend that is pushing more toward hypofractionated treatments for patient convenience and to reduce costs. Additionally, new technology has improved the accuracy of dose delivery.

3. **A** In the early time of RT, the impacts of normal tissue complications were not clearly understood; thus hypofractionation was used.

4. **B** Normal tissue complication creates a dilemma in radiotherapy as lower doses cannot kill the disease but using higher doses can cause normal tissue complications.

5. **B** BED calculated with the LQ model can only be applied for the "shoulder" part of the cell survival curve. The LQ model fails in the high-dose region of the curve.

6. **A** So far no radiobiological explanation is available for the late effects of NTC.

7. **C** Ribosomes synthesize proteins in cells.

8. **C** The dose from an x-ray radiograph for the chest is around 10 mrem. According to the NRC, Americans receive a radiation dose of approximately 620 mrem per year. So the dose from an x-ray radiograph for the chest is equivalent to $365 \times (10/620) = 6$ (days).

9. **C** The margin for SRS is quite small and sometimes is zero. Since the margin is so small, the normal tissue complication can be reduced. One area of current research is the dose limits to critical structures during SRS. The current method uses much lower tolerance limits than conventional fractionation knowing that the normal tissues do not have a chance to repair damage between fractions.

10. **D** SBRT uses the high-dose region of the cell survival curve, so the BED method may be used, but very carefully as the LQ model fails in the high-dose region.

Radiation Safety

Contents

7.1	Maximum Permissible Dose Equivalent (Questions)	450
7.2	Time, Distance, and Shielding (Questions)	457
7.3	Brachytherapy Source Handling and Storage (Questions)	459
7.4	Dose Survey and Exposure Monitoring (Questions)	469
7.5	Nuclear Medicine Procedures (Questions)	474
7.6	Structural Shielding Design (Questions)	476
7.7	Radioactive Material Shipping (Questions)	481
7.8	Summary (Questions)	483
7.9	Maximum Permissible Dose Equivalent (Answers)	488
7.10	Time, Distance, and Shielding (Answers)	493
7.11	Brachytherapy Source Handling and Storage (Answers)	494
7.12	Dose Survey and Exposure Monitoring (Answers)	500
7.13	Nuclear Medicine Procedures (Answers)	504
7.14	Structural Shielding Design (Answers)	506
7.15	Radioactive Material Shipping (Answers)	509
7.16	Summary (Answers)	510

Like radiotherapy, radiation safety is also based on radiobiology but focuses more on the practical application of radiobiology in any environment with radioactive material. Any medical center or institution that uses radioactive material will have a radiation safety program led by a radiation safety officer (RSO).

CMD or ABR candidates need to remember a lot of detailed information about radiation safety but learning this information can help to keep you safe. Much of radiation safety is common sense, but the more you know about the rules and regulations, the less you are at risk of having an accident happen.

7.1 Maximum Permissible Dose Equivalent (Questions)

Quiz 1 (Level 2)

1. The biological effects of radiation depend on:
   A. I, II, and III.
   B. I and III only.
   C. II and IV only.
   D. IV only.
   E. All are correct.
   I. Organ
   II. Dose received
   III. Tissue
   IV. Type of radiation received

2. Which of the following is the dose equivalent formula?
   A. $H = D \times Q$
   B. $H1/H2 = d2^2/d1^2$
   C. $X = \Gamma \times A \times t/d^2$
   D. $H = D/Q$

3. What is the SI unit for both dose and dose equivalent?
   A. Becquerel (Bq)
   B. Joules per kilogram
   C. Rem
   D. Gray

4. What does the quality factor used to calculate dose equivalent depend on?
   A. I, II, and III.
   B. I and III only.
   C. II and IV only.
   D. IV only.
   E. All are correct.
   I. Organ
   II. Tissue
   III. Biologic endpoint under consideration
   IV. Type of radiation

5. Match the following radiation type with its quality factor:
   A. X-ray, γ-rays, and electrons
   B. Thermal neutrons
   C. Neutrons and heavy particles (α)
   I. Q = 5
   II. Q = 20
   III. Q = 1

7.1 Maximum Permissible Dose Equivalent (Questions)

6. The effective dose equivalent is defined as:
A. The energy absorbed from an ionizing radiation beam per unit mass of absorber
B. The sum of the weighted dose equivalents for irradiated tissues or organs
C. The dose modified by quality or weighting factor
D. A graph of dose distribution produced by passing a dosimeter across the beam

7. Which of the following organization is a US group of radiation experts who make recommendations in the area of ionization radiation and develop standards for the use of radiation in this country?
A. International Commission on Radiological Protection (ICRP)
B. US Nuclear Regulatory Commission (USNRC)
C. National Council on Radiation Protection and Measurements (NCRP)
D. Individual states

8. What is an "agreement state"?
A. A state that has entered into an agreement with the USNRC in which they assume responsibility for enforcing the regulations specific to the by-product material as well as accelerator-produced nuclides
B. An independent group of experts from a wide range of disciplines who have a vested interest in the safe use of all types of radiation sources
C. The federal agency charged with the regulation of radioactive materials produced in nuclear reactors
D. A state that has entered into an agreement not to use radioactive material in excess so that radiation incidents are kept below average

9. Which of the following statements is *not* true?
A. The weighting factor represents the different risk of each tissue to mortality from cancer and hereditary effects in the first two generations.
B. The effective dose equivalent is the sum of the weighted dose equivalents for all irradiated tissues.
C. Different types of radiation (photons, neutrons, protons) have different biological effectiveness for equal absorbed doses.
D. Different types of radiation (photons, neutrons, protons) have equal biological effectiveness for equal absorbed doses.

10. What is the dose equivalent to a person who receives an average whole body dose of 150 mrem from thermal neutrons?
A. 30 mrem
B. 750 mrem
C. 145 mrem
D. 155 mrem

11. As per NCRP recommendations, what is the maximum accumulated dose a 50-year-old occupational worker can have?
A. I, II, and III.
B. I and III only.
C. II and IV only.
D. IV only.
E. All are correct.
I. 500 mSv
II. 10 mSv
III. 50 rem
IV. 1 mSv

12. A deterministic effect is defined as an effect in which:
A. The probability of occurrence of an effect is higher for higher doses, but the severity of the effect is independent of dose.
B. The severity of a particular effect in an exposed individual increases with dose above the threshold for the occurrence of the effect.
C. The specific dose equivalent an individual is permitted to receive annually from working with radiation on the job.
D. The probability of occurrence of the effect is the same for any dose received.

13. Determine if the following are deterministic or stochastic effects (answers can be used more than once):
A. Deterministic effect
B. Stochastic effects
I. Nausea
II. Reddening of the skin
III. Hereditary effects
IV. Leukemia
V. Congenital malformations of the embryo

14. Which of the following are considered background radiation?
A. I, II, and III.
B. I and III only.
C. II and IV only.
D. IV only.
E. All are correct.
I. Terrestrial radiation
II. Cosmic radiation
III. Radioactive elements in our bodies
IV. Medical procedures

15. Which of the following statements is *not* true?
A. Terrestrial radiation varies over the earth.
B. Cosmic radiation levels change with elevation.

7.1 Maximum Permissible Dose Equivalent (Questions)

C. The internal irradiation arises mainly from ^{40}K in our body.
D. Background radiation is contributed by terrestrial, cosmic, medical, and radioactive elements in our body.

16. Which of the following is the most common hazardous naturally occurring radioactive material?
A. Lead
B. Uranium
C. Radon
D. Thorium

17. Which of the following statements are true?
A. I, II, and III.
B. I and III only.
C. II and IV only.
D. IV only.
E. All are correct.
I. Large doses of radiation produce identifiable effects within a relatively short period.
II. Large doses of radiation produce identifiable effects within a relatively long period.
III. Low doses of radiation effects are difficult to ascertain due to low frequency with which these effects might occur.
IV. Low doses of radiation are easy to measure.

18. Exposures to low-level radiation may produce:
A. I, II, and III.
B. I and III only.
C. II and IV only.
D. IV only.
E. All are correct.
I. Genetic effects
II. Neoplastic diseases
III. Effects on growth and development
IV. Effects on life span and cataracts

19. The harmful effects of radiation may be classified into:
A. I, II, and III.
B. I and III only.
C. II and IV only.
D. IV only.
E. All are correct.
I. Stochastic effects
II. Occupational factor
III. Nonstochastic effects
IV. Use factor

20. A stochastic effect is defined as:
A. The probability of occurrence increases with increasing absorbed dose, but the severity in affected individuals does not depend on the magnitude of the absorbed dose.
B. The probability increases in severity with increasing absorbed dose in affected individuals.
C. The probability of occurrence decreases with increasing absorbed dose, but the severity in affected individuals does not depend on the magnitude of the absorbed dose.
D. The probability of occurrence increases with decreases in absorbed dose as well as severity in affected individuals.

21. Examples of nonstochastic effects are:
A. I, II, and III.
B. I and III only.
C. II and IV only.
D. IV only.
E. All are correct.
I. Organ atrophy
II. Fibrosis
III. Cataracts
IV. Blood changes

22. NCRP recommendations on exposure limits of radiation workers are based on:
A. I, II, and III.
B. I and III only.
C. II and IV only.
D. IV only.
E. All are correct.
I. At low radiation levels the nonstochastic effects are essentially avoided.
II. The predicted risk for stochastic effects should not be greater than the average risk of accidental death among workers in industries.
III. The ALARA principle should be followed.
IV. At any radiation level, all effects must be avoided.

23. Occupational and public dose limits include:
A. I, II, and III.
B. I and III only.
C. II and IV only.
D. IV only.
E. All are correct.
I. Exposure received from medical procedures
II. Exposure received by a worker pursuing his/her occupation
III. Natural background radiation
IV. Exposure received by a member of the public

7.1 Maximum Permissible Dose Equivalent (Questions)

24. The ALARA principle states:
A. Keep radiation exposure as low as reasonably achievable, considering the economic and social factors.
B. Maximum permissible levels should be kept low.
C. A level of average annual excess risk of fatal health effects can be attributed to irradiation.
D. Keep radiation exposure as low as reasonably achievable outside the work area.

25. Exposure incurred by patients as part of their own medical or dental diagnosis or treatment is the definition of?
A. Occupational exposure
B. Medical exposure
C. Public exposure
D. Volunteers' exposure

26. Which of the following are the main physical quantities used in safety standards?
A. I, II, and III.
B. I and III only.
C. II and IV only.
D. IV only.
E. All are correct.
I. Activity
II. Equivalent dose
III. Absorbed dose
IV. Effective dose

27. What is the definition of organ dose?
A. The sum of the weighted dose equivalents for all irradiated tissues
B. The mean dose in a specified tissue or organ of the human body
C. Total dose received throughout the period of time during which the radionuclide remains in the body
D. The summation of the product of the mean dose in the various groups of exposed people and the number of individuals in each group

28. How often should a personnel radiation monitoring device be changed?
A. Biweekly
B. Monthly
C. Biannually
D. Yearly

29. What is the yearly occupational maximum permissible dose (MPD) for the whole body?
A. 50 mSv or 5 rem/year
B. 1 mSv or 0.1 rem/year
C. 5 mSv or 0.5 rem/year
D. 500 mSv or 50 rem/year

30. The lifetime or cumulative occupational limit exposure is:
A. 10 mSv or 0.1 rem×age (years)
B. 5 mSv or 0.5 rem×age (years)
C. 10 mSv or 1 rem×age (years)
D. 1 mSv or 0.1 rem×age (years)

31. What is the annual occupational maximum permissible dose (MPD) for the lens of the eye?
A. 50 mSv or 5 rem
B. 15 mSv or 150 rem
C. 5 mSv or 0.5 rem
D. 150 mSv or 15 rem

32. What is the monthly maximum permissible dose (MPD) for a pregnant woman worker?
A. 0.01 mSv or 0.001 rem
B. 0.5 mSv or 0.05 rem
C. 5 mSv or 0.5 rem
D. 1 mSv or 15 rem

33. The occupational effective dose limit in any year based on the NCRP recommendations should not exceed:
A. 50 mSv (5 rem)
B. 5 mSv (0.5 rem)
C. 1 mSv (0.1 rem)
D. 10 mSv×age

34. The nonoccupational (public) effective dose to the extremities, skin, and lens in any year based on the NCRP recommendations should not exceed:
A. 500 mSv (50 rem)
B. 150 mSv (15 rem)
C. 50 mSv (5 rem)
D. 15 mSv (1.5 rem) education and training exposure lens

35. Which of the following statements are true?
A. I, II, and III.
B. I and III only.
C. II and IV only.
D. IV only.
E. All are correct.
I. Dose limits are subject to the concept of ALARA.
II. Since radiation is potentially harmful, exposure to it should be monitored continually and controlled.
III. Exposure of personnel and the public should be kept to a minimum.
IV. The reduction in exposure to personnel is considered reasonable based on the expense used to reduce the exposure.

36. Once a pregnancy is declared, the NCRP recommends a monthly limit to the embryo or fetus of:
A. 1 mSv (0.1 rem)
B. 0.5 mSv (0.05 rem)
C. 15 mSv (1.5 rem)
D. 0.1 mSv (0.01 rem)

7.2 Time, Distance, and Shielding (Questions)

Quiz 1 (Level 2)

1. Which of the following statements are true?
A. I, II, and III.
B. I and III only.
C. II and IV only.
D. IV only.
E. All are correct.
I. Maximizing the distance will reduce the dose to a greater degree than minimizing time for equal changes.
II. Radiation dose is proportional to time.
III. Dose is inversely related to the distance squared.
IV. Time, distance, and shielding are not considered in radiation protection.

2. Which of the following laws is used to calculate dose versus distance?
A. Equivalent square field
B. Direct square law
C. Inverse square law
D. Half-value layer

3. ALARA stands for:
A. As low as radiation association
B. At lower absolute radiation achievable
C. As low as reasonably achievable
D. As longer as radiation acquired

4. Which of the following is the best method to use for radiation protection?
A. Using the appropriate radiation monitor
B. Using the personnel monitoring device at all times on the collar
C. Using a lead apron around radioactive patients
D. Maximizing distance from the source

5. Radiation exposure to employees can be reduced by:
A. I, II, III, and IV.
B. I and III only.
C. II and IV only.
D. IV only.
E. All are correct.
I. Reducing the time around radioactive patients or procedures
II. Increasing distance from the source of radiation
III. Using appropriate shielding
IV. Using personnel monitoring devices (film badge)

6. Why is a long forceps used in handling LDR sources?
A. To increase time of exposure
B. To extend the distance from the source
C. To keep the source aseptic
D. To keep the hands clean

7. What actions are taken to reduce the exposure to the environment while shipping a radioactive source?
A. Use a shielded container.
B. Try to reduce the exposure time to the public while shipping.
C. Put exposure rate warning on package surface to reduce the distance to the public.
D. All of the above.

8. What is level 1 of ALARA?
A. 10 % of the exposure limit
B. 30 % of the exposure limit
C. 50 % of the exposure limit
D. 70 % of the exposure limit

9. What actions are normally taken to reach level 1 ALARA?
A. Reduce time
B. Increase shielding
C. Extend distance
D. All of the above

10. Which of the following items should a radiographer use for protection against scattered radiation?
A. Gloves
B. Lead apron
C. Thyroid shield
D. All of the above

7.3 Brachytherapy Source Handling and Storage (Questions)

Quiz 1 (Level 2)

1. Which of the following are considered safety systems on an HDR unit?
A. I, II, and III.
B. I and III only.
C. II and IV only.
D. IV only.
E. All are correct.
I. Interlocks prevent initiation of treatment if the door is open.
II. Backup batteries are provided to take over operation in case of power failure.
III. A manual source retraction mechanism is available to withdraw the source into the storage safe if it gets stuck.
IV. The treatment is aborted if the system detects blockage or excessive friction during source transit.

2. The shielding and safety requirements for the HDR room are mandated by:
A. International Commission on Radiation Protection (ICRP)
B. Nuclear Regulatory Commission (NRC)
C. National Council on Radiation Protection and Measurements (NCRP)
D. Committee on Biologic Effects of Ionizing Radiation (BEIR)

3. Which of the following safety features must be present on an HDR room to comply with NRC mandate?
A. I, II, and III.
B. I and III only.
C. II and IV only.
D. IV only.
E. All are correct.
I. Electrical interlock system
II. Inaccessibility of console keys to unauthorized persons
III. A permanent radiation monitor and continuous viewing and intercom systems
IV. Restricted area controls

4. Restricted area controls include:
A. I, II, and III.
B. I and III only.
C. II and IV only.
D. IV only.
E. All are correct.

I. Signs and door warning lights indicating "Radiation ON"
II. Locks
III. Visible/audible alarms
IV. Radiation safety officer present to avoid unauthorized personnel to be around the HDR unit

5. In order to be licensed for HDR according to NCR, the applicant requirements are:
A. I, II, and III.
B. I and III only.
C. II and IV only.
D. IV only.
E. All are correct.
I. Source description
II. Manufacturer's name and model of the HDR unit
III. Intended use and authorized users
IV. Quality assurance program

6. A high-dose rate (HDR) quality management program must include:
A. I, II, and III.
B. I and III only.
C. II and IV only.
D. IV only.
E. All are correct.
I. A written directive
II. Patient identification
III. Treatment plan verification
IV. Documentation

7. The identity of the patient must be verified by:
A. Asking the patient his/her name
B. Checking the patient's identification bracelet or hospital identification card
C. Two independent methods
D. Asking your coworker

8. HDR pretreatment safety checks must be performed:
A. Once a week
B. On any day that the HDR procedure is scheduled
C. Once a month
D. Before each patient's treatment

9. Prior to the initiation of HDR treatment, the authorized operator must verify:
A. I, II, and III.
B. I and III only.
C. II and IV only.
D. IV only.
E. All are correct.

7.3 Brachytherapy Source Handling and Storage (Questions)

I. Name of the patient under treatment
II. Dose to be delivered to a patient
III. Site of administration
IV. Times for each dwell location

10. Which of the following statement(s) is *not* true about the quality management program for HDR?
A. Immediately after each treatment, a survey of the afterloading device and the patient must be performed.
B. Calibration of the source must be performed by an authorized physicist before the first patient treatment.
C. Records for each treatment along with a completed checklist will be maintained in an auditable form for a minimum of 3 years.
D. During all patient treatments, both the authorized physician user and the authorized medical physicist must be in any satellite clinic to be called if needed.

11. Brachytherapy cases will be reviewed by an authorized physician and/or physicist at intervals:
A. No greater than 24 months
B. No greater than 12 months
C. Of 3 years
D. No greater than 2 weeks

12. If a recordable event or misadministration is uncovered during the periodic review:
A. The HDR unit will be locked in the off position and not used until further notice.
B. All personnel involved in the treatment are liable.
C. The number of cases to be reviewed will be expanded to include all cases for that calendar year.
D. One recordable event or misadministration is not of great concern.

13. Which of the following statements is true about the quality management program review for an HDR machine?
A. I, II, and III.
B. I and III only.
C. II and IV only.
D. IV only.
E. All are correct.
I. The quality management program will be reviewed on an annual basis.
II. A written summary of the review must be submitted to the RSO and the radiation safety committee.
III. Any modification made to the program must be reported to the NRC regional office or state if governed by an agreement state within 30 days after modification has been made.
IV. The quality management program will be reviewed every 2 years if the committee had more than 10 HDR units to review.

14. Immediately after each use of the HDR device, the physicist will ensure the source has been returned to the full-shielded position by:
A. Survey of the device only
B. Survey of the connectors only
C. Survey of the afterloader and the patient
D. Survey of the HDR room door

15. Full calibration measurements of a teletherapy unit must be done:
A. I, II, and III.
B. I and III only.
C. II and IV only.
D. IV only.
E. All are correct.
I. Before the first medical use of the unit
II. If the spot check measurements indicate that the output differs more than 5 % from the output obtained at the last full calibration
III. Following replacement of source or relocation of the unit
IV. Following repair of the unit

16. Periodic spot checks for teletherapy units must be done:
A. Once a year
B. Once in each calendar month
C. Every 2 years
D. Every 5 years

17. Radiation surveys for teletherapy units must be done:
A. I, II, and III.
B. I and III only.
C. II and IV only.
D. IV only.
E. All are correct.
I. Before medical use
II. After each installation of a teletherapy source
III. After making any change for which an amendment is required
IV. When the room is built, before placement of the teletherapy machine

18. What is the leakage limit from the source head with the beam in the off position?
A. 2 mrem/h on average and 10 mrem/h maximum at a distance of 1 m from the source
B. 4 mrem/h on average and 20 mrem/h maximum at a distance of 1 m from the source
C. 2 mrem/h on average and 10 mrem/h maximum at a distance of 5 m from the source
D. 4 mrem/h on average and 10 mrem/h maximum at a distance of 1 m from the source

7.3 Brachytherapy Source Handling and Storage (Questions)

19. How often must a teletherapy unit be fully inspected?
A. During teletherapy source replacement or at intervals not to exceed 3 years, whichever comes first
B. During teletherapy source replacement or at intervals not to exceed 5 years, whichever comes first
C. At intervals not to exceed 5 years only
D. During teletherapy source replacement or whenever major upgrades are complete

20. Which of the following must be included as the appropriate emergency equipment on an HDR unit?
A. I, II, and III.
B. I and III only.
C. II and IV only.
D. IV only.
E. All are correct.
I. Two pairs of long-handled forceps and a pair of long-handled scissors
II. A shielded container
III. Stopwatch or timer
IV. Portable survey meter

21. HDR simulation films must include:
A. I, II, and III.
B. I and III only.
C. II and IV only.
D. IV only.
E. All are correct.
I. Patient name and date
II. Catheter identification and length
III. Magnification factor and marker seeds consecutively from the distal end of each catheter
IV. Anatomical structures where dose contribution is to be calculated

22. Some methods used to calculate dose distribution around a linear ^{192}Ir source are:
A. I, II, and III.
B. I and III only.
C. II and IV only.
D. IV only.
E. All are correct.
I. TG-43 formalism
II. Monte Carlo
III. Sievert integral
IV. Triple A (AAA)

23. Which of the following are reports published by AAPM for HDR quality assurance irradiation therapy?
A. I, II, and III.
B. I and III only.
C. II and IV only.
D. IV only.
E. All are correct.
I. TG-59
II. TG-56
III. TG-40
IV. TG-43

24. When choosing lead-lined safes with lead-filled drawers for storing brachytherapy sources, the physicist in charge must consider:
A. I, II, and III.
B. I and III only.
C. II and IV only.
D. IV only.
E. All are correct.
I. Adequacy of shielding
II. Distribution of sources
III. Time required for personnel to remove sources from, and return sources to, the safe
IV. Person who handles the sources

25. The storage area for radium, encapsulated powdered sources, or sources containing microspheres:
A. Should be ventilated by the main air conditioning of the hospital or building
B. Should be ventilated by a direct filtered exhaust to the outdoors
C. Should be ventilated by a direct filtered exhaust to the hall
D. Should be hermetically closed to the outdoors

26. Which of the following appliances is usually provided in the storage room?
A. A refrigerator to freeze the radionuclides
B. A washing machine to wash the cloths used by the physicist who remove the radionuclides
C. A sink to clean source applicators
D. A purifier to sterilize the return sources

27. Which of the following should be included in the storage room for source preparation?
A. I, II, and III.
B. I and III only.
C. II and IV only.
D. IV only.
E. All are correct.
I. A source preparation bench close to the safe
II. A protective L-block barrier constructed of lead

7.3 Brachytherapy Source Handling and Storage (Questions)

III. A lead glass viewing window
IV. Suitably short forceps

28. Which of the following actions must be taken by the operator working with a brachytherapy source?
A. Minimize the time in the vicinity of the sources, as well as minimize the distance from the sources.
B. Maximize the time in the vicinity of the sources and minimize the distance from the sources.
C. Minimize the time in the vicinity of the sources and maximize the distance from the sources.
D. Time and distance are not effective since there are various kinds of protective shielding available in the vicinity of the source.

29. A source is considered to be leaking if a presence of:
A. 0.5 µCi or more of removable contamination is measured.
B. 0.05 µCi or more of removable contamination is measured.
C. 0.005 µCi or more of removable contamination is measured.
D. 0.0005 µCi or more of removable contamination is measured.

30. As per NRC rules, how often must the source be leak tested?
A. Once a year
B. Every 6 months
C. Every month
D. Quarterly

31. According to applicable state or federal regulations, how often should the brachytherapy storage area be surveyed?
A. Every week
B. Every 6–12 months
C. Every month
D. Every day

32. The Nuclear Regulatory Commission (NRC) requires that:
A. I, II, and III.
B. I and III only.
C. II and IV only.
D. IV only.
E. All are correct.
I. Immediately after implanting and removing sealed sources from a patient, the patient and the area must be surveyed.
II. Safety instructions must be provided to all personnel caring for the implanted patient.
III. An inventory describing the number of sources removed and number of sources returned to the safe must be performed.
IV. The patient can share a room with another patient as long as both use the same radioactive source.

33. Which of the following is a "violation" of NRC regulations for housing a patient with radioactive sources?
A. Signs posted indicating the presence of radioactive materials in the room.
B. Permitted visiting times posted in the room.
C. Visitors must stand at least 6 ft from the patient.
D. Items leaving the room do not need to be surveyed.

34. Which of the following devices should be used when handling radioactive sources?
A. Any kind of gloves.
B. It can be touched with the hands if 2 mrem/h or less is detected.
C. Long forceps.
D. Lead apron and special gowns.

35. Which of the following statements are true about safety features for the storage and preparation of radioactive sealed sources for manual brachytherapy?
A. I, II, and III.
B. I and III only.
C. II and IV only.
D. IV only.
E. All are correct.
I. Rooms should be used only for source storage.
II. Rooms should be provided with a locked door.
III. A radiation sign should be posted on the door.
IV. There should be shielded storage (safe) available for all sources.

36. Which of following are correct about brachytherapy patient treatment rooms?
A. I, II, and III.
B. I and III only.
C. II and IV only.
D. IV only.
E. All are correct.
I. Shielding should be provided for nurses and visitors of brachytherapy patients.
II. Prior to each treatment, movable shields should be placed close to the patient's bed.
III. Treatment room should contain a shielded storage container.
IV. An area monitor should be placed at the treatment room entrance.

37. Quality controls need to be carried out:
A. I, II, and III.
B. I and III only.
C. II and IV only.
D. IV only.
E. All are correct.

7.3 Brachytherapy Source Handling and Storage (Questions)

I. Periodically under normal operating conditions
II. After the source has been installed or replaced
III. After repairs or maintenance
IV. After 5 % source decay

38. Sealed sources should be subject to leak tests:
A. I, II, and III.
B. I and III only.
C. II and IV only.
D. IV only.
E. All are correct.
I. Prior to the first use
II. Before each use
III. At regular intervals thereafter the first use
IV. Before repair

39. A leak test should be capable of detecting the presence of:
A. 2 Bq of removable contamination from a sealed source
B. 0.02 µBq of removable contamination from a sealed source
C. 0.2 kBq of removable contamination from a sealed source
D. 2 mBq of removable contamination from a sealed source

40. Match the following brachytherapy procedures with its correct test (answers can be used more than once):
A. Manual brachytherapy sources
B. Teletherapy
C. Remote afterloader brachytherapy
D. 226Ra sources
I. Indirect wipe test of the nearest accessible surface
II. Direct wet wipe test
III. Immersion test

41. The proper use of survey equipment should include:
A. I, II, and III.
B. I and III only.
C. II and IV only.
D. IV only.
E. All are correct.
I. Checking the battery
II. Checking the monitor response with a check source
III. Turning the instrument on and starting to monitor from outside the room in which the source is located
IV. Starting monitoring from higher dose rate to lower dose rate areas

42. For safe operation of brachytherapy units, which of the following actions are to be taken?
A. I, II, and III.
B. I and III only.
C. II and IV only.
D. IV only.
E. All are correct.
I. The source strength of each source should be determined individually before it is used on a patient.
II. The source documentation should be checked carefully.
III. The unit of activity used for source calibration should be the same as the unit of activity used in the TPS.
IV. After verification of the source strength, the source holder does not need to be marked.

43. Specific precautions during the cutting and handling of ^{192}Ir ribbons should include:
A. I, II, and III.
B. I and III only.
C. II and IV only.
D. IV only.
E. All are correct.
I. Forceps, cutting devices, magnifying glasses, and good illumination of the work surface are available.
II. A container to hold cut lengths should be provided and labeled.
III. Surfaces and tools are properly decontaminated.
IV. Radioactive waste can be collected and stored in the bag as long as they are inside the cutting room.

44. What should a female worker who becomes pregnant do?
A. I, II, and III.
B. I and III only.
C. II and IV only.
D. IV only.
E. All are correct.
I. Notify the employer
II. Work at home or not be allowed in the radiation department
III. Adapt to working conditions in respect to occupational exposure
IV. Work on brachytherapy as soon as she has two monitors to ensure that the embryo or fetus is protected

45. Medical exposures should be justified:
A. By weighting the diagnostic or therapeutic benefits they produce against the radiation detriment they might cause
B. By keeping exposure of normal tissue during radiotherapy as low as reasonably achievable consistent with delivering the required dose to the planned target volume

C. As soon as a qualified expert in diagnostic therapy or radiotherapy approved the study or treatment of the patient
D. As soon as the health professional who prescribed the treatment has the necessary training

46. Which of the following factors should be considered when irradiating a pregnant woman?
A. I, II, and III.
B. I and III only.
C. II and IV only.
D. IV only.
E. All are correct.
I. Fetal doses below 100 mGy should not be considered a reason for terminating a pregnancy.
II. Any therapeutic procedure for pregnant women should be planned to deliver the minimum dose to any embryo or fetus.
III. Radiotherapeutic procedures causing exposure of the abdomen or pelvis of women who are pregnant or likely to be pregnant should be avoided unless there are strong clinical indications.
IV. The magnitude and type of fetal damage depends on the radiation dose and the stage of the pregnancy.

7.4 Dose Survey and Exposure Monitoring (Questions)

Quiz 1 (Level 2)

1. Which of the following radiation monitoring instruments is best suited to search for lost clinical radioactive implant sources?
A. Survey meter
B. Thermoluminescent dosimeters (TLD)
C. Photographic film
D. Geiger-Müller counters

2. Disadvantages of Geiger-Müller counters are:
A. I, II, and III.
B. I and III only.
C. II and IV only.
D. IV only.
E. All are correct.
I. The electrical field needs to be reestablished after every event.
II. They have a dead time.
III. It is not a dose-measuring device.
IV. In a very high-intensity radiation field, it can actually read zero.

3. Which of the following radiation monitoring instruments is best suited to measure dose rate around an implanted patient?
A. Geiger-Müller counters
B. Well chamber
C. Survey meter
D. Proportional counters

4. Match the appropriate detector with its potential situation for use:
A. Well chambers
B. Survey meters
C. Proportional counters
D. G-M counters
I. Measure dose rate around an implanted patient and patient room. It is used to survey in and around the storage area in which radioactive materials are kept and survey areas around radiation-producing machines such as ^{60}Co units.
II. Survey the operating room, personnel, and instruments after implant procedures. Find lost radioactive seeds, monitor incoming radioactive source material packages, search for holes in the walls of the linear accelerator room, and are used as an in-room radiation monitor in the treatment room.
III. Measure the activity of brachytherapy sources.
IV. Discriminate the type of contamination in a survey (β, γ, α), count radioactive spills, and are used as a detector in some CT scanners.

5. According to applicable state or federal regulations, how often are survey meters routinely calibrated?
A. Once every 2 years
B. Every 6–12 months
C. Every month
D. Quarterly

6. Which of the following statements are true about the use of a survey meter?
A. I, II, and III.
B. I and III only.
C. II and IV only.
D. IV only.
E. All are correct.
I. The battery supplying the high voltage to the detector must be verified before each day of use.
II. The detector should not be used if a weak battery is detected.
III. The detector must be tested with a calibration source of radioactivity that produces a known reading before each day of use.
IV. Survey meters should have a sticker indicating its date of calibration and an indication of the measurement point of the detector.

7. Which of the following devices can be used as personal dosimeters?
A. I, II, and III.
B. I and III only.

7.4 Dose Survey and Exposure Monitoring (Questions) 471

C. II and IV only.
D. IV only.
E. All are correct.
I. Thermoluminescent dosimeters (TLDs)
II. Parallel-plate chamber
III. Film badges
IV. Geiger-Müller counters

8. Personnel monitoring devices should be worn:
A. On the front pants pocket
B. On the front of the upper torso
C. On the front of the lower torso
D. On the neck area (collar)

9. In the radiotherapy departments, the personal dosimeters should be exchanged at regular intervals:
A. Not exceeding 1 month
B. Not exceeding 6 months
C. Not exceeding 3 months
D. Once a year

10. What if an individual's dosimeter is lost?
A. I, II, and III.
B. I and III only.
C. II and IV only.
D. IV only.
E. All are correct.
I. The licensee shall perform and document an assessment of the dose received.
II. The licensee shall estimate the individual's dose by using his or her recent dose history if nothing unusual occurred in the period.
III. The licensee shall add the estimated dose to the worker's dose record.
IV. The licensee shall wait until the next period and record a double dose.

11. Which of the following statements are true about monitoring?
A. I, II, and III.
B. I and III only.
C. II and IV only.
D. IV only.
E. All are correct.
I. Monitoring of the source storage and handling area is to be conducted with a survey meter immediately following the removal from or return to storage of brachytherapy sources.
II. A survey should be made of exposure rates in the vicinity of the patient soon after implantation of the sources.
III. A survey is to be performed after removal of the sources from a patient to confirm removal from the patient and return to shielding of all sources.
IV. The transport container should be surveyed before and after brachytherapy procedures.

12. Which of the following can be used for monthly exposure monitoring?
I. Film badge
II. TLD
III. OSL
IV. MOSFET
A. I and II
B. I, II, and III
C. I, II, and IV
D. All of the above

Quiz 2 (Level 3)

1. When the "latent image" in a computer radiograph (CR) is read by the laser, what kind of process happens?
A. Fluorescence
B. Phosphorescence
C. Luminescence
D. Photoelectric

2. In the film badge or OSL badge, there are three small pieces of metals inside (copper, tin, and aluminum). What are the functions of these metal pieces?
A. To attenuate the radiation
B. To monitor the energy or type of the radiation
C. To frame the badge
D. To generate secondary particles for imaging

3. When the exposure information in an OSL badge is read, what kind of process happens?
A. Fluorescence
B. Phosphorescence
C. Luminescence
D. Photoelectric

4. Are diode arrays used for absolute dose measurements or for relative dose measurements?
A. Both, since they are very sensitive and very stable
B. Only for relative dose, since they are very sensitive but not stable enough
C. Only for absolute dose since they are very stable
D. Neither, since they are neither stable nor sensitive

7.4 Dose Survey and Exposure Monitoring (Questions)

5. If an OSL dosimeter is used to monitor individual exposure, how frequently should it be replaced?
A. 2 weeks
B. 1 month
C. 2 months
D. 3 months

6. In the glow curve for a TLD, which peaks are used for dose information?
A. Peaks 1 and 2
B. Peaks 2 and 3
C. Peaks 4 and 5
D. Peaks 6 and 7

7. What is the *G* value for a chemical dosimetry?
A. Constant to indicate the change of molecules versus dose
B. Constant to indicate the change of mass versus dose
C. Constant to indicate the change of color versus dose
D. Constant to indicate the change of time versus dose

8. What is the general principle of MOSFET?
A. It is a circuit of a diode connected reversely, which can be conducted by irradiation.
B. It is a circuit of a field effect transistor, in which the irradiation changes the threshold voltage.
C. It is a circuit of two diodes connected reversely, which can be conducted by irradiation.
D. It is a semiconductor transistor connected reversely, which can be conducted by irradiation.

9. What is the operation range of ^{10}B neutron detector?
A. Ionization region
B. Proportional region
C. Geiger-Müller region
D. Continuous discharge region

10. In a typical superheated drop detector (also called "bubble detector") for neutron detection, how do you get rid of the bubbles after reading?
A. It cannot be removed because a bubble detector is not reusable.
B. Release the pressure a little, and the bubbles will be gone.
C. Apply a little more pressure, and the bubbles will be gone.
D. Either release the pressure or apply more pressure, and the bubbles will be gone.

7.5 Nuclear Medicine Procedures (Questions)

Quiz 1 (Level 2)

1. Which of the following is *not* true with regard to ^{131}I given to a patient?
   A. Contaminated linens and disposable food trays must be collected and stored for radioactive decay.
   B. Patient vomiting within the first 24 h after administration can pose a radiation problem.
   C. After patient discharge the room must be decontaminated.
   D. After discharge, the patient is not a radiation problem to his/her household members and the public.

2. What is the dose limit of leakage in locations surrounding the patient's room (hallway, adjacent patient room, etc.)?
   A. 2 mrem/h.
   B. 2 rem/h.
   C. 10 mrem/h.
   D. The dose rate surrounding the patient's room is never of concern.

3. What does "thyroid bioassay" mean?
   A. A test done to the patient who receives administration of ^{131}I
   B. A test done to equipment used in the preparation of radioactive thyroid substance
   C. A test done to all personnel involved in the administration and/or preparation of ^{131}I
   D. A test done to all personnel involved in the administration and/or preparation of ^{125}I

4. Which of the following statements are true about the thyroid bioassay test?
   A. I, II, and III.
   B. I and III only.
   C. II and IV only.
   D. IV only.
   E. All are correct.
   I. It measures the uptake of ^{131}I in the thyroid of the workers.
   II. The detector used for thyroid bioassay test is the NaI crystal detector.
   III. Very little activity detected is enough to receive a significant dose to the thyroid.
   IV. The test must be performed within 72 h after the administration.

5. Which of the following radionuclides are used to treat thyroid cancer?
   A. I, II, and III.
   B. I and III only.

C. II and IV only.
D. IV only.
E. All are correct.
I. ^{131}I
II. ^{125}I
III. ^{32}P
IV. ^{103}P

6. Which actions should be taken if a radionuclide spills from the vial or syringe during administration?
A. I, II, and III.
B. I and III only.
C. II and IV only.
D. IV only.
E. All are correct.
I. Throw an absorbent paper, such as hospital chux, on the spill area.
II. Warn others not to enter the area of the spill.
III. Notify the radiation safety officer.
IV. Clean the spill right away.

7. When can a radioactive source be discarded into a regular landfill?
A. It should never be discarded into a regular landfill.
B. When the landfill is in a rural area.
C. If it has decayed at least ten half-lives.
D. If its activity was measured.

8. When can a patient with a temporal or permanent implant be discharged?
A. I, II, and III.
B. I and III only.
C. II and IV only.
D. IV only.
E. All are correct.
I. After temporal implant, when sources have been removed and patient surveyed
II. After permanent implant, when dose rate at 1 m is <2 mrem/h
III. After permanent implant, when dose rate at 1 m is <5 mrem/h
IV. After temporal implant, when sources have been removed

9. The appropriate device to check a spill area is:
A. Geiger-Müller counters
B. Ionization chambers
C. Cutie pie
D. Proportional counters

10. Which of the following is the right TG report for ^{90}Y microsphere therapy?
A. TG-137
B. TG-144
C. TG-201
D. TG-119

11. Is the workload of a busy PET/CT center higher than that of a busy CT only center?
A. Comparable.
B. CT alone has a higher workload because PET/CT needs two scans.
C. CT alone has a higher workload because patients in PET/CT need to wait for 30–60 min before the scans.
D. PET/CT center has a higher workload.

12. To calculate the shielding of a PET/CT room, which of the shielding should be considered?
A. Both CT and PET shielding are considered.
B. Only PET because the energy of CT is too low.
C. Do the shielding as if all workload are CTs.
D. Either is fine since they are comparable.

13. During the time of uptake and waiting, a patient to take a PET/CT scan should void to clear the activity in the bladder by urinating, and this amount is about what percentage of total activity?
A. 5 %
B. 15 %
C. 25 %
D. 35 %
E. 45 %

14. How many PET/CT patients can a technician/therapist scan in a year without exceeding the annual limit of 50 mSv?
A. 500
B. 1,000
C. 1,500
D. 2,000
E. 2,400

7.6 Structural Shielding Design (Questions)

Quiz 1 (Level 2)

1. Structural shielding design for radiation therapy installations is discussed in:
A. TG-43 recommendations
B. NCRP report 34
C. NCRP report 151
D. TG-40

7.6 Structural Shielding Design (Questions)

2. Radiation protection barriers are designed:
A. To ensure that the dose equivalent received by any individual does not exceed the applicable maximum permissible value
B. To ensure that the dose equivalent received by radiation workers only does not exceed the applicable maximum permissible value
C. To ensure that no one is standing in a controlled area
D. To protect against scatter radiation only

3. A controlled area is designated as:
A. I, II, and III.
B. I and III only.
C. II and IV only.
D. IV only.
E. All are correct.
I. An area under the supervision of a radiation protection supervisor
II. An area where some form of personnel monitoring is required
III. An area that has physical boundaries
IV. An area in which occupational exposure conditions are kept under review though protective measures and safety provisions are not needed

4. Which of the following statements are true?
A. I, II, and III.
B. I and III only.
C. II and IV only.
D. IV only.
E. All are correct.
I. For calculations, the dose equivalent limit is assumed 0.1 mSv/week for the controlled areas.
II. Protection is required against primary, scattered, and leakage radiation.
III. For calculations, the dose equivalent limit is assumed 0.02 mSv/week for the uncontrolled areas.
IV. The areas surrounding the room are designated as controlled or uncontrolled areas.

5. A secondary barrier is:
A. I, II, and III.
B. I and III only.
C. II and IV only.
D. IV only.
E. All are correct.
I. A barrier sufficient to attenuate the useful beam to the required degree
II. A barrier sufficient to attenuate leakage and scatter radiation
III. A barrier capable to attenuate neutron radiation
IV. A barrier sufficient to attenuate stray radiation

6. Which of the following factors must be considered in calculating barrier thickness?
A. I, II, and III.
B. I and III only.
C. II and IV only.
D. IV only.
E. All are correct.
I. Workload
II. Use factor
III. Occupancy factor
IV. Distance

7. Use factor (U) is defined as:
A. Fraction of the operating time during which the area of interest is occupied by the individual
B. Distance in meters from the radiation source to the area to be protected
C. Fraction of the operating time during which the radiation under consideration is directed toward a particular barrier
D. Weekly dose delivered at 1 m from the source

8. Which of the following are considered full occupancy areas?
A. I, II, and III
B. I and III only
C. II and IV only
D. IV only
E. All
I. Nurse stations
II. Restrooms
III. Work areas
IV. Outside areas used for pedestrians or vehicular traffic

9. Which of the following *cannot* be used as a barrier material?
A. Steel
B. Concrete
C. Plywood
D. Lead

10. Match the following materials with its corresponding density:
A. Concrete   I.   7.8 g cm^3
B. Lead   II. 2.3 g cm^3
C. Steel   III. 11.3 g cm^3
D. Polyethylene IV. 0.9 g cm^3

7.6 Structural Shielding Design (Questions)

11. Which of the following are usually used to calculate the equivalent thickness of various materials?
A. I, II, and III
B. I and III only
C. II and IV only
D. IV only
E. All
I. Tenth-value layers (TVL)
II. Half-value layers (HVL)
III. Relative densities
IV. Transmission factor

12. The amount of scattering from the patient depends on:
A. I, II, and III
B. I and III only
C. II and IV only
D. IV only
E. All
I. Beam intensity incident on the patient
II. The quality of radiation
III. The field size of the beam at the scattered radiation
IV. The scattering angle

13. Which of the following statements are true?
A. I, II, and III
B. I and III only
C. II and IV only
D. IV only
E. All
I. Unless a maze entranceway is provided, the treatment door must provide shielding equivalent to the wall surrounding the door.
II. The door on megavoltage treatment rooms requires a motor drive as well as a means of manual operation in case of emergency.
III. A maze arrangement drastically reduces the shielding requirements for the door.
IV. With proper maze design, the door is exposed mainly to scattered radiation of significantly reduced intensity and energy.

14. The function of the maze is to:
A. Prevent excess exposure to therapists working on the console
B. Prevent direct incidence of radiation at the treatment door
C. Minimize radiation to the control area
D. Prevent radiation to affect workers and equipment in the console area

15. If the proper maze is built in a treatment room, what happens to the radiation outside the door?
A. I, II, and III
B. I and III only
C. II and IV only
D. IV only
E. All
I. It will be significantly reduced.
II. It will not be minimized at the door.
III. It will be scattered at least twice before incidence on the door.
IV. Scatter will be stopped totally on the maze and will not reach the door.

16. Which of the following beams will contain neutron contamination?
A. 6 MV
B. 20 MeV
C. 15 MV
D. 12 MeV

17. Neutron contamination is produced by:
A. I, II, and III.
B. I and III only.
C. II and IV only.
D. IV only.
E. All are correct.
I. High-energy photons
II. Electrons incident on target and flattening filter material
III. >10 MV photon beam incident on collimators and other shielding components
IV. 6 MV incident on air

18. The proper material used in the door of a linac machine to thermalize and further reduce neutron dose is:
A. Concrete
B. Steel
C. Polyethylene
D. Lead

19. The best method to reduce the neutron influence incident at the door is:
A. By building a maze of any dimension
B. By building a maze longer than 5 m
C. By adding lead shielding to the door
D. By adding steel shielding to the door

7.7 Radioactive Material Shipping (Questions)

Quiz 1 (Level 3)

1. What body governs radioactive material shipping and handling?
A. National Council on Radiation Protection and Measurements (NCRP)
B. US Department of Transportation (DOT)
C. National Research Council Committee on Biological Effects of Ionizing Radiation (NRC-BEIR)
D. Nuclear Regulatory Commission (NRC)

2. What is transportation index (TI)?
A. Reading in mrem/h at surface of package
B. Reading in mrem/min at surface of package
C. Reading in mrem/h at 1 m from the surface of package
D. Reading in mrem/min at 1 m from the surface of package

3. What is the range of a TI?
A. 1–100
B. 1–20
C. 1–10
D. 1–5

4. Which of the following are normally used in shipping radioactive material in radiotherapy?
I. Strong tight container
II. Type A package
III. Type B package
IV. NRC special handling
A. II and III
B. I, II, and III
C. IV only
D. I and II
E. All of the above

5. At what range of A value is a strong tight container used for shipping?
A. 0–0.001A
B. 0–0.01A
C. 0–0.1A
D. 0–1A

6. Due to DOT rules, what are the A values (in Ci) for ^{192}Ir, ^{125}I, and ^{60}Co, respectively?
   A. 540, 27, and 10.8
   B. 27, 540, and 10.8
   C. 27, 10.8, and 540
   D. 10.8, 27, and 540
   E. 10.8, 540, and 27

7. For prostate case, an order of 100 ^{125}I seeds is shipped; assuming the seed strength is 0.5 U, what type of package is used?
   A. Strong tight container
   B. Type A package
   C. Type B package
   D. NRC special handling

8. At what range of A value is a Type A package needed for shipping?
   A. 0.001–1 A
   B. 0.01–1 A
   C. 0.1–1 A
   D. 1–10 A
   E. 1–100 A

9. What is the problem if a White I label is stamped on a package and there is no TI information on the label?
   A. No problem at all.
   B. The TI information should be always indicated.
   C. It depends; if the reading at 1 m is zero, then there is no need to show TI information.
   D. The label should be changed to Yellow.

10. If TI=2, can this package be carried as a passenger-carrying box onto the airplane?
    A. Nope, radioactive materials can never be carried that way.
    B. Yes, since the maximal TI allowed is 3.
    C. Yes, as long as TI <10, it can be carried as a passenger-carrying box.
    D. Nope, only White I package can be carried that way.

11. For standard ^{60}Co source change, all 201 sources of 6,600 Ci in total need to be replaced. What type of shipping package is needed?
    A. NRC has to handle this since the activity is too strong.
    B. Type C package
    C. Type B package
    D. Type A package
    E. Strong tight container

7.8 Summary (Questions)

12. Leakage is found in a single (out of 201) ^{60}Co source and the source needs changing. What type of package is used in shipping?
A. Type C package
B. Type B package
C. Type A package
D. Strong tight container

13. At what range of A values is a Type B package required for shipping?
A. 1–100 A
B. 1–1,000 A
C. 1–3,000 A
D. 1–5,000 A
E. 1–10,000 A

14. A professor asks one of his graduate students to ship a source from one lab to another lab. The student puts the source into the trunk of his car. Is this *ok*?
A. Nope. The professor should always ship the source himself.
B. Yes. It is always fine to use private transportation vehicles.
C. Only if the student has the proper training on radioactive material handling.
D. The package should never be handled by a student.

15. How many types of radioactive labels are used by DOT?
A. 2
B. 3
C. 5
D. 10

7.8 Summary (Questions)

Quiz 1 (Level 3)

1. A radiation therapist's daily work includes taking CT scans for patients and treating patients with linear accelerators. If a radiation therapist is pregnant, what should she do considering her baby in the current working environment?
A. She definitely needs to change to a job of less exposure.
B. Her annual exposure is negligible; thus, she does not need to do anything.
C. Her baby should be within ALARA limit. However, she should be more careful to avoid any unnecessary exposure.
D. Small exposure is beneficial to baby's intelligence development.

2. In the annual report, the radiation safety officer (RSO) found that most of the medical physicists had exposure of 5.5 mSv. What will he do?
A. Nothing, since the tolerance is 50 mSv.
B. Reexamine the ALARA program, find out the reason, and improve it if possible.
C. Erase the records while reporting to high level.
D. Suggest an immediate adjourn of the radiation program.

3. A pregnant woman moved into a new customized luxury home which was constructed with a lot of stone materials during the last month of her pregnancy. One week later the house was discovered to have a radiation level 2 orders higher than the background, and the family moved out immediately. What would possibly happen to the baby and the mother?
A. Termination of pregnancy
B. Mental development difficulty for the baby
C. Increase in the probability of a difficult birth
D. Leukemia in early childhood for the baby

4. A clinic plans to start an HDR program. The room for HDR therapy used to be a vault for routine 6 MV linear accelerator. What major construction is needed in order to fit the HDR requirement?
A. All the secondary walls need more shielding because in HDR treatment all walls are considered primary.
B. Physicists need to do a careful survey outside the room when an HDR treatment (with a full strength source) is on and then find out what to do.
C. Nothing is needed, although a routine check is normally performed.
D. Destroy the vault and rebuild for HDR requirement.

5. A new vault for 6 and 15 MV linear accelerator has no door, but it contains an "L"-shaped maze, i.e., this is a double maze vault. A state officer went for the inspection of this new vault. What would the officer possibly do?
A. Fail the inspection because a door is absolutely necessary for neutron shielding.
B. Examine the workload for 15 MV. It is fine if current workload for 15 MV is less than 20 %.
C. It might be sufficient because the number of neutrons reaching the door is minimal due to multiple scatterings in the maze although a real-time survey is required.
D. Approve the inspection, but ask the clinic to turn off the 15 MV energy.

7.8 Summary (Questions)

6. A clinic ordered 20 seeds of I-125 loaded into an eye plaque to treat a patient's retinoblastoma. The source strength is around 10 mCi, which is about 20 times larger than the seeds for prostate implant. Due to the DOT rules, what type of package is needed for shipping?
   A. A Type A package.
   B. A Type B package.
   C. Strong tight container.
   D. Regular box with radioactive label.
   E. Insufficient information. It could be anything depending on the source strength.

7. An HDR unit could not retract its source after the treatment. The emergency program was activated and the patient was escorted outside the treatment room. The physician removed the applicator and put it in the lead pig with tools and then left the room. It took him 5 min to complete everything. What level of exposure did he have? Assume that the exposure rate constant for Ir-192 is 4.69 R cm^2/h×mCi and his arm length is 1 m:
   A. 0.5 cGy
   B. 5 cGy
   C. 50 cGy
   D. 0.5 Gy

8. A linear accelerator vault used for 3D-CRT is upgraded to IMRT treatment. Is it necessary to increase the shielding on the walls?
   A. Not really. IMRT does not increase the dose to the patient, i.e., the workload is unchanged, and so neither the primary nor the secondary walls need more shielding.
   B. Not really. The vault was built at ALARA standard; thus, the change due to IMRT is still within the tolerance.
   C. Yes. One-half layer of shielding at primary energy is needed.
   D. Yes. One-half layer of shielding at scattering energy is needed.

9. Here are the energies for a linear accelerator: 4 and 6 MV and 6, 9, 12, 16, and 20 MeV. What shielding is needed for the door?
   A. A sandwich shielding for neutrons and corresponding photons.
   B. No need to consider neutron shielding in door design since the X-ray energy is low.
   C. No door is needed.
   D. Find out the workload of using 20 MeV and then design the door shielding for neutrons.

10. After being exposed to radiation, cell A has three single-strand breaks in DNA, and cell B has one double-strand break in DNA. What will happen to those two cells?
A. Both have mitotic death.
B. Cell A survives, whereas cell B has mitotic death.
C. Cell B survives, whereas cell A has mitotic death.
D. Both survive.

11. In the past, all radiotherapy treatments were hypo-fractionated, i.e., patients were treated with 1–2 fractionations. Many patients died of corresponding normal tissue complications and this spurred the popularity of hyper-fractionation later. Now, hypo-fractionated treatments are becoming popular again with many fewer problems. The reason for this is:
A. Hypo-fractionation is better for tumor control but also makes normal tissue complications increase. In the past, the energy was low, causing more NTC.
B. There is minimal evidence that hypofractionation is good for tumor control. The reason for NTC in the past was that the beam energy was low.
C. Hypo-fractionation is better for tumor control but also increases NTC. Modern technology has better delineation of tumors and better precision in targeting.
D. There is minimal evidence that hypofractionation is good for tumor control, but it better for patients since they only have a few treatments. In addition, modern technology has more accurate delineation of tumors and better precision in targeting.
E. Modern technology significantly reduces the radiation safety issue.

12. A patient under treatment for thyroid cancer with I-131 was released from the hospital. The patient's exposure rate measured at 1 m is 7 mrem/h. The patient chose to take a public bus and did not tell other passengers sitting close to him. It took the bus 1 h to reach his home. What should other passengers do?
A. Nothing. This amount of exposure is within the 500 mrem annual tolerance of the public.
B. Keep the right to sue the hospital only for releasing such a patient who exposed the public.
C. Keep the right to sue the patient only because he should take a private vehicle or notify other passengers.
D. Keep the rights to sue both the hospital and patient together.

7.8 Summary (Questions)

13. The *A* value for ^{125}I is 540 Ci, whereas for ^{192}Ir is only 27 Ci. Why are they so different?
    A. Those are arbitrary numbers by DOT regulations.
    B. Because a single ^{192}Ir source is already 10 Ci, whereas a single ^{125}I source is only 0.4 mCi.
    C. Because the average energy of photons produced by ^{192}Ir is much higher than ^{125}I.
    D. Because the air kerma rate constants are so different.

14. A linear accelerator vault is designed to be within ALARA level 1. As a rule of thumb, what is the normal shielding on walls?
    A. 1 TVL or 3.2 HVLs
    B. 2 TVLs
    C. 3 TVLs
    D. 4 TVLs

15. A PET/CT center is constructed to shield radiation from ^{18}F-labeled fluorodeoxyglucose (FDG). Other radioisotopes such as ^{124}I-labeled drugs are used later. The energy for the positrons emitted by ^{124}I is much larger than those by ^{18}F. If the workload remains unchanged, should any extra shielding be considered as there is an increase in the positron energy?
    A. Yes, gamma photons annihilated from electron-positron pairs have more energy.
    B. No, positron energy alone has nothing to do with the shielding.
    C. No, previous shielding should be sufficient of any change of radioisotopes.
    D. Yes, but only the waiting room needs more shielding.

16. What is the general thickness of Pb for PET/CT shielding based on ALARA level 1?
    A. There is no such criterion, everything should be calculated.
    B. A conservative thickness is 5 cm (2 in.) for walls.
    C. A conservative thickness is 2.5 cm (1 in.) for walls.
    D. A conservative thickness is 1.3 cm (0.5 in.) for walls.

7.9 Maximum Permissible Dose Equivalent (Answers)

Quiz 1 (Level 2)

1. **C** The biological effects of radiation depend on the dose and the type of radiation received by the individual.

2. **A** Dose equivalent is $H = D \times Q$, where D is the absorbed dose and Q is the quality factors for the radiation. The quality factor accounts for the fact that not all radiation deposits dose in the same manner which makes some radiation more or less effective at damaging DNA. $H1/H2 = d_2^2/d_1^2$ is the inverse square law as the dose is inversely proportional to the distance squared. $X = \Gamma \times A \times t/d^2$ is the exposure formula used for calculating the exposure from a radioactive source.

3. **B** The SI unit for both dose and dose equivalent is joule per kilogram. The special name for the SI unit of dose equivalent is Sievert (Sv). The Becquerel (Bq) is the SI unit of activity of a radionuclide. The non-SI unit for dose is the rad, and for dose equivalent, it is rem. The unit for absorbed dose in SI units is the gray (Gy). Remember that a Sv is just the dose in Gy times a quality factor.

4. **D** The quality factor used to calculate dose equivalent depends on the type of radiation, and it is independent of the organ, tissue, or biologic endpoint under consideration.

5. The higher the quality factor, the more effective the radiation is at creating DNA damage. Heavy charged particles have the highest linear energy transfer (LET) and therefore have a higher Q.
   A. III. X-ray, γ-rays, and electrons ($Q=1$)
   B. I. Thermal neutrons ($Q=5$)
   C. II. Neutrons and heavy particles (α) ($Q=20$)

6. **B** The effective dose equivalent is defined as the sum of the weighted dose equivalents for irradiated tissues or organs. The reason that effective dose is used is that usually exposures are not to the total body, so to quantify the potential risks involved with an exposure to the gonads versus an extremity, an additional weighting factor for the specific organ is included. The definition of dose is the energy absorbed from an ionizing radiation beam per unit mass of absorber. Dose modified by quality or weighting factor is the definition of dose equivalent, and a graph of dose distribution produced by passing a dosimeter across the beam is the definition of dose profile.

7.9 Maximum Permissible Dose Equivalent (Answers)

7. C The National Council on Radiation Protection and Measurements (NCRP) is a national group of radiation experts from the United States that make recommendations in the area of ionization radiation and develop standards for the use of radiation in this country. The International Commission on Radiological Protection (ICRP) is an independent group of international experts who are interested in the safe use of all types of radiation. They provide recommendations for protection against ionization radiation. The US Nuclear Regulatory Commission (USNRC) and the individual states establish regulations that are incorporated into federal and state laws. The recommendations by the ICRP and NCRP can be reviewed by the USNRC and the individual states and put into law. Until the process happens, the recommendations by NCRP and ICRP are only that, a recommendation.

8. A An agreement state is defined as a state that has entered into an agreement with the USNRC in which they assume responsibility for enforcing the regulations specific to a by-product material as well as accelerator-produced nuclides. Most states are agreement states and this means that inspections are done by the state's inspectors. In a nonagreement state, inspections would be done using NRC inspectors.

9. D Only A, B, and C are true. The weighting factor represents the different risk of each tissue to mortality from cancer and hereditary effects in the first two generations. The effective dose equivalent is the sum of the weighted dose equivalents for all irradiated tissues, and different types of radiation (photons, neutrons, protons) have *different* biological effectiveness for *equal* absorbed doses. Remember that the biological effect is going to depend on how the specific radiation deposits dose in tissue.

10. B The formula for dose equivalent is $H = D \times Q$, where D is the absorbed dose and Q is the quality factors for a particular radiation. If a person receives an average whole body dose of 150 mrad from thermal neutrons, then the dose equivalent is 750 mrem. This means that the same dose from thermal neutrons is equivalent to a higher dose of photons or electrons.
Dose received $(D) = 150$ mrad
Quality factor for thermal neutrons $(Q) = 5$
Dose equivalent formula:
$H = D \times Q$
$H = 150 \text{ mrad} \times 5$
$H = 750$ mrem

11. B As per NCRP recommendations, the cumulative exposure for occupational workers should not exceed the age times 10 mSv. Thus, a 50-year-old worker should not have accumulated more than 500 mSv = 50,000 mrem = 50 rem.

12. **B** A deterministic effect is defined as an effect where the severity increases with dose above the threshold for the occurrence of the effect. A stochastic effect is when the probability of the occurrence is higher for higher doses, but the severity is independent of dose. An example of a stochastic effect is cancer where any occurrence of cancer is bad.

13. Deterministic or stochastic effect:
    A. I, II, and V are deterministic effects
    B. III and IV are stochastic effects
    As a quick example, reddening of the skin is considered a deterministic effect because the redness of the skin increases with dose above specific value (threshold). The more doses the individual receives above the threshold, the more the skin will be affected. If the individual received a dose below the threshold value, then the skin will not get red.

14. **A** Background radiation is part of the natural environment and includes terrestrial radiation, cosmic radiation, and radioactive elements in our bodies. Medical procedures are not considered natural, so it is not a background radiation.

15. **D** Terrestrial radiation varies over the earth because of differences in the amount of naturally occurring elements in the earth's surface. Cosmic radiation levels change with elevation since the higher you are, the amount of shielding from the atmosphere diminishes. The internal irradiation arises mainly from ^{40}K in our body which is the most abundant natural isotope that humans have in their body. Remember that medical procedures are not considered natural, so it is not a background radiation.

16. **C** Radon is the most common hazardous naturally occurring radioactive material. Many buildings may have elevated levels of radon emitted by naturally occurring uranium-238 in the soil. It has been estimated that the average annual dose equivalent to bronchial epithelium from radon decay products is approximately 24 mSv (2.4 rem). A way to reduce the exposure from radon is to ensure basements are well ventilated.

17. **B** Large doses of radiation produce identifiable effects within a relatively short period, but low doses of radiation are difficult to measure due to low frequency with which these effects might occur and the sensitivity of the measuring devices.

18. **E** Exposures to low-level radiation may produce genetic effects such as radiation-induced gene mutations, chromosome breaks, and anomalies. Neoplastic diseases such as leukemia, thyroid tumors, and skin lesions can also be produced by low levels of radiation although it is difficult to determine if these are a result of genetic abnormalities or the low radiation dose. Low doses of radiation can also affect growth and development especially if the exposure is during the fetal stage of development. The life span can

7.9 Maximum Permissible Dose Equivalent (Answers)

also be shortened or premature aging induced after low doses of radiation, and cataracts can also form although there is a threshold for these to occur. The major difficulty with assessing the effects of low doses of radiation is being able to measure the actual dose and separate the effect from the natural background incidence of the effect.

19. B The harmful effects of radiation may be classified into stochastic and nonstochastic (or deterministic) effects.

20. A A stochastic effect is defined as an effect in which the probability of occurrence increases with increasing absorbed dose, but the severity in affected individuals does not depend on the magnitude of the absorbed dose.

21. E Examples of nonstochastic effects include organ atrophy, fibrosis, cataracts, blood changes, and decrease in sperm count. Remember that these effects have a threshold and that the severity is proportional to the dose.

22. A NCRP recommendations on exposure limits of radiation workers are based on the fact that at low radiation levels, nonstochastic effects are essentially avoided. Additionally, the predicted risk for stochastic effects should not be greater than the average risk of accidental death among workers in industries. For all situations, the ALARA principle (as low as reasonably achievable) should be followed.

23. C Occupational and public dose limits include exposure received by a worker pursuing his/her occupation as well as exposure received by a member of the public. They exclude exposures received from medical procedures and natural background radiation.

24. A The ALARA principle states that one should keep radiation exposure as low as reasonably achievable, considering the economic and social factors. This means that one should reduce their exposure as low as possible while still performing one's duties. An example would be a shield for a linac vault. The wall could be built thick enough to reduce the dose to basically 0 Sv, but this would result in an extremely thick wall which would be very expensive. The level of average annual excess risk of fatal health effects attributable to irradiation is the definition of negligible individual risk level (NIRL).

25. B Medical exposures are incurred by patients as part of their own medical or dental diagnosis or treatment and also by persons, other than those occupationally exposed, knowingly helping in the support and comfort of a patient, that is, has radioactive material in them. Another example of a medical exposure is one incurred by volunteers in a research program. Occupational exposures are all exposures of workers incurred in the course of their work, and public exposures are exposures incurred by members of the public from radiation sources, excluding any occupational or medical exposure and the normal local natural background radiation but including exposure to authorized sources and practices and from intervention situations.

26. B The main physical quantities used in safety standards are the activity and absorbed dose. Equivalent dose account for physical effects but also for the biological effects of radiation upon tissues and effective dose accounts for physical effects but also for the biological effects of radiation upon tissues.

27. B The organ dose is defined as the mean dose in a specified tissue or organ of the human body. The sum of the weighted dose equivalents for all irradiated tissues is the definition of effective dose equivalent and the total dose received throughout the period of time during which radionuclide remains in the body is the definition of committed dose. Finally, the summation of the product of the mean dose in the various groups of exposed people and the number of individuals in each group is the definition of collective dose.

28. B NRC or state laws require that personnel monitoring devices must be worn at all times while working with radiation or radiation machines. Each authorized user is responsible for ensuring proper wearing of dosimetry and timely exchange of radiation badges at the end of each month.

29. A The yearly occupational maximum permissible dose (MPD) for the whole body is 50 mSv or 5 rem/year. 1 mSv or 0.1 rem/year is the effective dose equivalent limit for continuous or frequent exposure for the public and educational and training personnel. 5 mSv or 0.5 rem/year is the total dose equivalent limit for embryo/fetus exposures, and finally, 500 mSv or 50 rem/year is the annual occupational exposure for the organs, extremities, and skin.

30. C The lifetime or cumulative occupational exposure limit is 10 mSv or 1 rem × age (years).

31. D The annual occupational maximum permissible dose (MPD) for the lens of the eye is 150 mSv or 15 rem; 50 mSv or 5 rem is the effective dose equivalent limit for the lens of the eye for the public and educational and training personnel.

32. B The monthly maximum permissible dose (MPD) for a pregnant woman worker is 0.5 mSv or 0.05 rem. 0.01 mSv or 0.001 rem is the annual effective dose equivalent per source or practice. 5 mSv or 0.5 rem is the total dose equivalent limit to an embryo/fetus during the gestation term. 1 mSv or 15 rem is the annual effective dose equivalent limit for the public and education and training exposures.

33. A The effective dose in any year for occupational exposure based on the NCRP should not exceed 50 mSv (5 rem). The cumulative for occupational

7.10 Time, Distance, and Shielding (Answers)

exposure is 10 mSv × age. 5 mSv (0.5 rem) is the maximum permissible annual effective dose equivalent limit for nonoccupational infrequent exposure, and for nonoccupational continuous or frequent exposure, the annual effective dose should not exceed 1 mSv (0.1 rem).

34. C The nonoccupational (public) effective dose to the extremities, skin, and lens in any year should not exceed 50 mSv (5 rem) based on the NCRP recommendations.

35. E All are correct since radiation is potentially harmful; exposure to it should be monitored continually and controlled, and exposure of personnel and the public should be kept to a minimum. As a rule of thumb in the nuclear power industry in the United States, ALARA has a cash value of about $1,000 per 10 mSv (1 rem). If the exposure of person to 10 mSv (1 rem) can be avoided by the expenditure of this amount of money, it is considered reasonable. If the cost is more, it is considered unreasonable and the exposure is allowed for low dose levels. For higher doses, a cash value of about $10,000 per 10 mSv (1 rem) is established.

36. B Once a pregnancy is declared, the NCRP recommends a monthly limit to the embryo or fetus of 0.5 mSv (0.05 rem). The concept of declaring pregnancy is very important. In the eyes of the NRC or state, a woman is not pregnant until she declares herself to be pregnant IN WRITING. The reason for this is if the worker feels that she cannot perform her duties with the limitations enforced by the NRC or state, she does not have to declare her pregnancy. This is a decision made by the mother.

7.10 Time, Distance, and Shielding (Answers)

Quiz 1 (Level 2)

1. A Maximizing the distance will reduce the dose to a greater degree than minimizing time for equal changes because of the inverse square law. Radiation dose is proportional to time and dose is inversely related to the distance squared. Time, distance, and shielding are the three ways to reduce the exposure to radiation. One can increase the distance from the source, reduce the time near the source, and place a shield to reduce the exposure.

2. C Mathematically, the dose is inversely related to the distance squared. The intensity of radiation becomes weaker as it spreads out from the source.

$$\frac{I_1}{I_2} = \frac{D_2^2}{D_1^2}$$

where I_1 = intensity 1 at D_1, I_2 = intensity 2 at D_2, D_1 = distance 1 from the source, and D_2 = distance 2 from the source.

3. C ALARA is a philosophy of maintaining personnel radiation exposure as low as reasonably achievable.

4. D Maximizing the distance is the best method used on radiation protection to take advantage of the inverse square law. The other answers here are also good to follow in terms of radiation protection.

5. A Radiation exposure to employees can be reduced by time, distance, and shielding. Personnel monitoring devices do not protect from radiation but measure radiation exposure received by workers.

6. B Forceps are used mainly to extend the distance between the source and fingers.

7. D The US Department of Transportation (DOT) governs the rules and regulations for shipping radioactive material. To ship radioactive material, both the shipper and receiver must have the proper training.

8. A ALARA in general means much lower dose than the limit. For instance, the annual exposure limit for an occupational work is 50 mSv, at level 1 ALARA; the worker should receive no more than 5 mSv annually.

9. B Level 1 ALARA normally refers to the amount of shielding required to reduce the dose to 10 % of the annual limit.

10. D Typically the gloves have lead in them as well. One can also use glasses with lead in them to protect the eyes.

7.11 Brachytherapy Source Handling and Storage (Answers)

Quiz 1 (Level 2)

1. E HDR safety systems include interlocks to prevent initiation of treatment if the door is open and backup batteries to take over operation in case of power failure. A manual source retraction mechanism is available to withdraw the source into the storage safe if it gets stuck, and the treatment is aborted if the system detects blockage or excessive friction during source transit.

2. B The shielding and safety requirements for the HDR room are mandated by the Nuclear Regulatory Commission (or the state if an agreement state).

7.11 Brachytherapy Source Handling and Storage (Answers)

Remember that the ICRP and NCRP just provide recommendations. The Committee on Biologic Effects of Ionizing Radiation (BEIR) is an arm of the National Academy of Sciences.

3. **E** All are correct.

4. **A** Only I, II, and III are correct. Restricted area controls include signs, door warning lights indicating "Radiation ON," locks, and visible/audible alarms. The appropriate signage is defined by the NRC (or state) regulations. The RSO responsibilities do not include being present to avoid unauthorized personnel to be around the HDR unit.

5. **E** All are correct. In order to be licensed for HDR unit use according to NCR, the applicant is required to provide proof of source description, manufacturer's name and model of the HDR unit, the intended use, and the authorized users; a description of the quality assurance program; an outline of initial training of authorized users and device operators; a description of radiation detection and survey instruments to be used; a floor plan of the facility identifying room(s), doors, windows, conduits, density, and thickness of shielding materials; a shielding calculation; calibration procedures and frequency; the training and frequency of retraining of individual operators; the training or certification of individuals performing source changes; the personal radiation monitoring program; emergency procedures; postings; locations; the disposal arrangements of decayed sources; the operating procedures and manuals; and inspection and servicing of HDR equipment.

6. **E** A high-dose rate (HDR) quality management program must include a written directive, patient identification, treatment plan verification, pretreatment safety checks, treatment delivery, post-treatment survey, source replacement and calibration check, recording, supervision, recordable event or misadministration, and periodic reviews.

7. **C** The identity of the patient must be verified by two independent methods. This may be accomplished by asking the patient his/her name and confirming the name by comparison with patient's identification bracelet or hospital identification card.

8. **B** HDR pretreatment safety checks must be performed before treatment on any day that the HDR procedure is scheduled.

9. **E** Prior to the initiation of HDR treatment, the authorized operator must verify the name of the patient under treatment, the dose to be delivered to a patient, the site of administration, and the times for each dwell location. These are all included in the written directive.

10. D All are true expect D. During all patient treatments, both the authorized physician user and the authorized medical physicist must be physically present within audible range of normal human speech.

11. B Brachytherapy cases will be reviewed by an authorized physician and/or physicist at intervals no greater than 12 months. A representative number of cases will undergo this review which will consist of checking that the delivered radiation dose was in accordance with the written directive and plan of treatment.

12. C If a recordable event or misadministration is uncovered during the periodic review, the number of cases to be reviewed will be expanded to include all cases for that calendar year.

13. A The quality management program will be reviewed on an annual basis and a written summary of the review must be submitted to the RSO and the radiation safety committee, and any modification made to the QMP must be reported to the NRC regional office (or state) within 30 days after modification has been made.

14. C Immediately after each use of the HDR device, the physicist will ensure that the source has been returned to the full-shielded position by performing a survey of the afterloader and the patient including the connectors, applicator, and the full length of guide tubes.

15. E Full calibration measurements of a teletherapy unit must be done before the first medical use of the unit, if the spot check measurements indicate that the output differs more than 5 % from the output obtained at the last full calibration, following replacement of source or relocation of the unit, following repair of the unit, and always at intervals not exceeding 1 year.

16. B Periodic spot checks for teletherapy units must be done once in each calendar month and must include timer constancy and linearity, on/off error, light field versus radiation field coincidence, accuracy of all distance measuring and localization devices, door interlock, and beam condition indicator lights.

17. A Radiation surveys for teletherapy units must be done before medical use, after each installation of a teletherapy source, and after making any change for which an amendment is required.

18. A The leakage from the source head with the beam in the off position cannot exceed 2 mrem/h on average and 10 mrem/h maximum at a distance of 1 m from the source.

7.11 Brachytherapy Source Handling and Storage (Answers)

19. B Teletherapy units must be fully inspected during teletherapy source replacement or at intervals not to exceed 5 years, whichever comes first.

20. E All are correct. The shielded container is used to contain the applicator and source if it cannot be retracted. The forceps and scissors are used to help the physician remove the applicator from the patient. The stopwatch is used to time how long each person is in the treatment room to calculate the exposure to the personnel.

21. E HDR simulation films must include patient name and date, catheter identification and length, magnification factor, and marker seeds consecutively from the distal end of each catheter, and anatomical structures where dose contribution is to be calculated must be drawn.

22. A Some methods used to calculate dose distributions around a linear 192-Ir source are the TG-43 formalism, the Monte Carlo, and the Sievert integral. The TG-43 formalism is a modular dose calculation algorithm that uses multiple components to model the dose distribution.

23. A TG-59, TG-56, and TG-40 are reports published by AAPM for HDR quality assurance. TG-43 is described as a formalism for calculating dose distributions in brachytherapy.

24. A When choosing lead-lined safes with lead-filled drawers for storing brachytherapy sources, the physicist in charge must consider adequacy of shielding including the number of sources and the source activity and energy, the distribution of sources, and the time required for personnel to remove sources from, and return sources to, the safe. The individual who handles the sources is independent of the drawer selected.

25. B The storage area for radium, encapsulated powdered sources, or sources containing microspheres should be ventilated by a direct filtered exhaust to the outdoors because of the possibility of radon leaks or as a precaution if a source ruptures to prevent the radionuclide from being drawn into the general ventilation system of the building.

26. C The storage rooms are usually provided with a sink of cleaning source applicators. The sink should be provided with a filter or trap to prevent the loss of a source.

27. A A source preparation bench should be provided closest to the safe so that the time handling the source is minimized. The preparation of source applicators should be carried out behind a protective L-block barrier constructed of lead to shield the operator, and a lead glass viewing window provides some protection by providing shielding and distance between the face of the operator and the sources. Brachytherapy sources should never be touched directly with the hands, so a suitably *long* forceps should be used to provide as much distance as practical between sources and the operator.

28. C Besides various kinds of protective shielding available for brachytherapy applications, the operator must be aware of the effectiveness of time and distance in radiation protection. Exposures can be reduced by minimizing the time in the vicinity of the sources and maximizing the distance from the sources.

29. C A source is considered to be leaking if a presence of 0.005 µCi or more of removable contamination is measured. The source should be returned to a suitable agency for disposal of radioactive material. Wipe tests are done by taking a small piece of paper and physically wiping the outside of the source or source container. The paper is then planed in a well chamber and measured to see if there is any contamination.

30. B As per NRC rules, radioactive sources must be leak tested every 6 months. If there is 0.005 µCi or more of removable contamination, the source should be taken out of the department and sent back for repair or disposal.

31. A According to applicable state or federal regulations, the brachytherapy storage area must be surveyed every week.

32. A The Nuclear Regulatory Commission (NRC) requires that immediately after implanting and removing sealed sources from a patient, the patient and the area must be surveyed, safety instructions must be provided to all personnel caring for the implanted patient, and an inventory describing the number of sources removed and number of sources returned to the safe must be performed. The patient shall be in a private room and only people 18 years of age and older are allowed in the room, not including pregnant women.

33. D Items leaving the room of a patient with sources must be surveyed at all times. Additionally, there must be signs posted indicating the presence of radioactive materials in the room, permitted visiting times, and that visitors must stand at least 6 ft from the patient.

34. C When handling radioactive sources, long forceps should be used at all times. Unless the gloves are leaded, they do not provide much protection against photon-emitting sources.

35. E The room should be used only for source storage as well as provided with a lock. A radiation sign should be posted on the door, there should be shielded storage (safe) available for all sources, the safe should have compartments for different source activities, the workbench should be provided with an L-block shielding, the source handling area should be well illuminated, forceps should be available, sources should be readily identifiable by sight, and there should be a clear indication of the radiation level in the room.

36. E Brachytherapy patient treatment rooms must have shielding for nurses and visitors, and prior to each treatment, movable shields should be placed close to the patient's bed, the treatment room should contain a shielded storage container, and an area monitor should be placed at the treatment room entrance.

37. A Quality controls need to be carried out periodically under normal operating conditions, after the source has been installed or replaced and after repairs or maintenance.

38. B Sealed sources should be leak tested prior to the first use and at regular intervals thereafter. If the source is broken, it should be sent to the appropriate agency

39. C A leak test should be capable of detecting the presence of 0.2 kBq of removable contamination from a sealed source.

40. Brachytherapy procedures with its correct test
A. II. Manual brachytherapy sources (direct wet wipe test)
B. I. Teletherapy (indirect wipe test of the nearest accessible surface)
C. I. Remote afterloader brachytherapy (indirect wipe test of the nearest accessible surface)
D. III. ^{226}Ra sources (immersion tests). An immersion test checks for bubbles meaning that the source is leaking radon gas.

41. A The proper use of survey equipments should include checking the battery, checking the monitor response with a check source and turning the instrument on, and starting to monitor from outside the room in which the source is located.

42. A For safe operation of brachytherapy units, the source strength of each source should be determined individually before it is used on a patient, the source documentation should be checked carefully, the unit of activity used for source calibration should be the same as the unit of activity used in the TPS, and after verification of the source strength, the source holder should be marked with unique identifiers (like different colors).

43. A Specific precautions during the cutting and handling of ^{192}Ir ribbons should include forceps and cutting devices, magnifying glasses and good illumination of the work surface should be available, a container to hold cut lengths should be provided and labeled, and surfaces and tools should be properly decontaminated. Radioactive waste can be collected and stored only in adequate containers.

44. B A female worker who became pregnant should notify the employer as soon as possible so that the employer can adapt her to working conditions in respect to occupational exposure so as to ensure that the embryo or fetus is afforded the same broad level of protection as required for members of the public. Remember though that a female is not considered pregnant until she declares her pregnancy IN WRITING. Again, this is to protect the employee from potentially having to stop working due to the limits placed on the fetus.

45. A Medical exposures should be justified by weighting the diagnostic or therapeutic benefits they produce against the radiation detriment they might cause, taking into account the benefits and risks of available alternative techniques that do not involve medical exposure.

46. E All of the following factors are true: fetal doses below 100 mGy should not be considered a reason for terminating a pregnancy although this must be a discussion between the parents and the physician. Any therapeutic procedure for pregnant women should be planned to deliver the minimum dose to any embryo or fetus, and radiotherapeutic procedures causing exposure of the abdomen or pelvis of women who are pregnant or likely to be pregnant should be avoided unless there are strong clinical indications. The magnitude and type of fetal damage depends on the radiation dose and stage of the pregnancy. The dose to various locations on the mother (fundus, umbilicus and pelvis) should be measured during the first treated fraction to assess the total dose to the fetus.

7.12 Dose Survey and Exposure Monitoring (Answers)

Quiz 1 (Level 2)

1. D A Geiger-Müller counter is a very sensitive type of ionization chamber. Any detected radiation will be recorded which makes it well suited for finding lost sources. It does not quantify the amount of radiation like a survey meter; it only alerts the operator to the presence of radiation.

2. E Geiger-Müller counters produce a large signal even after a small event because of the very high operating voltage. This makes them very sensitive but also limits them because they have a dead time where they cannot respond to radiation until the electric field is reestablished. Also, G-M counters are not a dose-measuring device, and in a very high-intensity

7.12 Dose Survey and Exposure Monitoring (Answers) 501

radiation field, it can actually read zero. Remember that G-M detectors are used to search for lost clinical radioactive implant sources like ^{125}I seeds, ^{198}Au, ^{137}Cs, ^{226}Ra, or ^{192}Ir; they are not used for routine surveys around linear accelerators as they cannot quantify the dose or exposure.

3. C A survey meter (or portable ionization chamber) can measure dose rate around an implanted patient. Remember that the Geiger-Müller counter is not a dose-measuring device. Well chambers are used in measuring the activity of brachytherapy sources, and proportional counters are typically used to measure alpha and beta radiation.

4. Appropriate detector
A. III. Well chambers: measure the activity of brachytherapy sources.
B. I. Survey meters: measure dose rate around an implanted patient and patient room. It is used to survey in and around the storage area in which radioactive materials are kept and survey areas around radiation-producing machines such as ^{60}Co units.
C. IV. Proportional counters: discriminate the type of contamination in a survey (β, γ, α), count radioactive spills, and are used as a detector in some CT scanners.
D. II. G-M counters: survey operating room, personnel, and instruments after implant procedures, find lost radioactive seeds, monitor incoming radioactive source material packages, search for holes in the walls of the linear accelerator room, and are used as an in-room radiation monitor in the treatment room.

5. B According to applicable state or federal regulations, survey meters are routinely calibrated every 6–12 months by a calibration laboratory.

6. E All statements are true about the use of a survey meter.

7. B Thermoluminescent dosimeters (TLDs) and film badges are devices used as personal dosimeters. Optically stimulated luminescence dosimeters and some special neutron detectors like the bubble detector can also be used. Parallel-plate chambers allow measurements practically at the surface of a phantom without significant wall attenuation, so it is used to measure dose as a function of depth at shallow depths where cylindrical chambers are unsuitable because of their large volume. Geiger-Müller counters are radiation monitoring instruments used to detect individual photons or individual particles that can aid in finding a radioactive source or a crack in shielding.

8. B Personnel monitoring devices should be worn on the front of the upper torso at all times while in the department. In most radiotherapy exposures the whole body is assumed to be uniformly exposed.

9. **C** In the radiotherapy departments the personal dosimeters should be changed at regular intervals not exceeding 3 months. Moreover, the reports should become available as soon as possible but no later than within 3 months after the exchange.

10. **A** If an individual's dosimeter is lost, the licensee shall perform and document an assessment of the dose received and add the estimated dose to the worker's dose record. The individual's dose can be estimated by using his or her recent dose history if nothing unusual occurred in the period. A new badge will be ordered and replace the old badge.

11. **E** All statements are correct.

12. **B** MOSFET is not typically used for monthly exposure monitoring. A MOSFET is a metal oxide semiconductor field effect transistor and can be used as an in vivo dosimeter in radiation therapy. When it is exposed, the semiconductor material becomes ionized and changes. This change can be measured by detecting the voltage required to allow a charge to flow through the material. The voltage can be related to the absorbed dose.

Quiz 2 (Level 3)

1. **B** The computed radiograph is generated using a photostimulable phosphor (PSP). It uses laser light to read the "latent image" generated during the X-ray exposure. The laser converts the latent image into light photons through the process of phosphorescence. The light photons can be detected and converted into the digital computed radiograph.
Fluorescence is X-ray-induced prompt light, whereas phosphorescence has time delay. Luminescence in general means cold light (not from a heated body).

2. **B** After the attenuation of different metals, the reading from the dosimeter will be different. By analyzing the differences, one may properly estimate the energy or type of radiation. Since those three metals are quite different, a large energy range can be covered.

3. **C** OSL = optically stimulated luminescence. Just like a TLD, an OSL dosimeter will gain trapped electrons when irradiated. To release these electrons, a TLD uses heat but an OSL uses light, hence "optically stimulated."

4. **B** Diodes are extremely sensitive, however, not quite stable for absolute dose measurements.

5. **C** An OSL dosimeter can be replaced every 2 months, whereas a film badge dosimeter should be replaced monthly. This is due to the wider dose range

7.12 Dose Survey and Exposure Monitoring (Answers)

of the OSL material. This being said, if OSLs are being used for personnel monitoring, they are usually replaced every month.

6. C When a TLD is heated, the trapped electrons are held at different energy levels which will release the electron at a different temperature. Some of these traps will release the electron at room temperature, so they are very unstable and not suited for dosimetry. These are the low number peaks and they have a lifetime in the order of minutes or seconds. The lifetime for peaks 4 and 5 is over 70 years meaning the traps are very stable, which is good for dosimetry, and are commonly used.

7. A G value = number of molecules/100 eV (dose).
The general principle of chemical dosimetry is that the color of the solution changes with irradiation, and the change in color is read by spectrophotometry.
For a given solution, the G value is roughly constant and slightly different for different beam qualities.

8. B MOSFET = MOS + FET.
MOS = metal oxide semiconductor.
FET = field effect transistor.
A MOSFET consists of a semiconductor material (silicon, just like a diode), but it has three terminals, a source, a gate, and a drain. The functioning of a MOSFET was discussed in an earlier question, but to repeat, the current in a MOSFET is induced by applying an external voltage between the source and the drain. The threshold of the external voltage required is changed by irradiation; thus, the dose is recorded by the voltage change.

9. B Proportional region. Ion chambers display different properties depending on the operating voltage. For dosimetry in radiation therapy, the operating voltage is typically 300 V. This is the "ion chamber" region because the response of the chamber at this voltage is flat regardless of energy. This is a desirable characteristic because the ion chamber is energy independent. Below 300 V is a region called the recombination region. In this region, the electric field is not strong enough to cause the ions and electrons to separate and be detected; rather, they recombine in the sensitive volume of the chamber. Above 300 V, there is a region called the proportional region. In this region, the response of the chamber is proportional to the energy. This is useful when trying to discriminate between different radiation types like alphas and betas. This is why neutron detectors operate in the region. A boron neutron detector detects neutrons because the incoming neutron reacts with the boron and produces an alpha particle. This is then detected. Around 1,000 V, an ion chamber is in the Geiger-Müller region. In this region, an interaction causes a huge avalanche of charged particles that is detected. A single photon will cause this avalanche, so it is useful for detecting a small amount of radiation but not quantifying the amount. Above 1,000 V, the ion chamber has an electric field that is strong enough to create ionizations without radiation. This is the continuous discharge region and at this level the ion chamber will break.

10. **C** Apply more pressure, and the bubbles will be removed.
A bubble detector uses liquid gas drops, which means the gas is in a liquid state because of pressure. After neutron irradiation, some liquid will become gas which can be visualized as bubbles; however, they can be removed by applying more pressure and becoming liquid again. In this way, a bubble detector can be reused.

7.13 Nuclear Medicine Procedures (Answers)

Quiz 1 (Level 2)

1. **D** With regard to ^{131}I given to a patient, contaminated linens and disposable food trays must be collected and stored for radioactive decay because the patient's secretions are radioactive. Patient vomiting within the first 24 h after administration can pose a radiation problem, and after patient discharge, the room must be decontaminated. After discharge the patient must be provided with radiation safety guidance that will help keep radiation dose to household members and the public as low as reasonably achievable.

2. **A** The dose rate in locations surrounding the patient's room (hallway, adjacent patient room, etc.) cannot exceed 2 mrem/h.

3. **C** "Thyroid bioassay" is a test done to all personnel involved in the administration and/or preparation of ^{131}I used for thyroid cancer treatment.

4. **E** All the statements are correct. The test must be performed within 72 h after the administration, and it measures the uptake of ^{131}I in the thyroid of the workers using a NaI crystal detector positioned close to the thyroid. Because of the volatility of ^{131}I liquid even when encapsulated, the potential exists for airborne release and subsequent ingestion by personnel during preparation and/or administration. Very little activity detected is enough to receive a significant dose to the thyroid. NaI is a scintillation crystal that emits light when a photon interacts in the crystal. By using photomultiplier tubes, the light produced in the crystal can be detected, and the amount and type of radiation present can be determined.

5. **B** ^{131}I and ^{32}P radionuclides are used for the treatment of thyroid cancer. Prior to administration there is always the chance of spilling from the vial or

7.13 Nuclear Medicine Procedures (Answers)

syringe, so radiation precautions should be applied at all times even though ^{32}P only emits beta particles. One must carefully watch for drainage from the injection site by checking the dressing because one can receive an extensive dose to the hands. ^{125}I and palladium-103 are used in the treatment of early stage prostate cancer with permanent implants.

6. A If a radionuclide spills from the vial or syringe upon administration, the worker should throw an absorbent paper, such as hospital chux, on the spill area and warn others not to enter the area of the spill. The radiation safety officer should be immediately notified. The therapist should not attempt to clean the spill without supervision from the RSO. If the spill occurs on the hands, wash with a mild soap and water.

7. C A radioactive source can be discarded into regular landfill once they have decayed at least ten half-lives. At this point, the radioactivity is indistinguishable from the background.

8. B A patient can be discharged after temporal implant, when sources have been removed and patient surveyed, and after a permanent implant when the dose rate at 1 m is <5 mrem/h.

9. A The appropriate device to check a spill area is the Geiger-Müller (G-M) counters.

10. B

11. C It takes much longer (30–40 min) to do a PET/CT scan. In a PET scan, the patient is translated though the ring of detectors and each slice is measured individually which takes significantly longer than a normal CT scan (<5 s). Therefore, many more patients can be scanned if only CT is being used.

12. B The energy of a CT scanner is usually 150 keV maximum. Remember that a CT scanner uses a diagnostic X-ray tube which emits a bremsstrahlung spectrum, so the mean energy is about 1/3 of the max energy. PET imaging, on the other hand, utilized 511 keV annihilation photons. If the shielding is sufficient for the 511 keV photons, it is more than enough for the CT component.

13. B 15 % on average. During a PET scan, a patient is typically injected with fluorodeoxyglucose which will be taken up in tissue that is highly metabolic (tumor tissue is highly metabolic). This uptake occurs over time, so the patient must wait from the injection to the scan.

14. D The maximal number of patients that a therapist can scan is around 2,000. However, this number is calculated from 50 mSv, which is for non-ALARA consideration.

7.14 Structural Shielding Design (Answers)

Quiz 1 (Level 2)

1. **C** Structural shielding design for radiation therapy installations is discussed in NCRP report 151. TG-43 describes a dose calculation formalism for brachytherapy. NCRP report 34 is used for structural shielding design and evaluation of medical X-ray and gamma-ray protection for energies up to 10 MeV. TG-40 describes periodic linac QA.

2. **A** Radiation protective barriers are designed to ensure that the dose equivalent received by any individual does not exceed the applicable maximum permissible value. They are designed to protect against primary radiation as well as scatter and leakage radiation.

3. **A** The designation of controlled or uncontrolled radiation areas depends on the level of radiation exposure in that area. Uncontrolled areas are designated as any area which is not under the supervision of a radiation protection supervisor, so it does not require any physical boundaries. On the other hand, a controlled area is an area under the supervision of a radiation protection supervisor. A controlled area should be labeled appropriately and should have physical boundaries. A supervised area is an area in which occupational exposure conditions are kept under review though protective measures and safety provisions are not needed. The permissible dose level is higher in a controlled area than in an uncontrolled area. The benefit of having a higher dose limit is that less shielding is required but monitoring of those areas is required. Before a vault is built, the uncontrolled and controlled areas must be clearly understood and defined.

4. **E** All statements are true.

5. **C** Secondary barrier is a barrier sufficient to attenuate stray radiation (leakage and scatter radiation). A barrier sufficient to attenuate the useful beam to the required degree is the primary barrier.

6. **E** Workload (W), use factor (U), occupancy factor (T), and distance (d) are all factors to be considered when calculating the barrier thickness. These will be addressed in the next few questions. The equation to calculate the primary barrier thickness is

$$B = Pd^2 / WUT$$

where B is the transmission of the primary barrier and P is the permissible dose limit per week. The number of TVLs $= -\log(B)$.
For scattered radiation the equation is

$$B = P d_{sca}^2 d_{sec}^2 / aWT \times 400 / F$$

7.14 Structural Shielding Design (Answers)

where dsca is the distance from the source to the patient and dsec is the distance from the patient to the point of interest. a is the scatter fraction that depends on the scattering angle. F is the field size incident on the patient. Notice there is no use factor because scatter is considered to be isotropic (all directions).

For leakage radiation:

$$B = 1{,}000 \times \mathrm{Pd}^2 / WT$$

The factor of 1,000 is used because this is the typical level of leakage radiation from a linac. Usually for a primary barrier, the leakage and scattered components are much smaller than the primary component.

7. C The use factor (U) is defined as the fraction of the operating time during which the radiation under consideration is directed toward a particular barrier. The use factor is usually assumed to be ¼ as there are four primary walls in a linac vault. This might not be true if a special procedure like TBI is performed often with the gantry directed at a single barrier. To be conservative, a use factor of 1 can be used. The occupancy factor (T) is the fraction of the operating time during which the area of interest is occupied by the individual. The occupancy factor is based on a 40 h week, so if a worker is operating the linac all week, the occupancy factor would be 1 (40/40). In an area like a storage closet, the occupancy factor could be as low as 1/40. To be conservative, an occupancy factor of 1 can be used. The distance (d) is the distance in meters from the radiation source to the area to be protected, and the workload (W) is the weekly dose delivered at 1 m from the source. The workload depends on how many patients are treated and what is the delivered dose at the isocenter. If high-dose SBRT procedures are common, the workload can increase.

8. B Full occupancy ($T=1$): work areas, offices, and nurse station.
Partial occupancy ($t=¼$): corridors, restrooms,, and elevators with operators.
Occasional occupancy ($t=1/8–1/16$): waiting rooms, restrooms, stairways, unattended elevators, and outside areas used only for pedestrians or vehicular traffic. The reason for the occupancy factor is to allow for thinner shielding. With the thinner shielding, the instantaneous dose rate might exceed the limit, but averaged over the course of the week, the likelihood of some individual standing in a hallway for 40 h is unlikely. This all plays into the ALARA principle.

9. C Concrete, lead, and steel can be used as barrier materials. The choice of barrier material depends on structural and spatial considerations. Concrete is the most used material because it is relatively cheap and easy to work with. Lead and steel can be used where space is at a premium as the density is much higher, so the TVL is much less.

10. Material density

A.	II.	Concrete	(2.3 g cm³)
B.	III.	Lead	(11.3 g cm³)
C.	I.	Steel	(7.8 g cm³)
D.	IV.	Polyethylene	(0.9 g cm³)

11. B The equivalent thickness of various materials is usually calculated using tenth-value layers (TVL) for the given beam energy. If such information is not available specifically for a given material, relative densities can be used in most cases.

12. E The amount of radiation scattered from the patient depends on the beam intensity, the quality of radiation, the area of the beam at the isocenter, and the scattering angle.

13. E All statements are correct. Unless a maze entranceway is provided, the treatment door must provide shielding equivalent to the wall surrounding the door. The door on megavoltage treatment rooms requires a motor drive as well as a means of manual operation in case of emergency, and a maze arrangement drastically reduces the shielding requirements for the door. With the proper maze design, the door is exposed mainly to scattered radiation of significantly reduced intensity and energy. The longer the maze and the thicker the wall separating the maze from the linac, the thinner the door can be. Typically the door is borated polyethylene layered with steel or lead. The borated polyethylene is used to attenuate neutrons that scatter down the maze. This is not a concern if the maximum energy of the linac is 10 MV or less.

14. B The function of the maze is to prevent direct incidence of radiation at the treatment door.

15. B With the proper maze design, the door is exposed mainly to multiply scattered radiation where the radiation is scattered at least twice before interacting with the door.

16. C Only high-energy X-ray beams (>10 MV) are contaminated with neutrons as the threshold for photons to generate neutrons in different materials is around 10 MeV.

17. B Neutron contamination is produced by high-energy photons incident on the target, flattening filter material, collimators, and other shielding components.

18. C The proper material for use at the door of a linac machine to thermalize and further reduce neutron dose is a few inches of a hydrogenous material such

as polyethylene. Remember that the most effective neutron shield is a hydrogenous material since the electrons are slowed down through elastic collisions with the hydrogen. High-Z materials do not effectively shield neutrons. A steel or lead sheet may be added to the door to protect against scattered X-rays.

19. B A longer maze (>5 m) is desirable in reducing the neutron fluence at the door, as well as a few inches of a hydrogenous material such as polyethylene added to the door to thermalize the neutrons and reduce the neutron dose further. The TVL of neutrons in air is around 4 m.

7.15 Radioactive Material Shipping (Answers)

Quiz 1 (Level 3)

1. B The US Department of Transportation (DOT) regulations 49CFR are the rules to follow in radioactive material shipping. NRC regulations 10CFR guide shipping for radioactive material of extremely strong activity, normally nuclear fuels, which would not be used in radiotherapy.

2. C TI = transportation index. This is the reading in mrem/h at 1 m from the package surface.

3. C Packages should never have a reading more than 10 mrem/h at 1 m from the surface, per DOT regulations. Thus, the reading for TI is between 1 and 10. If the reading at 1 m is less than 1 mR/h, it should not be labeled.

4. B A strong tight container and Type A and Type B packages are normally used for radioactive material. The type of container is determined by the amount of activity being shipped. All containers must have a radioactive type 7 label.

5. A A strong tight container can be used in normal transportation, which can survive in small accident. For this reason, the activity inside the container cannot be too strong in order to reduce the potential pollution to the environment in case of an accident. The maximal tolerance is 0.001A.

The A value is the activity limit for a particular radionuclide.
The A value is the criteria on which the package is chosen for shipping. Here are the definitions for package choosing:
  0–0.001 A: strong tight container
  0.001–1 A: Type A package
  1–3,000 A: Type B package
  Above 3,000 A: NRC will handle it – too strong to be implemented in radiotherapy

6. **B** Notice how as the energy of the radionuclide increases, the *A* value decreases. This means that less material is able to be shipped in a particular container.

   Please note that for ^{60}Co the *A* value is only 10.8 Ci, whereas a source in Gamma Knife is about 33 Ci, so ^{60}Co sources cannot be shipped by Type A package, not even a single ^{60}Co source! A Type B package must be used to ship any number of ^{60}Co source for Gamma Knife.

7. **A** A strong tight container is always used to ship prostate implant seeds due to the low energy of I-125. The total activity for a seed implant is typically 40–50 mCi.

8. **A** Type A package can handle activity less or equal to 1A. Beyond this level a Type B package is normally used.

9. **A** White I label means zero reading at 1 m from package surface, that is, TI=0. Since there is no exposure at 1 m, there is no need to indicate a TI.

10. **B** The maximal TI is 3 if the package is carried with passenger.

11. **C** Type B package is for ^{60}Co shipment. There is no Type C package.

12. **B** A single source ^{60}Co is about 33 Ci, so a Type B package is still needed.

13. **C** The upper limit for Type B package is 3,000A. The upper limit for Type A package is 1A.

14. **C** A student is qualified if he/she has the proper training on how to handle radioactive materials.

15. **B** There are three labels for radioactive packages: White I, Yellow II, and Yellow III. The label is dependent on the TI.

7.16 Summary (Answers)

Quiz 1 (Level 3)

1. **C** The ALARA limit is essentially 10 %, i.e., 5 mSv in 12 months. It is rare that a therapist has more than 5 mSv annually. Nevertheless, she should be careful during the daily work. For instance, try to avoid the door of the vault if high-energy X-ray beam is on. It is also important to remember that she is not considered pregnant unless she declares it IN WRITING.

7.16 Summary (Answers)

2. B The ALARA limit is 10 % of the annual limit, which is 5 mSv. Under a good ALARA program, a reading of 2–3 mSv would be considered normal for medical physicists who handled a lot of brachytherapy cases. A reading of 5.5 mSv is a little too high. The RSO should examine the program, find out the reasons, and make improvements to reduce the exposure if possible.

3. D The time of pregnancy is important. At a very early time, e.g., 4 weeks, the exposure could cause a miscarriage. In the middle of pregnancy, mental development problem is the major concern. In the late pregnancy, the baby is more likely to have disease in the early childhood.

4. C The shielding for linear accelerator is normally much more than what is required for HDR treatments. It is true that the HDR source is isotropic, so there are only primary barriers, but even the secondary barriers in a linac vault will be sufficient for an HDR unit. Following installation, a documented shielding survey must be completed to verify that everything is as expected.

5. C A double maze design significantly reduces the probability of scattered neutrons at the door because the neutrons have to scatter at least twice before they reach the door. This being said, an "L" maze without a door is uncommon.

6. C A strong tight container is sufficient. The maximum strength per seed is normally less than 10 mCi. Type A is normally for HDR Ir-192 sources.

7. A For a full strength of 10 Ci, the exposure should be at 0.5 cGy level if a physician stays for 5 min. The arm is normally 1 m long, and a tool of at least 10 cm effective length is normally used; thus, the distance is approximated to be 1 m.

8. C IMRT increases the leakage at the "treatment head" of the linear accelerator by about three to five times. IMRT delivers about the same dose as conventional treatments but the number of MUs is much higher. Leakage radiation is dependent on the number of MUs whereas the primary and scatter radiation is dependent on the delivered dose. The energy for leakage is the same energy as primary X-rays. Thus, a HVL at primary energy level is sufficient to account for this increase. The HVL at scattering energy is much thinner because the energy is lower and hence is insufficient.

9. B High-energy electrons cannot produce neutrons. Only high-energy photons can produce neutrons.

10. B This is most likely the case as double-strand breaks are much more difficult for the cell to repair.

11. C   Larger dose per fraction is better for local control, and this is also the idea of radiosurgery.

12. A   It might be a little unlucky to sit with a patient who was just released to the public; however, this amount of exposure is within the public limit and could not cause any deterministic damage.

13. D   Air kerma rate constant is the reason. The air kerma rate for Ir-192 is much higher than I-125 due to the higher specific activity and energy. Answer C tells partially the truth but still not the exact answer.

14. C   3 TVLs are the rule of thumb for vault shielding.

15. B   If the positrons are more energetic, they will have more "free path" before they eventually annihilate with electrons; therefore, the image quality will be worse than ^{18}F-labeled images. However, the gamma photons from annihilations have the same energy of 0.511 MeV as before, simply because those annihilated positrons are at thermal level – only at this energy level they can be captured by electrons. In other words, the positron energy affects the image quality, but they do not exit the patient and therefore do not affect the shielding. When designing a facility to shield a positron emitter, the 511 keV photons are the radiation that needs consideration.

16. C   Although everything needs to be calculated, a conserved thickness of 1 in. is needed for all walls. Sometimes 0.5 in. is acceptable; however, this is not a conservative value.

Quality Assurance

Contents

8.1 QA Guidance and Protocols (Questions) 513
8.2 Requirements and Tolerance for QA Procedures (Questions) 516
8.3 QA for Treatment Planning System (Questions) 525
8.4 Equipment or Devices for Measurement (Questions) 527
8.5 QA Procedures (Questions) 532
8.6 QA Guidance and Protocols (Answers) 534
8.7 Requirements and Tolerance for QA Procedures (Answers) 535
8.8 QA for Treatment Planning System (Answers) 541
8.9 Equipment or Devices for Measurement (Answers) 542
8.10 QA Procedures (Answers) 545

8.1 QA Guidance and Protocols (Questions)

Quiz-1 (Level 2)

1. Which of the following associations set minimum standards of QA required for hospitals seeking accreditations?
   A. American College of Radiology (ACR)
   B. American Association of Medical Physics (AAPM)
   C. Nuclear Regulatory Commission (NRC)
   D. Joint Commission for Accreditation of Health Care Organization (JCAHO)

2. The Intersociety Council for Radiation Oncology (ISCRO) specifies in the blue book that:
   A. I, II, and III only
   B. I and III only
   C. II and IV only

D. IV only
E. All are correct
I. At least one dosimetrist must cover a center for up to 300 patients treated annually.
II. At least one physicist must cover a center for up to 400 patients treated annually.
III. At least one radiation oncologist must cover a center for up to 200–250 patients treated annually.
IV. Dosimetrists can perform physics work as long as a physicist established the procedures, directs the activities, and reviews the results.

3. Which of the following statements is NOT true?
A. Dosimetrists can perform calibration of radiation generators or sources.
B. Calibration of radiation generators or sources is the exclusive responsibility of the medical physicist.
C. The radiation oncologist undoubtedly has the overall responsibility for the conduct of the entire treatment process.
D. A dual-energy linear accelerator can provide all the beams necessary for modern radiotherapy.

4. What is the primary physicist's role when radiotherapy equipment is purchased?
A. Write technical specifications.
B. Share responsibilities between the radiation oncologist and administrator.
C. Decide the budget.
D. Select the location to be installed.

5. A radiotherapy equipment acceptance test is done to:
A. I, II, and III only
B. I and III only
C. II and IV only
D. IV only
E. All are correct
I. Demonstrate that the product meets the specifications of the manufacturer
II. Prove that the product arrives on specified date and time at the hospital or institution
III. Satisfies the legal requirements of equipment safety
IV. Train the physicist on the new equipment or product

6. A qualified medical physicist must:
A. I, II, and III only
B. I and III only
C. II and IV only
D. IV only
E. All are correct

I. Have a MS or PhD degree in physics, medical physics, or a closely related field.
II. Have a minimum of a high school diploma.
III. Have a certification in radiation oncology physics by the American Board of Radiology, the American board of Medical Physics, or another appropriate certifying body.
IV. Have a certification by the American Association of Medical Dosimetrists

7. Which of the following are responsibilities of the physicist?
A. I, II, and III only
B. I and III only
C. II and IV only
D. IV only
E. All are correct
I. Acceptance testing of new equipment
II. Commissioning of new equipment
III. Calibration of equipment
IV. Installation of new equipment

8. Which of the following parameters are considered during the radiation survey performed by the physicist after installation of new equipment?
A. I, II, and III only
B. I and III only
C. II and IV only
D. IV only
E. All are correct
I. Dose rate output
II. Machine on time
III. Use factor
IV. Occupancy factor

9. Which of the following is NOT included on a formal radiation protection survey after completion of new equipment installation?
A. Measurement of head leakage and area survey
B. Tests of interlocks and warning lights
C. Emergency switches
D. Radiation dose received by installation workers

10. Which of the following is the comprehensive guidance for radiation oncology QA from the AAPM?
A. TG-40
B. TG-43
C. TG-51
D. TG-21

11. Since new technologies such as IMRT were developed in recent decades, AAPM generated another QA guideline for linear accelerators as an important amendment to meet the new needs. Which of the following is that report of AAPM?
A. TG-135
B. TG-142
C. TG-144
D. TG-101

12. What is the protocol of AAPM for absolute dosimetry QA for high-energy photon and electron beams after year 1999?
A. TG-40
B. TG-43
C. TG-51
D. TG-21

13. What is the difference between acceptance testing and commissioning of equipment?
A. They are essentially the same.
B. They are totally irrelevant.
C. Acceptance test runs a small portion of dataset of commissioning.
D. Commissioning runs a small portion of dataset of acceptance test.

8.2 Requirements and Tolerance for QA Procedures (Questions)

Quiz-1 (Level 2)

1. The approximately overall uncertainty to a point when using wedges in a treatment field is:
A. 1.6 %
B. 2.0 %
C. 3.0 %
D. 5.5 %

2. Which of the following is NOT a method used to check jaw symmetry?
A Graph paper
B. Film
C. Machinist's dial indicator
D. Front pointer

3. Which of the following gantry angles should be used when checking light versus x-ray field alignment for acceptance testing of a linac?
A. I, II, and III only
B. I and III only

C. II and IV only
D. IV only
E. All are correct
I. 0° gantry angle
II. 90° gantry angle
III. 180° gantry angle
IV. 270° gantry angle

4. According to the AAPM guidelines, the alignment between the light field and the x-ray field should be:
A. 2 mm diameter circle
B. ±2 mm or 1 % on a side
C. ±1 mm or 1 % on a side
D. ±5 mm or 1 % on a side

5. Which of the following QA tests are done using films that show star patterns with a dark central region?
A. II, III, and IV only
B. I and III only
C. II and IV only
D. IV only
E. All are correct
I. Field symmetry
II. Collimator rotation
III. Table rotation
IV. Gantry rotation

6. The split-field test is used to detect:
A. I, II, and III only
B. I and III only
C. II and IV only
D. IV only
E. All are correct
I. Focal spot displacement
II. Asymmetry of collimator jaws
III. Displacement in the collimator or gantry rotation axis
IV. Light field with x-ray field alignment

7. The most practical method of specifying clinical beam energy is:
A. Depth-dose distribution
B. Sandwiched film between buildup sheets
C. Machinist's dial indicator
D. Clarkson's method

8. Which of the following should be considered in order to determine clinical beam energy?
A. I, II, and III only
B. I and III only

C. II and IV only
D. IV only
E. All are correct
I. Ion chamber diameter should be larger than 3 mm diameter.
II. Ion chamber diameter should be smaller than 3 mm diameter.
III. Absolute values of the percent depth dose should be used for comparing depth-dose distribution with published data.
IV. Depth-dose ratios for depths beyond the depth of Dmax should be used for comparing depth-dose distribution with published data.

9. The depth-dose distribution for photon clinical beam energy is specified at:
A. 10×10 cm field size, 100 cm SAD, 10 cm depth
B. 40×40 cm field size, 100 cm SSD, 10 cm depth
C. 10×10 cm field size, 100 cm SSD, 10 cm depth
D. 10×10 cm field size, 100 cm SAD, Dmax

10. Which is the difference in the depth-dose ratio or ionization ration acceptance from the published values data when performing photon beam energy measurement?
A. ±1 %
B. ±2 %
C. ±3 %
D. ±4 %

11. For acceptance testing, photon beam flatness should be checked for which of the following situations?
A. I, II, and III only
B. I and III only
C. II and IV only
D. IV only
E. All are correct
I. For a 10×10 field size at least at 10 cm and Dmax depth
II. For the maximum field size at least at 10 cm and Dmax depth
III. For a 10×10 field size at a depth of 10 cm
IV. Using diagonal scans

12. Which of the following methods are used for electron beam energy measurements?
A. Depth-dose or depth ionization curve for a broad beam
B. Depth-dose distribution measured at depth 10 cm using a 10×10 cm field size at 100 SSD
C. Using a radiographic film to measure the distribution of activity
D. Depth-dose curve in a water phantom for a broad beam at Dmax

13. Match the following QA test with the correct tolerance:
A. Optical distance indicator
B. Gantry and collimator angles

8.2 Requirements and Tolerance for QA Procedures (Questions)   519

C. Sag of couch
D. Jaw symmetry
E. Light beam with x-ray beam
F. Collimator rotation
G. Beam flatness and symmetry
I. ±1 mm from baseline
II. 1°
III. 1 mm diameter circle
IV. 2 mm
V. ±1 % change from baseline
VI. 2 mm from baseline
VII. 2 mm or 1 % on a side

14. Which of the following statements is NOT true?
A. Short-lived interstitial sources in the form of seeds, wires, or seed-loaded ribbons can be tested by visual inspection behind a leaded glass window.
B. A standard seed of a different isotope should be used to calibrate the well ionization chamber.
C. For a batch of a large number of sources, a randomly selected sample of three or four ribbons of a given strength should be check for calibration.
D. ^{125}I seeds are difficult to calibrate because of the low energy of the emitted photons.

15. Acceptance procedures for a HDR remote afterloading unit should include:
A. I, II, and III only
B. I and III only
C. II and IV only
D. IV only
E. All are correct
I. Operational testing of the afterloader unit
II. Radiation safety check of the facility
III. Checking of source calibration and transport
IV. Checking of treatment planning software

16. A linear accelerator is ready to be used for patient treatments:
A. After acceptance testing is done, reviewed, and approved
B. After commissioning is done, reviewed, and approved
C. After QA is done, reviewed, and approved
D. After the vendor installation is completed

17. Linear accelerator commissioning is completed:
A. After calibration of all modalities and energies according to current protocols
B. After a transverse, longitudinal, and diagonal dose profiles for all modalities and energies at Dmax for electrons and selected depths for photons are acquired

C. After the beam data has been input into the treatment planning computer and the computer generated dose distributions have been checked
D. After all output factors as a function of field size for all photon energies and all electrons as a function of cones and standard insets are complete

18. Acceptance testing and commissioning of the treatment planning computer system include:
    A. I, II, and III only
    B. I and III only
    C. II and IV only
    D. IV only
    E. All are correct
    I. Checking the accuracy and linearity of input digitizers, output plotters, and printers
    II. Checking the accuracy of dose distributions for a selected set of treatment conditions against measured distributions or manual calculations
    III. Checking the algorithm accuracy, precision, limitations, and special features
    IV. Checking the treatment planning computer system's company records

19. Which of the following QA tests must be done daily on a linear accelerator?
    A. Emergency off switches check
    B. Door interlock check
    C. Light/radiation field coincidence check
    D. Tabletop sag check

20. Which of the following QA test must be done daily on a simulator?
    A. Fluoroscopic image quality
    B. Field size indicator
    C. Distance indicator (ODI)
    D. Exposure rate

21. The NRC requires full calibration of a teletherapy unit:
    A. I, II, and III only
    B. I and III only
    C. II and IV only
    D. IV only
    E. All are correct
    I. Before the first medical use of the unit and at intervals not exceeding 1 year
    II. Whenever spot-check measurements differ by more than 5 % from the output at the last full calibration
    III. Following replacement of the source or relocation of the unit
    IV. Following repairs that could affect the source exposure assembly

22. Some calibration checks of a teletherapy units required by NRC include:
    A. I, II, and III only
    B. I and III only

C. II and IV only
D. IV only
E. All are correct
I. Output being within ±3 %
II. On-off error
III. Uniformity of radiation field and its dependence on the orientation of the radiation field
IV. Timer constancy and linearity over the range of use

23. As per ICRP recommendations, simulator annual QA tube leakage must not exceed:
A. 1 R/h at 1 m
B. 0.1 R/min at 1 m
C. 0.1 R/h at 1 m
D. 1 R/h at 10 m

24. When performing simulator annual QA tube leakage tests:
A. I, II, and III only
B. I and III only
C. II and IV only
D. IV only
E. All are correct
I. Measurement of tube leakages must be done using highest kVp setting.
II. Measurement of tube leakages should be done using any combination of kVp and mA.
III. Measurement of tube leakages must be done using the highest mA.
IV. Measurement of tube leakage should be done with the machine in the off position.

25. Simulator kVp accuracy must be:
A. Within 10 kVp from selected at control panel
B. Within 5 kVp from selected at control panel
C. Within 3 kVp from selected at control panel
D. Within 15 kVp from selected at control panel

26. Simulator mA linearity is done:
A. I, II, and III only
B. I and III only
C. II and IV only
D. IV only
E. All are correct
I. To measure the mA setting versus the exposure rate proportionality
II. To measure the exposure at different mA settings
III. To measure exposure as a function of mA setting
IV. To measure exposure as a function of tube current and time setting

27. Ionization chamber and electrometer systems must be sent to an ADCL for calibration at intervals not exceeding:
A. Every six months
B. One year
C. Two years
D. Five years

28. Instruments used to measure relative dose or dose distribution (diodes, TLD, films) should be calibrated by an ADCL every:
A. Six months
B. One year
C. Two years
D. No required calibration

29. Calibration of survey meters must be done at intervals not exceeding:
A. Every six months
B. One year
C. Two years
D. Five years

30. Closed-circuit television and audio monitoring systems:
A. I, II, and III only
B. I and III only
C. II and IV only
D. IV only
E. All are correct
I. Are required in treatment rooms
II. Should be checked daily for proper operation
III. Should be turned on for all treatments
IV. Are not necessary if any tracking system (calypso, respiratory gating, etc.) is used

31. Which of the following statements is NOT correct?
A. Port films must be approved by the physician before the second treatment fraction.
B. MLC inter-leaf leakage should be <3 %.
C. If only one 0.5 cm leaf is retracted when it is supposed to be extended, the treatment can be done because the radiation through 0.5 cm is minimal.
D. The MLC pattern must be checked by the therapist for each fraction.

32. Percentage depth-dose QA should be done:
A. I, II, and III only
B. I and III only
C. II and IV only
D. IV only

8.2 Requirements and Tolerance for QA Procedures (Questions) 523

E. All are correct
I. At the time of commissioning
II. Following repair
III. Monthly check
IV. Annually check

33. QA acceptance tolerance for beam flatness and symmetry are:
A. Both beam flatness and symmetry at depth 10 cm should be <3 %.
B. Flatness at depth 10 cm should be 3 %, and symmetry at depth 10 cm should be 2 %.
C. Flatness at depth 10 cm should be 2 %, and symmetry at depth 10 cm should be 3 %.
D. Flatness at Dmax should be 3 %, and symmetry at Dmax should be 2 %.

34. Which of the following CT-simulator QA tests are correct?
A. I, II, and III only
B. I and III only
C. II and IV only
D. IV only
E. All are correct
I. HU or CT number for water should be checked daily with a tolerance of ±5 HU.
II. CT image noise should be checked daily.
III. Electron density to CT number conversion should be checked annually or after calibration.
IV. Spatial and contrast resolution should be checked annually.

35. Which of the following gantry CT-simulator statements are correct?
A. I, II, and III only
B. I and III only
C. II and IV only
D. IV only
E. All are correct
I. The digitally indicated angle of the CT-scanner gantry with respect to the nominal vertical imaging plane should be accurate within 1°.
II. A ready-pack film taped to a square acrylic or water-equivalent plastic sheet is used for CT-scanner gantry angle accuracy test.
III. After the gantry is tilted for test purposes, it should return to the nominal vertical imaging plane.
IV. A CT scan for a brain can be done using a 5° caudal gantry tilt.

36. Which of the following statements are true about CT image noise?
A. I, II, and III only
B. I and III only
C. II and IV only
D. IV only

E. All are correct
I. The standard deviation of pixel values in a region of interest (ROI) within a uniform phantom is an indication of image noise.
II. CT image noise can be expressed in terms of standard deviation of the CT numbers in Hounsfield units (HU).
III. CT image noise can be expressed as a percent of the linear attenuation coefficient of water.
IV. CT image noise determines the lower limit of subject contrast that can be distinguished by the observer.

37. Which of the following is the standard for representing and exchanging medical imaging data?
A. Digital Image Communications in Medicine (DICOM)
B. National Electrical Manufacturers Association (NEMA)
C. Picture archiving and communication system (PACS)
D. Hewlett Packard (HP) image transfer

38. Some of the QA for CT-simulation software includes:
A. I, II, and III only
B. I and III only
C. II and IV only
D. IV only
E. All are correct
I. Image input test
II. Structure delineation
III. Multimodality image registration
IV. Image reconstruction

39. Complete calibration of a linac should be performed:
A. Daily
B. Quarterly
C. Every 6 months
D. Annually

40. All electron energy QA must be done at least:
A. Daily
B. Twice a weekly
C. Quarterly
D. Semiannually

41. A test of the constancy of dose per MU when using photon beams QA must be done at least:
A. Daily
B. Weekly
C. Quarterly
D. Semiannually

8.3 QA for Treatment Planning System (Questions)

42. If a dual-energy linac accelerator uses 6 and 18 MV:
A. Only the highest energy should be checked daily.
B. The output of both photon energies must be checked daily.
C. Neither photon energy must be checked daily.
D. Only the lower energy should be checked daily.

43. The accuracy of the mechanical isocenter can be checked by:
A. Using a film to measure coincidence between light beam and radiation beam
B. Using a front pointer positioned at the isocenter and a horizontal rod with a fine point held in a ring stand
C. Rotating the gantry 360° and looking at the light field projection
D. Moving the couch in-out, side to side, and up and down while the gantry is in a fixed position

44. The output of cobalt-60 units must be checked:
A. Daily
B. Weekly
C. Monthly
D. Annually

8.3 QA for Treatment Planning System (Questions)

Quiz-1 (Level 2)

1. Which of the following components should be tested periodically in the treatment planning system?
A. I, II, and III only
B. I and III only
C. II and IV only
D. IV only
E. All are correct
I. Measure data
II. Data entry
III. Data output
IV. Algorithm

2. IMRT QA involves:
A. I, II, and III only
B. I and III only
C. II and IV only
D. IV only
E. All are correct
I. The irradiation of a phantom to verify the delivered dose distribution versus the planned dose distribution
II. Verification with hand MU calculations

III. Verification of treatment safety parameters
IV. Verification that the calculation point is not close to the MLC edge or in high dose gradient region

3. Which of the following instruments can be used for IMRT QA?
A. I, II, and III only
B. I and III only
C. II and IV only
D. IV only
E. All are correct
I. Film
II. Diode
III. Ion chamber
IV. Personal dosimetry

4. Which of the following treatment modalities cannot be used in the treatment of stereotactic radiosurgery?
A. Linear accelerator
B. Gamma Knife
C. CyberKnife
D. HDR

5. Which of the following are acceptance tests done on a TPS?
A. I, II, and III only
B. I and III only
C. II and IV only
D. IV only
E. All are correct
I. Beam description
II. Dose display, DVH
III. Electron beam dose calculation
IV. Hard copy output

6. What are the criteria for gamma analysis for IMRT QA?
A. 5 mm distance, 5 % in dose difference
B. 4 mm distance, 4 % in dose difference
C. 3 mm distance, 3 % in dose difference
D. 2 mm distance, 2 % in dose difference

7. What measurements are input to commission the TPS?
A. Data from annual QA
B. Data from machine commissioning
C. Data from monthly QA
D. Gold data provided by vendor

8. What can be used for enhance dynamic wedge (EDW) commissioning?
A. Ion chamber and water tank
B. Film, chamber, and solid-water phantom
C. Ion chamber and solid wedges
D. MOSFET and solid-water phantom

9. Can gold data be used for planning?
A. Never, since gold data has a lot uncertainty.
B. No, gold data is from vendor thus cannot be used even though very likely they have less than 2 % uncertainty.
C. Yes, since gold data always has less than 2 % uncertainty.
D. Yes, but only if it is commissioned and less than 2 % uncertainty.

8.4 Equipment or Devices for Measurement (Questions)

Quiz-1 (Level 2)

1. In what year did the international commission on radiation units and measurements (ICRU) adopt the Roentgen as the unit of measuring x and γ radiation exposure?
A. 1895
B. 1896
C. 1898
D. 1828

2. Electronic equilibrium is said to exist if:
A. I, II, and III only
B. I and III only
C. II and IV only
D. IV only
E. All are correct
I. The ionization lost in a free-air chamber is compensated by the ionization gained.
II. The electrons deposit their energy outside the free-air chamber volume.
III. The ionization lost at the end of the specified volume is compensated for ionization gained at the beginning of the specified volume in a free-air chamber.
IV. Electrons produced by photons in a specified volume spend all their energies by ionization in air outside the region of ion collection or volume.

3. Which of the following ionization chambers is an instrument used in the measurement of the Roentgen and generally used for calibration of secondary instruments designed for field use?
A. Thimble chambers
B. Free-air ionization chamber

C. Farmer chamber
D. Parallel-plate chamber

4. What is the maximum energy that a free-air ionization chamber can accurately measure?
A. 6 MeV
B. 2 MeV
C. 3 MeV
D. 10 MeV

5. The thimble chamber walls are:
A. I, II, and III only
B. I and III only
C. II and IV only
D. IV only
E. All are correct
I. Air equivalent material
II. Made so that electronic equilibrium occurs inside the cavity
III. Effective atomic number same as that of air
IV. A solid shell

6. Which of the following wall materials cannot be used on a thimble chamber?
A. Graphite
B. Tungsten
C. Bakelite
D. Mixture of graphite and Bakelite

7. Chambers desirable characteristics include:
A. I, II, and III only
B. I and III only
C. II and IV only
D. IV only
E. All are correct
I. Minimal variation in sensitivity or exposure calibration factor over a wide range of photon energies
II. Suitable volume to allow measurements for the expected range of exposures
III. Minimal variation in sensitivity with the direction of incident radiation
IV. Minimal stem leakage

8. Which of the following chambers are used to measure surface dose?
A. I, II, and III only
B. I and III only
C. II and IV only
D. IV only
E. All are correct

8.4 Equipment or Devices for Measurement (Questions)

I. Parallel-plate chamber
II. Farmer chamber
III. Extrapolation chamber
IV. Thimble chamber

9. An instrument used to search for lost clinical radioactive implant source is a:
A. Survey meter
B. Thimble chamber
C. Geiger-Muller counters
D. Extrapolation chamber

10. A survey meter:
A. I, II, and III only
B. I and III only
C. II and IV only
D. IV only
E. All are correct
I. Is used to measure dose rate around an implanted patient and patient room
II. Is used to survey in and around the storage area in which radioactive materials are kept
III. Is used to survey areas around radiation producing machines such as ^{60}Co units
IV. Is used to calibrates linear accelerators or ^{60}Co units

11. Proportional counters are NOT used to:
A. Discriminate the type of contamination in a survey (β, γ, α)
B. Count radioactive spills
C. Measure dose around an implanted patient
D. Generate a CT image

12. Which detector will you used if your department receives a radioactive source material package and you are called to monitor the package?
A. Ionization chamber
B. Survey meter
C. Proportional counter
D. G-M counter

13. Which of the following are true about G-M detectors?
A. I, II, and III only
B. I and III only
C. II and IV only
D. IV only
E. All are correct
I. Used to survey operating rooms, personnel, and instruments after procedures with radioactive material
II. Find lost radioactive seeds or ribbons
III. Search for holes in the walls of the linear accelerator room
IV. Use as an in-room radiation monitor for treatment room (not in beam)

14. Ionization chambers are used to:
A. I, II, and III only
B. I and III only
C. II and IV only
D. IV only
E. All are correct
I. Calibrate linear accelerators or ^{60}Co treatment units
II. Measure treatment beam characteristics
III. Used in a linear accelerator monitor chamber
IV. Search for holes in the walls of the linear accelerator room

15. Unsealed ion chambers must be corrected for temperature and pressure changes because:
A. Density or mass of air in the chamber volume will increase or decrease.
B. The ions collected will increase.
C. The ion chamber will expand.
D. The dose buildup effect.

16. The density or mass of air in the ion chamber or the chamber reading for a given exposure will increase as:
A. Temperature increases and pressure increases.
B. Temperature decreases and pressure decreases.
C. Temperature increases and pressure decreases.
D. Temperature decreases and pressure increases.

17. Temperature-pressure correction factor is given by:
A. $C_{tp} = (760/p) \times (273+t/295)$
B. $F = [(SSD_2 + d_m/SSD_1 + d_m)(SSD_1 + d/SSD_2 + d)]^2$
C. $s = 4A/p$
D. $C_{tp} = (760/t) \times (273 + p/295)$

18. If the temperature is 22 °C and the pressure is 750 mm of mercury, the correction needed to an ionization chamber would be:
A. 0.8622
B. 119.79
C. 1.0133
D. 0.0133

19. The standard laboratories calibrate chambers under the conditions present at the time of calibration and then converted to specific atmospheric conditions of:
A. Pressure of 760 mmHg and temperature of 22 °C
B. Temperature of 760 mmHg and pressure of 22 °C
C. Pressure of 760 mmHg and temperature of 295.2 °C
D. Temperature of 273.2 mmHg and pressure of 22 °C

8.4 Equipment or Devices for Measurement (Questions)

20. Which of the following types of radiation can be detected by a Geiger counter?
A. I, II, and III only
B. I and III only
C. II and IV only
D. IV only
E. All are correct
I. Alpha particles
II. Beta particles
III. Gamma rays
IV. X-rays

21. Which of the following are considered portable radiation survey instruments?
A. I, II, and III only
B. I and III only
C. II and IV only
D. IV only
E. All are correct
I. Pocket dosimeter
II. Survey meter
III. Film badge
IV. Geiger-Muller counter

22. The reason that diodes cannot be used for absolute dosimetry is:
A. Not sensitive enough
B. Easy to brake
C. Too many dependencies on other factors
D. Cannot be used in water

23. Which of the following can be used for EPID QA?
A. Water phantom
B. Solid-water phantom
C. Las Vegas phantom
D. keV cubic phantom

24. Does the electrometer need to be calibrated with ion chamber in ADCL?
A. Yes, they should be calibrated together.
B. Not necessary, although normally they are.
C. They should be calibrated separately.
D. Only the chamber is calibrated; there is no need to calibrate electrometer.

25. Which of the following can be used for on-patient measurements?
I. TLDs
II. Radiochromatic film
III. Ion chamber
IV. MOSFETs

A. I and II
B. I, III, and IV
C. I and IV
D. All of them

8.5 QA Procedures (Questions)

Quiz-1 (Level 3)

1. If the barometer is broken, what should the physicist do during the QA?
A. Use the number of last QA, since the pressure will not change much.
B. Call the nearby airport to find out.
C. Stop the QA.
D. Make the correction of pressure to be 1.0.

2. After completing TG-51 measurement if the result is 3 % off, what should be done next?
A. Call the vendor to fix the machine.
B. Nothing, this is within the tolerance.
C. Adjust the corresponding linac to ensure the calibration is correct.
D. Change the parameters in TPS since the machine output changes.

3. How would you check the collimator angle accuracy?
A. Use a film and a level.
B. Use a level, and rotate gantry 90°.
C. Use a ruler and a level.
D. Use a graph paper and a level.

4. How would you check the alignment of the light versus radiation field?
A. Use the laser to define the field and irradiate the field.
B. Use field light to define the field, mark the field size on the film, and then irradiate the field.
C. Use field light to define the field on a film, mark the field size, and then irradiate the field and measure with a diode.
D. Use field light to define the field on a phantom, put an ion chamber at the edge of the field, and irradiate the field.

5. What is the general idea for monthly output check QA?
A. Measure the output in a given solid phantom geometry with an ion chamber, correct for temperature and pressure, and compare the result to a baseline measurement.

8.5 QA Procedures (Questions)

B. Measure the output in water phantom with a diode, correct for temperature and pressure, and compare the result to a baseline measurement.
C. Measure the output in a given solid phantom geometry with film, and compare the result to a baseline film.
D. Measure the output in a given solid phantom geometry with a diode array, correct for temperature and pressure, and compare the result to a baseline measurement.

6. What is the general idea for monthly energy check QA?
A. Spot-check the PDD with an ion chamber in solid water or water and compare to the baseline.
B. Measure the PDD with chamber in a water phantom and compare to baseline.
C. Measure the TMR with chamber in a water phantom and compare to baseline.
D. Measure the TMR with film in a solid phantom and compare to baseline.

7. What does a "picket fence" test check?
A. It is a QA for mechanical accuracy of the dynamic MLC position.
B. It is a QA for mechanical accuracy of the enhanced dynamic wedge position.
C. It is a QA for mechanical accuracy of the static MLC positions.
D. It is a QA for mechanical accuracy of a static wedge position.

8. How could you check the centricity of the cross hair?
A. Use cross hair aligned with graph paper and rotate couch.
B. Use cross hair aligned with graph paper and rotate collimator.
C. Use cross hair aligned with graph paper and rotate gantry.
D. Use cross hair aligned with film and rotate couch.

9. How would you QA the couch motion and readout accuracy?
A. Use graph paper and the digital console.
B. Use jaw-defined field, graph paper, and film.
C. Use lasers and digital console.
D. Use film and digital console.

10. What is the general idea to test MU linearity of a linear accelerator?
A. Compare the chamber readouts ratio for a series of known MUs.
B. Compare the chamber readouts for a certain MUs to that of the same MUs but being interrupted several times in the middle of delivery.
C. Compare the chamber readouts for 2 identical time intervals set by personal clock with long beam times.
D. Compare the chamber readout for a certain MUs to the baseline readout.

8.6 QA Guidance and Protocols (Answers)

Quiz-1 (Level 2)

1. **D** Joint Commission for Accreditation of Health Care Organization (JCAHO) sets minimum standards of QA required for hospital seeking accreditations. The American College of Radiology (ACR) and American Association of Medical Physics (AAPM) are organizations that develop models for QA programs in radiation oncology. In addition, mandatory programs with QA components have been instituted by the Nuclear Regulatory Commission (NRC) and the individual states.

2. **E** All of the statements are correct.

3. **A** Calibration of radiation generators or sources is the exclusive responsibility of the medical physicist, but the radiation oncologist has the overall responsibility for the conduct of the entire treatment process.

5. **A** The purchase of radiotherapy equipment is a shared responsibility between the radiation oncologist, the physicist, and the hospital administrators. The physicist's role is primarily to write technical specifications although all groups participate in the decision process.

6. **B** A radiotherapy equipment acceptance test is done by the manufacturer with the physicist to demonstrate that the product meets the specifications contained in its brochures and satisfies the legal requirements of equipment safety. Following acceptance testing, a legal document is signed by both the physicist and the manufacturer stating that the device meets all the requirements.

7. **B** A qualified medical physicist must have a M.S or PhD degree in physics, medical physics, or a closely related field and a certification in radiation oncology physics by the American Board of Radiology, the American board of Medical Physics, or another appropriate certifying body. A qualified medical dosimetrist must have a minimum of a high school diploma and a certification by the American Association of Medical Dosimetrists.

8. **A** Roles and responsibilities of the medical physicist include acceptance testing of new equipment, commissioning and beam data measurement of new equipment, calibration of equipment, selection and specifications of equipment, and periodic quality assurance testing. Installation of new equipments is carried out by the vendor personnel. Acceptance testing and commissioning follows installation.

8.7 Requirements and Tolerance for QA Procedures (Answers)   535

9. **E** As soon as the installation of the new radiation producing device has been done, the physicist must perform a radiation survey around the room to ensure that during the testing and use of the device, the exposure levels outside the room will not exceed permissible limits considering the dose rate output, machine on time, use factors, and occupancy factors for the surrounding areas. This survey must be documented in a written report as required by the state regulatory agency.

10. **D** After completion of the installation, a formal radiation protection survey will measure the head leakage, the radiation levels in the surrounding areas. And tests will check the functionality of interlocks, warning lights, and emergency switches.

11. **A** AAPM TG-40 contains general guidance.

12. **B** AAMP TG-142 addresses QA needs of new equipment that has been developed such as IMRT, VMAT, the MLC, and on-board imaging.

13. **C** AAPM TG-51. The report replaced TG-21. TG-51 simplified the overall calibration process by standardizing the equipment needed and the setup geometry.

14. **C** Acceptance test is done when new device is delivered or installed, which contains only a portion of commissioning procedures. In addition, acceptance testing is the *legally binding* tests done with the vendor and physicist that demonstrate that the equipment meets the standards stated by the vendor. Commissioning is the acquisition of the extra data required to safely implement the machine clinically. An example of commissioning data would be the PDDs and profiles required to model the linac in the treatment planning system.

8.7 Requirements and Tolerance for QA Procedures (Answers)

Quiz-1 (Level 2)

1. **B** When delivering a certain dose to a patient at a reference point such as at the isocenter, uncertainty is in the range of 1.6–3 %. Remember that the overall dosimetric accuracy needs to be within 5 % with spatial accuracy of 5 mm. To achieve this overall accuracy, each component (like a wedge) must have greater accuracy as each additional component will increase the uncertainty.

2. **D** There are several methods to check jaw symmetry. One of the methods of checking jaw symmetry is with a machinist's dial indicator. Graph paper can also be used with a ruler. Graph paper can also be used to check

collimator axis and cross-hairs accuracy. Film placed on the table is used for light field with x-ray field alignment and can also be used to check the jaw symmetry. The front pointer is used to determine the mechanical isocenter and check SSD.

3. E The alignment between the x-ray field edges and the light field can be checked visually or by optical density profiles. For acceptance testing, the process should be repeated at all four cardinal gantry angles to test the affects of gravity.

4. B According to the AAPM guidelines, the alignment between the light field and the x-ray field should be within ±2 mm or 1 % on a side.

5. A To test the accuracy of the collimator, gantry, and table rotation, star shots are obtained. For each component, a film is irradiated with thin slits with the component rotated to various angles. The combination of the different angles creates the star pattern. The intersection of the different slits demonstrates the accuracy of the rotation. The tolerance for the star shot films is ±1 % from the baseline measurement obtained during acceptance testing. For field symmetry, the most common method is a cross-beam profile.

6. A A split-field test is performed to detect simultaneously three general causes of beam misalignment: focal spot displacement, asymmetry of collimator jaws, and displacement in the collimator or gantry rotation axis. It consists of double-exposing a film with beams 180° apart. The relative shift of the two images is indicative of the misalignment. The alignment between the x-ray beam edges and the light beam can be checked visually using a film or by cross-beam optical density profiles.

7. A The most practical method of specifying clinical beam energy is by verification of the depth-dose distribution. A central axis depth-dose curve measured with a suitable ion chamber in a water phantom can be compared with published data to specify the energy. The change in the PDD indicates a change in the beam energy.

8. C In order to determine the clinical beam energy, the ion chamber diameter should be smaller than 3 mm diameter to minimize displacement correction. Also, it is preferable to compare depth-dose ratios for depths beyond the Dmax as it is difficult to accurately measure doses at depths shallower than Dmax due to the steep dose buildup and electron contamination.

9. B

9. C According to AAPM TG-51, the photon clinical beam energy is usually specified in terms of depth dose for a 10×10 cm field size, 100 cm SSD at 10 cm depth. Although less common, a SAD setup is also acceptable, but the depth is still 10 cm.

8.7 Requirements and Tolerance for QA Procedures (Answers) 537

10. A A difference of ±1 % from baseline in the depth-dose ratio or ionization ratio from the published values is acceptable.

11. C For acceptance testing, photon beam flatness should be checked for a maximum field size at least at 10 cm and Dmax depths. In addition to the profiles along the principal axes of the field, diagonal scans should be obtained.

12. A The method used for electron beam energy measurement is the depth-dose or depth ionization curve for a broad beam with a suitable ion chamber in a water phantom.

13.
- **A.** IV. Optical distance indicator (2 mm)
- **B.** II. Gantry and collimator angles (1°)
- **C.** VI. Sag couch (2 mm from baseline)
- **D.** I. Jaw symmetry (±1 mm from baseline)
- **E.** VII. Light beam with x-ray beam (2 mm or 1 % on a side)
- **F.** III. Collimator rotation (1 mm diameter circle)
- **G.** V. Beam flatness and symmetry (±1 % change from baseline)

14. B Short-lived interstitial sources in the form of seeds, wires, or seed-loaded ribbons can be tested by visual inspection behind a leaded glass window. For a batch of a large number of sources, a randomly selected sample of three or four ribbons (or 10 % of the seeds) of a given strength should be checked for calibration. In some cases, ^{125}I seeds are difficult to calibrate because of the low energy of the emitted photons or because they come sterilized, so the institution may accept the vendor's calibration. A standard seed of SAME isotope and manufacturer should be used to calibrate the well ionization chamber.

15. E All are correct.

16. B Some equipment is ready for clinical use after acceptance testing; however linear accelerators should not be used for patient treatments until the physicist has declared it commissioned. Commissioning is important because it sets the baselines for all subsequent QA and also verifies that all clinical parameters have been set appropriately.

17. C Commissioning is complete only after the beam data have been input into the treatment planning computer and the computer generated dose distributions have been checked and approved by a physicist.

18. A The acceptance testing and commissioning of the treatment planning computer system includes testing of both hardware and software as well as algorithm verification.

19. B The type and frequency of testing are dictated primarily by the probability of occurrence of a particular performance error, its clinical impact, and the time required for performing the test. Door interlock checks must be performed daily along with output checks, field size checks, audio/visual monitor checks, radiation monitor checks, and laser checks. Emergency off switches and light/radiation field coincidence are done monthly, and a tabletop sag check is done during annual QA.

20. C The optical distance indicator (ODI) test is perform daily. Fluoroscopic image quality and field size indicators are checked monthly, and the exposure rate is checked annually. Again, the frequency of the test is determined by the potential clinical effect and the time required to complete the test. Daily tests should check the most critical components and should be quick. Annual tests should be more rigorous and check all components.

21. E All are correct.

22. E All are correct.

23. C As per ICRP recommendations, simulator annual QA tube leakage must be not exceeding 0.1 R/h at 1 m.

24. B When performing simulator annual QA measurement of tube leakage, the highest kVp setting as well as highest mA setting should be used. The primary radiation reaching the console must be checked as well as visual inspection of the whole x-ray tube.

25. B Simulator kVp accuracy must be within 5 kVp from the kVp chosen at control panel.

26. A Simulator mA linearity measures the mA setting versus the exposure rate proportionality or the exposure as a function of mA setting. Remember that as the x-ray tube current (mA) increases, exposure rate increases proportionally. This can be tested by measuring the exposure at different mA settings. Exposure as a function of tube current and time setting determines mAs linearity.

27. C Ionization chamber and electrometer systems must be sent to an ADCL for calibration at intervals not exceeding 2 years. These can be calibrated separately or as a unit.

28. D Instruments used to measure relative dose or dose distribution such as diodes, TLD, or films do not require an absolute calibration but should be checked frequently (usually monthly) to ensure that they have not drifted from the relative calibration.

29. B Calibration of survey meters must be done at intervals not exceeding 1 year. All battery-operated survey meters must be tested before each use.

8.7 Requirements and Tolerance for QA Procedures (Answers)   539

30. A Closed-circuit television and audio monitoring systems are required in treatment rooms; they should be turned on for all treatments and must be checked daily for proper operation.

31. C If one leaf is retracted or not in correct position, treatment should be stopped until fixed as this indicates a mechanical problem with the leaf.

32. E Percentage depth-dose QA should be done at time of commissioning, following repair, during monthly QA, and during annual QA. The PDD check is to ensure that the energy has not changed. Typically monthly, the PDD is spot-checked at a single depth, while annually, the scanning tank is used to acquire the entire PDD.

33. B From TG-40 QA acceptance tolerance for beam flatness and symmetry are measured at 10 cm depth. Beam flatness must be within 3 % and beam symmetry within 2 %. In TG-142, the terminology and tests were changed slightly. For the monthly QA, the test now checks beam profile constancy meaning you compare the current profile to your baseline profile to check flatness and symmetry. The tolerance is 1 %. For annual QA, the test is to check the flatness and symmetry change from baseline. The tolerances are 1 % for flatness and ±1 % for symmetry.

34. E All are correct. CT-simulator tests are as important as linac QA. HU or CT number for water should be checked daily with a tolerance of ±5 HU. Four to five different materials HU values should be checked monthly. CT image noise should be also checked daily as well as laser accuracy with a tolerance of ±2 mm. Electron density (ED) to CT number conversion as well as spatial and contrast resolution should be checked annually or after calibration. The CT to ED conversion is critical to accurate heterogeneity corrections in the planning system.

35. A The majority of CT scanners are capable of acquiring non-orthogonal CT scans by tilting the gantry. This is used for acquiring diagnostic images through certain anatomical structures which are not parallel with the imaging plane. However, for radiation oncology purposes and treatment planning, the CT-simulation gantry should be vertical at all times.

36. E The standard deviation of pixel values in a region of interest (ROI) within a uniform phantom is an indication of image noise. CT image noise can be expressed in terms of standard deviation of the CT numbers in Hounsfield units (HU) or as a percent of the linear attenuation coefficient of water. CT image noise determines the lower limit of subject contrast that can be distinguished by the observer so noise should be reduced as much as possible. One way of reducing noise is to acquire at a higher mAs, but this also increases patient dose. There is always a tradeoff in imaging.

37. **A** The standard for representing and exchanging medical imaging data is the Digital Image Communications in Medicine (DICOM). The National Electrical Manufacturers Association (NEMA) holds the copyright of DICOM. Picture archiving and communication system (PACS) is a medical imaging technology that provides storage and access to images from multiple modalities. Hewlett Packard (HP) image transfer is used to transfer pictures but not related to medical images.

38. **E** Some of the QA for CT-simulation software includes an image input test which verifies that image transfer from the CT simulator or other modality has the correct image geometry such as pixel size, spatial fidelity, slice thickness, and spacing. The correct image orientation is also critical because of treatment planning (i.e., patient prone vs. supine or head first vs. feet first). Structure delineation QA is used to test that anatomical structures and contouring are geometrically and spatially accurate. Multimodality image registration is often part of CT-simulation process, and proper operation of software and image transfer must be verified. Finally, image reconstruction is used to aid and evaluate beam placement and block design in 3D views. The tests should verify that the software accurately reconstructs these displays and that beam and block projections on these views are accurate.

39. **D** Complete calibration (TG-51) should be done annually or if any major repair needs to be done on the linac.

40. **B** One electron energy needs be checked at least daily, but all electron energies are to be checked at least twice a week. It depends on the frequency of use and how comfortable the physicist feels about the QA test.

41. **A** All photon energy output must be checked daily.

42. **C** All photon energy output must be checked daily on a linac accelerator. This is a critical component that could seriously affect patient treatment.

43. **B** The mechanical isocenter is the intersection point of the axis of rotation of the collimator, gantry, and couch. Due to its heavy weight, the gantry frame may flex during rotation, so a front pointer positioned at the isocenter and a horizontal rod with a fine point held in a ring attached to the couch. The gantry is moved through 360°, and the displacement between the front pointer and the horizontal rod point is visually noted and measured. The tolerance of the isocenter motion with full gantry rotation is ±1 mm.

44. **C** The output of cobalt-60 units must be checked monthly and the tolerance is 2 %.

8.8 QA for Treatment Planning System (Answers)

Quiz-1 (Level 2)

1. E All of these components should be tested. One way to test the accuracy of the treatment planning system is an end-to-end test. This is a test where a phantom is scanned, transferred to the planning system, a plan is generated, the dose to a point is calculated, and then the plan is actually delivered to the phantom at the linac and the dose is measured and compared to the planning system dose.

2. E IMRT QA must be done prior to each treatment. It involves validating radiation safety parameters, treatment planning calculations, machine characteristics, and patient-specific dosimetric verification. Typically it is done using a phantom that is irradiated to verify the delivered dose distribution versus the planned dose distribution. In addition, a secondary calculation is done as well, and the verification point should be in a low-dose gradient region away from the MLC edge.

3. A Films, diodes, or ion chambers are instruments used for IMRT QA. There are different methods used to accurately perform IMRT QA depending on the resources available in the clinic. Common phantoms contain an array of diodes or ion chambers that can measure the overall dose distribution.

4. D Stereotactic radiosurgery can be accomplished via linear accelerator, Gamma Knife, or CyberKnife. HDR can be used to deliver hypofractionated treatments, but they do not use stereotactic localization.

5. E Acceptance tests done on a TPS include CT input; anatomical description; beam description to verify that all beam techniques work; photon, electron, and brachytherapy beam dose calculations; dose display; DVH display; dose calculation results; and hardcopy output.

6. C 3 mm and 3 % are recommended with a 90–95 % pass rate usually signifying an acceptable plan. Gamma analysis is a combination of the dose difference and distance-to-agreement tests. The dose difference simply takes the absolute (or relative) dose difference between the measured and calculated points. This test works well in low-gradient regions, but it tends to fail in steep-gradient regions where the dose changes quickly. The other test is the distance to agreement where the algorithm searches around the measurement point to see how far away it has to look to find a planned dose point that is the same. This works well in high gradient regions, but does not work well in low-gradient regions where the dose does not change quickly. Gamma analysis combines these two tests, so there is no bias toward a plan with high or low-gradient regions.

7. B To commission the TPS, an exhaustive set of measurements are required. The more data acquired, the better the beam model in the planning system, and also there is more data to establish baselines for future periodic QA. The more comprehensive the commissioning data, the easier it is in the future to determine if a parameter has changed. Gold data provided by the vendor provides a comparison to see if your commissioned data is reasonable or not. The gold data is an average of similar linacs commissioned by other institutions. Your linac should be close, but not necessarily identical to the gold beam data provided by the vendor. Therefore it is usually recommended to use your own commissioned data rather than the gold data.

8. B Film or a chamber array needs to be used to commission an EDW. A single ion chamber or diode can be used, but only point measurements could be acquired not an entire profile because both the chamber and jaw would have to be in motion resulting in an inaccurate measurement.

9. D It is recommended to not use the gold beam data, but if all of the commissioning measurements are within 2 % of the gold data, to save time in the beam modeling process, the gold beam data can be used.

8.9 Equipment or Devices for Measurement (Answers)

Quiz-1 (Level 2)

1. D In 1928, the international commission on radiation units and measurements (ICRU) adopted the Roentgen as the unit of measuring x and γ radiation exposure. I In 1895 Wilhelm Roentgen discovered x-ray, and 1 year after, in 1896, Henri Becquerel discovered radioactivity. In 1898 Marie Curie and her husband Pierre Curie discovered the element radium.

2. B I and III are correct. Electronic equilibrium is said to exist if the ionization loss in a free-air chamber is compensated by the ionization gained or the ionization loss at the end of the specified volume is compensated for ionization gain at the beginning of the specified volume in a free-air chamber. Remember that electrons produced by photons in a specified volume must spend all their energies by ionization in air enclosed by the plates or region of ion collection.

3. B The free-air ionization chamber is the instrument used in the measurement of the Roentgen and generally used for calibration of secondary instruments designed for field use. This device is generally only used in laboratories and is limited to photons with energies <3 MeV. Thimble chambers

are used directly to measure exposure, and farmer chambers and parallel-plate chambers are used for electron and photon beam dosimetry.

4. **C** The limit on the photon energy above which free-air ionization chamber cannot be accurately measured is about 3 MeV. This occurs because as the photon energy increases, the range of the electrons liberated in air increases rapidly which affects electronic equilibrium in the chamber. Additionally, air attenuation, photon scatter, and reduction in the efficiency of ion collection contribute to this problem. Above this energy, it is almost impossible to create a chamber with a uniform electric field large enough to establish electronic equilibrium.

5. **E** All of them are correct. Although the thimble chambers walls is solid, it is air equivalent material, typically graphite; therefore its effective atomic number is the same as that of air, and it is made so that electronic equilibrium occurs inside the cavity.

6. **B** The most commonly used wall material on a thimble chamber are graphite, bakelite, or a mixture of both. Remember that the wall must be air equivalent; those materials are a little less than that of air but the greater atomic number of the central electrode compensates for the lower Z number of the wall. Tungsten is of high Z number used as a target material to generate Bremsstrahlung photons.

7. **E** All are desirable chamber characteristics.

8. **B** The only true method to measure surface dose is to use an extrapolation chamber. Because these are very rare, parallel-plate chambers are typically used in the clinic as they are the next best alternative. Farmer chambers are used to measure absolute photon and electron dosimetry, and thimble chambers are used directly to measure exposure. Care should be taken when using cylindrical chambers to measure electron beams because they may produce significant perturbations in the electron field. TG-51 recommends parallel-plate chamber be used for energies <10 MeV, and they must be used for energies <6 MeV.

9. **C** G-M detectors are used to search for lost clinical radioactive implant sources due to their high sensitivity. Remember that they cannot be used for quantitative measurements.

10. **A** A survey meter is used to measure dose rate around an implanted patient and patient room, survey in and around the storage area in which radioactive materials are kept, and survey areas around radiation producing machines such as ^{60}Co units. Farmer ionization chambers are used to calibrate linear accelerators or ^{60}Co units.

11. C Proportional counters are used to discriminate the type of contamination in a survey (β, γ, α), to count radioactive spills, and as a detector in some CT scanners. They can also be used for thermal neutrons detection.

12. D A G-M counter is used to monitor incoming radioactive source material packages to ensure there is no contamination.

13. E All are correct about G-M counter detector.

14. E Ionization chambers are used to calibrate linear accelerators or ^{60}Co treatment units, measure treatment beam characteristics, and used in a linear accelerator monitor chamber. Remember that G-M counters are a type of ionization chamber that are operating at a high voltage, around 1,000 V.

15. A Unsealed ion chambers must be corrected for temperature and pressure because density or mass of air in the chamber volume will change which results in a change in the charge collected. The chamber is calibrated at standard temperature and pressure so to accurately measure dose, these factors need to be accounted for.

16. D The density or mass of air in the ion chamber or the chamber reading for a given exposure will increase as temperature decreases and pressure increases. Remember that exposure is given by the ionization charge collected per unit mass of air.

17. A Temperature-pressure correction factor is given by $C_{tp} = (760/p) \times (273 + t/295)$. $F = [(SSD_2 + d_m/SSD_1 + d_m)(SSD_1 + d/SSD_2 + d)]^2$ is the formula of Mayneord F-factor used to calculate PDD at a new SSD. $s = 4A/p$ is the equation for equivalent square, where s is the side of equivalent square, A is the area of the rectangular field, and P is the perimeter of the rectangle. Answer D in incorrect because the t and p are incorrectly placed in the formula.

18. C If the temperature is 22 °C and the pressure is 750 mm of mercury, the correction needed to an ionization chamber would be 1.0133.
$C_{tp} = (760/p) \times (273 + t/295)$
$C_{tp} = (760/750) \times (273 + 22/295)$
$C_{tp} = 1.0133$
If the placement of the pressure and temperature is inverted, the answer is 119.79, which is wrong. Also if the – sign is replaced by the + sign, the answer is 0.8622. So be careful and remember to memorize the correct formula.

19. A The standard laboratories calibrate chambers under the conditions present at the time of calibration and then convert to specific atmospheric conditions of pressure of 760 mmHg and temperature of 22 °C (standard temperature and pressure).

8.10 QA Procedures (Answers)

20. E Geiger-Muller counters (G-M tube) can detect individual photons or individual particles. It can be used to detect alpha and beta particles as well as gamma ray, x-rays, and neutrons.

21. C Detector survey meter is typically used to make accurate determinations of leakage and scatter radiation around machines and radiation levels around patients with radioactive sources in them. Geiger-Muller counters (G-M) are used to detect the presence of low levels of radiation. Film badge and pocket dosimeter are personal monitoring devices so they are portable, but cannot provide instantaneous readings.

22. C Diodes are very sensitive, robust, and capable for measurement in air and water. However, the performance of diodes depends on a lot factors: temperature, orientation, energy of beam, and the performance changes with damage caused by irradiation.

23. C The aluminum Las Vegas phantom is normally used for EPID QA. It consists of a pattern of different thickness and diameter aluminum circles. The number of visible circles can be counted to ensure the EPID image quality has not degraded. Due to the qualitative nature of this test, more recent EPID QA phantoms use line pair phantoms and contrast objects that can be analyzed with software and provide quantitative image quality results.
(EPID = Electric Portal Image Device)

24. B Electrometer and ion chamber can be calibrated separately. In that case, each will have a separate calibration coefficient.
(ADCL = *Accredited Dosimetry Calibration Laboratory*)

25. C Both TLD and MOSFETs are typically used for on-patient measurements. Ion chambers can be used, but it is usually avoided because ion chambers are fragile and expensive.

8.10 QA Procedures (Answers)

Quiz-1 (Level 3)

1. B The airport has the updated pressure, which is roughly a constant in the same city. Care must be taken because sometime the airport corrects the pressure back to sea level. In this case, the pressure at the airport must be correct back to the elevation of the clinic.

2. C   Since the output of the machine is 3 % off, something must be done because the tolerance is 1 %. The physicist should adjust the output and ensure the new MU output is consistent with the planning system with is typically 1 cGy per MU at 100 cm SSD, 10×10 cm field size at Dmax.

3. B   One has to rotate the gantry to 90° and then use a level to check the collimator angle accuracy.

4. B   The general idea is to mark the light field on a film and then irradiate the field to compare the edge of field defined by light and by the radiation. They should correspond to within 2 mm or 1 % on a side.

5. A   Both output and energy QA are comparison of measurement to a baseline value set immediately following TG-51 calibration. The test is done using a small water tank or solid water which is much quicker than setting up the large scanning tank. The important thing to remember is that the geometry set during the baseline should be identical to the geometry set during the monthly QA; this includes correcting for temperature and pressure differences on that particular day.

6. A   Typically the PDD is spot-checked at one depth for each energy monthly with an ion chamber, either in solid water or water, and compared to the baseline value set annually. The important thing is that the geometry must be identical to that set during the baseline measurement. TMR can also be measured, but this is not typically done.

7. A   The "picket fence" is the QA done to check the positional accuracy of the dynamic MLC. A plan is delivered where the MLCs move across the field and stop at various locations to form vertical slits. The resulting image looks like a series or vertical strips, hence the name picket fence. Any deviation in MLC position appears as a bump in the vertical slit. Typically the test is run at the cardinal gantry angles or in an arc delivery to test the affects of gravity.

8. B   To test the centricity of the cross hair, align a piece of graph paper to the cross hair with the gantry vertical and mark the center. Rotate the collimator 90°, mark the center, rotate to 270°, and mark the center. Draw a circle that contains all three marks and determine the diameter. The tolerance for the diameter is 1 mm.

9. A   A simple test is to align a piece of graph paper with the cross hair. Record the table position from the digital readout. Now move the couch exactly some distance in the lateral and longitudinal direction using the graph paper (or a ruler) as a reference. Record the digital position of the table and make sure it is within 2 mm of the expected shift. The same can be done in the vertical direction by using the laser and a ruler.

8.10 QA Procedures (Answers)

10. B   The idea for MU linearity of a linear accelerator is to see whether the output is stable if the same dose is delivered in one long delivery or several short deliveries.

This is important in treatment because in case there is an issue in the machine during a treatment, not all of the MUs have been delivered; the remaining MUs are delivered once the issue has been fixed.

Fundamentals of Computer Technologies

Contents

9.1 Basic Computer Terminology (Questions) 549
9.2 Internet and Telecommunication (Questions) 553
9.3 Medical Images (Questions) 554
9.4 Basic Computer Terminology (Answers) 556
9.5 Internet and Telecommunication (Answers) 558
9.6 Medical Images (Answers) 559

9.1 Basic Computer Terminology (Questions)

Quiz-1 (Level 1)

1. LAN stands for?
A. Large application network
B. Line added network
C. Local area network
D. License analytical network

2. One bit is equal to?
A. A binary digit (0 or 2)
B. A single digit (1)
C. A binary digit (0 or 1)
D. A decimal digit (0 to 9)

3. One byte equals?
A. 8 bits
B. 16 bits
C. 1 field
D. 32 bits

4. A group of bytes is?
A. A bit
B. A field
C. A file
D. A record

5. How many combinations of 0s and 1s can a byte have?
A. 150
B. 200
C. 256
D. 500

6. Which of the following is the most used scheme to represent text, letters, punctuations, and other symbols?
A. IBM
B. ISO
C. ANSI
D. ASCII

7. PACS stands for?
A. Picture active computer systems
B. Printer analog computer systems
C. Picture archiving and communication systems
D. Projection access communication systems

8. The systems and programs that process data and turn that data into information is called?
A. Software
B. Hardware
C. Network
D. Data and information

9. CPU stands for?
A. Central primary utility
B. Computer program unit
C. Central processing unit
D. Computer provide utility

10. The principal components of the CPU is/are?
A. I, II, and III only
B. I and III only
C. II and IV only
D. IV only
E. All are correct

I. The processor or control unit
II. Registers
III. Primary storage
IV. External hard drive

11. Which of the following computer components transmit data from one part of a computer to another?
A. RAM
B. Buses
C. ALU
D. Registers

12. Which of the following is not a computer input device?
A. Keyboard
B. Mouse
C. Microphone
D. Printer

Quiz-2 (Level 2)

1. How much data can be transmitted at one time is determined by?
A. The bus speed
B. The RAM size
C. The bus size
D. The primary storage

2. The common metric prefixes used with computers are?
A. I, II, and III only
B. I and III only
C. II and IV only
D. IV only
E. All are correct
I. Kilo
II. Mega
III. Giga
IV. Tera

3. One kilobyte equals?
A. 1,048,576 bytes
B. 1,024 bytes
C. 1,073,741,824 bytes
D. 32 bytes

4. A file containing 510 KB equals?
A. 510×1,024 bytes of data
B. 5,010×1,024 bytes of data
C. 510×32 bytes of data
D. 50,010×1,024 bytes of data

5. Which of the following is a set of programs that provides the instructions for telling a computer what to do and how to do it?
A. Software
B. Hardware
C. Optical disk drive
D. Central processing unit

6. Which of the following is also call CRT?
A. Computer hardware
B. Computer software
C. Computer monitor
D. External processor

7. A binary digit use by computer's operating system is referred to as?
A. Byte
B. Bit
C. Bin
D. Megabyte

8. The difference between RAM and ROM is/are?
A. I, II, and III only
B. I and III only
C. II and IV only
D. IV only
E. All are correct
I. RAM can be written to and read while ROM is used only for reading.
II. RAM stays on only as long as the computer is running and gets deleted as soon as compute is switched off while ROM generally cannot be written to.
III. RAM is random access memory, while ROM stands for read-only memory.
IV. RAM is lost when the computer is switched off, while ROM is permanent.

9. What is cache in a computer?
A. Part of the RAM
B. Part of ROM
C. A small memory unit attached to CPU
D. A small external drive

10. How is the number 12 represented in binary?
A. 1,010
B. 1,100
C. 1,001
D. 1,111

9.2 Internet and Telecommunication (Questions)

Quiz-1 (Level 2)

1. Which of the following is the communication protocol of computer networks?
A. ISDN
B. TCP/IP
C. HTTP
D. SS7

2. Which of the following is a group of searching engines for the Internet?
A. Netscape, Bing, Google, Yahoo
B. Netscape, IE, Firefox
C. Bing, Google, Yahoo, Webopedia
D. Facebook, YouTube, Amazon

3. Which of the following is a group of web navigators?
A. Netscape, Bing, Google, Yahoo
B. Netscape, IE, Firefox, Chrome
C. Bing, Google, Yahoo, Webopedia
D. Facebook, YouTube, Amazon, Chrome

4. Which of the following technologies is the most rapid in data transportation?
A. Modem
B. ISDN
C. DSL
D. SS7

5. Which of the following is the key device to form a LAN on a series of computers, iPhones, and printers?
A. Phone lines
B. Router
C. Operating system for multiple users
D. Outlets

6. Which is the standard protocol for file transfer from one host to another through TCP-based network?
A. HTTP
B. IP
C. FTP
D. UDP

7. Which language is designed to search specific entries in a relational database?
A. C/C++
B. SQL
C. Visual Basic
D. SAS

8. A fatal virus is destructive to a Windows-based LAN; what would most likely happen if it attacks a UNIX system?
A. Same damages as to Windows system
B. More severe damages
C. No damage at all
D. Small damages

9. A local phone uses standard SS7 system to route; what about a cell phone?
A. I only
B. II only
C. II and IV
D. I and III
E. IV only
I. SS7 system
II. Internet
III. Cell phone-specific network, e.g., PCS network
IV. Voice over IP (VoIP)

10. Dialing a local phone may reach a cell phone which is on. Why is this possible?
A. Because the cell phone can be searched by satellites
B. Because the cell phone's registration is stored in its local SS7 database
C. Because the cell phone is connected to the Internet wirelessly
D. Because the cell phone emits signals detectable by its service network

9.3 Medical Images (Questions)

Quiz-1 (Level 2)

1. In a typical CT image, how many bytes are required in each pixel?
A. 2
B. 1
C. 3
D. 8

9.3 Medical Images (Questions)

2. In a typical ultrasound image, how many bytes are required in each pixel?
A. 2
B. 1
C. 3
D. 8

3. About how much storage is required for a typical 100-slice diagnostic CT image set?
A. 50 KB
B. 50 MB
C. 50 GB
D. 50 TB

4. About how much storage is required for a typical 50-slice diagnostic MRI image set?
A. 6 KB
B. 6 MB
C. 6 GB
D. 6 TB

5. How many pixels are in a typical computed or digital radiograph?
A. 512×512
B. 128×128
C. $2,048 \times 2,048$
D. $10,000 \times 10,000$

6. Which of the following influence image visualization?
A. I only
B. II only
C. II and IV
D. I, II, and III
E. All are correct
I. Image dimension
II. Grayscale levels
III. Resolution
IV. Image modality

9.4 Basic Computer Terminology (Answers)

Quiz-1 (Level 1)

1. **C** LAN stands for local area network, a computer network that interconnects computers in a limited area such as work, home, school, etc. It permits shared data among computers within a limited area.

2. **C** One bit is equal to a binary digit of two possible values, 0 or 1. All computer data is stored like this.

3. **A** One byte is equal to 8 bits. A byte is a group of 8 bits that can represent a number or a letter.

4. **B** A field is a group of bytes in which a specific data element such as a name is stored; a record is a group of fields that represents the data that is being stored for a particular entity; a file is a collection of related records.

5. **C** A byte contains eight consecutive 0 s and 1 s or combinations of bits. Therefore, each byte contains one of 256 different combinations of 0 s and 1 s. Another way to look at it is there are 2^8 possible combinations.

6. **D** American Standard Code for Information Interchange (ASCII) is the most used scheme to represent text, letters, punctuations, and other symbols.

7. **C** PACS stands for picture archiving and communication systems. This is an electronic information system used for acquiring, sorting, transporting, storing, and electronically displaying medical images, and it is designed to allow physicians and medical workers to view digital images of diagnostic tests.

8. **A** Software is the systems and programs that process data and turn that data into information; examples are WordPerfect or Microsoft Word. Hardware is the actual physical computer or computer peripheral device; examples are PC, workstation, disk drive, etc. A network is the communication media that allows multiple computers to share data and information simultaneously and data is a set of variables and information is organized and processed data that is meaningful to somebody.

9. **C** CPU stands for central processing unit, and it is the control center of the computer system.

10. **A** The main components of a CPU are the processor or control unit which directs and coordinates most of the operations within the computer; the

arithmetic/logic units (ALU) which perform arithmetic, comparison, and logic functions; and the register that stores the data. An external hard drive is a secondary storage device and not part of the actual computer.

11. B Buses are the information highway for the CPU. They consist of two parts, the address bus which transfers information about where the data should go and the data bus which transfers actual data. Buses transmit data from one part of a computer to another.

12. A Input devices supply the data to be processed. Examples are keyboards, mice, touch screens, scanners, and microphones. Output devices transfer data from the processing unit to various output media. Examples are printers, speakers, and plotters.

Quiz-2 (Level 2)

1. C The size of the bus determines how much data can be transferring at one time. A 16-bit bus can transmit 16 bits of data, while a 32-bit bus can transmit 32 bits of data.

2. E All of them are common metric prefixes used with computers. Kilo (K), 2^{10} (1,024); mega (m), 2^{20} (1,048,576); giga (g), 2^{30} (1,073,741,824); and tera (t), 2^{40} (1,099,511,627,776), are all used to quantify the number of bytes in a computer. Typical hard drives now store gigabytes or even terabytes of data.

3. B One kilobyte equals 1,024 bytes, one megabyte equals 1,048,576 bytes, one gigabyte equals 1,073,741,824 bytes, and one terabyte equals 1,099,511,627,776 bytes.

4. A Abbreviations are used to describe the prefixes; in this case a file containing 510 KB refers to a file containing 510 kilobytes which is the same as 510×1,024 bytes of data.

5. A Software is a set of programs that provides the instructions for telling a computer what to do and how to do it. Computer hardware refers to the physical parts or components of a computer, and an optical disk drive is a device that uses laser light as part of the reading or writing data. The central processing unit (CPU) is the hardware within a computer system which carries out the instructions of a computer program.

6. C CRT stands for cathode ray tube and it was used on the first computer monitors. Now most monitors are liquid crystal displays (LCD) or light-emitting diodes (LED) which provide higher contrast and better viewing angles than LCDs.

7. **B** A binary digit is the smallest unit of information on a computer, and it is referred to as bit; a single bit can hold only one of two values (0 or 1); a byte is composed of eight bits.

8. **E** All of them are correct.

9. **C** A cache is used to store data in a separate location so if it is needed again, it can be retrieved in less time since it does not have to come from the main memory.

10. **B** Remember that in a binary number, the only possible digits are 1 or 0. This is useful in computers because the 0 can be represented by a switch being off and a 1 can be represented by a switch being on. To convert a number to binary, the following process is used.
    It is important to realize how a binary number is represented. Take the following binary number: 111 (remember this in not one hundred eleven). This number can be represented like
    $(1 \times 2^2)+(1 \times 2^1)+(1 \times 2^0)=(1 \times 4)+(1 \times 2)+(1 \times 1)=7$
    Try another example: 10,010 bin
    $(1 \times 2^4)+(0 \times 2^3)+(0 \times 2^2)+(1 \times 2^1)+(0 \times 2^0)=(1 \times 16)+(0 \times 8)+(0 \times 4)+(1 \times 2)+(0 \times 1)=18$
    To solve the problem here, the same process can be used:
    $(1 \times 2^3)+(1 \times 2^2)+(0 \times 2^1)+(0 \times 2^0)=(1 \times 8)+(1 \times 4)+(0 \times 2)+(0 \times 1)=11$

9.5 Internet and Telecommunication (Answers)

Quiz-1 (Level 2)

1. **B** TCP/IP is the communication protocol.

2. **C** Google is mainly used for searching purpose, whereas Yahoo contains integrated information. They are all called search engines.

3. **B**

4. **C** DSL and cable modems are much faster than modem or ISDN; however, the speed of a cable modem also depends on the number of current users.

5. **B** A router is a popular choice for now.

6. **C** FTP (file transfer protocol) is the protocol for file transferring. An advantage of FTP is that it can be secured or encrypted.

7. **B** SQL is specially developed for searching databases.

8. C UNIX is completely different. Viruses normally attack the *.dll files which do not exist in UNIX system.

9. D Once a cell phone is turned on, it will search the local service network for a cell which is connected to the local SS7 network for local phone service. If a cell phone finds a local network (normally at a certain frequency), the cell phone number is automatically registered to the local SS7 database which means this cell phone can be treated as a local phone for now.

Cell phone uses both the SS7 network and the local service network. Cell phone service is essentially based on the local phone service.

10. B See the explanation in answer 9.

9.6 Medical Images (Answers)

Quiz-1 (Level 2)

1. A The number of bits per pixel defines the range of grayscale values used in the image. The more levels of grayscale, the more contrast there is available in the image. At the same time, above a certain level, the human eye cannot distinguish between different gray levels if the difference is minimal. Therefore, typically in CT imaging, 12 bits per pixel are used. This allows for 4,096 different gray levels. Remember that 1 byte is 8 bits so 2 bytes are required for each pixel. Another disadvantage of adding more gray levels is that adding more bytes increases the size of the image and this will be looked at in the next few questions.

2. B Ultrasound images do not have the dynamic range of CT, so only 8 bits (1 byte) are required. MRI and digital radiography also use 12 bit pixels like CT. When color is added to images, typically 24 bits (3 bytes) are required.

3. B To calculate how much space is required for an image set, you need to know several things. The first is the number of pixels in each image, the second is the number of bytes in each pixel, and the third is the number of images in the set. Here we are told that we have 100 slices and that we have a diagnostic CT. You have to know that a CT is 512×512 pixels and that each pixel is 12 bits (2 bytes). Now we can calculate the storage space required:

Number of pixels per image × number of images × bytes per pixel = bytes per image

$512 \times 512 \times 100 \times 2 = 52,428,800$ bytes

Remember that 1 KB = 1,024 bytes (2^{10}) and 1 MB = 1,048,576 bytes (2^{20}).

Therefore, the image set required is 50 MB of storage space.

This example shows why a large hospital requires a huge amount of storage in their PACS system to be able to hold all of these images.

4. B This can be calculated in the same manner as the previous problem. The difference is that a typical MR image is only 256×256 pixels:
$256 \times 256 \times 50 \times 2 = 6{,}553{,}600$ bytes $= 6.25$ MB
Nuclear medicine scans typically only have 128×128 pixels per image.

5. C A typical digital radiograph has 4,194,304 pixels. This is because the detail required in these images for a radiologist to diagnose a problem is extremely high. Remember that they might be looking for a hairline fracture or a small pneumothorax. This means that these images also require a large amount of storage space:
$2{,}048 \times 2{,}048 \times 2$ bytes $= 8{,}388{,}608$ bytes $= 8$ MB

6. D The image dimension (number of pixels), the number of grayscale levels, and the resolution (pixels per inch) all influence the visualization of an image. The image modality does not affect this.

Professional Responsibilities 10

Contents

10.1 Working as Professionals at Health System (Questions) 561
10.2 Professional Medical Dosimetrists (Questions) 570
10.3 Working as Professionals at Health System (Answers) 574
10.4 Professional Medical Dosimetrists (Answers) 581

This part includes (1) the lawful knowledge related to professional work in a health system which applies to nurses, therapists, dosimetrists, medical physicists, and physicians and (2) the essential lawful knowledge of being professional medical dosimetrists. It is useful to understand how the health system works to have a big picture view of why we do what we do and how to do it with the best interest of the patient in mind.

10.1 Working as Professionals at Health System (Questions)

Quiz 1 (Level 2)

1. Which of the following is the discipline dealing with what is good or bad and right or wrong and moral principles that apply values and judgments to the practice of medicine?
   A. Legal concepts
   B. Ethics
   C. Moral ethics
   D. Fidelity

2. Beneficence means:
A. The ethical principle of doing no harm to a patient by a medical professional.
B. Patients who are independent and have freedom or self-government.
C. Health-care professionals must act in the best interest of a patient, even at some inconvenience and sacrifice to themselves. The state or quality of being kind, charitable, or beneficial.
D. The principle of fairness and equity that is maintained for all individuals.

3. Paternalism is:
A. Doing what you think is best for the patient, against their will, right, or responsibilities.
B. Doing what is best for the patient using the patient consent or approval.
C. Doing harm to the patient without analyzing the consequences.
D. Making decisions for and not with the patient using the will of a family member.

4. Which of the following modes identify the caregiver as a scientist dealing only in facts and does not consider the human aspect of the patient?
A. Priestly model
B. Contractual model
C. Collegial model
D. Analytical model

5. What does the informed consent involve?
A. I, II, and III only
B. I and III only
C. II and IV only
D. IV only
E. All are correct
I. Every patient is entitled to informed consent before any procedure is performed.
II. Patients should be informed and educated about their medical facts and the risk involved.
III. Patients should understand and approve their treatments and participate responsibly in their own care.
IV. Every patient is entitled to informed consent after any procedure is performed.

6. When given an informed consent, the patient should be informed of:
A. I, II, and III only
B. I and III only
C. II and IV only
D. IV only
E. All are correct
I. The nature of the procedure, treatment, or disease
II. The expectation of the recommended treatment and the likelihood of success
III. Alternative available and probable outcome in absence of treatment
IV. The risks involved in procedure, treatment, or disease

10.1 Working as Professionals at Health System (Questions)

7. Which of the following are correct regarding informed consent?
A. I, II, and III only
B. I and III only
C. II and IV only
D. IV only
E. All are correct
I. It is a legal document.
II. It is entirely the responsibility of the physician.
III. It must be signed in front of a witness.
IV. It cannot be delegated to a third party.

8. Which of the following statements involving competency is *not* true?
A. Persons older than 18 years of age that can speak for themselves are considered competent.
B. Is the quality or condition of being legally qualified to perform an act or the minimum mental, cognitive, or behavioral ability required to assume responsibility.
C. Persons of age 18 years old or older are considered being competent, if no mental or physical condition is identified.
D. Persons of age younger than 18 years old are considered minors; therefore they are incompetent and parents or designated guardians must decide for them.

9. Which of the following statements are true about patient confidentiality?
A. I, II, and III only
B. I and III only
C. II and IV only
D. IV only
E. All are correct
I. Patient information should not be discussed with other departments unless in a direct line of duty.
II. Conversation about a patient between professionals should be kept in private.
III. Patient information should not be discussed with families and friends.
IV. Patient charts and computers with patient information should not be left unattended or unsecure.

10. Failure to take reasonable care or caution in doing something resulting in unintentional injury to a patient is the definition of:
A. Malpractice
B. Negligence
C. Bad ethics
D. Liability

11. Which of the following statements must be met in order for an incident to be considered negligence?
A. I, II, and III only
B. I and III only
C. II and IV only

D. IV only
E. All are correct
I. The plaintiff was owed a duty of care.
II. There was a dereliction or breach of that duty.
III. There was a direct injury caused by the breach of that duty.
IV. There was a proximate cause.

12. The difference between civil law and tort law is:
A. Civil law oversees rights between individuals in noncriminal actions, while tort law governs relationship between individuals.
B. Civil law generally provides for the legal relationships between persons, organizations, and the government, while tort law provides protection to each person from harm not intended to harm society as a whole.
C. Civil law provides protection to the government and each person from those who would intentionally harm that society (criminal law), while tort law provides protection to each person from harm not intended to harm society as a whole.
D. The result of violation of a civil law is usually becoming liable to pay for the damages that are caused to the victim, while tort law usually is punished by a fine or imprisonment.

13. Unlawful physical contact or touching of a person without permission is the definition of:
A. Assault
B. False imprisonment
C. Battery
D. Invasion of privacy

14. Which of the following is an example of false imprisonment?
A. A patient asks a professional about her breast cancer, and the professional starts palpating her breast without her permission.
B. A patient finished her treatment and wishes to go, but it is not allowed without seeing the doctor.
C. A professional threatens a patient by showing him/her a 10 gauge needle and states "if you do not allow me to palpate the supraclavicular nodes I have to get a blood sample with this needle," and the patient feels threatened.
D. A professional, who is examining a patient without clothes, leaves the room for 30 min, and several nurses enter and leave the room looking for utensils while the patient is exposed.

15. A false publication, as in writing, print, sign, or pictures, that damages the person's reputation is the definition of:
A. Libel
B. Slander
C. False imprisonment
D. Invasion of privacy

10.1 Working as Professionals at Health System (Questions)

16. Which is the doctrine stating that the thing speaks for itself?
A. Personal liability
B. Respondeat superior
C. Foreseeability
D. Res ipsa loquitur

17. Which of the following are correct about an incident report?
A. I, II, and III only
B. I and III only
C. II and IV only
D. IV only
E. All are correct
I. Should be consistent with the institution's policies and procedures.
II. Should have the facts of an injury to be valid.
III. Should contain only facts of the incident concerned.
IV. A copy of the incident report should be given to the patient involved.

18. Which of the following are correct regarding medical records?
A. I, II, and III only
B. I and III only
C. II and IV only
D. IV only
E. All are correct
I. Contain a chronological written account of a patient's examination and treatment that include the patient's medical history and complaints.
II. II. Should be maintained in independent departments from hospitals.
III. Must be signed and written in ink.
IV. Corrections should never be deleted, but a line should be placed over the incorrect entry and initialed with time and date.

19. Which of the following is *not* correct about HIPAA?
A. HIPAA stands for Health Insurance Portability and Accountability Act.
B. Makes health care more affordable and accessible for millions of Americans and for those who need its protections and benefits the most.
C. Broadens the scope of existing fraud and abuse provisions and increases penalties for fraud violations by health-care providers.
D. Protects privacy of health information.

20. Which of the following is *not* correct regarding patient's bill of rights?
A. It is a legal document that states a patient's wishes about medical decisions or names another person to make decisions for him/her.
C. The patient is always right because he/she is a customer.
B. It is a document describing the rights of patients and hospital's responsibilities.
D. The patient has the right to considerate and respectful care.

21. In order for billing to be valid, which of the following need(s) to be done?
A. I, II, and III only
B. I and III only
C. II and IV only
D. IV only
E. All are correct
I. Signed treatment plan (and DVH if applicable) is required.
II. MU calculations and/or QA must be signed and dated.
III. Each treatment device billed must be documented.
IV. Must be sent to the payee the same day the plan is signed.

22. Which of the following statements are true?
A. I, II, and III only
B. I and III only
C. II and IV only
D. IV only
E. All are correct
I. Gifts of small values are allowed by the AMA code of ethics.
II. II. A company who tries to make business with a physician or entity can give cash as a gift.
III. A physician should support access to medical care for all people.
IV. Principles adopted by the AMA is a law.

23. The AAMD board of directors is composed of:
A. I, II, and III only
B. I and III only
C. II and IV only
D. IV only
E. All are correct
I. President, president elect, and past president
II. II. Membership and recording secretaries
III. Treasurer
IV. Twenty regional directors

24. The mission statement of the AAMD is:
A. To foster the professional growth of radiologist technologist by expanding knowledge through education, research, and analysis; promoting exceptional leadership and service; and developing the radiology technology community through shared ethics and values.
B. To advance the science, education, and professional practice of medical physics.
C. To promote and support the medical dosimetry profession and provide opportunities for education, a forum for professional interaction, and a representative voice in the health-care community while seeking to promote the ideal of professional conduct to which its member should aspire and endorse the highest standard of patient care.

D. To enhance the quality of practice of medical physics, engage in professional activities for the benefit of the medical physics community, and promote the continuing competence of practitioners in medical physics.

25. Which of the following organizations is devoted to advance the practice of radiation oncology by disseminating the results of scientific research, promoting excellence in patient care, providing opportunities for educational and professional development of its members, developing policies, and representing radiation oncology in a rapidly evolving socioeconomic health-care environment?
A. ACR
B. AAMD
C. ACMP
D. ASTRO

26. What is the mission of MDCB?
A. To steer the advancement of the medical dosimetry profession by establishing certification and continuing education standards to enhance quality patient care
B. To elevate standards and advance the cause of medical dosimetry by encouraging its study and improving its practice
C. To recognize the continuing knowledge and skills of medical dosimetrists
D. To determine the certification eligibility of medical dosimetrists and conduct examinations to test the cognitive capability of voluntary candidates

27. The applicant for the MDCB exam can be eligible if:
A. I, II, and III only
B. I and III only
C. II and IV only
D. IV only
E. All are correct
I. Graduated from either a JRCERT-accredited program or a program of at least 12 or 18 months and completed at least 6 months of clinical medical dosimetry experience under the direction of a CMD or medical physicist
II. Owns a BS degree or holds an ARRT in radiation therapy and completed at least 24 months of clinical medical dosimetry experience under the direction of a CMD or medical physicist and 12 CE approved by the MDCB during his or her 24 months of clinical experience
III. Owns AAs, AS, or BS degree and completed at least 36 months of clinical medical dosimetry experience under the direction of a CMD or medical physicist and 24 CE approved by the MDCB during his or her 36 months of clinical experience
IV. Had been working as a radiation therapist for more than 10 years

28. Which of the following agencies promotes and supports the medical dosimetry profession?
A. The American College of Medical Physics (ACMP)
B. The American Association of Physicists in Medicine (AAPM)

C. The American Society of Radiologic Technologists (ASRT)
D. The American Association of Medical Dosimetrists (AAMD)

29. Which of the following is correct about the patient care partnership?
A. It is a legal document that informs patients about what they should expect during their hospital stay with regard to their rights and responsibilities.
B. It is a legal document which states that the patient has the right to considerate and respectful care.
C. It describes the systematic documentation of a single patient's medical history and care across time within one particular health-care provider's jurisdiction.
D. It is a form that is filled out in order to record details of an unusual event that occurs at the facility, such as an injury to a patient.

30. Which of the following should be included in a patient care partnership documents?
A. I, II, and III only
B. I and III only
C. II and IV only
D. IV only
E. All are correct
I. High-quality hospital care information
II. Clean and safe environment information
III. Protection of patient's privacy information
IV. Billing claims information

31. A document that contains instructions given by individuals specifying what actions should be taken for their health in the event that they are no longer able to make decisions due to illness or incapacity and appoints a person to make such decisions on their behalf is:
A. Patient care partnership documents
B. The patient's bill of rights
C. A living will
D. An incident report

32. Enforcement and penalties for noncompliance with HIPPA regulations include:
A. I, II, and III only
B. I and III only
C. II and IV only
D. IV only
E. All are correct
I. Civil money penalties
II. Death penalty
III. Criminal penalties
IV. Institution closed

10.1 Working as Professionals at Health System (Questions)   569

33. Which of the following professional organizations offers the certification in medical dosimetry?
A. AAMD
B. MDCB
C. ACMP
D. ARRT

34. Match the following organizations with its descriptions.
A. AAMD
B. MDCB
C. ACMP
D. ARRT
E. ABR
F. JCAHO
G. ACR
H. ASTRO
I. ASRT
J. AMA
K. HIPPA
L. AAPM
M. JRCERT
I. Devotes to advance the practice of radiation oncology
II. II. Oversees the certification and ongoing professional development of specialists in diagnostic radiology, radiation oncology, and medical physics
III. Serves patients and society by maximizing the value of radiology, nuclear medicine, and medical physics
IV. International society established to promote and support the medical dosimetry profession
V. Serves to steer the advancement of the medical dosimetry profession by establishing certification and continuing education standards to enhance quality patient care
VI. A USA-based not-for-profit organization that accredits over 19,000 healthcare organizations and programs in the USA
VII. Promotes high standards of patient care by recognizing qualified individuals in medical imaging, interventional procedures, and radiation therapy
VIII. Enhances the quality of practice of medical physics
IX. Fosters the professional growth of radiologist technologist
X. Seeks to advance the science, education, and professional practice of medical physics
XI. Dedicated to a body of ethical statements developed primarily for the benefit of the patient
XII. Protects privacy of health information
XIII. Promotes excellence in education and elevates the quality and safety of patient care through the accreditation of educational programs in radiography, radiation therapy, magnetic resonance, and medical dosimetry

10.2 Professional Medical Dosimetrists (Questions)

Quiz 1 (Level 2)

1. Which of the following organizations is *not* responsible for the medical dosimetry profession?
   A. MDCB
   B. ABR
   C. AAMD
   D. JRCERT

2. The MDCB code of ethics applies to?
   A. I, II, and III only
   B. I and III only
   C. II and IV only
   D. IV only
   E. All are correct
   I. Professionals holding certification credentials from the MDCB.
   II. All radiation oncology professionals.
   III. Persons applying for examination and certification by the MDCB in order to become certified medical dosimetrists.
   IV. Medical dosimetrists and medical physicists only.

3. Some of the MDCB code of ethics includes:
   A. I, II, and III only
   B. I and III only
   C. II and IV only
   D. IV only
   E. All are correct
   I. A CMD shall always promote the safety and welfare of his or her patients by performing medical dosimetry procedures safely and with reasonable skill.
   II. A CMD not under suspension, revocation, or other disciplinary action by any professional medical dosimetry organization, certifying body, licensing board, or credentialing agency.
   III. A CMD shall not make or file any report in connection with patient care, which report he or she knows to be false.
   IV. A CMD shall not practice beyond the scope he or she is competent to perform as defined in the Medical Dosimetry Scope and Standards of Practice Document.

4. Which of the following sanctions can be used by the MDCB against a certified medical dosimetrist?
   A. I, II, and III only
   B. I and III only

C. II and IV only
D. IV only
E. All are correct
I. The MDCB may deny, revoke, or suspend certification or re-certification when a CMD is found to be not in compliance with MDCB rules, regulations, and/or the foregoing Ethical Standards.
II. The MDCB may censure a CMD, issue public or private reprimands, place a CMD on probation for up to 5 years, or impose other sanctions related to the ethical violation.
III. The MDCB may refuse to allow the applicant to sit for the certification examination if an applicant for certification is not in compliance with MDCB Ethical Standards.
IV. In the event that the examination has been taken, The MDCB may refuse to release the examination results if not in compliance with MDCB Ethical Standards.

5. Which of the following statements are true about the MDCB code of ethics?
A. I, II, and III only
B. I and III only
C. II and IV only
D. IV only
E. All are correct
I. If the Chair of the Ethics Committee determines that there is evidence of a violation of the Ethical Standards, the Chair shall inform the respondent in writing that a complaint of ethical misconduct has been filed and a formal investigation will be conducted.
II. The respondent has thirty (30) days from the date of receipt of the notification letter or complaint of ethical misconduct to prepare and submit a response in writing.
III. The Ethics Committee shall evaluate all documentation pertaining to the matter and, within ninety (90) days of receiving all relevant evidence, determine whether the complaint is substantiated by clear and convincing evidence.
IV. A CMD or an applicant to whom the complaint of ethical misconduct notice is given shall have thirty (30) days from the date the notice is mailed to make a written request for a hearing.

6. The MDCB Scope of Practice is designed to:
A. I, II, and III only
B. I and III only
C. II and IV only
D. IV only
E. All are correct

I. Provide a statement of competence in medical dosimetry practice.
II. Define the practice of medical dosimetry.
III. Provide a useful guide for medical dosimetrists and others in evaluating the quality, effectiveness, and appropriateness of health-care service.
IV. Provide MDCB members to use the highest technology.

7. Which year was the MDCB Scope of Practice adopted?
A. 1996
B. 1997
C. 2000
D. 2001

8. Which of the following are correct about a medical dosimetrist?
A. I, II, and III only
B. I and III only
C. II and IV only
D. IV only
E. All are correct
I. A member of the radiation oncology team who has knowledge of the overall characteristics and clinical relevance of radiation oncology treatment and planning equipment.
II. Is a professional cognizant of procedures commonly used in brachytherapy.
III. Has the education and expertise necessary to generate radiation dose distributions and dose calculation.
IV. Frequently acts as liaison between medical physicists and other members of the radiation oncology team.

9. Which of the following should the medical dosimetrists have a clear understanding of?
A. I, II, and III only
B. I and III only
C. II and IV only
D. IV only
E. All are correct
I. Cancer, radiation biology, radiation therapy techniques
II. Radiation oncology physics, equipment technology, and radiation safety and protection
III. Anatomy, physiology, and mathematics
IV. Geography, foreign languages, and history

10. Which of the following should a medical dosimetrist do?
A. I, II, and III only
B. I and III only
C. II and IV only
D. IV only
E. All are correct

10.2 Professional Medical Dosimetrists (Questions)

I. Perform radiation treatment planning
II. Recognize and resolve equipment problems and treatment discrepancies
III. Recommend when treatment should be withheld until a physician and physicist can be consulted
IV. Sign radiation prescriptions if physician and/or physicists are not available

11. Which of the following statements are true?
A. I, II, and III only
B. I and III only
C. II and IV only
D. IV only
E. All are correct

I. It is recommended that the medical dosimetrist be certified by the Medical Dosimetry Certification Board (MDCB).
II. The medical dosimetrist has to be certified by the Medical Dosimetry Certification Board (MDCB) in order to perform his or her work.
III. The CMD must obtain 50 continuing education credits every five (5) years, as defined by the MDCB.
IV. The CMD must obtain 12 continuing education credits every year, as defined by the MDCB.

12. The purpose of the MDCB Scope of Practice is to define the scope of practice of medical dosimetrists in order to:
A. I, II, and III only
B. I and III only
C. II and IV only
D. IV only
E. All are correct

I. Delineate areas of technical service.
II. Educate professionals in the fields of health care, education, and other communities of interest regarding the expectations of medical dosimetrists.
III. Assist medical dosimetrists in their efforts to provide appropriate and high-quality services to those in need of radiation therapy.
IV. Establish a reference for curriculum review of educational programs in medical dosimetry.

13. Which of the following are tasks for medical dosimetrists?
A. I, II, and III only
B. I and III only
C. II and IV only
D. IV only
E. All are correct

I. Obtain and synthesize pertinent clinical data to facilitate the radiation oncology process.
II. Participate in the development of optimal treatment strategies. This includes but is not limited to the generation of radiation dose distributions and the performance of dose calculations.
III. Document treatment parameters associated with the radiation therapy process.
IV. Participate in implementation of prescribed treatment courses.

14. Which of the following performance standards defines the activities of the practitioner in the areas of education, interpersonal relationships, personal and professional self-assessment, and ethical behavior?
   A. Quality performance standard
   B. Professional performance standard
   C. Clinical performance standard
   D. Educational performance standard

15. Which of the following are correct regarding the CARE bill?
   A. I, II, and III only
   B. I and III only
   C. II and IV only
   D. IV only
   E. All are correct
   I. It stands for the Consistency, Accuracy, Responsibility, and Excellence in Medical Imaging and Radiation Therapy.
   II. It establishes federal minimum standards of education and certification for personnel who performs medical imaging examinations and plans or delivers radiation therapy treatment.
   III. It reduces health-care costs by lowering the number of radiologic examinations that must be repeated due to improper positioning or poor technique.
   IV. It improves the safety of radiologic procedures.

10.3 Working as Professionals at Health System (Answers)

Quiz 1 (Level 2)

1. **B** Ethics is the discipline dealing with what is good or bad and right or wrong and moral principles that apply values and judgments to the practice of medicine. Legal concepts are the sum of rules and regulations by which society is governed in any formal and legally binding manner. Moral ethics focuses in a concept of right or wrong as it relates to conscience, and fidelity is the act to perform what is right, remaining faithful and loyal to the patient and their well-being.

2. **C** Beneficence means that health-care professionals must act in the best interest of a patient, even at some inconvenience and sacrifice to themselves.

The state or quality of being kind, charitable, or beneficial; non-maleficence involves the ethical principle of doing no harm to a patient by a medical professional. Autonomy is defined as the a patient who has a condition of independence, freedom, or self-government. Justice is defined as the principle of fairness and equity that is maintained for all individuals.

3. A Paternalism is doing what you think is best for the patient, against their will, right, or responsibilities.

4. D The analytical model identifies the caregiver as a scientist dealing only in facts and does not consider the human aspect of the patient. The priestly model provides a caregiver with a godlike paternalism attitude that makes decisions for and not with the patient. The contractual model maintains a business relationship between the provider and the patient, and the collegial model is a more cooperative method of pursuing health care for the provider and patient. There is also a covenant model that recognizes areas of health care not covered by a contract.

5. A Every patient is entitled to informed consent *before* any procedure is performed. They should be informed and educated about their medical facts and the risk involved; they should understand and approve their treatments and participate responsibly in their own care.

6. E When given an informed consent, the patient should be informed of the nature of the procedure, treatment, or disease and the risk involved, the expectation of the recommended treatment and the likelihood of success, and, finally, alternative available and probable outcome in absence of treatment.

7. E Informed consent is a legal document which cannot be delegated to a third party, the physician is solely responsible, and a witness must be present and sign at the time of consent.

8. A Competency is the quality or condition of being legally qualified to perform an act or the minimum mental, cognitive, or behavioral ability required to assume responsibility. A person of age 18 years or older is considered to be competent if no mental or physical condition is identified, and a person of age younger than 18 years is considered a minor; therefore they are incompetent, and parents or designated guardians must decide for them..

9. E Every professional must not divulge confidential information from a patient without the consent of the patient. Patient information should not be discussed with other departments unless a direct line of duty; also, conversation about a patient between professionals should be kept in private. Patient information should not be discussed with families and friends, and patient charts and computers with patient information should not be left unattended or unsecure.

10. B Negligence describes the failure to take reasonable care or caution in doing something resulting in unintentional injury to a patient. Malpractice refers to negligence or misconduct by a professional. Ethics is the discipline dealing with what is good or bad and right or wrong and the moral principles that apply values and judgments to the practice of medicine. Liability means the legal responsibility of one's act or omission because a professional or entity failed to meet his or her responsibility to open a lawsuit for any resulting damages.

11. E All statements must be met in order for an incident to be considered negligence. The plaintiff was owed a duty of care which was neglected or breached by a professional; there has to be a direct injury caused by the breach of that duty, and there was a proximate cause meaning that proof must be shown that the harm was caused by the tort you are suing.

12. B Civil law generally provides for the legal relationships between persons, organizations, and the government, and it is usually punished by reimbursement to the plaintiff for losses caused by the defendant behavior. Tort law provides protection to each person from harm not intended to harm society as a whole, and it is usually becoming liable to pay also for the damages that are caused to the victim. In criminal law the defendant can be punished to incarceration, death penalty, or a fine.

13. C Battery refers to unlawful physical contact or touching of a person without permission which is different from assault which refers to the fear of such touch or an unlawful threat or attempt to do bodily injury to another person. False imprisonment refers to the restraint of a person in a bounded area without justification or consent. Invasion of privacy refers to the intrusion into the personal life of another without cause, the confidentiality of information has not been maintained, or the patient's body has been improperly exposed or touched.

14. B False imprisonment refers to a restrain of a person in a bounded area without justification or consent; therefore answer B is correct. Answer A is an example of battery, answer C is an example of assault, and answer D is an example of invasion of privacy.

15. A Libel is defined as a false publication, as in writing, print, sign, or pictures, that damages the person's reputation. Slander is similar but is spoken. Slander is defined as oral communication of false statements injurious to a person's reputation.

16. D Res ipsa loquitur means "the thing speaks for itself." This means that there might not have to be direct proof or evidence to convict the defendant of a

breach of care. Personal liability means that persons are liable for their own negligent conduct. Respondent superior means "let the master answer" and refers to a case where the employer can be responsible for things that employees do while working directly under orders from the employer. Foreseeability is a principle of law that someone is responsible for all consequences of a single action.

17. **B** An incident report should be consistent with the institution's policies and procedures, and an injury does not have to occur for an incident report to be filled. It could be any event which is not consistent with the desire, normal, or unusual operation of the department, and it should contain only facts of the incident in concern. All copies should be retained in the risk manager's office. Incident reports should not be copied, photocopied, or retained by individuals or given to patients.

18. **E** Medical records contain a chronological written account of a patient's examination and treatment that include the patient's medical history and complaints. It should be maintained in independent departments from hospitals. After every entry, it must be signed in ink (or a digital signature). Corrections should never be deleted, but a line should be placed over the incorrect entry and initialed with time and date; it should never include inappropriate comments about staff or the patient.

19. **B** The Health Insurance Portability and Accountability Act (HIPAA) broadens the scope of existing fraud and abuse provisions and increases penalties for fraud violations by health-care providers. It protects privacy of health information while allowing the flow of health information needed to provide high-quality health care and reduces cost of administrative. The Affordable Care Act (ACA) is a law that makes health care more affordable and accessible for millions of Americans and for those who need its protections and benefits the most.

20. **C** The patient's bill of rights is a legal document which states that the patient has the right to considerate and respectful care and has the right to obtain relevant, current, and understandable information concerning diagnosis, treatment, and prognosis. Additionally, the patient has the right to make decisions about the plan of care, has the right to have an advance directive or a legal document that states patient's wishes about medical decisions or names another person to make decisions for him/her, has the right of privacy and confidentiality, has the right to review his or her records, and has the right to consent or decline to participate in studies.

21. **A** The bill is not required to be sent to the payee the same day the plan is signed.

22. B The American Medical Association (AMA) is an association dedicated to a body of ethical statements developed primary for the benefit of the patient. Physicians must recognize responsibilities to patients even though the principles adopted by the AMA are not a law but standard of conduct which defines the essentials of honorable behavior for the physician. Some of these values include that gifts of small values are allowed by the AMA code of ethics, a company who tries to make business with a physician or entity cannot offer cash as a gift, a physician should support access to medical care for all people, and any incentive from companies should be not accepted by a physician.

23. A The AAMD board of directors is composed of the president, the president elect, past president, membership and recording secretaries, the treasurer, and six regional directors. http://medicaldosimetry.org

24. C The mission statement of the AAMD is to promote and support the medical dosimetry profession and provide opportunities for education, a forum for professional interaction, and a representative voice in the health-care community while seeking to promote an ideal of professional conduct to which its member should aspire and endorse the highest standard of patient care. The American Society of Radiologic Technologists (ASRT) is a society that fosters the professional growth of radiologic technologists by expanding knowledge through education, research, and analysis; promoting exceptional leadership and service; and developing the radiology technology community through shared ethics and values. The American Association of Physicists in Medicine (AAPM) is a professional organization seeking to advance the science, education, and professional practice of medical physics. The American College of Medical Physics (ACMP) is an organization that enhances the quality of practice of medical physics; it is also engaged in professional activities for the benefit of the medical physics community and promotes the continuing competence of practitioners in medical physics.

25. D The American Society of Therapeutic Radiology and Oncology (ASTRO) is devoted to advance the practice of radiation oncology by disseminating the results of scientific research, promoting excellence in patient care, providing opportunities for educational and professional development of its members, developing policies, and representing radiation oncology in a rapidly evolving socioeconomic health-care environment. The American College of Radiology (ACR) is an organization that serves patients and society by maximizing the value of radiology, nuclear medicine, and medical physics.

26. A The mission statement of the MDCB is to steer the advancement of the medical dosimetry profession by establishing certification and continuing

10.3 Working as Professionals at Health System (Answers) 579

education standards to enhance quality patient care. The purpose of the MDCB is to elevate standards and advance the cause of medical dosimetry by encouraging its study and improving its practice, recognize the continuing knowledge and skills of medical dosimetrists, determine the certification eligibility of medical dosimetrists and conduct examinations to test the cognitive capability of voluntary candidates, grant and issue certificates to successful candidates, and offer a registry service to CMDs.

27. A The applicant for the MDCB exam can be eligible if he/she complies with one out of the three routes. Route 1: graduated from either a JRCERT-accredited program or a program of at least 12 or 18 months or completed at least 6 months of clinical medical dosimetry experience under the direction of a CMD or medical physicist. Route II: own a BS degree or hold an ARRT in radiation therapy and completed at least 24 months of clinical medical dosimetry experience under the direction of a CMD or medical physicist and 12 CE approved by the MDCB during his or her 24 months of clinical experience. Route III: own AAs, AS, or BS degree and completed at least 36 months of clinical medical dosimetry experience under the direction of a CMD or medical physicist and 24 CE approved by the MDCB during his or her 36 months of clinical experience.

28. D The American Association of Medical Dosimetrists (AAMD) is an agency that promotes and supports the medical dosimetry profession.

29. A A patient care partnership is a legal document that informs patients about what they should expect during their hospital stay with regard to their rights and responsibilities. The patient's bill of rights is a legal document which states that the patient has the right to considerate and respectful care. A medical record describes the systematic documentation of a single patient's medical history and care across time within one particular healthcare provider's jurisdiction. An incident report is a form that is filled out in order to record details of an unusual event that occurs at the facility, such as an injury to a patient.

30. E All are correct.

31. C An advance health-care directive, also known as a living will, personal directive, advance directive, or advance decision, is instructions given by individuals specifying what actions should be taken for their health in the event that they are no longer able to make decisions due to illness or incapacity and appoints a person to make such decisions on their behalf.

32. B Entities (person) that fail to comply voluntarily with HIPPA standards may be subject to civil money penalties and or criminal prosecution. The entity

(person) may be fined from a minimum of $100 to $50,000 or more per violation not to exceed $1,500,000 per calendar year cap. If criminal charges are filed, the institution (person) may face fines up $250,000 and/or 10 years imprisonment.

33. **B** The Medical Dosimetry Certification Board (MDCB) offers the certification in medical dosimetry. The American Association of Medical Dosimetrists (AAMD) is an agency that promotes and supports the medical dosimetry profession. The American College of Medical Physics (ACMP) is an organization that enhances the quality of practice of medical physics, and the American Registry of Radiologic Technologists (ARRT) promotes high standards of patient care by recognizing qualified individuals in medical imaging, interventional procedures, and radiation therapy.

34. Match the following:
   A. (IV)   The American Association of Medical Dosimetrist (AAMD) is an international society established to promote and support the medical dosimetry profession.
   B. (V)   The Medical Dosimetry Certification Board (MDCB) serves to steer the advancement of the medical dosimetry profession by establishing certification and continuing education standards to enhance quality patient care.
   C. (VII) The American College of Medical Physics (ACMP) is an organization that enhances the quality of practice of medical physics.
   D. (VII) The American Registry of Radiologic Technologists (ARRT) promotes high standards of patient care by recognizing qualified individuals in medical imaging, interventional procedures, and radiation therapy.
   E. (II)   The American Board of Radiology (ABR) oversees the certification and ongoing professional development of specialists in diagnostic radiology, radiation oncology, and medical physics.
   F. (VI)   The Joint Commission on Accreditation of Healthcare Organizations (JCAHO) is a USA-based not-for-profit organization that accredits over 19,000 health-care organizations and programs in the USA.
   G. (III) The American College of Radiology (ACR) is an organization that serves patients and society by maximizing the value of radiology, nuclear medicine, and medical physics.
   H. (I)   The American Society of Therapeutic Radiology and Oncology (ASTRO) is devoted to advance the practice of radiation oncology.
   I. (IX)   The American Society of Radiologic Technologists (ASRT) is a society that fosters the professional growth of a radiologist technologist.

10.4 Professional Medical Dosimetrists (Answers)

J. (XI) The American Medical Association (AMA) is an association dedicated to a body of ethical statements developed primary for the benefit of the patient.

K. (XII) The Health Insurance Portability and Accountability Act (HIPAA) protects the privacy of health information.

L. (X) The American Association of Physicists in Medicine (AAPM) is an organization seeking to advance the science, education, and professional practice of medical physics.

M. (XIII) The Joint Review Committee on Education in Radiologic Technology (JRCERT) promotes excellence in education and elevates the quality and safety of patient care through the accreditation of educational programs in radiography, radiation therapy, magnetic resonance, and medical dosimetry.

10.4 Professional Medical Dosimetrists (Answers)

Quiz 1 (Level 2)

1. **B** MDCB, AAMD, and JRCERT are responsible for the medical dosimetry profession.

2. **B** The MDCB code of ethics applies to professionals holding certification credentials from the MDCB and persons applying for examination and certification by the MDCB in order to become certified medical dosimetrists. http://mdcb.org/about/ethics

3. **E** A CMD shall always promote the safety and welfare of his or her patients by performing medical dosimetry procedures safely and with reasonable skill. A CMD shall not engage in conduct likely to deceive, defraud, or harm the public. Irrespective of whether a patient is actually injured or otherwise harmed, a CMD shall not demonstrate a willful or reckless disregard for the health, welfare, or safety of a patient.

    A CMD may not be convicted of, or enter a plea of nolo contendere to, regardless of adjudication, a crime, in any jurisdiction, which the crime either directly relates to the provision of patient care or involves fraud, dishonesty, or moral turpitude, including without limitation in the context of the CMD's employment.

    A CMD shall not, without the prior express written consent of the MDCB, use or reproduce, in whole or in part, or aid another in using or reproducing, in any manner or fashion, any MDCB examination materials (or the contents thereof), certificates, logos, abbreviations, emblems, or other documents or property of the MDCB.

A CMD shall not misuse the MDCB name or any MDCB certificate, title, logo, or emblem.

A CMD may not be under suspension, revocation, or other disciplinary action by any professional medical dosimetry organization, certifying body, licensing board, or credentialing agency.

A CMD shall not, without authorization to do so, possess, use, or have access to any MDCB examination documents or materials, nor shall a CMD receive any unauthorized assistance prior to or during the conduct of any portion of a CMD examination. A CMD shall not divulge to others information gained from his or her CMD examination experience.

A CMD shall not make any material misrepresentation of fact during application for MDCB certification or re-certification and shall not fail to disclose any material fact where the disclosure of which is necessary to avoid having other statements be misleading. A CMD shall not engage in any act or omission to obtain or assist another in obtaining MDCB certification or re-certification by fraud, misrepresentation, or deception.

A CMD having knowledge and evidence of a violation of any ethical standard by another CMD shall report such violation promptly by filing a written complaint with the MDCB. Any such complaint shall include specific detail and documentation regarding the identity of the person(s) involved in the alleged ethical violation. The identity of the complainant must be disclosed, as well as the identities of others known to have knowledge of the facts and circumstances surrounding the alleged ethical violation.

A CMD shall not, knowingly, falsely accuse another CMD of violating these Ethical Standards.

A CMD shall not make or file any report in connection with patient care, which report he or she knows to be false.

A CMD's ability to practice medical dosimetry with reasonable skill and safety shall not be materially impaired by reason of illness; use of alcohol, drugs, narcotics, chemicals, or any other type of material; or as a result of any mental or physical condition.

A CMD shall not practice beyond the scope he or she is competent to perform as defined in the Medical Dosimetry Scope and Standards of Practice Document.

A CMD shall cooperate with, and shall not obstruct, the MDCB in connection with any investigation or hearing under the Ethical Standards. http://mdcb.org/about/ethics

4. E The MDCB may deny, revoke, or suspend certification or re-certification when a CMD is found to be not in compliance with MDCB rules, regulations, and/or the foregoing Ethical Standards. In addition, the MDCB may censure a CMD, issue public or private reprimands, place a CMD on probation for up to 5 years, or impose other sanctions related to the ethical violation. A CMD placed on probation may continue to use the certification credential but shall be subject to revocation of his or her certified

status in the event of another ethical violation during the period of probation. If an applicant for certification is not in compliance with these Ethical Standards, the MDCB may refuse to allow the applicant to sit for the certification examination, or, in the event that the examination has been taken, the MDCB may refuse to release the examination results. http://mdcb.org/about/ethics

5. **E** If the Chair of the Ethics Committee determines that there is evidence of a violation of the Ethical Standards, the Chair shall inform the respondent in writing that a complaint of ethical misconduct has been filed and a formal investigation will be conducted; the respondent has thirty (30) days from the date of receipt of the notification letter or complaint of ethical misconduct to prepare and submit a response in writing; the ethics committee shall evaluate all documentation pertaining to the matter and, within ninety (90) days of receiving all relevant evidence, determine whether the complaint is substantiated by clear and convincing evidence; and a CMD or an applicant to whom the complaint of ethical misconduct notice is given shall have thirty (30) days from the date the notice is mailed to make a written request for a hearing. http://mdcb.org/about/ethics

6. **A** The MDCB Scope of Practice is designed to provide a statement of competence in medical dosimetry practice, define the practice of medical dosimetry, and provide a useful guide for medical dosimetrist and others in evaluating the quality, effectiveness, and appropriateness of health-care service.

7. **D** The final MDCB Scope of Practice document was adopted on March 13, 2001. In 1996, the medical dosimetrist scope of practice research committee was formed, and in 1997 the medical dosimetrist scope of practice data began to be collected. In 2000, the medical dosimetrist scope of practice first committee was held, and the document was made available to important institutions for comment.

8. **E** All are correct.

9. **A** The medical dosimetrist must demonstrate an understanding of topics including, but not limited to, cancer, radiation biology, radiation therapy techniques, radiation oncology physics, equipment technology, radiation safety and protection, anatomy, physiology, mathematics, and the psychosocial aspects of cancer.

10. **A** The medical dosimetrist must perform radiation treatment planning, recognize and resolve equipment problems and treatment discrepancies, and recommend when treatment should be withheld until a physician and physicist can be consulted. The only professional allowed to sign radiation prescriptions is the physician.

11. B   Up to now, the medical dosimetrist does not has to be certified by the Medical Dosimetry Certification Board (MDCB) in order to perform his or her work, but it is recommended that the medical dosimetrist be certified by the Medical Dosimetry Certification Board (MDCB). To maintain MDCB certification, a level of expertise and awareness of changes and advances in practice must be acquired. The CMD must obtain 50 continuing education credits every five (5) years, as defined by the MDC.

12. E   All are correct.

13. E   All are correct.

14. B   The professional performance standards define the activities of the practitioner in the areas of education, interpersonal relationships, personal and professional self-assessment, and ethical behavior. The quality performance standards define the activities of the practitioner in the technical areas of performance including equipment and material assessment, safety standards, and total quality management. The clinical performance standards define the activities of the practitioner in the care of patients and delivery of therapeutic treatment planning by incorporating patient assessment and management with procedural analysis, performance, and evaluation.

15. E   The CARE bill stands for the Consistency, Accuracy, Responsibility, and Excellence in Medical Imaging and Radiation Therapy. This act established federal minimum standards of education and certification for personnel who perform medical imaging examinations and plan or deliver radiation therapy treatment. In addition, it attempts to reduce health-care costs by lowering the number of radiologic examinations that must be repeated due to improper positioning or poor technique, improves the safety of radiologic procedures, and ensures that quality information is presented for diagnosis and that quality radiation therapy treatments are delivered, leading to accurate diagnosis, treatment, and cure. http://www.asrt.org/CAREBILL

Radiation Oncology

11

Contents

11.1	The Brain (Questions)	585
11.2	The Head and Neck Region (Questions)	591
11.3	The Thorax (Questions)	607
11.4	The Abdomen (Questions)	619
11.5	The Pelvis (Questions)	622
11.6	The Spinal Canal (Questions)	631
11.7	Children (Questions)	633
11.8	Benign Diseases (Questions)	642
11.9	The Skin (Questions)	643
11.10	Soft Tissue Sarcomas (Questions)	645
11.11	Extras (Questions)	646
11.12	The Brain (Answers)	647
11.13	The Head and Neck Region (Answers)	650
11.14	The Thorax (Answers)	658
11.15	The Abdomen (Answers)	666
11.16	The Pelvis (Answers)	668
11.17	The Spinal Canal (Answers)	672
11.18	Children (Answers)	673
11.19	Benign Diseases (Answers)	678
11.20	The Skin (Answers)	679
11.21	Soft Tissue Sarcomas (Answers)	680
11.22	Extras (Answers)	681

11.1 The Brain (Questions)

The Brain, Brainstem, and Cerebellum

1. Some of the clinical presentations of a brain neoplasm are:
A. I, II, and III only
B. I and III only

C. II and IV only
D. IV only
E. All are correct
I. Edema
II. Focal neurological dysfunction
III. Intracranial pressure
IV. Hydrocephalus

2. Tumors of the cranial and spinal nerves include:
A. I, II, and III only
B. I and III only
C. II and IV only
D. IV only
E. All are correct
I. Schwannoma
II. Malignant lymphomas
III. Neurofibroma
IV. Pituitary adenoma

3. Which of the following will decrease cerebral edema preoperatively, postoperatively, and during irradiation? Administration of:
A. Glucocorticoid (dexamethasone)
B. Phenytoin (Dilantin)
C. Carbamazepine (Tegretol)
D. Phenobarbital

4. Which of the following modalities are used to deliver radiation to CNS patients?
A. I, II, and III only
B. I and III only
C. II and IV only
D. IV only
E. All are correct
I. External beam radiation therapy
II. Radiosurgery (stereotactic irradiation)
III. Interstitial brachytherapy
IV. LDR brachytherapy

5. Criteria for CNS brachytherapy include:
A. I, II, and III only
B. I and III only
C. II and IV only
D. IV only
E. All are correct
I. Tumor confined to one hemisphere
II. No transcallosal or subependymal spread
III. Tumor size less than 5–6 cm
IV. Tumor well circumscribed on CT or MRI

11.1 The Brain (Questions)

6. Which of the following anatomic landmarks can be used for cranial radiation therapy techniques?
A. I, II, and III only
B. I and III only
C. II and IV only
D. IV only
E. All are correct
I. The external acoustic meatus
II. The sella turcica
III. The cribriform plate
IV. The mandibular angle

7. The sella turcica is used as a landmark for:
A. I, II, and III only
B. I and III only
C. II and IV only
D. IV only
E. All are correct
I. The inferior border of whole-brain irradiation fields
II. The hypothalamus
III. The pineal body
IV. The optic canal

8. The most common error in head and neck treatment setup is:
A. Head rotation and/or tilting
B. Head rotation and/or in/out position
C. Tilting and/or anterior/posterior position
D. Anterior/posterior and/or in/out position

9. Irradiation techniques of the entire intracranial contents include:
A. I, II, and III only
B. I and III only
C. II and IV only
D. IV only
E. All are correct
I. Parallel-opposed lateral portals
II. Inferior border 0.5–1 cm inferior to the cribriform plate, middle cranial fossa, and foramen magnum
III. Anterior border 3 cm posterior to the ipsilateral eyelid
IV. Superior and posterior flash

10. Which of the following tumor locations in the brain is best treated with parallel-opposed lateral portals?
A. I, II, and III only
B. I and III only
C. II and IV only
D. IV only
E. All are correct

I. Bilateral or medial cerebral hemispheric tumors
II. Brainstem, posterior parietal, occipital, or frontal lesions/tumors
III. Midcerebral tumors
IV. Craniopharyngiomas and pituitary, optic nerve, hypothalamic, and brainstem tumors

11. When irradiating brain tumor on a pregnant patient:
A. I, II, and III only
B. I and III only
C. II and IV only
D. IV only
E. All are correct
I. The fetal exposure should be less than **0.**10 Gy.
II. Brain irradiation should be avoid due to the high risk of fetal death.
III. Leukemia risk in the child must be considered.
IV. The fetal exposure can exceed 20 Gy when high doses are used.

12. Which of the following statements is true about CNS irradiation?
A. I, II, and III only
B. I and III only
C. II and IV only
D. IV only
E. All are correct
I. The patient may be irradiated with a helmet field and one or two spine fields followed by a brain boost.
II. Patients can be treated supine or prone.
III. Collimator and couch angles are critical for setup reproducibility.
IV. Couch angle must be used on helmet brain and collimator angles on spine fields.

13. Which of the following statements is true about CNS irradiation?
A. I, II, and III only
B. I and III only
C. II and IV only
D. IV only
E. All are correct
I. The junctions are moved every 20 Gy of tumor dose.
II. The junctions are moved every 10 Gy of tumor dose.
III. The gap used should be located between the helmet brain and superior spine field.
IV. Three or four junctions are typically used on CNS cases.

14. The most serious late reaction to irradiation of CNS is:
A. Nausea and vomiting
B. Alopecia
C. Mucositis and esophagitis
D. Necrosis

11.1 The Brain (Questions)

15. Most brainstem gliomas are:
A. High-grade astrocytomas
B. Ependymoma
C. Medulloblastoma
D. Meningiomas

16. The most common primary brain tumor is:
A. Astrocytomas
B. Gliomas
C. Medulloblastoma
D. Meningiomas

17. Which of the following are considered benign brain tumors?
A. I, II, and III only
B. I and III only
C. II and IV only
D. IV only
E. All are correct
I. Astrocytomas
II. Acoustic neuroma
III. Glioblastomas
IV. Meningiomas

18. An acoustic neuroma is also called:
A. Astrocytomas
B. Gliomas
C. Schwannoma
D. Meningiomas

The Pituitary

1. The pituitary gland:
A. I, II, and III only
B. I and III only
C. II and IV only
D. IV only
E. All are correct
I. Is connected to the hypothalamus
II. Is located in the sella turcica
III. Secretes nine hormones that regulate homeostasis
IV. Produces a hormone that modulates the wake/sleep pattern

2. A patient treated for a pituitary tumor requires periodic assessment of:
A. I, II, and III only
B. I and III only
C. II and IV only
D. IV only
E. All are correct
I. Gonadal function
II. Thyroid function
III. Adrenal function
IV. Lacrimal gland function

3. Which of the following is true about pituitary radiation therapy techniques?
A. I, II, and III only
B. I and III only
C. II and IV only
D. IV only
E. All are correct
I. Lateral portals of 5×5 to 6×6 cm or shaped fields are used.
II. If photon energies below 10 MV are used, a vertex field is recommended to decrease the irradiation dose to the temporal lobes.
III. Special care must be taken to avoid exposure to the eyes.
IV. Bilateral coaxial wedge fields plus a coronal field, moving arc fields, and 360° rotational fields can be used.

4. In order to obtain a more homogeneous dose distribution and in decreasing the dose delivered to the optic chiasm:
A. I, II, and III only
B. I and III only
C. II and IV only
D. IV only
E. All are correct
I. Two parallel-opposed fields must be used with 40° wedges with heel placed posteriorly.
II. Two parallel-opposed fields and a vertex field must be used.
III. Two parallel-opposed fields must be used with 60° wedges with heel placed posteriorly.
IV. Two parallel-opposed fields must be used with 15° wedges with heel placed anteriorly.

5. Which of the following structures must be considered as critical when irradiating a pituitary tumor?
A. I, II, and III only
B. I and III only
C. II and IV only
D. IV only
E. All are correct

I. The optic chiasm
II. The temporal lobes
III. The brain stem
IV. The hypothalamus

6. The pituitary gland:
A. I, II, and III only
B. I and III only
C. II and IV only
D. IV only
E. All are correct
I. Is a middle structure situated in the body of the sphenoid bone
II. Is located superior to the sphenoid sinus and nasopharynx
III. Is composed of two lobes
IV. Is an endocrine gland

7. Which of the following hormones is produced by the pituitary gland?
A. I, II, and III only
B. I and III only
C. II and IV only
D. IV only
E. All are correct
I. Growth hormone
II. Thyroid-stimulating hormone
III. Prolactin
IV. Insulin

11.2 The Head and Neck Region (Questions)

The Hypopharynx

1. The hypopharynx is divided into:
A. I, II, and III only
B. I and III only
C. II and IV only
D. IV only
E. All are correct
I. The pyriform sinuses
II. The posterolateral pharyngeal wall
III. The postcricoid region
IV. Supraglottic

2. Which of the following parts of the hypopharynx has the highest incidence of tumor occurrence in the United States?
A. The pyriform fossa
B. The posterolateral pharyngeal wall
C. The postcricoid region
D. The pyriform sinuses

3. Most hypopharynx tumors are:
A. Carcinoma in situ
B. Squamous cell carcinoma
C. Malignant melanoma
D. Sarcoma

4. Preoperative irradiation of the hypopharynx is on the order of:
A. 65 to 70 Gy in 7–8 weeks
B. 60 to 66 Gy
C. 45 to 50 Gy in 4.5–5 weeks
D. 70 to 80 Gy in 10 weeks

5. If irradiation is given alone, the irradiated volume of the hypopharynx should encompass:
A. I, II, and III only
B. I and III only
C. II and IV only
D. IV only
E. All are correct
I. The nasopharynx
II. The oropharynx
III. The hypopharynx
IV. The upper cervical esophagus

6. Hypopharynx radiation treatment consists of:
A. Two parallel-opposed upper-neck lateral beams and one anterior photon field encompassing the lower neck plus a boost to the gross tumor
B. Two parallel-opposed upper-neck lateral beams and one anterior electron field encompassing the lower neck
C. Four oblique-field techniques (RAO, LAO, RPO, LPO) treating the upper and lower neck
D. PA/PA beams encompassing the upper and lower neck

7. The hypopharynx extends from:
A. I, II, and III only
B. I and III only
C. II and IV only
D. IV only
E. All are correct

11.2 The Head and Neck Region (Questions)

I. The level of the hyoid bone to the lower border of the cricoid cartilage.
II. The level of the thyroid to the lower esophagus
III. From cervical vertebra 4 to cervical vertebra 6
IV. From cervical vertebra 1 to cervical vertebra 2

The Larynx

1. The larynx is divided into:
A. I, II, and III only
B. I and III only
C. II and IV only
D. IV only
E. All are correct
I. Supraglottic area
II. Glottis
III. Subglottic area
IV. The pyriform sinuses

2. Which of the following is true about the subglottic area?
A. I, II, and III only
B. I and III only
C. II and IV only
D. IV only
E. All are correct
I. The subglottic area begins 5 mm below the vocal cord.
II. The subglottic area begins 5 cm below the vocal cord.
III. The subglottic area ends at the inferior border of the cricoid cartilage and the beginning of the trachea.
IV. The subglottic area ends at the inferior border of the true vocal cord.

3. The most common head and neck cancer occurs in the:
A. Hypopharynx
B. Larynx
C. Nasopharynx
D. Parotids

4. Cancer of the larynx is strongly related to:
A. Poor exercise
B. Alcohol
C. Cigarette smoking
D. Poor healthy food intake

5. Most of subglottic laryngeal lesions are:
A. I, II, and III only
B. I and III only
C. II and IV only
D. IV only
E. All are correct
I. Ipsilateral
II. Bilateral
III. Diagnosed early
IV. Diagnosed late

6. Some procedures to eradicate carcinoma of the larynx include:
A. I, II, and III only
B. I and III only
C. II and IV only
D. IV only
E. All are correct
I. Irradiation
II. Hemilaryngectomy
III. Cordectomy
IV. Total laryngectomy

7. Radiation therapy techniques for T1 laryngeal lesions generally include:
A. Field sizes from 10 cm × 10 cm to 15 cm × 15 cm.
B. Lateral field sizes extend from the thyroid notch superiorly to the inferior border of the cricoid cartilage and fall off anteriorly.
C. Lateral field sizes including the jugulodigastric and middle jugular lymph nodes.
D. Four oblique-field techniques (RAO, LAO, RPO, LPO) from 4 cm × 4 cm to 6 cm × 6 cm each.

8. Most laryngeal tumors are:
A. Carcinoma in situ
B. Squamous cell carcinoma
C. Malignant melanoma
D. Sarcoma

9. Which of the following nodes are mainly involved in carcinoma of the larynx?
A. The jugulodigastric nodes
B. The middle jugular nodes
C. The subdigastric nodes
D. The inferior jugular nodes

The Nasal Cavity and Paranasal Sinuses

1. A stage III nasal cavity or paranasal sinus has:
A. No extension out of the site of origin
B. Extension to orbit, nasopharynx, and paranasal sinuses
C. Extension to skin and pterygomaxillary fossa
D. Extension to the base of the skull or pterygoid plate and destruction and intracranial extension

2. The most common malignancy of the nasal cavity and paranasal sinuses is:
A. Carcinoma in situ
B. Squamous cell carcinoma
C. Malignant melanoma
D. Lymphoma

3. The preferred treatment for the nasal vestibule is:
A. Surgery
B. Chemotherapy
C. Radiation therapy
D. Chemoradiation

4. Nasal cavity and paranasal sinuses radiation therapy techniques include:
A. I, II, and III only
B. I and III only
C. II and IV only
D. IV only
E. All are correct
I. An anterior portal only
II. An anterior portal with one or two posterior tilted lateral portals, frequently using wedges
III. An anterior portal electron field and two opposed lateral fields, frequently using wedges
IV. A wedge-pair technique if the disease is ipsilateral only

5. When treating the nasal cavity and paranasal sinuses, complications of irradiation include:
A. I, II, and III only
B. I and III only
C. II and IV only
D. IV only
E. All are correct
I. Central nervous system damage
II. Unilateral or bilateral vision loss
III. Otitis media
IV. Chronic sinusitis

6. Which of the following statements is true about tumors in the nasal cavity and paranasal sinuses?
A. I, II, and III only
B. I and III only
C. II and IV only
D. IV only
E. All are correct
I. They are twice as common in males than in females.
II. They show a bimodal age distribution of 10–20 and 50–60 years of age.
III. They are considered rare tumors.
IV. Most tumors present at advance stage.

7. Which of the following nodes are mainly involved in nasal cavity and paranasal sinuses tumors?
A. I, II, and III only
B. I and III only
C. II and IV only
D. IV only
E. All are correct
I. Jugulodigastric nodes
II. Submandibular nodes
III. Inferior jugular nodes
IV. Subdigastric nodes

8. Which of the following areas of the nasal cavity and paranasal sinuses uses primary surgery followed by radiation therapy as the treatment of choice?
A. I, II, and III only
B. I and III only
C. II and IV only
D. IV only
E. All are correct
I. The nasal vestibule
II. The nasal cavity
III. The sphenoid sinus
IV. The maxillary sinus

The Nasopharynx

1. The most common site of distant metastasis from nasopharyngeal cancer is:
A. The bone
B. The lung
C. The liver
D. The brain

11.2 The Head and Neck Region (Questions)

2. The most common malignancy of the nasopharynx is:
A. Rhabdomyosarcoma
B. Lymphoma
C. Malignant melanoma
D. Epidermoid or undifferentiated carcinomas

3. The preferred treatment for the nasopharynx is:
A. Surgery
B. Chemotherapy
C. Radiation therapy
D. Chemoradiation

4. Which of the following statements is true about radiation therapy techniques for nasopharynx treatments?
A. I, II, and III only
B. I and III only
C. II and IV only
D. IV only
E. All are correct
I. The volume irradiated includes the nasopharynx, adjacent parapharyngeal tissues, and all of the cervical lymphatics.
II. The upper neck is treated using opposing lateral fields.
III. After 45 Gy, the lateral fields are modified to shield the spinal cord.
IV. Lower neck involvement is treated with anterior-posterior parallel-opposed fields.

5. Which of the following treatment modalities has been used for nasopharyngeal carcinoma?
A. I, II, and III only
B. I and III only
C. II and IV only
D. IV only
E. All are correct
I. Three-dimensional radiation therapy
II. Stereotactic irradiation
III. Brachytherapy
IV. Chemotherapy

6. Reirradiation techniques for the nasopharynx include:
A. I, II, and III only
B. I and III only
C. II and IV only
D. IV only
E. All are correct

I. External irradiation
II. Brachytherapy
III. Combination of external irradiation and brachytherapy
IV. Chemotherapy

7. Which of the following is true about nasopharyngeal carcinoma?
A. I, II, and III only
B. I and III only
C. II and IV only
D. IV only
E. All are correct
I. Children or young adults should be treated with irradiation alone.
II. For retreatment with external beams, relatively small fields must be used.
III. Irradiation dose depends on patient age and tumor stage.
IV. Hypopituitarism causing significant clinical signs and symptoms is commonly reported in children.

8. The nasopharynx is located:
A. I, II, and III only
B. I and III only
C. II and IV only
D. IV only
E. All are correct
I. At the level of the hyoid bone to the lower border of the cricoid cartilage
II. Anteriorly to the posterior choanae and posterior to cervical vertebrae 1 and 2 and the clivus
III. From cervical vertebrae 4–6
IV. Superior to the body of the sphenoid and inferior to the soft palate

9. Which of the following are common lymph nodes involved in carcinomas of the nasopharynx?
A. I, II, and III only
B. I and III only
C. II and IV only
D. IV only
E. All are correct
I. Deep posterior cervical lymph nodes
II. Submandibular nodes
III. Jugulodigastric lymph nodes
IV. Inferior jugular nodes

The Oral Cavity

1. The oral cavity consists of:
A. I, II, and III only
B. I and III only
C. II and IV only
D. IV only
E. All are correct
I. The upper and lower lips
II. The upper and lower gingiva
III. The hard palate
IV. The floor of mouth

2. The upper gingiva is composed of:
A. The orbicularis muscle
B. The alveolar ridge of the maxilla
C. Mucous membrane
D. Styloglossus, hyoglossus, and hyoid muscles

3. The treatment of choice for patients with clinically or radiographically ipsilateral positive neck nodes is:
A. Bilateral neck dissection followed by ipsilateral postoperative neck irradiation.
B. Ipsilateral neck dissection followed by bilateral postoperative neck irradiation.
C. Node removal and no further treatment is required other than observation.
D. Contralateral prophylactic neck dissection is required.

4. If radiation therapy is considered:
A. I, II, and III only
B. I and III only
C. II and IV only
D. IV only
E. All are correct
I. Optimal oral hygiene and pretreatment dental care must be completed.
II. Any potential surgical procedures and tooth extractions should be carried out before initiation of radiotherapy.
III. Approximately 8–10 days is needed for complete recovery before initiation of radiation therapy.
IV. After a course of irradiation, caution in tooth extraction or surgical procedure involving the gums is a lifelong commitment.

5. Which of the following statements is true about external irradiation of the oral cavity?
A. I, II, and III only
B. I and III only
C. II and IV only
D. IV only
E. All are correct

I. The most commonly used technique for carcinoma of the mobile tongue is opposed laterals.
II. A bite block is used to keep the tongue depressed away from the palate.
III. The radiation dose depends on the number of clonogenic cells.
IV. Every attempt should be made to avoid an excessive dose of radiation to the mandible.

6. The most common interstitial irradiation technique is:
A. Percutaneous afterloading with angiocatheters and iridium-192
B. Y-90
C. Manchester system
D. Surface mold

7. The best treatment for smaller, more anteriorly situated primary lesions of the oral tongue is:
A. External radiation alone
B. Interstitial implant or intraoral cone radiation therapy as a boost
C. Interstitial implant only
D. Combined surgery and irradiation

8. Which of the following is considered a risk factor for carcinoma of the oral cavity?
A. I, II, and III only
B. I and III only
C. II and IV only
D. IV only
E. All are correct
I. Alcohol
II. Smoking or chewing tobacco
III. Human immunodeficiency virus (AIDS)
IV. Vitamin deficiency

9. The most common malignancy of the oral cavity is:
A. Squamous cell carcinoma
B. Lymphoma
C. Malignant melanoma
D. Epidermoid or undifferentiated carcinomas

10. The level 2 lymphatic region in the head and neck includes:
A. The submental and submandibular triangle
B. The upper jugulodigastric
C. Deep jugular nodes of the middle and lower third of the neck
D. Spinal accessory and transverse cervical chains (posterior triangle)

11. Which of the following nodes are commonly included in radiation therapy portals of the oral cavity?
A. I, II, and III only
B. I and III only
C. II and IV only
D. IV only
E. All are correct
I. The submandibular nodes
II. The subdigastric nodes
III. The submental nodes
IV. The jugulodigastric nodes

The Oropharynx

1. The oropharynx is located:
A. From the level of the hyoid bone to the lower border of the cricoid cartilage, from cervical vertebrae 4 to 6
B. 5 mm below the vocal cord and ends at the inferior border of the cricoid cartilage and the beginning of the trachea
C. Between the soft palate and the hyoid bone
D. Anteriorly to the posterior choanae and posterior to cervical vertebrae 1 and 2 and the clivus. Also, superior to the body of the sphenoid and inferior to the soft palate

2. The oropharynx is composed of:
A. I, II, and III only
B. I and III only
C. II and IV only
D. IV only
E. All are correct
I. The soft palate
II. The tonsillar region
III. The base of the tongue
IV. The pharyngeal wall

3. Most oropharynx tumors are:
A. Melanomas
B. Sarcomas
C. Lymphomas
D. Keratinizing squamous cell carcinoma

4. The most common acute irradiation sequela when treating the oropharynx is:
A. I, II, and III only
B. I and III only
C. II and IV only
D. IV only
E. All are correct

I. Oropharyngeal mucositis
II. Fibrosis
III. Moderate-to-severe dysphagia
IV. Hearing loss

5. Which of the following modalities can be used to treat the base of the tongue?
A. I, II, and III only
B. I and III only
C. II and IV only
D. IV only
E. All are correct
I. External radiation alone (IMRT, conventional)
II. Combined surgery and irradiation
III. Brachytherapy
IV. Chemotherapy

The Ear

1. The ear is composed of:
A. I, II, and III only
B. I and III only
C. II and IV only
D. IV only
E. All are correct
I. The external ear
II. The middle ear
III. The internal ear
IV. The superficial ear

2. Which of the following anatomical parts belongs to the external ear?
A. I, II, and III only
B. I and III only
C. II and IV only
D. IV only
E. All are correct
I. The bony labyrinth
II. The tympanic membrane
III. The auditory ossicles
IV. The external auditory meatus (EAM)

3. The external ear involves:
A. I, II, and III only
B. I and III only
C. II and IV only
D. IV only
E. All are correct

I. The superficial parotid nodes
II. The retroauricular nodes
III. The superficial cervical group nodes
IV. No lymph node involvement

4. Basal cell carcinoma is the most common tumor type in what part of the ear?
A. The auditory canal
B. The middle ear
C. The mastoid area
D. The external ear

5. Tumors involving the pinna are best treated with:
A. Orthovoltage or electron fields
B. Chemotherapy only
C. Surgery
D. High-energy photons (23×)

6. The acoustic nerve is responsible for:
A. I, II, and III only
B. I and III only
C. II and IV only
D. IV only
E. All are correct
I. Auditory function
II. Temporal muscle function
III. Vestibular function
IV. Mastoid process function

7. Which of the following part of the ear does not contain lymphatics?
A. The external ear
B. The middle ear
C. The internal ear
D. The superficial ear

The Eye

1. The retina of the eye is located in:
A. The outer coat
B. The middle coat
C. The inner layer
D. The lens

2. The lens is:
A. I, II, and III only
B. I and III only
C. II and IV only
D. IV only
E. All are correct

I. Located posterior to the iris
II. Located anterior to the iris
III. Suspended from the ciliary body
IV. Suspended from the ocular muscles

3. Which of the following is the treatment of choice for basal and squamous cell carcinomas of the eyelid?
A. Surgery
B. Chemotherapy
C. Radiation therapy
D. Brachytherapy

4. The most common metastatic sites for tumors of the posterior uvea are:
A. I, II, and III only
B. I and III only
C. II and IV only
D. IV only
E. All are correct
I. In men, the prostate or lung
II. In men, the lung or GI track
III. In women, the bladder or breast
IV. In women, the breast or lung

5. An enucleation or exenteration is done for a malignant melanoma of the posterior uvea if:
A. I, II, and III only
B. I and III only
C. II and IV only
D. IV only
E. All are correct
I. The tumor exceeds 15 mm in diameter.
II. The tumor exceeds 10 mm in thickness.
III. There is extra-sclera extension at diagnosis.
IV. There are small growing melanomas.

6. Which of the following is the most common intraocular malignancy in children:
A. Malignant melanoma
B. Retinoblastoma
C. Rhabdomyosarcoma
D. Optic glioma

7. Which is the most common grouping system used for retinoblastoma?
A. Reese-Ellsworth classification system
B. TNM staging classification system
C. American Joint Committee staging system
D. Stage A, B, and C

8. Which of the following sources has been used on radioactive plaque retinoblastoma therapy?
A. I, II, and III only
B. I and III only
C. II and IV only
D. IV only
E. All are correct
I. Cobalt-60
II. Iodine-125
III. Iridium-192
IV. Ruthenium-109

9. Which of the following sources is the most common today for radioactive plaque retinoblastoma therapy?
A. Cobalt-60
B. Iodine-125
C. Iridium-192
D. Ruthenium-109

10. Which of the following statements is true about retinoblastoma tumors?
A. I, II, and III only
B. I and III only
C. II and IV only
D. IV only
E. All are correct
I. It is bilateral in one-third of patients.
II. It is unilateral in two-thirds of patients.
III. Most patients with hereditary form have bilateral disease.
IV. The common signs and symptoms are leukocoria (white papillary reflex) and strabismus (squint).

Salivary Glands

1. The salivary glands consist of:
A. I, II, and III only
B. I and III only
C. II and IV only
D. IV only
E. All are correct
I. The parotid gland
II. The submandibular gland
III. The sublingual gland
IV. The submaxillary gland

2. Which of the following is the largest salivary gland?
A. The parotid gland
B. The submandibular gland
C. The sublingual gland
D. The submaxillary gland

3. The most common malignant subtype of parotid tumors in children is:
A. Mucoepidermoid tumor
B. Adenoid cystic carcinoma
C. Pleomorphic adenoma
D. Astrocytomas

The Thyroid

1. Differentiated thyroid cancer consists of:
A. I, II, and III only
B. I and III only
C. II and IV only
D. IV only
E. All are correct
I. Papillary carcinoma
II. Mixed papillary-follicular carcinoma
III. Follicular adenocarcinoma
IV. Anaplastic cancer

2. Which of the following radioactive isotope is used in the treatment of thyroid cancer?
A. Iridium-192
B. Iodine-131
C. Iodine-125
D. Palladium-103

3. Which of the following statements about thyroid cancer is true:
A. I, II, and III only
B. I and III only
C. II and IV only
D. IV only
E. All are correct
I. Thyroid cancer is uncommon.
II. Thyroid cancer is more common in females than males.
III. There is higher risk after irradiation.
IV. Incidence is lowest in children.

4. The thyroid gland is composed of:
A. I, II, and III only
B. I and III only
C. II and IV only
D. IV only
E. All are correct
I. The right lobe
II. The pyramidal lobe
III. The left lobe
IV. The isthmus

5. Which of the following modalities best demonstrates thyroid function?
A. Nuclear medicine
B. CT
C. MRI
D. Ultrasound

Unusual Nonepithelial Tumors of the Head and Neck

1. Which of the following tumors are considered unusual nonepithelial tumors of the head and neck?
A. I, II, and III only
B. I and III only
C. II and IV only
D. IV only
E. All are correct
I. Hemangiopericytomas
II. Chordomas
III. Esthesioneuroblastomas
IV. Extramedullary plasmacytomas

11.3   The Thorax (Questions)

The Breast

1. Which of the following is considered early-stage breast cancer?
A. Tis, T1, and inflammatory only
B. Tis to T3 only
C. Tis, T1, T2 only
D. T4 and recurrent only

2. In the United States, the most common malignancy and the second most common cause of mortality in females is:
A. Colorectal cancer
B. Breast cancer
C. Lung cancer
D. Skin cancer

3. Risk factors associated with breast cancer include:
A. I, II, and III only
B. I and III only
C. II and IV only
D. IV only
E. All are correct
I. Sex
II. Genetic factors
III. Diet
IV. Endocrine factors

4. The mammary gland lies:
A. Over the pectoralis major muscle from the second to the sixth rib and from the sternum to the anterior or midaxillary line
B. Over the pectoralis minor muscle from the first to the twelfth rib and from the sternum to the anterior or midaxillary line
C. Under the pectoralis major muscle from the second to the sixth rib and from the sternum to the midaxillary line
D. Over the pectoralis minor muscle from the second to the sixth rib and from the sternum to the anterior or midaxillary line

5. Which of the following statements is true about breast cancer?
A. I, II, and III only
B. I and III only
C. II and IV only
D. IV only
E. All are correct
I. The lymphatic of the breast drains mainly superiorly and laterally.
II. The supraclavicular and internal mammary nodes are occasionally involved.
III. Metastases to the internal mammary nodes are more frequent form inner quadrant and central lesions.
IV. Vascular invasion and hematogenous metastases to the lungs, pleura, bone, and brain occur even with small tumors.

6. Most of the carcinomas of the breast occur in the:
A. Upper inner quadrant
B. Lower inner quadrant
C. Lower outer quadrant
D. Upper outer quadrant

7. Breast cancer spreads via:
A. I, II, and III only
B. I and III only
C. II and IV only
D. IV only
E. All are correct
I. Lymphatic vessels
II. Blood vessels
III. Direct invasion
IV. Mammary ducts

8. The best modality in detection of breast cancer is:
A. PET-CT
B. MRI
C. Mammography
D. CT scan

9. The most common type of breast cancer is:
A. Ductal carcinoma in situ (DCIS)
B. Invasive (infiltrating) ductal carcinoma
C. Lobular carcinoma in situ (LCIS)
D. Tubular carcinoma

10. Strong prognostic factors of breast cancer include:
A. I, II, and III only
B. I and III only
C. II and IV only
D. IV only
E. All are correct
I. Tumor size
II. Tumor location
III. Clinical stage
IV. PSA

11. Which of the following are genes associated with hereditary breast cancer?
A. I, II, and III only
B. I and III only
C. II and IV only
D. IV only
E. All are correct
I. BRCA3
II. BRCA1
III. BRCA4
IV. BRCA2

12. Axillary and supraclavicular nodal irradiation must be performed:
A. In patients with more than five positive axillary lymph nodes
B. In patients whom axillary dissection could not be performed
C. In patients with more than two or more positive axillary lymph nodes
D. All Tis patients

13. Adjuvant chemotherapy for breast cancer must be given to:
A. I, II, and III only
B. I and III only
C. II and IV only
D. IV only
E. All are correct
I. Node-negative patients with tumors less than 2 cm in diameter
II. Postmenopausal patients with positive nodes
III. Premenopausal patients with positive nodes
IV. All patients with positive nodes

14. General breast irradiation field borders include:
A. Superior, head of clavicles; inferior, 2–3 cm below the inframammary fold; medially, 1 cm over midline; lateral, 2 cm beyond palpable breast tissue
B. Superior, acromioclavicular joint; inferior, 1 cm below the inframammary fold; medially, 1 cm over midline; lateral, 2 cm beyond palpable breast tissue
C. Superior, head of clavicles; inferior, 1 cm below inframammary fold; medially, midline; lateral, 2 cm beyond palpable breast tissue
D. Superior, acromioclavicular joint; inferior, 2–3 cm below the inframammary fold, medially, 1 cm over midline; lateral, 1 cm beyond palpable breast tissue

15. Which of the following positions is recommended when treating a large pendulous breast?
A. I, II, and III only
B. I and III only
C. II and IV only
D. IV only
E. All are correct
I. Prone
II. Lateral decubitus
III. Modified lateral decubitus
IV. Supine

16. Which of the following is used for a breast planning to obtain a uniform dose distribution?
A. I, II, and III only
B. I and III only
C. II and IV only
D. IV only
E. All are correct

11.3 The Thorax (Questions)   611

I. Wedges
II. Compensating filters
III. Multileaf collimators
IV. Blocks

17. Which of the following irradiation techniques can be used for breast cancer?
A. I, II, and III only
B. I and III only
C. II and IV only
D. IV only
E. All are correct
I. Medial and lateral tangential fields
II. En face electron boost
III. Interstitial brachytherapy
IV. IMRT

18. Physical wedges must be avoided on medial tangent breast beams because:
A. The sternum is adjacent to the medial border.
B. The wedge can be dropped and injure the patient.
C. The contralateral breast will receive more doses due to scatter.
D. It is too heavy and difficult to position.

19. Most common intact breast, supraclavicular, and electron boost doses are:
A. Breast, 45 Gy; SCV, 50 Gy; electron boost, 10 Gy
B. Breast, 50 Gy; SCV, 45 Gy; electron boost, 10 Gy
C. Breast, 80 Gy; SCV, 50 Gy; electron boost, 10 Gy
D. Breast, 50 Gy; SCV, 45 Gy; electron boost, 45 Gy

20. Supraclavicular fields are angled 15–20° to:
A. Spare part of the spinal cord
B. Spare part of the lung
C. Properly match the breast tangents
D. Get more homogenous dose to the supraclavicular nodes

21. Which of the following anatomical parts is commonly blocked during a supraclavicular field irradiation?
A. I, II, and III only
B. I and III only
C. II and IV only
D. IV only
E. All are correct
I. The clavicle
II. The cord
III. The mandible
IV. The humeral head

22. Most supraclavicular fields are normalized:
A. At 5 cm depth
B. At 3 cm depth
C. At 7 cm depth
D. At body maximum because depth is not important

23. The most common method of treatment when a supraclavicular field is needed is:
A. Tangent fields with a table kick and collimator rotation
B. ARC IMRT technique
C. Monoisocentric technique
D. Mini-tangents with supraclavicular angled 15–20°

24. Axillary lymph nodes field borders are:
A. Superior, head of clavicles; inferior, 2–3 cm bellow inframammary fold; medially, 1 cm over midline; lateral, 2 cm beyond palpable breast tissue (breast irradiation)
B. Inferior, matching superior fields with tangent fields; superior, cover acromioclavicular joint; medially, 1 cm across the midline, following the medial border of the sternocleidomastoid muscle; lateral, vertical line at the level of the anterior axillary fold, splitting the humeral head (SCV)
C. Medially, allow **1.**5–2 cm of the lung to show on the portal field; inferior, at the same level as the inferior border of the supraclavicular field; lateral, blocks falloff across the posterior axillary field; superior, splits the clavicles
D. Medial, midline; lateral, usually 5 cm lateral to the midline; superior, abuts the inferior border of the supraclavicular field; inferior, at the xiphoid process

25. Which of the following calculation points is used for the axillary lymph nodes?
A. I, II, and III only
B. I and III only
C. II and IV only
D. IV only
E. All are correct
I. At 3 cm depth
II. At 2 cm depth inferior to the midportion of the clavicle
III. At 5 cm depth
IV. At a point midplane to the axilla

26. Internal mammary lymph nodes are irradiated:
A. I, II, and III only
B. I and III only
C. II and IV only
D. IV only
E. All are correct
I. On patients with primary tumors in the inner quadrants
II. On patients with primary tumors in the outer quadrants
III. On patients with tumors on the periareola that are larger than 3 cm in diameter
IV. All T3 patients

11.3 The Thorax (Questions)

27. Which of the following is the most common male breast cancer?
A. Infiltrated ductal carcinoma or invasive ductal carcinoma (IDC)
B. Invasive lobular carcinoma or infiltrative lobular carcinoma (ILC)
C. Lobular carcinoma in situ or lobular neoplasia (LCIS)
D. Ductal carcinoma in situ or intraductal carcinoma (DCIS)

28. Methods to treat the internal mammary chain (IMC) include:
A. I, II, and III only
B. I and III only
C. II and IV only
D. IV only
E. All are correct
I. Deep tangents
II. En face IM field
III. Shallow tangents matched to breast tangents
IV. Brachytherapy

29. The most important prognostic factor for breast cancer is:
A. Tumor size
B. Stage
C. Axillary node status
D. Patient age

30. Which of the following is considered a PAB (post axillary boost) field?
A.

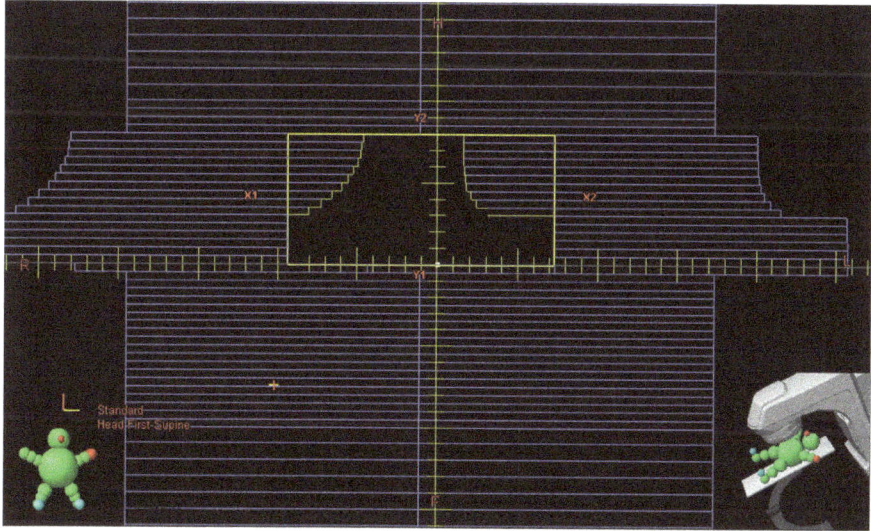

Fig. 11.3.1

B.

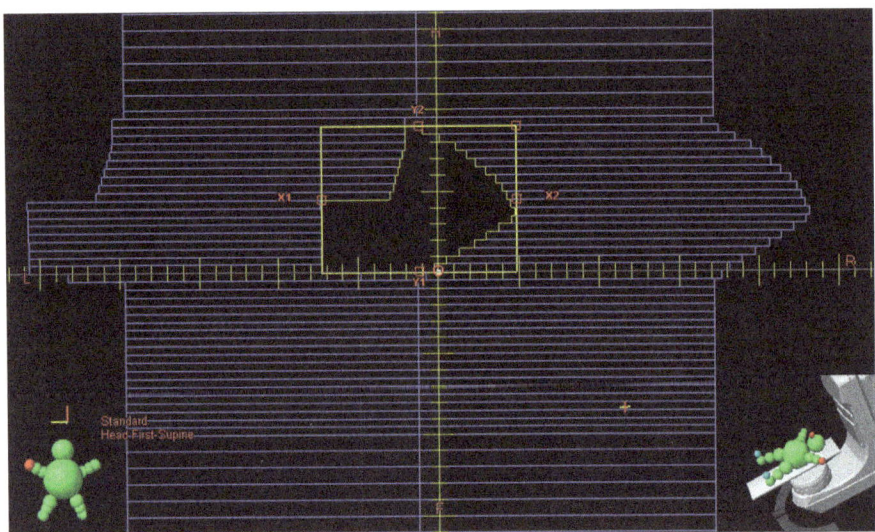

Fig. 11.3.2

C.

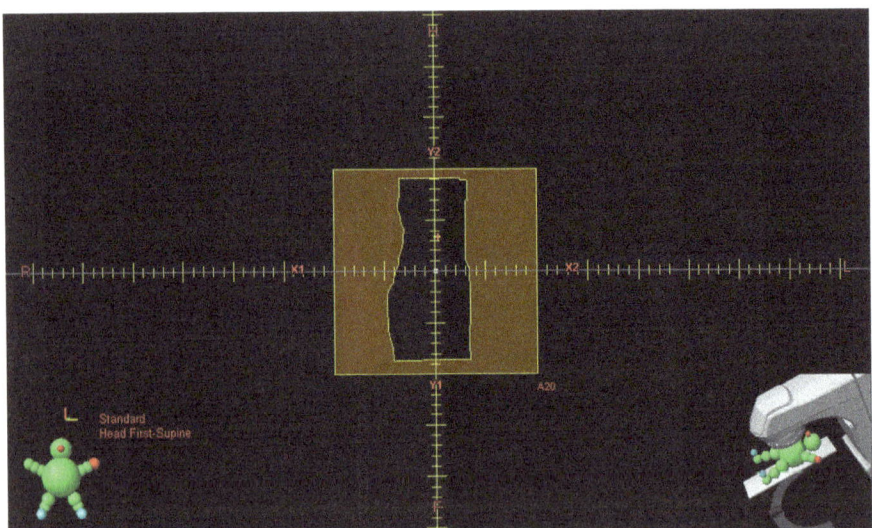

Fig. 11.3.3

11.3 The Thorax (Questions)

D.

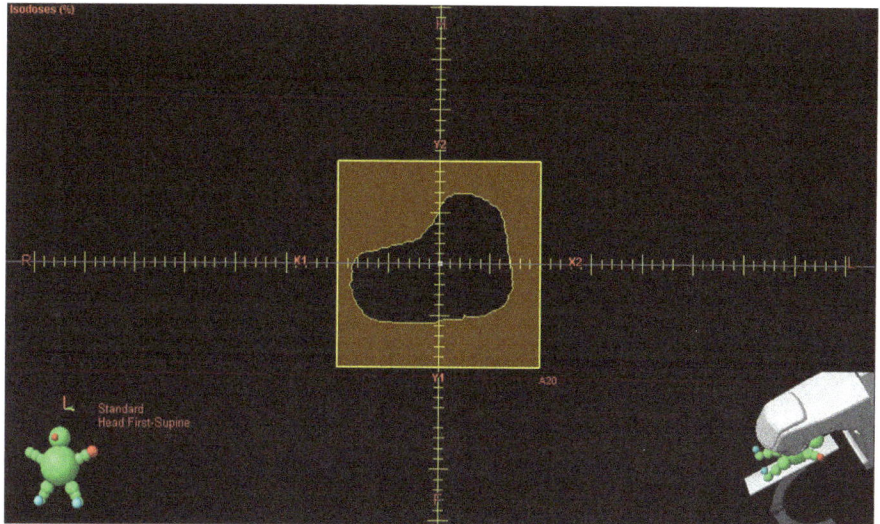

Fig. 11.3.4

31. Which of the following are dose-limiting organs for irradiation of the left breast and SCV fields?
A. I, II, and III only
B. I and III only
C. II and IV only
D. IV only
E. All are correct
I. The lungs
II. The heart
III. The spine
IV. The pancreas

The Esophagus

1. The esophagus:
A. I, II, and III only
B. I and III only
C. II and IV only
D. IV only
E. All are correct
I. Measures approximately 25 cm long
II. Metastasizes to the brain
III. Is located between C7 to T11
IV. Has no lymphatic risk

2. The esophagus is composed of which parts?
A. I, II, and III only
B. I and III only
C. II and IV only
D. IV only
E. All are correct
I. Cervical
II. Upper thoracic
III. Mid-thoracic
IV. Lower thoracic

3. Which anatomical area of the esophagus has the highest incidence of squamous cell carcinoma?
A. Upper one-third of the esophagus.
B. Middle one-third of the esophagus.
C. Lower one-third of the esophagus.
D. All areas have the same incident.

4. Which of the following conditions is most commonly associated with adenocarcinoma of the esophagus?
A. Barrett's esophagus
B. Gastric acid reflux
C. Hiatal hernia
D. Achalasia

5. Which study is best in diagnosing esophageal cancer?
A. I, II, and III only
B. I and III only
C. II and IV only
D. IV only
E. All are correct
I. Ultrasound
II. Computer tomography
III. Diagnostic X-rays
IV. Positron-emission tomography

The Lungs

1. The right lung is composed of:
A. One lobe
B. Two lobes
C. Three lobes
D. Four lobes

11.3 The Thorax (Questions)

2. The bifurcation of the trachea (carina) is approximately at:
A. The level of the seventh cervical vertebra
B. The level of the first thoracic vertebra
C. The level of the third thoracic vertebra
D. The level of the fifth thoracic vertebra

3. The most common metastatic sites of lung cancer are:
A. I, II, and III only
B. I and III only
C. II and IV only
D. IV only
E. All are correct
I. The lung
II. The liver
III. The brain
IV. The bone

4. Which of the following is the major symptom in lung cancer?
A. Hemoptysis
B. Dyspnea
C. Cough
D. Dysphagia

5. The most common lung cancer is:
A. Non-small and small-cell carcinomas
B. Astrocytoma
C. Malignant melanoma
D. Ductal carcinoma in situ (DCIS)

6. Which of the following areas should be treated prophylactically when small-cell carcinoma of the lung is diagnosed?
A. The lumbar spine
B. The thoracic spine
C. The pelvic area
D. The brain

7. Superior vena cava syndrome:
A. I, II, and III only
B. I and III only
C. II and IV only
D. IV only
E. All are correct
I. Is a medical emergency seen in patients with malignant neoplasia
II. Results from bronchogenic carcinoma
III. Requires an initial high dose of radiation
IV. Should include the mediastinum, hilar, and adjacent pulmonary parenchyma lesions

8. The second most common malignancy in males in the United States is:
A. Breast cancer
B. Lung cancer
C. Prostate cancer
D. Colorectal cancer

9. The highest risk factor associated with lung cancer is due to:
A. Diet
B. Genetic factors
C. Radon
D. Cigarette smoking or inhalation

10. The hila contain:
A. I, II, and III only
B. I and III only
C. II and IV only
D. IV only
E. All are correct
I. The bronchi
II. The pulmonary arteries and veins
III. The bronchial arteries and veins
IV. The lymphatics

11. What is the name of the bifurcation of the trachea?
A. The carina
B. The alveoli
C. The hilum
D. The sternal notch

The Mediastinum and Trachea

1. The mediastinal boundaries include:
A. I, II, and III only
B. I and III only
C. II and IV only
D. IV only
E. All are correct
I. The first thoracic vertebra
II. The diaphragm
III. The parietal pleura
IV. The vertebral column

2. Most of mediastinal lymphomas are located in the:
A. Anterior compartment
B. Posterior compartment
C. Medial compartment
D. Lateral compartment

3. The most common tumor of the anterior mediastinum is:
A. Neurogenic tumor
B. Thymoma
C. Cyst
D. Endocrine tumor

4. The most common primary carcinoma of the trachea is:
A. Chondroma
B. Hemangioma
C. Squamous cell and adenoid cystic carcinoma
D. Papilloma

11.4 The Abdomen (Questions)

The Pancreas and Hepatobiliary Track

1. The pancreas lies approximately:
A. At the level of T9–T12
B. At the level of L1–L2
C. At the level of the bifurcation
D. At the level of the sacrum

2. The head of the pancreas is located anatomically:
A. On the right side of the abdomen
B. On the left side of the abdomen
C. On the right side of the pelvis
D. On the left side of the pelvis

3. The majority of pancreatic cancers are:
A. Lymphomas
B. Giant-cell carcinoma
C. Adenocarcinoma
D. Sarcomas

4. The majority of pancreatic cancers occur:
A. In the head of the pancreas.
B. In the body of the pancreas.
C. In the tail of the pancreas.
D. All are equal.

5. The common hepatic duct is composed of:
A. I, II, and III only
B. I and III only
C. II and IV only
D. IV only
E. All are correct

I. The right hepatic duct
II. The cystic duct
III. The left hepatic duct
IV. The common bile duct

6. Which of the following are dose-limiting organs for irradiation of the pancreas?
A. I, II, and III only
B. I and III only
C. II and IV only
D. IV only
E. All are correct
I. The small intestine
II. The stomach
III. The liver
IV. The kidneys

7. Which of the following statements is true about conformal radiation treatment of the pancreas?
A. I, II, and III only
B. I and III only
C. II and IV only
D. IV only
E. All are correct
I. When treating the head of the pancreas, the entire duodenal loop with margin is included.
II. When treating the body of the pancreas, two-thirds of the left kidney is excluded.
III. When treating body or tail lesions, at least 50 % of the left kidney may need to be included.
IV. When treating the head of the pancreas, at least 50 % of the right kidney may need to be included.

8. Which of the following is the anatomical part of the pancreas that extends toward the spleen?
A. The head
B. The body
C. The neck
D. The tail

The Stomach

1. The stomach is divided into:
A. I, II, and III only
B. I and III only
C. II and IV only
D. IV only
E. All are correct

I. The fundus
II. The body
III. The pylorus
IV. The tail

2. The most common sites of distant metastases of stomach cancer are:
A. I, II, and III only
B. I and III only
C. II and IV only
D. IV only
E. All are correct
I. The pancreas
II. The liver
III. The spleen
IV. The lungs

3. The majority of gastric cancers are:
A. Lymphomas
B. Giant-cell carcinoma
C. Adenocarcinoma
D. Gastric sarcomas

4. Most stomach cancers originate in:
A. The cardiac sphincter
B. The outermost lining
C. The pylorus
D. The innermost lining

The Kidney, Renal Pelvis, and Ureter

1. Which of the following statements is true about the kidneys?
A. I, II, and III only
B. I and III only
C. II and IV only
D. IV only
E. All are correct
I. They are located between the eleventh rib and the third lumbar vertebral body.
II. They move vertically as much as 4 cm during normal respiration.
III. The right kidney is slightly more inferior than the left.
IV. They are located in the retroperitoneal space.

2. The left kidney drains to:
A. The paracaval lymph nodes
B. The interaortocaval lymph nodes
C. The paraaortic lymph nodes
D. The external iliac lymph nodes

3. The most common sites of distant metastases of renal cellv carcinoma is/are:
A. I, II, and III only
B. I and III only
C. II and IV only
D. IV only
E. All are correct
I. The lungs
II. The bones
III. Soft tissue
IV. The liver

4. Carcinoma of the ureter occurs most often:
A. In the proximal third of the ureter
B. In the distal third of the ureter
C. Multifocally
D. In the mid-ureter

5. The majority of renal cancers are:
A. Lymphomas
B. Transitional cell carcinomas
C. Squamous cell carcinomas
D. Adenocarcinoma

6. Which of the following malignant neoplasm of the kidney occurs in children?
A. Medulloblastoma
B. Neuroblastoma
C. Wilms' tumor
D. Adenocarcinoma

11.5 The Pelvis (Questions)

The Anal Canal

1. The anal canal:
A. I, II, and III only
B. I and III only
C. II and IV only
D. IV only
E. All are correct
I. Is 3–4 cm long
II. Is 10–15 cm long
III. Extends from the level of the pelvic floor to the anal verge
IV. Extends from the sigmoid colon to the anal canal

11.5 The Pelvis (Questions)

2. Which of the following are considered risk factors for anal cancer?
A. I, II, and III only
B. I and III only
C. II and IV only
D. IV only
E. All are correct
I. History of anal warts
II. Cervical dysphasia
III. Gonorrhea
IV. More than ten sexual partners in a lifetime

3. The most common carcinoma of the anal canal is:
A. Squamous cell carcinomas
B. Mucoepidermoid carcinomas
C. Adenocarcinoma
D. Undifferentiated cancers

4. The major lymphatic pathways of the anal canal drain to:
A. I, II, and III only
B. I and III only
C. II and IV only
D. IV only
E. All are correct
I. The external iliac system
II. The internal iliac system
III. The mesenteric system
IV. The preauricular node system

The Colon and Rectum

1. Risk factors associated with colorectal cancer include:
A. I, II, and III only
B. I and III only
C. II and IV only
D. IV only
E. All are correct
I. Environmental
II. Genetic factors
III. Diet
IV. Sex

2. Which of the following is the most common colorectal cancer?
A. Adenocarcinoma
B. Squamous cell carcinomas
C. Astrocytomas
D. Malignant melanoma

3. Which of the following is true about the rectal anatomy?
A. I, II, and III only
B. I and III only
C. II and IV only
D. IV only
E. All are correct
I. The rectum starts at S3.
II. The rectum measures about 15 cm in length.
III. The rectum is composed of three valves.
IV. The rectum follows the sigmoid colon anatomically.

4. The colon is composed of:
A. I, II, and III only
B. I and III only
C. II and IV only
D. IV only
E. All are correct
I. The ascending colon
II. The descending colon
III. The transverse colon
IV. The splenic and hepatic flexures

5. On a 3D conformal rectal external beam treatment plan:
A. Three-field techniques are typically used with the patient in a supine position.
B. Four-field techniques are typically used with the patient in a supine position.
C. Three-field techniques are typically used with the patient in a prone position.
D. Eight-field techniques are typically used with the patient in either a prone or supine position.

The Bladder

1. The apex of the bladder is:
A. Located toward the pubic symphysis
B. The largest part of the bladder
C. The most inferior part of the bladder
D. Posteriorly located in the bladder

2. Ureters enter the bladder:
A. At the neck, inferiorly and laterally
B. At the apex or vertex, inferiorly and anteriorly
C. At the base or fundus, superiorly and dorsally
D. At the body, superiorly and dorsally

11.5 The Pelvis (Questions)

3. The urinary bladder is composed of:
A. I, II, and III only
B. I and III only
C. II and IV only
D. IV only
E. All are correct
I. The neck
II. The body
III. The trigone
IV. The tail

4. The trigone of the urinary bladder is formed by the:
A. Apex, vertex, and fundus
B. Neck, body, and tail
C. Urethral opening and ureteral exits
D. Ureteral opening and urethral exits

5. The most common sites of bladder tumor development are:
A. I, II, and III only
B. I and III only
C. II and IV only
D. IV only
E. All are correct
I. The trigone
II. The lateral and posterior walls
III. The neck
IV. The apex

6. The most common sites of distant metastases of bladder cancer are:
A. I, II, and III only
B. I and III only
C. II and IV only
D. IV only
E. All are correct
I. The lung
II. The bone
III. The liver
IV. The spleen

7. The majority of bladder cancers are:
A. Lymphomas
B. Transitional cell carcinomas
C. Squamous cell carcinomas
D. Adenocarcinoma

8. The highest risk factor associated with bladder cancer is:
A. Diet
B. Genetic factors
C. Sex
D. Cigarette smoking or inhalation

The Female Urethra

1. The primary lymphatics associated with the urethra are:
A. I, II, and III only
B. I and III only
C. II and IV only
D. IV only
E. All are correct
I. The obturator nodes
II. The internal iliac nodes
III. The external iliac nodes
IV. The suprapancreatic nodes

The Penis and Male urethra

1. Most malignant penile tumors are:
A. Undifferentiated or mixed carcinomas
B. Transitional cell carcinomas
C. Well-differentiated squamous cell carcinomas
D. Adenocarcinoma

The Prostate

1. The prostate is divided into:
A. I, II, and III only
B. I and III only
C. II and IV only
D. IV only
E. All are correct
I. The anterior lobe
II. The posterior lobe
III. The median lobe
IV. The lateral lobes

11.5 The Pelvis (Questions)

2. The most useful tool in diagnosing prostate cancer is:
A. The Gleason score
B. Prostate-specific antigen (PSA)
C. Nodal involvement
D. Rectal digital examination

3. The most common sites of distant metastases of prostate cancer are:
A. The lung
B. The bone
C. Soft tissue
D. The liver

4. Most malignant prostate tumors are:
A. Sarcomas
B. Lymphomas
C. Squamous cell carcinomas
D. Adenocarcinoma

5. Which of the following is used as prostate cancer treatment?
A. I, II, and III only
B. I and III only
C. II and IV only
D. IV only
E. All are correct
I. Surgery
II. Hormonal therapy
III. Radiation therapy
IV. Chemotherapy

6. Which of the following organs can be treated prophylactically before hormonal therapy for prostate cancer?
A. The liver
B. The rectum
C. The breast
D. The kidneys

7. Radioactive source used for prostate temporal implant includes:
A. Iodine-125
B. Iridium-192
C. Palladium-103
D. Gold-198

The Testis

1. Testis nodes crossover are common:
A. From left to right side
B. From right to left side
C. From superior to inferior side
D. From inferior to superior side

2. The most common testicular cancer is:
A. Adenocarcinoma
B. Lymphoma
C. Sarcoma
D. Germ cell tumor

3. Most testicular cancer patients receive radiation to:
A. I, II, and III only
B. I and III only
C. II and IV only
D. IV only
E. All are correct
I. The hepatic nodes
II. The paraaortic lymph nodes
III. The contralateral pelvic nodes
IV. The ipsilateral pelvic nodes

4. Testicular cancer is most commonly found in males:
A. Age 70 and above
B. Age 50–70
C. Age 15–30
D. Newborn babies

The Endometrium

1. The uterus is divided into:
A. I, II, and III only
B. I and III only
C. II and IV only
D. IV only
E. All are correct
I. The corpus
II. The body
III. The cervix
IV. The tail

2. The most common gynecologic malignancy is:
A. Cervical cancer
B. Endometrial cancer
C. Ovarian cancer
D. Vaginal cancer

3. The most common presenting symptom of endometrial cancer is:
A. Back pain
B. Enlarged uterus
C. Vaginal bleeding
D. Urgency or frequent urination

4. The most common form of carcinoma of the endometrium is:
A. Serous carcinoma
B. Clear-cell carcinoma
C. Pure squamous cell carcinoma
D. Adenocarcinoma

The Ovary

1. The most common ovarian carcinoma is:
A. Germ cell
B. Epithelial
C. Sex cord
D. Stromal

The Uterine Cervix

1. The most common metastatic site of uterine cervix cancer is:
A. The bones
B. The paraaortic nodes
C. The lungs
D. The liver

2. Which of the following staging is most used on gynecologic cancer?
A. FIGO
B. TNM
C. AJCC
D. Chang

3. The majority of uterine cervix cancers are:
A. Adenoid cystic carcinomas
B. Squamous cell carcinomas
C. Clear-cell carcinomas
D. Adenocarcinomas

4. Which of the following isotopes is used for HDR brachytherapy of uterine cervix cancer?
A. Cesium-137
B. Iridium-192
C. Iodine-125
D. Gold-192

5. Intracavitary brachytherapy techniques of the uterine cervix include the use of:
A. I, II, and III only
B. I and III only
C. II and IV only
D. IV only
E. Tandem
I. Ovoid/ring
II. Cylinder
III. Balloon catheter
IV. Endobronchial catheter

The Vagina

1. Most vaginal cancers occur:
A. On the anterior wall of the upper third of the vagina
B. On the posterior wall of the lower vagina
C. On the posterior wall of the upper third of the vagina
D. On the anterior wall of the lower vagina

2. The majority of vaginal cancers in adults are:
A. Adenoid cystic carcinomas
B. Epidermoid carcinomas
C. Sarcomas
D. Adenocarcinomas

3. The majority of vaginal cancers in children under 5 years old are:
A. Leiomyosarcomas
B. Epidermoid carcinomas
C. Rhabdomyosarcomas
D. Lymphomas

4. Which of the following is the preferred treatment for most carcinomas of the vagina?
A. I, II, and III only
B. I and III only
C. II and IV only
D. IV only
E. All are correct

I. Surgery
II. Hormonal therapy
III. Combination of radiation and surgery
IV. Radiation therapy

5. Which of the following modalities of treatment is used for vaginal tumors?
A. I, II, and III only
B. I and III only
C. II and IV only
D. IV only
E. All are correct
I. Surgery
II. Intracavitary and interstitial LDR or HDR
III. Chemotherapy
IV. External beam radiation therapy

6. Which of the following is true when performing brachytherapy for a vaginal treatment?
A. I, II, and III only
B. I and III only
C. II and IV only
D. IV only
E. All are correct
I. Vaginal surface dose and tumor dose should be calculated.
II. The largest diameter cylinder possible should be used.
III. The strength of the sources in the ovoids should be 15 mgRaeq.
IV. Dome cylinders can be used for homogeneous irradiation of the vaginal cuff.

11.6 The Spinal Canal (Questions)

The Spinal Cord

1. Spinal canal tumors are classified as:
A. I, II, and III only
B. I and III only
C. II and IV only
D. IV only
E. All are correct
I. Intramedullary
II. Extramedullary
III. Intradural-extramedullary
IV. Medullary

2. Which of the following tumors arise intramedullary?
A. I, II, and III only
B. I and III only
C. II and IV only
D. IV only
E. All are correct
I. Astrocytomas
II. Oligodendrogliomas
III. Ependymomas
IV. Meningiomas

3. Which of the following is true about the spinal cord?
A. I, II, and III only
B. I and III only
C. II and IV only
D. IV only
E. All are correct
I. The spinal cord is composed of 31 pairs of nerves.
II. The white matter is located in the periphery and surrounds the central gray matter.
III. The spinal cord ends near the level of the L1 vertebral body.
IV. The lower lumbar, sacral, and coccygeal nerves form the cauda equina.

4. Which of the following radiation therapy techniques is most used in the treatment of cervical spinal canal?
A. Direct posterior field
B. Opposed anteroposterior and posteroanterior portals
C. Opposed lateral fields
D. Paired set of oblique-wedged fields combined with PA field

5. The arachnoid mater:
A. I, II, and III only
B. I and III only
C. II and IV only
D. IV only
E. All are correct
I. Is the innermost lining and covers the spinal cord and its blood vessels
II. Is located between the pia mater and the dura mater
III. Forms a dense, fibrous barrier between the bony spinal canal and the spinal cord
IV. Encloses the subarachnoid space filled with cerebrospinal fluid (SPF)

6. Traditionally, the field borders used for treating a spinal cord tumor are:
A. I, II, and III only
B. I and III only
C. II and IV only
D. IV only
E. All are correct

I. Superior and inferior to encompass two vertebral bodies above and below the tumor.
II. Superior and inferior to encompass 2 cm above and below the tumor.
III. Width is typically 4–8 cm with the anterior border including the vertebral foramen.
IV. Width is typically covering half of the spinous process with the anterior border including the vertebral foramen.

7. Which of the following structures contains cerebrospinal fluid?
A. The subarachnoid
B. The dura mater
C. The pia mater
D. The dural sac

8. Where does the spinal cord end?
A. L3–L5
B. Sacrum
C. L1–L2
D. Coccyx

11.7 Children (Questions)

Brain Tumors in Children

1. Which of the following is a brain tumor in children?
A. Rhabdomyosarcoma
B. Neuroblastoma
C. Medulloblastoma
D. Wilms' tumor

2. Radiation treatment of medulloblastoma is best accomplished via:
A. Two lateral opposed brain fields
B. AP/PA spine fields
C. Total body irradiation
D. CNS irradiation

3. Which of the following organs is boosted for medulloblastoma irradiation?
A. The posterior fossa
B. The occipital lobe
C. The corpus callosum
D. The temporal lobes

4. Infants and young children tumors include:
A. I, II, and III only
B. I and III only
C. II and IV only
D. IV only
E. All are correct
I. Low-grade gliomas
II. Malignant gliomas
III. Brainstem gliomas
IV. Craniopharyngiomas

Hodgkin's Disease

1. Hodgkin's disease occurs:
A. In the liver
B. In the pancreas
C. In the lymph nodes
D. In the lungs

2. Which nodal area is most commonly involved in Hodgkin's disease?
A. Paraaortic nodes
B. Cervical nodes
C. Inguinal nodes
D. Mediastinal nodes

3. Which of the following staging system is used for Hodgkin's disease?
A. FIGO
B. TNM
C. AJCC
D. Ann Arbor

4. Stage III Hodgkin's disease includes:
A. Involvement of a single lymph node region
B. Involvement of two or more lymph node regions on the same side of the diaphragm
C. Involvement of lymph node regions on both sides of the diaphragm
D. Disseminated involvement of one or more extralymphatic organs or tissues

5. Which of the following are subtypes of Hodgkin's disease?
A. I, II, and III only
B. I and III only
C. II and IV only
D. IV only
E. All are correct

11.7 Children (Questions)

I. Lymphocyte-predominant HD (LPHD)
II. Nodular sclerosis HD (MSHD)
III. Mixed-cellularity HD (MCHD)
IV. Lymphocyte-depleted HD (LDHD)

6. Which of the following subtypes of Hodgkin's disease is the most common and often involves the mediastinum?
A. Lymphocyte-predominant HD (LPHD)
B. Nodular sclerosis HD (MSHD)
C. Mixed-cellularity HD (MCHD)
D. Lymphocyte-depleted HD (LDHD)

7. Which of the following fields is used to treat Hodgkin's disease with radiation?
A. I, II, and III only
B. I and III only
C. II and IV only
D. IV only
E. All are correct
I. Mantle fields
II. Preauricular fields
III. Subdiaphragmatic fields
IV. Medial and lateral tangential fields

8. Waldeyer's fields are used for Hodgkin's disease irradiation:
A. To treat the retroperitoneal and pelvic lymph nodes
B. To treat the submandibular, preauricular, occipital, and high cervical nodes
C. To treat pulmonary hilar nodes
D. High cervical nodes only

9. Common areas blocked during Hodgkin's disease irradiation include:
A. I, II, and III only
B. I and III only
C. II and IV only
D. IV only
E. All are correct
I. The lungs
II. The occipital region
III. The spinal cord
IV. The humeral head

10. Which of the following symptoms seen in Hodgkin's disease are considered as B symptoms?
A. I, II, and III only
B. I and III only
C. II and IV only
D. IV only
E. All are correct

I. Fever
II. Night sweats
III. 10 % weight loss in the past months
IV. Painless lymphadenopathy

Non-Hodgkin's Lymphoma

1. Non-Hodgkin's lymphoma can be found in:
A. I, II, and III only
B. I and III only
C. II and IV only
D. IV only
E. All are correct
I. Lymph nodes
II. The spleen
III. The bone marrow
IV. Waldeyer's ring

2. Non-Hodgkin's lymphoma:
A. I, II, and III only
B. I and III only
C. II and IV only
D. IV only
E. All are correct
I. Has a lymphatic contiguity much weaker than Hodgkin's lymphoma
II. Commonly involves Waldeyer's ring
III. Commonly involves epitrochlear and brachial nodes
IV. Increases incidence of bone marrow and mesenteric lymph node

3. Which of the following staging system is used on non-Hodgkin's lymphoma?
A. FIGO
B. TNM
C. AJCC
D. Ann Arbor

4. Which of the following is considered a non-Hodgkin's lymphoma?
A. I, II, and III only
B. I and III only
C. II and IV only
D. IV only
E. All are correct
I. MALT
II. Mantle cell
III. Peripheral T cell
IV. Anaplastic large cell

Neuroblastoma

1. The most common site of neuroblastoma origin is:
A. The thoracic
B. The head and neck
C. The adrenal medulla
D. The paraspinal ganglia

2. Which of the following organs is the most common site of distant metastasis of neuroblastoma?
A. I, II, and III only
B. I and III only
C. II and IV only
D. IV only
E. All are correct
I. The lymph nodes
II. The bones
III. The bone marrow
IV. The skin

3. The most common presenting symptom of neuroblastoma is:
A. Pain
B. Weight loss
C. Fever
D. Malaise

Rhabdomyosarcoma

1. Rhabdomyosarcoma may occur in the:
A. I, II, and III only
B. I and III only
C. II and IV only
D. IV only
E. All are correct
I. The head and neck
II. The orbit
III. The extremity
IV. The genitourinary tract

2. The most common site of gynecologic rhabdomyosarcoma is:
A. The vagina
B. The cervix
C. The uterus
D. The vulva

Wilms' Tumor

1. The most common metastatic sites of Wilms' tumor is:
A. The bones
B. The paraaortic nodes
C. The lungs
D. The liver

2. Which of the following statements is true about Wilms' tumor?
A. I, II, and III only
B. I and III only
C. II and IV only
D. IV only
E. All are correct
I. It is often localized at diagnosis.
II. It is curable in most children.
III. It is spread throughout the peritoneal cavity.
IV. Abdominal swelling on one side of the abdomen is felt.

3. Wilms' tumor patients should start radiation treatment:
A. Immediately after surgery.
B. Within 10 days after surgery.
C. 10 days before surgery.
D. Radiation treatment timing is not important after surgery.

The Bone

1. Most common skeletal bone tumors include:
A. I, II, and III only
B. I and III only
C. II and IV only
D. IV only
E. All are correct
I. Osteosarcoma
II. Ewing's sarcoma
III. Chondrosarcomas
IV. Chordoma

2. Chondrosarcomas most often involve:
A. The femur
B. The tibia
C. The shoulder girdle
D. The base of the skull

11.7 Children (Questions)

3. Which of the following staging system is used for bone sarcomas?
A. FIGO
B. TNM
C. Enneking
D. Ann Arbor

4. Osteosarcoma occurs most often:
A. In the diaphyseal region of the humerus or radius
B. In the diaphyseal region of the distal femur or proximal tibia
C. In the epiphyseal region of the distal femur or proximal tibia
D. In the epiphyseal region of the humerus or radius

Ewing's Sarcoma

1. Which of the following is most commonly involved in Ewing's sarcoma?
A. I, II, and III only
B. I and III only
C. II and IV only
D. IV only
E. All are correct
I. The femur
II. The metaphysis
III. The diaphysis
IV. The epiphysis

2. The main or midsection (shaft) of a long bone is:
A. The metaphysis
B. The diaphysis
C. The epiphysis
D. The medullary cavity

3. Which of the following Ewing's sarcoma tumors have the worst prognosis?
A. I, II, and III only
B. I and III only
C. II and IV only
D. IV only
E. All are correct
I. Tumors of the distal bones
II. Tumors of the long bones
III. Tumors of the proximal bones
IV. Tumors of the pelvis area

4. Which of the following malignant tumors occur in young children?
A. Ewing's sarcomas
B. Multiple myelomas
C. Small-cell carcinomas
D. Adenocarcinomas

Leukemia

1. Which of the following are types of leukemia?
A. I, II, and III only
B. I and III only
C. II and IV only
D. IV only
E. All are correct
I. Acute lymphoblastic leukemia
II. Chronic myelogenous leukemia
III. Acute myelogenous leukemia
IV. Chronic lymphocytic leukemia

2. The most common type of pediatric leukemia is:
A. ALL (acute lymphoblastic leukemia)
B. CML (chronic myelogenous leukemia)
C. AML (acute myelogenous leukemia)
D. CLL (chronic lymphocytic leukemia)

3. Acute lymphocytic leukemias are classified into:
A. I, II, and III only
B. I and III only
C. II and IV only
D. IV only
E. All are correct
I. B cell acute lymphoblastic leukemia
II. T cell acute lymphoblastic leukemia
III. Non-B cell, non-T cell acute lymphoblastic leukemia
IV. L cell acute lymphoblastic leukemia

4. The most common treatment options for leukemia patients include:
A. I, II, and III only
B. I and III only
C. II and IV only
D. IV only
E. All are correct
I. Radiation therapy
II. Chemotherapy
III. Bone marrow transplantation (BMT)
IV. Surgery

5. Acute myelogenous leukemia (AML) is most commonly seen in:
A. Patients between ages 5 and 6
B. Patients over 40 years old
C. Patients over 50 years old
D. Patients younger than 4 years old

6. Which of the following organs is considered to be hematopoietic:
A. I, II, and III only
B. I and III only
C. II and IV only
D. IV only
E. All are correct
I. Blood
II. The liver
III. The bone marrow
IV. The lymph nodes

7. Which of the following staging system is used for chronic lymphocytic leukemia (CLL)?
A. FIGO staging system
B. TNM staging system
C. Ann Arbor staging system
D. Rai staging system

8. Which of the following organs must be prophylactically irradiated due to potential shelter site for leukemic cells?
A. I, II, and III only
B. I and III only
C. II and IV only
D. IV only
E. All are correct
I. The liver
II. The CNS
III. The pancreas
IV. The testis

Multiple Myeloma and Plasmacytoma

1. Which of the following is true about multiple myeloma and plasmacytoma?
A. I, II, and III only
B. I and III only
C. II and IV only
D. IV only
E. All are correct

I. It is a disease associated with plasma cells.
II. The main presentation is bone pain.
III. Both chemotherapy and radiation therapy are effective in palliation.
IV. Hemibody irradiation relieves pain in 80–90 % of patients within 48 h.

2. Common clinical presentations of multiple myeloma include:
A. I, II, and III only
B. I and III only
C. II and IV only
D. IV only
E. All are correct
I. Bone pain
II. Bone fracture
III. Hypercalcemia
IV. Multifocal swelling

3. Which of the following malignant tumors can produce paraplegia due to spinal column pressure on the spinal cord?
A. Leukemia
B. Thymomas
C. Multiple myeloma
D. Lymphoma

4. Which of the following is the most common primary malignant bone tumor?
A. Ewing's sarcoma
B. Osteosarcoma
C. Multiple myeloma
D. Chondrosarcomas

11.8 Benign Diseases (Questions)

1. Which of the following are considered benign diseases that are treated with radiation therapy:
A. I, II, and III only
B. I and III only
C. II and IV only
D. IV only
E. All are correct
I. Pterygium
II. Keloids
III. Heterotopic bone formation
IV. Thymomas

2. Arteriovenous malformations (AVMs) of the brain is best treated using:
A. Low-dose rate brachytherapy
B. Linac external radiation therapy
C. Stereotactic radiosurgery
D. High-dose rate brachytherapy

3. Which of the following statements is true about plantar warts?
A. I, II, and III only
B. I and III only
C. II and IV only
D. IV only
E. All are correct
I. A single radiation treatment of 10 Gy using close lead shielding to define the treatment field.
II. The wart usually separates and falls off in 3–4 weeks without sequelae after radiation treatment.
III. Liquid nitrogen cryosurgery can be used with cure rates of 90 %.
IV. Surgical treatment is the best approach.

4. Which of the following radioactive materials is used after percutaneous transluminal coronary angioplasty (PTCA) when treating stenotic lesions?
A. Gold-198
B. Cesium-137
C. Iodine-125
D. Iridium-192

5. Which of the following is true regarding heterotopic bone formation?
A. I, II, and III only
B. I and III only
C. II and IV only
D. IV only
E. All are correct
I. Radiation treatment is given immediately following the postoperative period.
II. Doses in a single fraction of 7 or 10 Gy in 4–5 fractions.
III. Occurs in 30 % of patients undergoing hip arthroplasty.
IV. Treatment can be given 1 month after surgery.

11.9 The Skin (Questions)

1. The skin is composed of:
A. I, II, and III only
B. I and III only
C. II and IV only
D. IV only
E. All are correct

I. The epidermis
II. The dermis
III. The subcutaneous tissue
IV. The metaphysis

2. Which of the following is true about carcinoma of the skin?
A. I, II, and III only
B. I and III only
C. II and IV only
D. IV only
E. All are correct
I. It is the most common malignancy in the United States.
II. The most common cause is exposure to solar radiation.
III. Most commonly occurring in patients over 40 years of age.
IV. The skin complexion type is not a risk factor.

3. The most common skin carcinoma is:
A. I, II, and III only
B. I and III only
C. II and IV only
D. IV only
E. All are correct
I. Basal cell carcinoma
II. Melanomas
III. Squamous cell carcinoma
IV. Lymphomas

4. Which of the following are malignant tumors of the skin?
A. I, II, and III only
B. I and III only
C. II and IV only
D. IV only
E. All are correct
I. Basal cell carcinoma
II. Melanomas
III. Squamous cell carcinoma
IV. Kaposi's sarcoma

5. Which of the following surgical techniques is used for skin cancer?
A. I, II, and III only
B. I and III only
C. II and IV only
D. IV only
E. All are correct

I. Curettage
II. Electrodesiccation
III. Mohs' microsurgery
IV. Cryotherapy

6. Radiation therapy skin treatments include:
A. I, II, and III only
B. I and III only
C. II and IV only
D. IV only
E. All are correct
I. Use of electron beams in most cases
II. Use of the 80–90 % isodose line for the prescription dose with electrons
III. Use of bolus to enhance surface dose
IV. Use of 23 MV photon beams, common for large tumors

7. Which of the following is true about radiation therapy of non-AIDS-associated Kaposi's sarcoma?
A. I, II, and III only
B. I and III only
C. II and IV only
D. IV only
E. All are correct
I. Local irradiation includes the lesion plus a normal tissue border of **1.5–2.0** cm.
II. Thin, cutaneous lesions can be treated effectively with low-energy electrons or superficial X-ray beams.
III. Eyelid lesions are treated most easily by superficial X-rays with shields over the optic lens.
IV. If edema is present, parallel-opposed fields and megavoltage therapy are needed to treat deep tissues.

11.10 Soft Tissue Sarcomas (Questions)

1. A soft tissue sarcoma is:
A. A disease of the nervous system
B. A disease of the digestive system
C. A disease of the respiratory system
D. A disease of the musculoskeletal system

2. The most common subsite of origin of soft tissue sarcomas is:
A. The chest
B. The head and neck
C. The thigh
D. The upper extremities

3. The most common metastatic sites of soft tissue sarcomas is:
A. The bones
B. The paraaortic nodes
C. The lungs
D. The liver

4. The most common soft tissue sarcoma is:
A. Liposarcoma
B. Malignant fibrous histiocytomas
C. Rhabdomyosarcoma
D. Myofibrosarcoma

11.11 Extras (Questions)

1. The spread of cancer from its primary site of origin to a distant site is known as:
A. Metastasis
B. Hyperplasia
C. Metaplasia
D. Necrosis

2. Which of the following are characteristics of the radiopaque contrast used in CT simulation?
A. I, II, and III only
B. I and III only
C. II and IV only
D. IV only
E. All are correct
I. Increase organ density
II. High atomic number
III. Increase absorption of X-rays
IV. Aid with visualization of the lymph nodes

3. Which of the following documents must be obtained from all patients before injecting a patient with a contrast agent in the CT simulation?
A. I, II, and III only
B. I and III only
C. II and IV only
D. IV only
E. All are correct
I. Informed consent
II. Pregnancy test result
III. Allergic history
IV. Family history

4. Which of the following is considered minor iodine contrast reaction?
A. I, II, and III only
B. I and III only
C. II and IV only
D. IV only
E. All are correct
I. Claustrophobia
II. Feeling of warmth
III. Anaphylaxis
IV. Nausea and vomiting

5. Which of the following tests is ordered before iodine contrast injection when performing a CT scan study?
A. I, II, and III only
B. I and III only
C. II and IV only
D. IV only
E. All are correct
I. Blood urea nitrogen test (BUN)
II. PSA
III. Creatine
IV. Alpha-fetoprotein (AFP)

6. The function of contrast media is to:
A. Increase tissue contrast
B. Increase tissue density
C. Increase sharpness
D. Increase latitude

11.12 The Brain (Answers)

The Brain, Brainstem, and Cerebellum

1. **E** Some of the clinical presentations of a brain neoplasm are edema, focal neurological dysfunction, intracranial pressure, and hydrocephalus. The patient might also present with headaches, optic atrophy and blindness, seizures, and lumbar back pain or bladder dysfunction which may suggest CSF metastasis in the lumbar cistern.

2. **B** Tumors of the cranial and spinal nerves include schwannoma and neurofibroma. Malignant lymphomas are a hemopoietic (blood) neoplasm, and a pituitary adenoma is a sellar tumor.

3. **A** Administration of glucocorticoid (dexamethasone) preoperatively, postoperatively, and during irradiation decreases cerebral edema. Phenytoin

(Dilantin), carbamazepine (Tegretol), and phenobarbital are administered to patients for generalized seizures.

4. A Radiation therapy can be delivered within the CNS by fractionated external beam radiation therapy, small-field stereotactic irradiation, or interstitial brachytherapy.

5. E All are correct.

6. E Some of the anatomic landmarks used for cranial radiation therapy techniques are the external acoustic meatus, the sella turcica, the cribriform plate, the mandibular angle, the anterior cranial fossa, and the two anterior parts of the middle cranial fossa floors.

7. C The sella turcica is used as a landmark for the lower border of the median telencephalon and diencephalon. The hypothalamic structures are located 3 cm superior to the sellar floor, and the optic canal runs, at the most, 1 cm superior and 1 cm anterior to that point. The cribriform plate is an important landmark for the inferior border of whole-brain irradiation fields, and the pineal body usually sits approximately 1 cm posterior and 3 cm superior to the external acoustic meatus.

8. A The head should be positioned so that its major axes are parallel and perpendicular to the central axis. The most common error in head and neck treatment setup is head rotation and/or longitudinal axis deviation (tilting).

9. E All are correct about whole-brain irradiation techniques. The beam can also be angled about 5 or 7° against the frontal plane so that the anterior beam border traverses the head in a frontal plane about 0.5 cm posterior to the lenses. Superior and posterior flash (extra space beyond the patient skin added to account for possible motion) is used to encompass the whole brain.

10. B Bilateral or medial cerebral hemispheric tumors or midcerebral tumors are best treated with parallel-opposed lateral portals. Brainstem, posterior parietal, occipital, or frontal lesions/tumors can be treated using anterior and/or posterior lateral perpendicular beams (wedge pair). Craniopharyngiomas and pituitary, optic nerve, hypothalamic, and brainstem tumors are deep and centrally located tumors so they may be treated using a three or four isocentric portal technique or arc.

11. B If irradiation of a brain tumor is needed during pregnancy, fetal exposure should be less than 0.10 Gy even at high doses. This may confer an increased but acceptable risk of leukemia in the child but has no other deleterious effects to the fetus after the fourth week of gestation. Because of the long distance from the field, the dose to the fetus is usually low and can be reduced even further using a shield.

12. A On CNS irradiation the patient can be treated supine or prone using helmet brain lateral fields and one or two spine fields followed by a brain boost. When the setup is done, both collimator and couch angles are critical for reproducibility and matching fields. A couch angle must be used on spine fields to match with the inferior border of the helmet brain fields, and collimator angles on helmet brain fields are used to match the divergence of the upper spine field.

13. C CNS irradiation requires junction shifts every 10 Gy of tumor dose to avoid hot or cold spots. On adult patients two spine fields are required because of the length of the spine; if this is the case, a gap should be located between the inferior border of the upper spine field and the superior border of the lower spine field. The inferior border of the lower spine field stays at S3 level (dural sac and subarachnoid space) in most cases.

14. D The most serious late reaction to irradiation of the CNS is necrosis (tissue death), which may appear 6 months to many years after treatment. Nausea and vomiting, dermatitis, alopecia, mucositis, and esophagitis are early reactions.

15. A Most brainstem gliomas are high-grade astrocytomas. Ependymomas are tumors that may arise anywhere within the brain or spinal cord, medulloblastoma is a posterior fossa tumor, and meningiomas occur in the cerebral convexities, falx cerebri, tentorium cerebelli, cerebellopontine angle, and sphenoid ridge.

16. B The most common primary brain tumor is glioma 50 %, followed by meningiomas 21 %, and pituitary adenomas 15 %.

17. C Benign brain tumors represent half of all primary brain tumors and they do not metastasize. Some of them are meningiomas, acoustic neuroma, pituitary adenoma, and craniopharyngiomas.

18. C A schwannoma is also called acoustic neuroma; this is a benign tumor in the 8th cranial nerve arising from Schwann cells and account for about 9 % of all brain tumors. This tumor may be observed in order to monitor its growth, or surgery can be performed. Another option is radiosurgery.

The Pituitary

1. A The pituitary gland is connected to the hypothalamus, is located in the sella turcica, and secretes nine hormones that regulate homeostasis (the property of the system that regulates its internal environment and tends to maintain

2. A For all patients treated for pituitary tumors, periodic assessment of gonadal, thyroid, and adrenal function is necessary because hypopituitarism may occur as a result of irradiation or surgery.

3. E All are correct.

4. D Fifteen-degree wedges, with the heel placed anteriorly, assist in obtaining a more homogeneous dose distribution and in decreasing the dose delivered to the optic chiasm.

5. E All of them are considered critical structures when irradiating a pituitary tumor due to the proximity. Therefore, when planning a pituitary tumor irradiation, calculation of dose to adjacent structures must be well established.

6. E The pituitary gland is an endocrine gland composed of two lobes and a middle structure situated in the sella turcica in the body of the sphenoid bone. It is located superior to the sphenoid sinus and nasopharynx.

7. A The anterior pituitary or adenohypophysis synthesizes and secretes a growth hormone also referred to as the human growth hormone which stimulates growth, cell reproduction, and regeneration. It also produces thyroid-stimulating hormone which stimulates the thyroid gland to produce thyroxine to stimulate the metabolism of almost every tissue in the body. Prolactin is another important hormone created by the pituitary gland that, among other functions, regulates the immune system. Other hormones are adrenocorticotropic hormone, beta endorphin, luteinizing hormone, and follicle-stimulating hormone. Insulin and glucagon are produced by the pancreas and they maintain the blood glucose level within an acceptable range.

11.13 The Head and Neck Region (Answers)

The Hypopharynx

1. A The hypopharynx is divided into the pyriform sinuses, the posterolateral pharyngeal wall, and the postcricoid region. The supraglottic region is part of the larynx.

2. A More than 65 % of tumors occurring in the hypopharynx in the United States are in the pyriform fossa followed by the postcricoid (20 %) and the hypopharyngeal wall (0–15 %).

3. B Over 95 % of tumors of the hypopharynx are squamous cell carcinomas.

11.13 The Head and Neck Region (Answers)   651

4. C Small lesions are controlled with irradiation alone on the order of 65–70 Gy in 7–8 weeks. When using adjuvant irradiation postoperatively, 60–66 Gy is recommended, but if irradiation is given preoperatively, 45–50 Gy in 4.5–5 weeks is suggested.

5. E If irradiation is delivered alone, the irradiated volume of the hypopharynx should encompass the nasopharynx, oropharynx, hypopharynx, and upper cervical esophagus because of the propensity of hypopharynx cancer to spread submucosally.

6. A Historically, hypopharynx radiation treatment consists of two parallel-opposed upper-neck lateral beams and one anterior photon field encompassing the lower neck plus a boost to the gross tumor after 60 Gy up to an additional 10–15 Gy. More and more, IMRT and VMAT are being used for head and neck cancers due to its ability to spare critical structures while still delivering a high dose.

7. B The hypopharynx extends from the level of the hyoid bone to the lower border of the cricoid cartilage which coincide with cervical vertebrae 4 to 6; the nasopharynx is located anteriorly to the posterior choanae and posterior to cervical vertebrae 1 and 2 and the clivus, also superior to the body of the sphenoid and inferior to the soft palate.

The Larynx

1. A The larynx is composed of the supraglottic, glottis, and subglottic regions. The supraglottis is composed of the epiglottis, false vocal cords, ventricles, aryepiglottic folds, and arytenoids. The glottis is composed of the true vocal cords and anterior commissure, and the subglottis is located below the vocal cords.

2. B The subglottis begins 5 mm below the vocal cords and ends at the inferior border of the cricoid cartilage and the beginning of the trachea.

3. B The larynx is the most common head and neck cancer location excluding the skin.

4. C Cancer of the larynx is strongly related to cigarette smoking, even though alcohol can play an important role.

5. C Because early diagnosis is uncommon, most subglottic laryngeal lesions are bilateral or circumferential at discovery.

6. E All are correct. Irradiation is the initial treatment for T1 and T2 lesions, while surgery is reserved for salvage after radiation therapy failure. Hemilaryngectomy or cordectomy produces comparable cure rates for

selected T1 and T2 lesions but irradiation generally is preferred. Favorable lesions are advised of the alternatives to irradiation with surgical salvage or immediate total laryngectomy.

7. **B** T1 laryngeal lesions are treated so that the field sizes extend from the thyroid notch superiorly to the inferior border of the cricoid cartilage and fall off anteriorly. The posterior border depends on the posterior extension of the tumor. Most field sizes range from 4 cm × 4 cm to 6 cm × 6 cm plus flash anteriorly. T3 and T4 lesions require larger portals, which include the jugulodigastric and middle jugular lymph nodes.

8. **B** Most laryngeal tumors are squamous cell carcinomas.

9. **C** Subdigastric nodes are mainly involved in carcinoma of the larynx, and more than half of patients have positive nodes at the time of diagnosis.

The Nasal Cavity and Paranasal Sinuses

1. **D** A stage III nasal cavity and paranasal sinus tumor has extension to the base of the skull or pterygoid plate and destruction and intracranial extension. Stage I is limited to site of origin and stage II has extension to the orbit, nasopharynx and paranasal sinuses, skin, and pterygomaxillary fossa.

2. **B** The most common malignancy of the nasal cavity and paranasal sinuses is squamous cell carcinoma. Malignant melanoma accounts for about 10 % of cancers of the nasal cavity.

3. **C** Radiation therapy is the preferred treatment for sphenoid sinus and nasal vestibule tumors with a 90 % local tumor control rate. Most nasal cavity and ethmoid sinus carcinomas are treated with surgery followed by postoperative irradiation. For unresectable lesions, high-dose irradiation remains the only alternative. Most malignancies of the maxillary sinus require radical maxillectomy including the entire maxilla and ethmoid sinus.

4. **C** Nasal cavity and paranasal sinuses radiation therapy techniques include an anterior portal with one or two posterior tilted lateral portals, frequently using wedges. Fields may be reduced to the initial gross disease, with a margin after 45–50 Gy. Also, if the disease is ipsilateral, a wedge-pair technique is usually used.

5. **E** Complications of irradiation include central nervous system damage, unilateral or bilateral vision loss, otitis media, and chronic sinusitis.

6. **E** Nasal cavity and paranasal sinus tumors are twice as common in males as in females and show a bimodal age distribution of 10–20 and 50–60 years of

age. Most tumors present at an advanced stage and are considered rare tumors because they account for only 3 % of upper respiratory track cancers.

7. **C** Lymph node metastases generally do not occur until the tumor has extended to areas that contain abundant capillary lymphatics. The submandibular and subdigastric lymph nodes are the most commonly involved.

8. **C** Nasal cavity, maxillary sinus, and ethmoid sinus treatments use primary surgery followed by radiation therapy as the treatment of choice. Nasal vestibule and sphenoid sinus treatments use radiation therapy alone as the treatment of choice.

The Nasopharynx

1. **A** The most common site of distant metastasis is the bone followed closely by the lungs and liver.

2. **D** Approximately 90 % of malignant tumors arising in the nasopharynx are epidermoid or undifferentiated carcinomas. The remaining 10 % are mainly lymphomas but also may be plasmacytomas, tumors of minor salivary gland origin, melanomas, rhabdomyosarcomas, and chordomas.

3. **C** Because the nasopharynx is immediately adjacent to the base of the skull, surgical resection with an acceptable margin is impossible. Radiation therapy has been the sole treatment for carcinoma of the nasopharynx.

4. **E** All are correct. More recently, IMRT and VMAT have become the modality of choice.

5. **E** All modalities mentioned have been used in the treatment of nasopharyngeal carcinoma. Brachytherapy has been used to deliver a higher dose to a limited volume of the nasopharynx. Frequently it is combined with external beam irradiation to treat extensive primary or recurrent carcinoma. Neoadjuvant or adjuvant chemotherapy has also been used to treat primary or recurrent nasopharyngeal cancer.

6. **A** Reirradiation techniques for the nasopharynx include external irradiation, brachytherapy (mold), or a combination of both.

7. **E** All are correct.

8. **C** The nasopharynx is located anteriorly to the posterior choanae and posteriorly to cervical vertebrae 1 and 2 and the clivus. It is superior to the body of the sphenoid and inferior to the soft palate. The hypopharynx extends

from the level of the hyoid bone to the lower border of the cricoid cartilage, from cervical vertebrae 4–**6.**

9. **C** The common lymph nodes involved in carcinomas of the nasopharynx are the deep posterior cervical lymph nodes and the jugulodigastric lymph nodes.

The Oral Cavity

1. **E** All are correct.

2. **B** The upper gingiva is formed by the alveolar ridge of the maxilla. The lips are composed of the orbicularis muscle, and the buccal mucosa is made up of mucous membrane. The floor of the mouth is bounded by the lower gingiva anteriorly and laterally, and the tongue is a muscular organ composed of the styloglossus, hyoglossus, and hyoid muscles.

3. **B** In patients with clinically or radiographically positive neck nodes, the treatment of choice for the neck is ipsilateral neck dissection followed by bilateral postoperative neck irradiation. In patients with small lesions resected with adequate margins, no further treatment other than observation is necessary. If neck dissection reveals only one positive node, radiation therapy is not recommended, but if it shows more than one a course of postoperative irradiation to the neck is indicated.

4. **E** If radiation therapy is considered optimal, oral hygiene and pretreatment dental care must be completed; any potential surgical procedures and tooth extractions should be carried out before initiation of irradiation, and approximately 8–10 days is needed for complete recovery before initiation of radiation therapy. After a course of radiotherapy, caution in tooth extraction or surgical procedure involving the gums is a lifelong commitment.

5. **E** All are correct.

6. **A** The most common interstitial irradiation technique used is percutaneous afterloading with angiocatheters and iridium-**192.** Most interstitial implants are done with a classic low-dose rate implant which delivers **4.5–5** Gy an hour.

7. **B** Smaller, more anteriorly situated primary lesions of the oral tongue are most suitable for interstitial implant or intraoral cone radiation therapy as a boost procedure. For advanced disease T3 and T4 lesions are best managed by planned, combined irradiation and surgery.

8. **E** All are correct. Others include but are not limited to age, sex, race, genetic factors, iron deficiency, poor dental hygiene, fungi, Epstein-Barr virus, herpes simplex virus, and radiation.

9. **A** The most common malignancy of the oral cavity is squamous cell carcinoma.

10. B Head and neck lymphatic regions are divided into levels: level I, submental and submandibular triangle; level 2, upper jugulodigastric; level 3 and 4, deep jugular nodes of the middle and lower third of the neck; and level 5, spinal accessory and transverse cervical chains (posterior triangle).

11. A Oral cavity radiation therapy portals commonly include the submandibular, subdigastric, and submental lymph nodes. Their coverage is especially important when the lesion is located at the tip of the tongue, anterior floor of the mouth, or lower lip.

The Oropharynx

1. C The oropharynx is located between the soft palate and the hyoid bone.

2. E All are correct.

3. D Most oropharynx tumors are keratinizing squamous cell carcinoma, but other types include malignant melanomas, sarcomas, and malignant lymphomas, usually non-Hodgkin's type.

4. B The most common acute irradiation sequelae when treating the oropharynx are oropharyngeal mucositis and moderate-to-severe dysphagia. Xerostomia also occurs in approximately 75 % of patients treated with conventional beam arrangements, but IMRT significantly reduces these other sequelae including laryngeal edema, fibrosis, and hearing loss.

5. E External radiation alone (IMRT or conventional) can be used on T1, T2, and T3 tumors to 60–75 Gy, with locoregional control of 70 %. Combined surgery and irradiation is best for larger tumors (T3–T4) that extend beyond the base of the tongue or infiltrate and partially fix the tongue. Chemotherapy and brachytherapy using catheters implanted in the patient and later loaded with radioactive sources are also options.

The Ear

1. A The ear is composed of the external, middle, and internal ear.

2. C The external ear consists of the auricle or pinna, external auditory meatus (EAM), and the tympanic membrane. The middle ear is the tympanic cavity and houses the auditory ossicles (bones). The inner or internal ear lies in the petrous portion of the temporal bone and is composed of the bony labyrinth and membranous labyrinth.

3. **A** The external ear involves the superficial parotid nodes, the retroauricular nodes, and the superficial cervical group nodes. The lymphatics in the middle ear are sparse, and the inner ear has no lymph node involvement.

4. **D** Basal cell carcinoma is common in the external ear, while squamous cell carcinoma is common in the auditory canal, middle ear, and mastoid area.

5. **A** Orthovoltage or electron beams are used in tumors involving the pinna as one does not want to treat to a deep point. Surgery depends on the stage and location of the tumor. Another method of treatment is interstitial radiation using iridium-192 for lesions <4 cm.

6. **B** The acoustic nerve, arising at the lateral termination of the internal acoustic meatus and ending in the brainstem between the pons and the medulla, is responsible for auditory and vestibular function.

7. **C** The internal ear is the only part of the ear that has no lymphatics.

The Eye

1. **C** The globe of the eye is composed of the inner layer which also contains the retina. The outer coat is composed of the cornea and sclera and the middle coat includes the uvea.

2. **B** The lens is located posterior to the iris and is suspended from the ciliary body.

3. **C** The treatment of choice for basal and squamous cell carcinoma of the eyelid is radiation therapy with a cure rate of higher than 90 %.

4. **C** The most common metastatic sites for tumors of the posterior uvea in men are the lung or GI track and in women the breast or lung.

5. **A** An enucleation or exenteration is done for a malignant melanoma of the posterior uvea if the tumor exceeds 15 mm in diameter and 10 mm in thickness and also if there is extra-sclera extension at diagnosis. For small growing melanomas brachytherapy is recommended.

6. **B** Retinoblastoma is the most common intraocular malignancy in children. Most children are diagnosed before 3–4 years of age and it is hereditary in approximately 40 % of diagnosed cases. Malignant melanoma represents 75 % of malignant tumors involving the eye. Rhabdomyosarcoma of the orbit is most often seen in young children, and optic glioma is more common in children younger than 15 years of age and more than 50 % of cases involve the optic chiasm.

11.13 The Head and Neck Region (Answers)

7. **A** The most widely used grouping system for retinoblastoma is the Reese-Ellsworth classification system.

8. **E** Radioactive plaque therapy offers another option for local treatment of retinoblastoma. Historically, all these sources have been used in the past, although I-125 is now the most common.

9. **B** The advantage of iodine-125 plaque therapy is related to its physical properties of low energy, adequate dose distribution, and ease of shielding.

10. **E** All are correct.

The Salivary Glands

1. **A** The salivary glands consist of three, large, paired major glands (the parotid, submandibular, and sublingual) and many smaller glands.

2. **A** The parotid gland is the largest of the three salivary glands and is located superficial to and partly behind the ramus of the mandible. The submandibular gland fills the triangle between the two bellies of the digastric and the lower border of the mandible and extends upward deeply to the mandible. The sublingual gland is the smallest of the three glands.

3. **A** The most common malignant subtype of parotid tumors in children is a mucoepidermoid tumor. Adenoid cystic carcinoma is the most common cancer of the submaxillary gland and in minor salivary glands, and pleomorphic adenoma is a benign mixed tumor and accounts for 65–75 % of all parotid epithelial tumors.

The Thyroid

1. **A** Differentiated thyroid cancer consists of papillary, mixed papillary-follicular, and follicular adenocarcinoma.

2. **B** Iodine-131 is used to treat follicular and papillary thyroid cancers. Iodine-131 is taken orally as a drink or capsule and travels to the bloodstream where thyroid cancer cells absorb the iodine preferentially. The patient is to stay in the hospital for a few days until radiation levels have fallen to acceptable levels.

3. **E** All are correct. Thyroid cancer is uncommon representing **1.2** % of all malignancies and accounts for **0.2** % of cancer deaths in the United States. It is more common in females than males (4,700 male and 12,500 female cases) and there is higher risk after irradiation.

4. **E** All of them are correct.

5. A Nuclear medicine is an imaging modality that uses radioactive material to diagnose a variety of diseases, including many types of cancers. The best modality to measure the function of the thyroid is a nuclear medicine study called the radioactive iodine uptake test (RAIU) or also known as a thyroid uptake. It is a measurement of thyroid structure and function.

Unusual Nonepithelial Tumors of the Head and Neck

1. E All are correct. Hemangiopericytoma is an unusual vascular tumor. Chordomas are rare neoplasms of the axial skeleton. Esthesioneuroblastomas are rare tumors thought to arise in the olfactory receptors in the nasal mucosa of the cribriform plate of the ethmoid bone, and extramedullary plasmacytoma is a rare tumor of plasma cell origin originating from the nasopharynx, nasal cavity, paranasal sinuses, and tonsils. Other unusual nonepithelial tumors include glomus, lethal midline granuloma, chloroma, nasopharyngeal angiofibroma, nonlentiginous melanoma, lentigo malignant melanoma, and sarcomas of the head and neck.

11.14 The Thorax (Answers)

The Breast

1. C Early-stage breast tumors include Tis (carcinoma in situ), T1, and T2. Late-stage or locally advanced breast tumors are (T3 and T4) inflammatory and recurrent tumors.

2. B In the United States, the most common malignancy and the second most common cause of mortality in females is breast cancer followed by lung and colorectal cancer.

3. E All are consider risk factors for breast cancer. Females are 146 times more likely to develop breast cancer than males. Male breast cancer only accounts for less than 1 % of cases. Genetic factors such as family history, familial syndromes, genetic abnormalities, diet, obesity, fat, and cholesterol play an important role as well. Endocrine factors and prolonged estrogen stimulation increases the risk of breast cancer.

4. A The mammary gland lies over the pectoralis major muscle from the second to the sixth rib and from the sternum to the anterior or midaxillary line and consists of glandular tissue arranged in multiple lobes composed of lobules connected in ducts, areola tissue, and blood vessels.

5. E All are correct.

11.14 The Thorax (Answers)

6. D Most of the carcinomas of the breast occur in the upper outer quadrant (48 %), upper inner quadrant (15 %), lower outer quadrant (11 %), and lower inner quadrant (6 %).

7. A Most common breast cancers spread via the lymphatic vessels and directly invade adjacent tissues. It is possible to spread through blood vessels as well.

8. C Mammography is invaluable in the detection of over 90 % of breast cancers. Ultrasonography is helpful in differentiating cysts from solid tumors, and MRI is being evaluated for breast imaging; however, cost and availability are major limitations. PET-CT using F-18 is more frequently used for detection of regional lymph node or distant metastases.

9. B The most common type of breast cancer is invasive (infiltrating) ductal carcinoma, accounting for more than 80 % of all cases. Ductal carcinoma in situ (DCIS) is a noninvasive lesion, lobular carcinoma in situ (LCIS) is a noninvasive proliferation of abnormal epithelial cells in the lobules of the breast, and tubular carcinoma has a nonaggressive growth pattern. Axillary lymph node involvement is reported in 10 % of cases.

10. B Strong prognostic factors of breast cancer include tumor size and stage. Tumor location in the breast does not affect prognosis.

11. C BRCA1 is a gene that maps to chromosome 17q21, and BRCA2 is a gene that maps to chromosome 13q12-**13**.

12. C Axillary and supraclavicular nodal irradiation must be performed in patients with more than two or more positive axillary lymph nodes.

13. B Adjuvant chemotherapy for breast cancer must be given to node-negative patients with tumors less than 2 cm in diameter and premenopausal patients with positive nodes. Postmenopausal patients with positive nodes are treated with tamoxifen.

14. A General breast irradiation field borders include the following: superior, head of clavicles or at the second intercostal space (angle of Louis); inferior, 2–3 cm bellow the inframammary fold; medially, 1 cm over midline, or if internal mammary field is used, the medial tangential is located at the lateral margin of the internal mammary field; and lateral, 2 cm beyond palpable breast tissue which coincides usually near the midaxillary line.

15. A To improve the dosimetry in patients with a large pendulous breast, the lateral decubitus, modified lateral decubitus with immobilization device, and primary prone position have been used. Supine position is not recommended due to the forward and unstable breast position.

16. A   Wedges, compensating filters, and multileaf collimators are used on a breast planning to obtain a uniform dose distribution.

17. E   All of the irradiation techniques mentioned can be used for breast cancer. Medial and lateral tangential fields are the standard. This is done to the lungs, heart, and spine. One to two centimeter of the lungs is recommended so that the entire chest wall is irradiated. En face electrons are typically used to boost the scar and the lumpectomy cavity after completion of the initial breast treatment. IMRT can be used in pendulous breasts to get more homogenous plans, and interstitial brachytherapy is also used for large breasts and deep tumors.

18. C   A physical wedge must be avoided on medial tangent breast fields because the contralateral breast will receive more doses due to scatter produced by the wedge. An alternative is to use a dynamic wedge.

19. B   Minimal intact breast dose of approximately 50 Gy is delivered to the entire breast in 5–6 weeks at **1.**8 or **2.**0 Gy per day. Supraclavicular nodes are taken to 45 Gy at 3 cm depth, and electron boost doses range from 10 to 20 Gy, depending on the size of the tumor and status of excision margins.

20. A   Supraclavicular fields are angled 15–20° in order to spare part of the spinal cord. Sometimes the medial border requires a corner MLC block on patients with scoliosis due to the curvature of the spine into the field.

21. C   Sometimes the medial SCV field border requires a corner MLC block on patients with scoliosis due to the curvature of the spine into the field. Also, the humeral head is blocked as much as possible without compromising coverage of the high axillary lymph nodes. The patient's head is tilted to the contralateral side so that the mandible is not in the SCV field. The field is usually half-beam blocked to match with the tangents without any divergence.

22. B   Most supraclavicular nodes run at 3 cm depth, so normalizing to 3 cm depth makes sense. The total dose is usually 45 Gy at **1.**8 Gy per day, or 46 Gy at 2 Gy per day, 5 fractions per week.

23. C   The most common method of treating when a supraclavicular field is needed is the monoisocentric technique so that the patient isocenter stays the same for both the breast and the SCV fields, minimizing setup errors. If the breast is too large for the monoisocentric technique, tangent fields with a table kick and a collimator rotation are used to match the fields. A VMAT technique delivers too much dose to the lungs, and mini-tangent breast fields are used when the lumpectomy is too deep so that en face electrons cannot be used.

11.14 The Thorax (Answers)

24. C Axillary lymph nodes field borders include the following: medially, allow **1.5–2** cm of the lungs to show on the portal field; inferior, at the same level as the inferior border of the supraclavicular field; lateral, blocks falloff across the posterior axillary field; superior, splits the clavicles.

Breast fields irradiation: superior, head of clavicles; inferior, 2–3 cm bellow the inframammary fold; medially, 1 cm over midline; lateral, 2 cm beyond palpable breast tissue.

Supraclavicular fields: inferior, matching superior fields of tangent fields; superior, cover acromioclavicular joint; medially, 1 cm across the midline, following the medial border of the sternocleidomastoid muscle; lateral, vertical line at the level of the anterior axillary fold, splitting the humeral head (SCV).

Internal mammary borders: medial, midline; lateral, usually 5 cm lateral to the midline; superior, abuts the inferior border of the supraclavicular field; inferior, at the xiphoid process.

25. C The dose to the midplane of the axilla from the supraclavicular field is calculated at a point approximately 2 cm inferior to the midportion of the clavicle. The dose to the midplane of the axilla is supplemented by a posterior axillary field. Supplemental dose to the axilla midplane is administered to deliver a full 45–46 Gy.

26. B Internal mammary lymph nodes are irradiated on patients with primary tumors in the inner quadrants and/or the periareolar region that are larger than 3 cm diameter.

27. A The most common men breast cancer is infiltrative ductal carcinoma or invasive ductal carcinoma (IDC). Invasive lobular carcinoma or infiltrative lobular carcinoma (ILC) is rare, and lobular carcinoma in situ or lobular neoplasia (LCIS) is not seen because the male breast does not have real lobules.

28. A Methods to treat internal mammary chain (IMC) include deep tangent fields used to cover the breast plus the IM nodes, but the disadvantage is the amount of lung area involved. En face electron IM fields are the most commonly used, although shallow tangents matched with the breast tangents can be used for large patients.

29. C The most important prognostic factor for breast cancer is axillary node status. Others include stage, tumor size, and patient age.

30. B Image B is a PAB field setup. Image A is a supraclavicular field setup. Image C is a tangent breast and an IMC field. Image D is an electron boost block.

A.

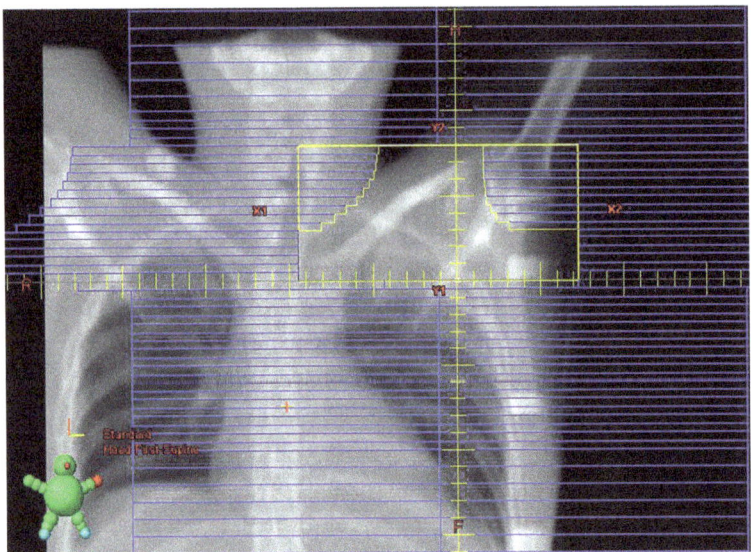

Fig. 11A.3.1

B.

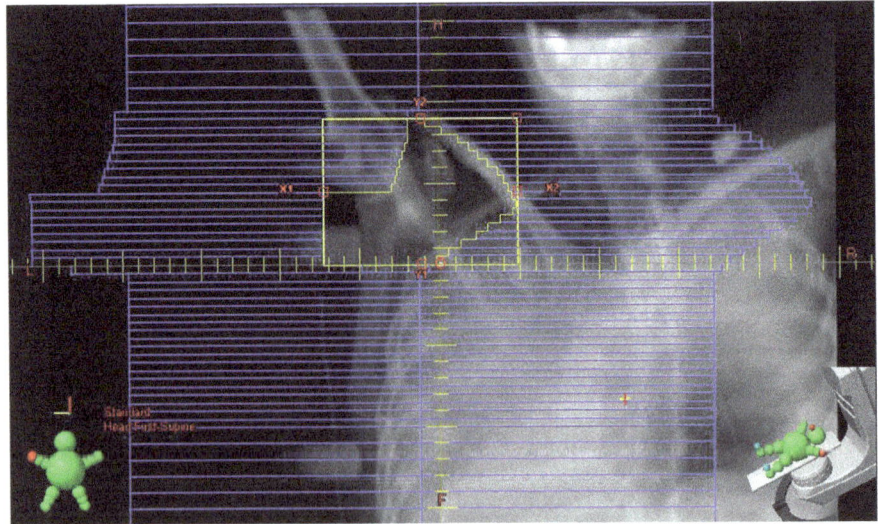

Fig. 11A.3.2

C.

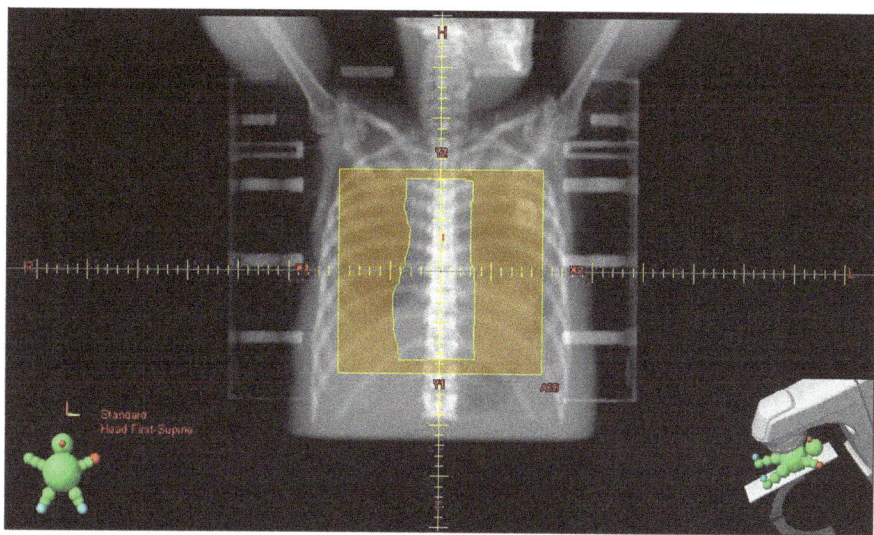

Fig. 11A.3.3

D.

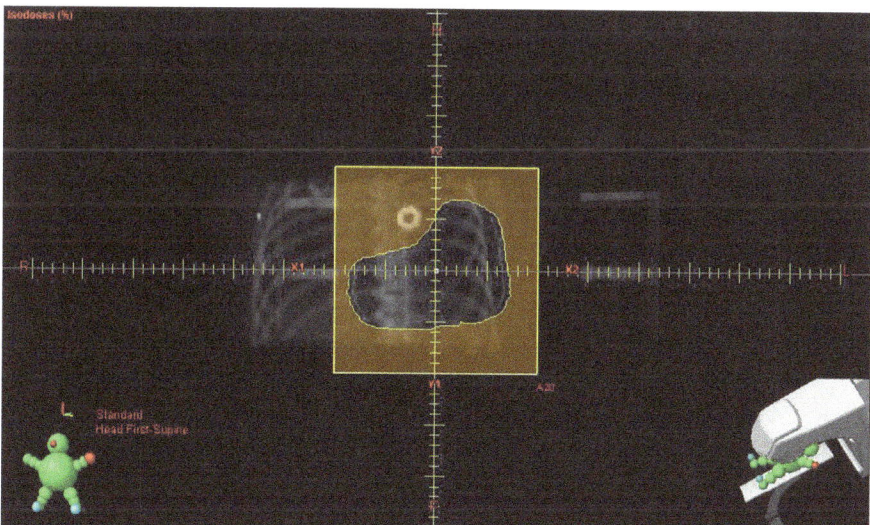

Fig. 11A.3.4

31. The lungs, heart, and spine are dose-limiting organs considered when irradiating the left breast and SCV fields. To help avoid the heart, a breath hold technique can be used when treating the left breast. If the right breast is to be treated, then the heart in most cases is not considered due to its left lateral position.

The Esophagus

1. **B** The esophagus measures approximately 25 cm long and can be located between C7 and T11. The most common sites of metastasis are the lungs, liver pleura, bone, kidney, and adrenal gland, and it is at risk of lymphatic metastasis.

2. **E** The American Joint Committee on Cancer divides the esophagus into four regions: cervical from C7 to T2, upper from T3 to T4, middle from T5 to T8, and lower thoracic from T9 to T11 approximately.

3. **B** 40–50 % of squamous cell carcinomas of the esophagus are detected in the middle 1/3. The upper 1/3 has the lowest incident with 10–25 %, and the lower 1/3 of the esophagus has between 25 and 50 % occurrence.

4. **A** Barrett's esophagus condition is most commonly associated with adenocarcinoma of the esophagus. Achalasia is associated with a 5 % incidence of squamous cell carcinoma of the esophagus.

5. **C** Computer tomography and positron-emission tomography are the best studies in the diagnoses of esophageal cancer. Most malignant tumors metabolize glucose at a higher rate which means a stronger signal from the FDG with PET imaging.

The Lungs

1. **C** The right lung is composed of three lobes; the upper, middle, and lower lobes. They are separated by the oblique and horizontal fissures. The left lung is composed of two lobes separated by a single fissure.

2. **D** The bifurcation of the trachea or carina is approximately at the level of the fifth thoracic vertebra.

3. **E** The most common metastatic sites of lung cancer are the lung, liver, brain, and bone.

4. **C** 75 % of patients have symptoms of cough (severe in 40 %). Hemoptysis occurs in 57 % of patients. Dyspnea, chest pain, hoarseness, Horner's syndrome, and dysphagia are other symptoms.

5. **A** The most common lung cancers are non-small-cell carcinoma (squamous cell, large-cell undifferentiated, and adenocarcinoma) and small-cell carcinomas.

6. **D** Prophylactic brain irradiation should be delivered when small-cell carcinoma of the lung is diagnosed because it decreases the overall incidence of intracranial metastasis.

7. **E** Superior vena cava syndrome is a medical emergency seen in patients with malignant neoplasia which requires immediate therapeutic treatment of initial high-dose radiation. Eighty percent of cases result from bronchogenic carcinoma, and portals should include mediastinal, hilar, and adjacent pulmonary parenchyma lesions.

8. **B** The second most common malignancy in males in the United States is lung cancer. Prostate cancer is the leading type and colorectal is the third. Breast cancer is the leading cancer for women in the United States followed by lung and colorectal cancer.

9. **D** All are risk factors associated with lung cancer, but cigarette smoking or inhalation is the leading risk factor associated with lung cancer. Tobacco smoking accounts for 85 % of all lung cancer cases, and the risk of developing lung carcinoma is directly proportional to the amount of tobacco smoked.

10. **E** The hila contain the bronchi, pulmonary arteries and veins, various branches from the pulmonary plexus, bronchial arteries and veins, and the lymphatics.

11. **A** The name of the area of bifurcation of the trachea is the carina which is found at the level of the fifth thoracic vertebra. The alveolus is the functional unit for gas exchange of oxygen and carbon dioxide in the lungs, and the hilum is an opening through which nerves, ducts, or blood vessels pass, as in the medial aspect of the lungs or the kidneys. The sternal notch is a human anatomical part found at the superior border of the manubrium of the sternum.

The Mediastinum and Trachea

1. **E** The mediastinal boundaries include the following: superior, the first thoracic vertebra; inferior, the diaphragm; anterior, the sternum; posterior: the vertebral column; lateral, the parietal pleura. It is divided into the anterior, medial, and posterior compartment.

2. **C** 50 % of mediastinal lymphomas are in the medial compartment.

3. **B** Thymomas are the most common tumors of the anterior mediastinum, accounting for approximately 20 % of all mediastinal tumors in adults.

Tumors of the middle mediastinum are congenital cysts, and tumors arising from the posterior mediastinum are often neurogenic tumors.

4. C   The most common primary carcinoma of the trachea is squamous cell and adenoid cystic carcinomas. Chondromas are the most common benign tumors.

11.15 The Abdomen (Answers)

The Pancreas and Hepatobiliary Track

1. B   The pancreas lies in the retroperitoneal space, approximately at the level of the lumbar (L1–L2) spine.

2. A   The pancreas is composed of the head, body, and tail. The head of the pancreas is located anatomically on the right site of the abdomen and is connected to the duodenum, and the tail extends to the left side of the abdomen.

3. C   Approximately 80 % of pancreatic cancers are adenocarcinoma.

4. A   The majority of pancreatic cancers (75 %) occur in the head of the pancreas.

5. B   The common hepatic duct is composed of the right and left hepatic duct which originate from the liver. The cystic duct drains bile from the gallbladder into the common bile duct which is formed by the union of the common hepatic duct and the cystic duct.

6. E   The dose-limiting organs surrounding the pancreas include the small intestine, stomach, duodenum, liver, kidneys, and spinal cord. With IMRT techniques, the dose to these organs can be kept low enough to avoid late radiation injury.

7. E   When conformal radiation treatment of the pancreas is needed and the disease is on the head of the pancreas, the entire duodenal loop with margin is included because the disease may invade the medial wall of the duodenum and place the entire circumference at risk as well as 50 % of the right kidney. If the lesion is in the body or tail, two-thirds of the left kidney is excluded and at least 50 % of the left kidney may need to be included to achieve adequate margins and include node groups at risk.

8. D   The tail of the pancreas is located on the left site of the abdomen near the spleen.

The Stomach

1. **A** The stomach begins at the gastroesophageal junction and ends at the pylorus. The stomach is divided into the fundus, the body, and the pylorus.

2. **C** The most common sites of distant metastases from stomach cancer are the liver and the lungs.

3. **C** Adenocarcinoma accounts for 90–95 % of all gastric cancers and lymphomas are the second most common.

4. **D** The most common type of stomach cancer is adenocarcinoma and originates in the innermost lining of the stomach accounting for more than 90 % of tumors. The stomach is composed of the cardiac sphincter which controls movement of food from the esophagus into the stomach. The fundus is the upper expanded area of the stomach, and the pylorus is the terminal region where the stomach joins the small intestine.

The Kidney, Renal Pelvis, and Ureter

1. **E** The kidneys are located in the retroperitoneal space between the eleventh rib and the transverse process of the third lumbar vertebral body. The right kidney is slightly more inferior than the left because of its relationship to the right hepatic lobe, and both kidneys can move vertically as much as 4 cm during normal respiration.

2. **C** The left kidney drains exclusively to the paraaortic lymph nodes, while the right kidney drains to the paracaval and interaortocaval lymph nodes.

3. **E** The most common sites of distant metastases of renal cell carcinoma are the lungs (75 %), soft tissue (36 %), bone (20 %), liver (18 %), and central nervous system (8 %).

4. **B** Carcinoma of the ureter occurs most often in the distal third of the ureter.

5. **D** The majority of renal cancers are adenocarcinomas. More than 90 % of malignant tumors from the renal pelvis and ureter are transitional cell carcinomas and only 8 % are squamous cell carcinomas.

6. **C** Wilms' tumor occurs in children and it is curable in most of them. Malignant rhabdoid tumors of the kidney are the most lethal renal neoplasm in children. Neuroblastoma arises initially from any site along the sympathetic nervous system, and the most common site of origin is the adrenal medulla. Medulloblastoma is a tumor presenting in children that arises in the cerebellum.

11.16 The Pelvis (Answers)

The Anal Canal

1. **B** The anal canal is approximately 3–4 cm long and extends from the level of the pelvic floor to the anal verge. The average rectal length is 10–15 cm long and extends from the sigmoid colon to the anal canal.

2. **E** All are considered risk factors for anal cancer. Also, genital warts, history of genital warts, and HIV are all factors.

3. **A** Squamous cell carcinomas represent approximately 80 % of all malignant tumors of the anal canal. Mucoepidermoid carcinomas are rare, and the remaining include adenocarcinoma, small-cell cancers, and undifferentiated cancers.

4. **A** The major lymphatic pathways of the anal canal drain to the external and internal iliac system as well as the mesenteric system. The preauricular node system is a head and neck lymph node.

The Colon and Rectum

1. **B** Risk factors associated with colorectal cancer include environmental and dietary factors.

2. **A** Adenocarcinoma is the most common colorectal cancer.

3. **E** The rectal anatomy starts at S3 and measures about 15 cm in length. It is composed of three valves: the superior, middle, and inferior rectal valve. It is attached to the sigmoid colon at the rectosigmoid junction.

4. **E** The colon is composed of the ascending, transverse, and descending colon. The ascending colon is attached to the transverse colon by the splenic flexures, while the transverse colon is attached to the descending colon by the hepatic flexures.

5. **C** For rectal cancer treatments, a three-field technique is typically used with a PA and two opposed laterals fields with the patient in a prone position so that the bowel is removed as much as possible from the treatment area.

The Bladder

1. **A** The apex or vertex of the bladder is located toward the pubic symphysis, while the base or fundus lies posteriorly against the rectum or vagina in

females. The neck is the most inferior part of the bladder, and the body is the largest part located between the apex, fundus, and neck.

2. C   The ureters are thick-walled, narrow cylindrical tubes that carry urine from the kidneys to the bladder. They run inferior and medial in front of the psoas major muscles entering the pelvic cavity and open at the base or fundus, superiorly and dorsally.

3. A   The urinary bladder is composed of the neck which is attached to the pelvic diaphragm and it is continuous in the male with the prostate. The body is the largest part and the trigone is the part formed by the right and left ureter orifices and the internal urethral orifice.

4. D   The trigone of the urinary bladder is formed by the right and left ureteral orifices which receive the urine from the kidneys and the internal urethral orifice which releases the urine to the urethra.

5. A   The most common sites of bladder tumor development are the trigone, lateral and posterior walls, and bladder neck.

6. A   The most common sites of distant metastases of bladder cancer are the lungs, bone, and liver.

7. B   The majority of bladder cancers are transitional cell carcinomas accounting for 92 % of cases. Six to seven percent are squamous cell carcinomas and only 1–2 % are adenocarcinomas.

8. D   The highest risk factor associated with bladder cancer is cigarette smoking or inhalation. It is estimated that smoking is responsible for 30–40 % of all cases.

The Female Urethra

1. A   The primary lymphatics associated with the urethra are the obturator and internal and external iliac nodes.

The Penis and Male Urethra

1. C   Most malignant penile tumors are well-differentiated squamous cell carcinomas. Undifferentiated or mixed carcinomas, transitional cell carcinomas, and adenocarcinoma account for less than 15 % of penile tumors.

The Prostate

1. E The prostate is divided into the anterior, median, posterior, and two lateral lobes.

2. B Most carcinomas of the prostate are found because of elevated prostate-specific antigen (PSA). Rectal examination and Gleason score are important in diagnosis also.

3. B The most common sites of distant metastases of prostate cancer are the bones and, less frequently, the liver or lungs.

4. D Most malignant prostate cancers are adenocarcinoma arising from the peripheral acinar glands. It is graded as well, moderately, or poorly differentiated. Squamous cell carcinoma and lymphoma originating primarily in the prostate are extremely rare, and sarcomas are **0.**1 % of all primary neoplasms of the prostate.

5. A Surgery, hormonal therapy, and radiation therapy are the general management techniques for prostate cancer. Observation of low-risk prostate cancer is now considered an option as well.

6. C Before prostate hormonal therapy, breast irradiation is effective to prevent glandular hyperplasia.

7. B Prostate temporal implants are performed using iridium-**192**. HDR brachytherapy for the prostate is gaining popularity recently. Permanent implants used iodine-125, palladium-103, or gold-**198.**

The Testis

1. B Prostate lymph nodes have extensive intercommunicating lymphatic channels. Crossover from the right to the left side is constant but from the left to the right side is rare.

2. D Germ cell tumors (seminomas and nonseminomas) account for 95 % of all testicular tumors. Lymphomas account for less than 5 % of all testicular tumors.

3. C Most testicular cancer patients receive radiation to the paraaortic and ipsilateral pelvic nodes.

4. C Testicular cancer is a disease of young people and most commonly found in males aging from 15 to 30 years old. The incidence gradually decreases by the age of **70.**

The Endometrium

1. **A** The uterus is divided into the corpus, the body, and the cervix.

2. **B** The most common gynecologic malignancy is endometrial cancer.

3. **C** All of these are symptoms associated with endometrial cancer, but the most common presenting symptom is vaginal bleeding, which is reported by 70–80 % of patients.

4. **D** The most common form of carcinoma of the endometrium is adenocarcinoma (papillary, secretory, ciliated cells, and adenocarcinoma with squamous differentiation). The most aggressive ones are serous carcinoma, clear-cell carcinoma, and pure squamous cell carcinomas.

The Ovary

1. **B** Epithelial ovarian cancer is present in 85–90 % of patients, making it the most common ovarian carcinoma. Germ cell, sex cord, and stromal carcinomas are nonepithelial ovarian cancer seen in only 10 % of cases.

The Uterine Cervix

1. **C** The most common metastatic sites of uterine cervix cancer are the lungs (21 %), paraaortic nodes (11 %), mediastinal and supraclavicular lymph modes (7 %), and bones and liver with the lowest occurrence.

2. **A** The International Federation of Gynecologists and Oncologists (FIGO) is the most used staging for gynecologic cancer. The TNM system is not commonly used but it correlates with the FIGO stage grouping for ovarian malignancies.

3. **B** The majority of uterine cervix cancers are squamous cell carcinomas (90 %). Adenocarcinoma constitutes 7–10 % and clear-cell carcinomas only 1–2 %. Adenoid cystic carcinoma is a rare neoplasm of the cervix (less than 1 % incidence).

4. **B** Iridium-192 is used for HDR brachytherapy of uterine cervix cancer. Cesium-137 is a λ ray-emitting radioisotope used as a radium substitute in both interstitial and intracavitary brachytherapy. It is used for LDR brachytherapy of uterine cervix cancer.

5. **A** Brachytherapy of the uterine cervix can be delivered with intracavitary techniques using intrauterine tandem and vaginal colpostats (ovoids) or

ring. Vaginal cylinders may be used when necessary to cover large tumors.

The Vagina

1. **C** Vaginal cancers occur most commonly on the posterior wall of the upper third of the vagina.

2. **B** Epidermoid carcinoma accounts for approximately 90 % of primary vaginal tumors. Adenocarcinoma comprises approximately 5 %. Sarcomas are the most common mesenchymal tumor of the vagina in adults, and leiomyosarcomas comprise 68 % of vaginal sarcomas in adults. Adenoid cystic carcinoma of the vagina is rare.

3. **C** Rhabdomyosarcoma comprises approximately 90 % of female genital tract cases occurring in children under 5 years of age. Leiomyosarcomas account for 68 % of cases in adults, and epidermoid carcinoma accounts for approximately 90 % of primary vaginal tumors in adults.

4. **D** Radiation therapy is the preferred treatment for most carcinomas of the vagina. Surgery may be an appropriate treatment in young patients to preserve ovarian function, and a combination of radiation and surgery is suggested for extensive tumors.

5. **E** All are used. Surgery may be an appropriate treatment in young patients to preserve ovarian function. Intracavitary and interstitial LDR delivering 75–80 Gy to the involved vaginal mucosa is sufficient to control in situ lesions. For advanced tumors, whole-pelvis irradiation is used and systemic chemotherapy is recommended.

6. **E** All are correct.

11.17 The Spinal Canal (Answers)

The Spinal Cord

1. **B** Spinal canal tumors are classified as intramedullary (arising from the intrinsic substance of the spinal cord) or intradural-extramedullary (arising from connective tissues, blood vessels, or coverings adjacent to the cord or cauda equina).

2. **A** Astrocytomas, ependymomas, and oligodendrogliomas are intramedullary tumors. Ependymomas, nerve sheath tumors, meningiomas, and vascular tumors belong to intradural-extramedullary-type tumors.

11.18 Children (Answers)

3. **E** All are correct. The spinal cord is composed of 31 pairs of nerves: 8 cervical, 12 thoracic, 5 lumbar, 5 sacral, and 1 coccygeal. The white matter is located in the periphery and surrounds the central gray matter. By adulthood the spinal cord ends near the level of the L1 vertebral body and the lower lumbar, sacral, and coccygeal nerves form the cauda equina.

4. **C** Tumors involving the cervical spine can be treated with opposed lateral fields to avoid incidental irradiation of the hypopharynx and oral cavity. Primary tumors of the spinal canal can be easily treated with a direct posterior field, even though some lumbar region tumors may require opposed AP/PA portals because of the lumbar lordosis and the location of the vertebral bodies near the midline of the trunk. Finally, paired set of oblique-wedged fields combined with a PA field can be used in tumors involving the thoracic and lumbar spinal canal.

5. **C** The arachnoid mater is located between the pia mater and the dura mater and encloses the subarachnoid space filled with cerebrospinal fluid (SPF). The pia mater is the innermost lining and covers the spinal cord and its blood vessels. The dura mater forms a dense, fibrous barrier between the bony spinal canal and the spinal cord.

6. **B** Traditionally, the spinal cord borders are superior and inferior to encompass two vertebral bodies above and below the tumor, and the width is typically 4–8 cm with the anterior border including the vertebral foramen.

7. **A** Between the dura mater and the pia mater is the arachnoid mater, which encloses the subarachnoid space filled with cerebrospinal fluid (CSF).

8. **C** The spinal cord ends at the level of L1–L2. The lower lumbar, sacral, and coccygeal nerves form the cauda equina which is the collection of nerves that fill the thecal sac below **L1**.

11.18 Children (Answers)

Brain Tumors in Children

1. **C** Medulloblastoma is a primitive neuroectodermal tumor presenting in the posterior fossa of children. Wilms' tumor is cancer of the kidneys that typically occurs in children, rarely in adults. Neuroblastoma originates most frequently in the adrenal gland of children but can develop in the neck, chest, abdomen, and pelvis. Rhabdomyosarcoma is a soft tissue sarcoma that occurs in children and can develop in any site of the body.

2. **D** With medulloblastoma, the entire subarachnoid space is at risk, so full neuraxis irradiation is mandatory. Craniospinal irradiation (CSI) is required; two lateral craniocervical fields matched with a posterior or two adjacent spinal fields.

3. **A** The posterior fossa is typically boosted to encompass the entire infratentorial compartment.

4. **E** All are correct. Low-grade gliomas compose 40 % of pediatric brain tumors (astrocytomas, oligodendroglioma, mixed gliomas, and mixed neuroepithelial tumors). Malignant gliomas present in 7–10 % of pediatric CNS tumors. Brainstem gliomas occur predominantly in children between 3 and 9 years of age, and craniopharyngioma is a benign tumor present in children.

Hodgkin's Disease

1. **C** Hodgkin's disease nearly always begins in the lymph nodes.

2. **B** More than 80 % of patients with Hodgkin's disease present with cervical lymph node involvement followed by 50 % having mediastinal disease.

3. **D** The Ann Arbor staging system is used for Hodgkin's disease.

4. **C** Based on Ann Arbor staging classification, stage I Hodgkin's disease is involvement of a single lymph node region. Stage II disease includes involvement of two or more lymph node regions on the same side of the diaphragm, and stage III includes involvement of lymph node regions on both sides of the diaphragm. Stage IV is disseminated involvement of one or more extralymphatic organs or tissues.

5. **E** All of them are subtypes of Hodgkin's disease.

6. **B** Nodular sclerosis HD (MSHD) is the most common histological subtype and often involves the mediastinum. Lymphocyte-predominant HD (LPHD) is often diagnosed in young people, and most patients present with early-stage disease. This is the most favorable of the histological subtypes. Lymphocyte-depleted IID (LDHD) occurs in older patients and is associated with advanced disease. It has the worst prognosis of all. Finally, in mixed-cellularity HD (MCHD) patients more commonly present with advanced disease and is less favorable than NSHD.

7. **A** AP/PA mantel fields extend from the inferior portion of the mandible to the diaphragm. Blocks are placed over the occipital region, spinal cord posteriorly, larynx anteriorly, and humeral heads.

8. **B** Waldeyer's fields are used for Hodgkin's disease irradiation when there is a primary component of large cervical adenopathy to treat the submandibular, preauricular, occipital, and high cervical nodes. The retroperitoneal and pelvic lymph nodes are treated using a subdiaphragmatic field (inverted Y).

9. **E** Common areas blocked during Hodgkin's disease irradiation include the lungs, occipital region, spinal cord, larynx, humeral head, testicles, midline pelvic block, rectum, anus, ovaries, and genitalia.

10. **A** One-third of Hodgkin's disease patients present with one of the three B symptoms: fever, night sweats, or 10 % weight loss in the past 6 months. Patients with Hodgkin's disease generally present with painless lymphadenopathy.

Non-Hodgkin's Lymphoma

1. **E** Non-Hodgkin's lymphoma can arise in any area of lymphoid aggregation such as the lymph nodes, spleen, Waldeyer's ring, bone marrow, GI tract, and other tissues in which lymphoid cells may be circulating.

2. **E** All are correct.

3. **D** The Ann Arbor staging system is used for non-Hodgkin's lymphoma.

4. **E** All are considered non-Hodgkin's lymphomas. MALT lymphomas arise in the stomach, thyroid, salivary glands, breast, and bladder. Mantle cell lymphomas occur in older adults and arise in the spleen, bone marrow, and GI tract. Anaplastic large-cell lymphomas arise in the skin.

Neuroblastoma

1. **C** The most common site of neuroblastoma origin is the adrenal medulla (30–40 %) or paraspinal ganglia in the abdomen or pelvis (25 %). Thoracic (15 %) and head and neck primary tumors (5 %) are slightly more common in infants than in older children.

2. **E** More than 70 % of patients with neuroblastoma have metastatic disease at presentation. The most frequent sites are the lymph nodes, bone, bone marrow, skin, and liver. The lungs and central nervous system do not usually have metastatic involvement.

3. **A** The most common presenting symptom of neuroblastoma is pain due to bone, liver, or bone marrow metastases or local visceral invasion by the tumor. Other symptoms may include weight loss, anorexia, malaise, and fever.

Rhabdomyosarcoma

1. **E** Rhabdomyosarcoma is a highly malignant soft tissue sarcoma that arises in any site of the body.

2. **A** The most common site of gynecologic rhabdomyosarcoma is the vagina. Other sites are the vulva, cervix, and uterus which are approximately one-third as common as bladder and prostate primary tumors.

Wilms' Tumor

1. **C** The most common metastatic sites of Wilms' tumor are the lungs followed by the liver.

2. **E** Wilms' tumor is often localized at diagnosis and it is curable in most children. It is spread throughout the peritoneal cavity, and the classic presentation is that of a healthy child in whom abdominal swelling is discovered and a smooth, firm, non-tender mass on one side of the abdomen is felt.

3. **B** Irradiation does not need to be given immediately after operation, but treatment timing is important. Patients in whom irradiation was delayed for 10 days or more after surgery had a significantly higher chance of abdominal relapse

The Bone

1. **E** The most common skeletal bone tumors are osteosarcomas, Ewing's sarcomas, chondrosarcomas, fibrosarcomas, malignant fibrous histiocytomas of the bone, giant-cell tumors, aneurismal bone cysts, and chordomas.

2. **C** Chondrosarcomas involve most often the shoulder girdle, proximal shoulder, and humerus. Osteosarcomas occur in the diaphyseal region of tubular long bones like the distal femur or proximal tibia. Fibrosarcomas often occur in the femur or tibia also but, unlike osteosarcoma, most are in the metaphyseal or epiphyseal region. Finally, most chordomas originate in the sacrococcygeal region but also in the base of the skull and spine.

3. **C** There is no universally accepted staging system for primary bone sarcomas, but Enneking staging system classifies tumors according to grace, local extent, and presence or absence of distant metastases.

4. **B** Osteosarcoma occurs most often in the diaphyseal region of the distal femur or proximal tibia (75 %); 41 % of them occur in flat bones (Paget's disease association).

Ewing's Sarcoma

1. **B** Although any bone can be the site of a primary lesion in Ewing's sarcoma, the femur is the most common site at initial presentation and the diaphysis is more commonly involved than the metaphysis or the epiphysis. Lymph node metastases are rare.

2. **B** The main or midsection (shaft) of a long bone is the diaphysis. The metaphysis is the wider portion of a long bone adjacent to the epiphyseal plate and is the part of the bone that grows during childhood. The epiphysis is the rounded end of a long bone. The medullary cavity is the hollow center of the diaphysis.

3. **D** Ewing's sarcoma of the pelvic area has the worst prognosis followed by those involving other proximal bones such as the femur and humerus. Distal long bones have a better prognosis.

4. **A** Ewing's sarcoma is the second most common primary pediatric bone tumor after osteosarcoma. After the age of 20, the incidence decreases to nearly 0 by the age of **30.**

Leukemia

1. **E** All are types of leukemia.

2. **A** The most common type of pediatric leukemia is acute lymphoblastic leukemia (ALL).

3. **A** Acute lymphocytic leukemias are classified into B cell acute lymphoblastic leukemia which represents most adult leukemias. T cell acute lymphoblastic leukemia and non-B cell and non-T cell acute lymphoblastic leukemia are other classifications.

4. **A** The most common treatment options of leukemia patients include radiation therapy where cranial irradiation is indicated in patients with ALL following induction chemotherapy to reduce the incidence of CNS relapse. Males with ALL may require testicular irradiation as well. For CLL patients, splenic irradiation can be substituted for splenectomy in patients who are unable to have surgery. Total body irradiation for CLL has been found to have a complete response rate. Chemotherapy is used for both acute and chronic leukemia as well as bone marrow transplantation (BMT). Surgery plays essentially no role in the management of acute leukemia, and the only surgical option in patients with chronic leukemia is splenectomy, and it is indicated only for the palliation of symptomatic splenomegaly.

5. **B** Acute myelogenous leukemia (AML) is most commonly seen in patients over 40 years old while the incidence of ALL reaches an initial peak between ages 5 and **6.** More than 90 % of CLL cases occur in patients older than 50 years old. Ninety five percent of patients with juvenile CML (JCML) are younger than 4 years old at presentation whereas hairy cell leukemia (HCL) presents at a median age of 52 years.

6. **E** All of them are considered hematopoietic organs, meaning they are related to making blood cells.

7. **D** Although no TNM staging system can be applied to these hematologic malignancies, a staging system for CLL based on the extent of disease has been proposed by Rai. The Rai staging system was modified by Binet where the Binet staging system is based on the presence of adenopathy, splenomegaly, anemia, and thrombocytopenia.

8. **C** Cranial irradiation is indicated in patients with ALL to reduce the incidence of CNS relapse and may be required in patients with ANLL to reduce the likelihood of potentially fatal intracranial hemorrhage during therapy. Males with ALL may require testicular radiation.

Multiple Myeloma and Plasmacytoma

1. **E** All are correct.

2. **B** Common clinical presentations of multiple myeloma include bone pain in 68 % of the cases and hypercalcemia in 50 % of the patients. Infection, bleeding, easy fatigability, anemia, thrombocytopenia, and granulocytopenia are all symptoms. Radiographs show diffuse osteoporosis, well-demarcated lytic lesions, or localized cystic osteolytic lesions.

3. **C** Multiple myeloma can cause paraplegia due to pressure on the spinal cord.

4. **A** Multiple myeloma is the most common primary bone malignancy being ten times more prevalent than all other types of tumors combined. Ewing's sarcoma is predominantly a disease of children and is the second most common primary pediatric bone tumor after osteosarcoma.

11.19 Benign Diseases (Answers)

1. **A** Pterygium is a benign disease of the conjunctiva of the eye. It is thought to be caused by ultraviolet light, low humidity, and dust. The treatment of choice is surgery with postoperative radiation therapy to decrease the recurrence rate. Keloids are a benign disease of the skin where a scar overgrows. They are treated with surgery followed by radiation therapy started within

24 h after surgery. Heterotopic bone formation is a benign disease where the bone tissue grows outside the skeleton. This occurs in some patients after surgery, and the treatment of choice is postoperative radiation therapy. Thymomas are the most common tumor of the anterior mediastinum. Other benign diseases include exophthalmos, orbital pseudotumor, macular degeneration, plantar warts, keratoacanthomas, hemangiomas, AVMs, ocular angiomas, cavernous hemangioma of the liver, bursitis and tendinitis, desmoid tumor, Peyronie's disease, vascular restenosis, ameloblastoma, aneurysmal bone cyst, vertebral hemangioma, gynecomastia, ovarian castration, parotitis, and acute and chronic inflammatory disorders.

2. C   Arteriovenous malformations (AVMs) of the brain are sometimes treated with stereotactic radiosurgery using a single fraction of high-dose radiation to a stereotactically defined small volume to sclerose the AVM and prevent hemorrhage.

3. A   Plantar wart radiation therapy treatments are simple, safe, and effective using a single radiation treatment of 10 Gy using close lead shielding to define the treated field. The wart usually separates and falls off in 3–4 weeks without sequelae after radiation treatment. Liquid nitrogen cryosurgery can be used with cure rates of 90 %. Surgical treatment leads to incapacity during the long period of healing and may leave painful scars.

4. D   Percutaneous transluminal coronary angioplasty (PTCA) is used to treat coronary stenotic lesions by balloon dilatation in selected patients with atherosclerotic coronary artery disease. The use of intra-arterial iridium-192 afterloading after stent placement reduces considerable restenosis on patients.

5. A   Heterotopic bone formation occurs in 30 % of patients undergoing hip arthroplasty, so radiation treatment is given immediately following a postoperative period using doses in a single fraction of 7 or 10 Gy in 4–5 fractions.

11.20 The Skin (Answers)

1. A   The skin is composed of the epidermis which is composed of the outermost layer (the stratum corneum and the basal layer), the dermis which produces collagen and gives the skin strength, and finally the subcutaneous tissue which contains smooth muscles attached to the hair shaft and is responsive to cold and sweat.

2. A   Carcinoma of the skin is the most common malignancy in the United States, and the most common cause is exposure to solar radiation. It tends to occur

in patients over 40 years of age, and the skin complexion is a risk factor. Fair skin that freckles, green or blue eyes, red or light blond hair, and poor tanning ability are all correlated with an increased risk of skin cancer.

3. B The most common skin carcinomas are basal and squamous cell carcinomas. Melanomas are the most serious.

4. E All of them are malignant tumors of the skin. Basal and squamous cell carcinomas are the most common, and melanomas are the most serious. Others are Merkel cell carcinoma, adnexal tumors, connective tissue tumors, malignant lymphomas, mycosis fungoides, Kaposi's sarcoma, and keratoacanthomas.

5. E All of them are surgical techniques used on skin cancer. Curettage and electrodessication are used for small nodular basal cell carcinomas. Mohs' microsurgery is used for basal and squamous cell carcinomas and consists of taking frozen-section samples of residual tumors until negative margins are obtained. Cryotherapy is the use of liquid nitrogen on skin neoplasms causing necrosis of malignant cells by destruction of microvasculature.

6. A Typical radiation therapy skin treatments include the use of orthovoltage and supervoltage X-rays and electron beams. The choice of energy depends on the tumor size, depth, and anatomic location. To have proper coverage, the 80–90 % isodose line is used and bolus placement is used to enhance surface dose. Higher energies can be used for more advanced lesions with deep penetration and involvement of bone or cartilage, but not for larger tumors.

7. E Non-AIDS-associated Kaposi's sarcoma treatments include local irradiation of the lesion plus a normal tissue border of **1.5–2.0** cm. Thin, cutaneous lesions can be treated effectively with low-energy electrons or superficial X-ray beams. Eyelid lesions are treated most easily by superficial X-rays with shields over the optic lens, and if edema is present, parallel-opposed fields and megavoltage therapy are needed to treat deep tissues.

11.21 Soft Tissue Sarcomas (Answers)

1. D Soft tissue sarcomas can occur within any organ or any anatomic location within the musculoskeletal system.

2. C The most common subsite of origin of soft tissue sarcomas is the thigh.

3. C The most common metastatic site of soft tissue sarcomas is the lungs, and hematogenous metastasis is the most common pattern of metastatic disease; lymph nodes are uncommon.

11.22 Extras (Answers)

4. B The most common soft tissue sarcoma is malignant fibrous histiocytomas which occurs in 40 % of cases. Liposarcomas develop anywhere but appear in the deep fat tissues of limbs or the abdomen. Rhabdomyosarcoma is a rare cancer that begins in the muscles and occurs in children or young adults. It is most commonly found in the head and neck, bladder, vagina, prostate, testes, arms, or legs. Myofibrosarcomas are malignant tumors of myofibroblasts.

11.22 Extras (Answers)

1. A The spread of cancer from its primary site of origin to a distant site is known as metastasis. Hyperplasia is the increase in the number of cells in a tissue. Metaplasia is the transformation of one type of one mature differentiated cell type into another mature differentiated cell type. Necrosis is the death of body tissue.

2. E Radiopaque contrast or positive contrast used in CT simulation has a high atomic number so absorption of X-rays is increased. It also increases organ density; it is great for the visualization of lymph nodes as well. Examples are barium sulfate and iodine products. Radiolucent or negative contrasts are not radiopaque, and examples include air, oxygen, or carbon dioxide.

3. B Informed consent must be obtained from all patients before any procedure. If a contrast agent is to be used, the patient's allergic history must be obtained before the injection.

4. C Minor iodine contrast reactions include nausea and vomiting and a feeling of warmth. These occur in a very low percentage of people receiving the contrast. The symptoms occur only for a short period of time and do not require any type of treatment. Moderate reactions include severe vomiting, hives, and swelling and require treatment; most of the time Benadryl is used. Anaphylaxis is a severe life-threatening reaction to contrast media.

5. B Creatine and BUN are ordered before iodine contrast injection when performing a CT scan study. These tests asses kidney and liver functions. BUN normal levels are between 10 and 20 mg/dl for adults and 5–18 mg/dl for children. Creatine levels are between **0.5** and **1.1** mg/dl for an adult female and **0.6–1.2** mg/dl for an adult male. The most widely used biochemical blood test to detect liver cancer is alpha-fetoprotein (AFP)

6. A The function of a contrast agent is to increase or improve tissue contrast.

Anatomy

12

Contents

12.1 Brain (Questions) 683
12.2 Head and Neck (Questions). 685
12.3 Thorax (Questions) 687
12.4 Abdomen (Questions) 690
12.5 Pelvis (Questions) 693
12.6 Brain (Answers) 697
12.7 Head and Neck (Answers). 700
12.8 Thorax (Answers) 704
12.9 Abdomen (Answers) 709
12.10 Pelvis (Answers) 715

12.1 Brain (Questions)

Fig. 12.1.1

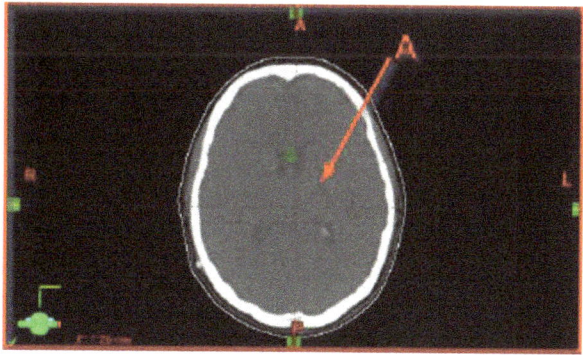

Courtesy of University of Miami, Sylvester Cancer Center
Innovative Cancer Institute

© Springer International Publishing Switzerland 2015
W. Amestoy, *Review of Medical Dosimetry: A Study Guide*,
DOI 10.1007/978-3-319-13626-4_12

Fig. 12.1.2

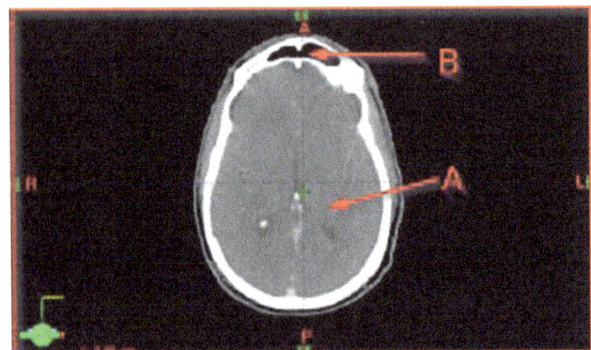

Fig. 12.1.3

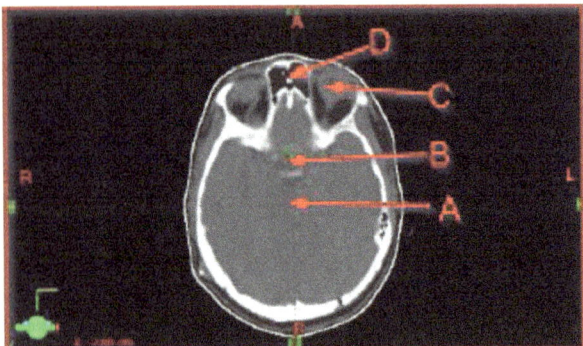

Fig. 12.1.4

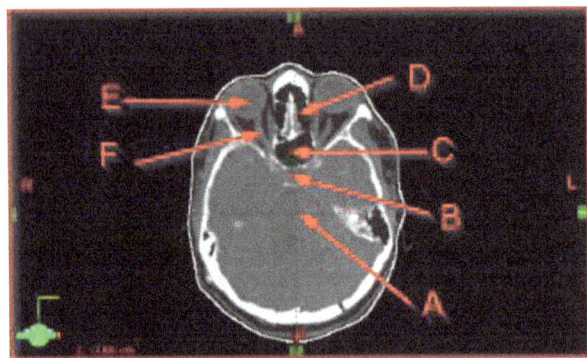

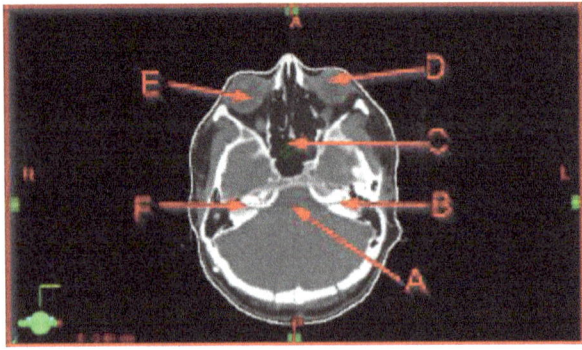

Fig. 12.1.5

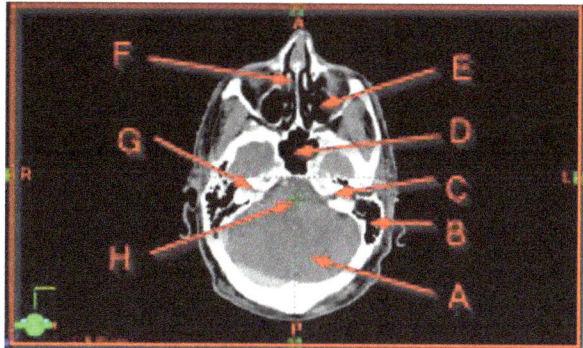

Fig. 12.1.6

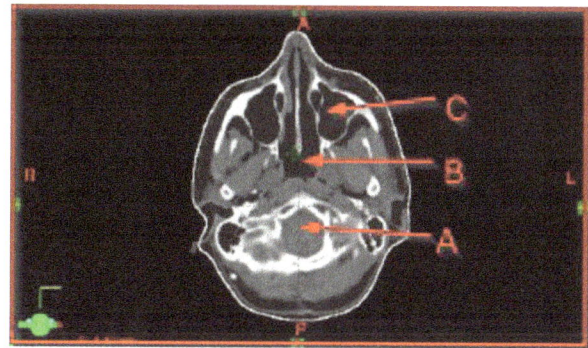

Fig. 12.1.7

12.2 Head and Neck (Questions)

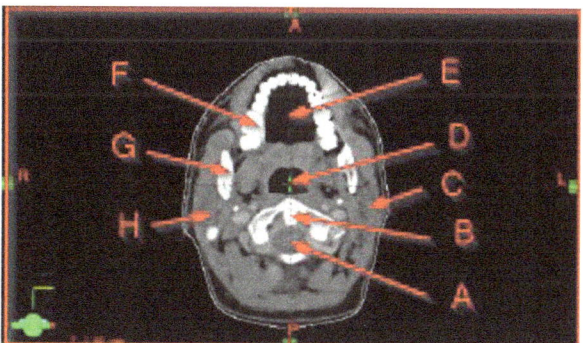

Fig. 12.2.1

Fig. 12.2.2

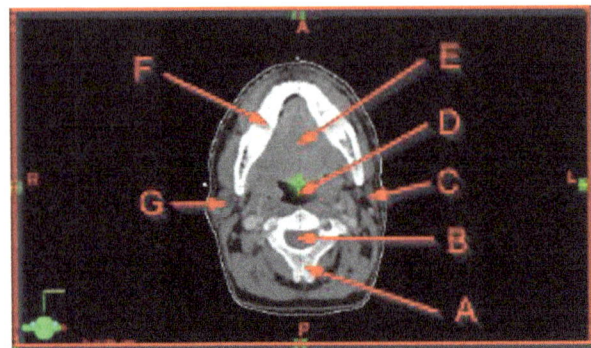

Fig. 12.2.3

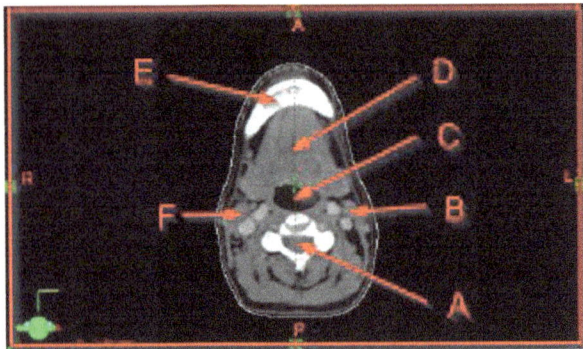

Fig. 12.2.4

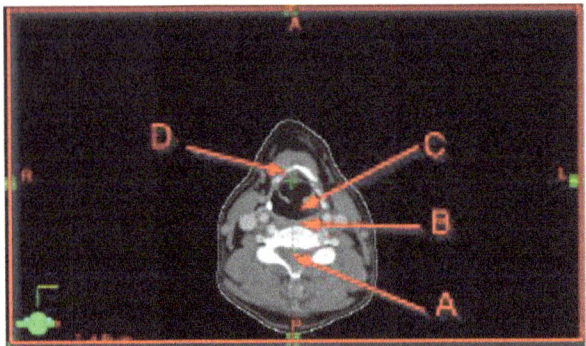

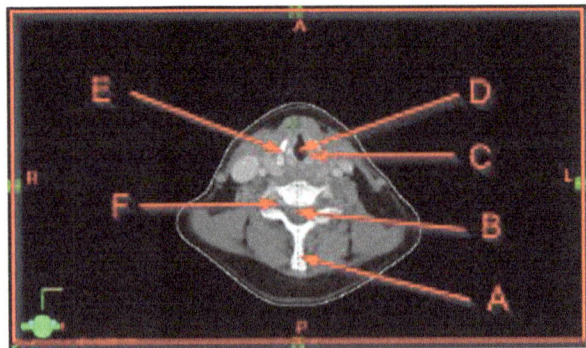

Fig. 12.2.5

12.3 Thorax (Questions)

Fig. 12.2.6

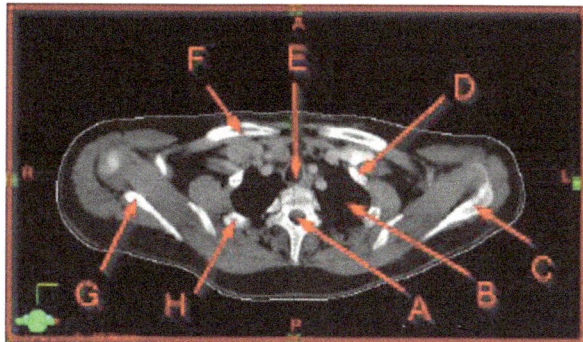

Fig. 12.2.7

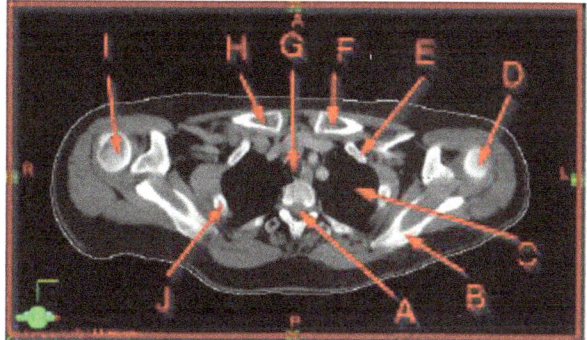

12.3 Thorax (Questions)

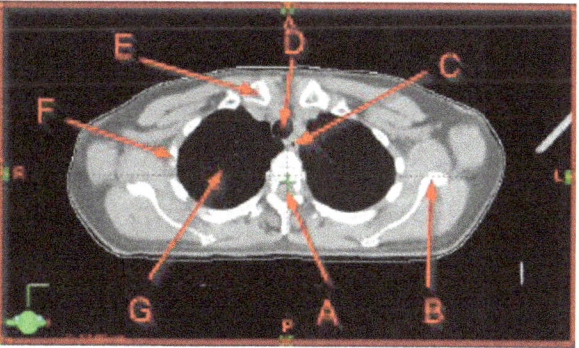

Fig. 12.3.1

Fig. 12.3.2

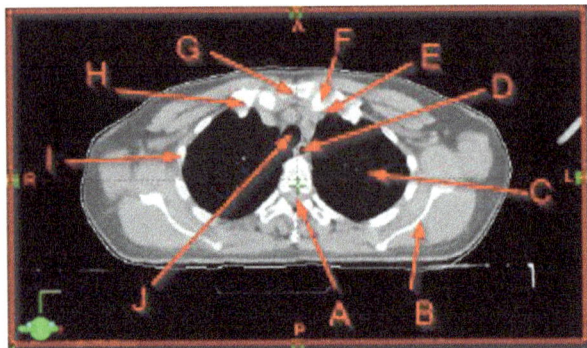

Fig. 12.3.3

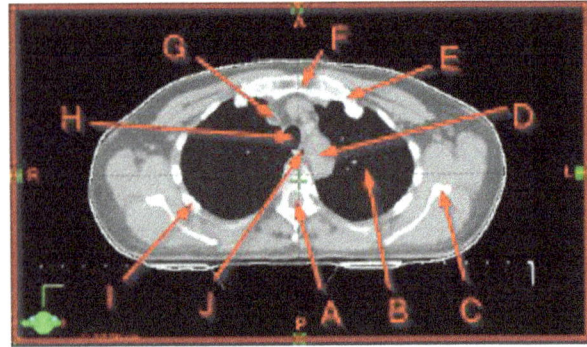

Fig. 12.3.4

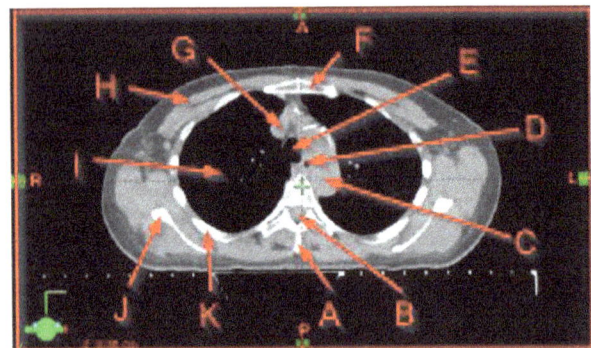

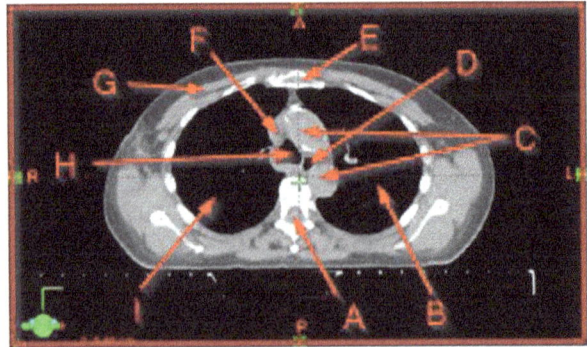

Fig. 12.3.5

12.3 Thorax (Questions)

Fig. 12.3.6

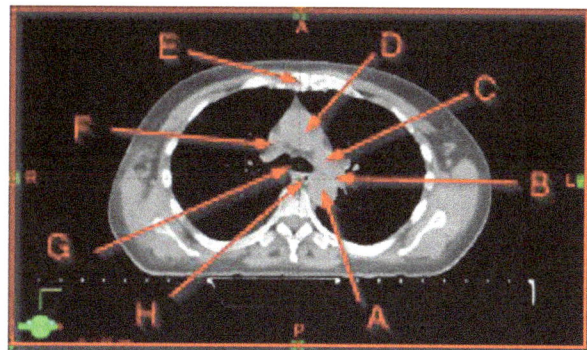

Fig. 12.3.7

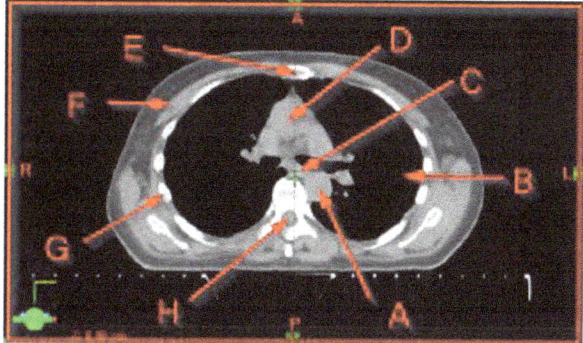

Fig. 12.3.8

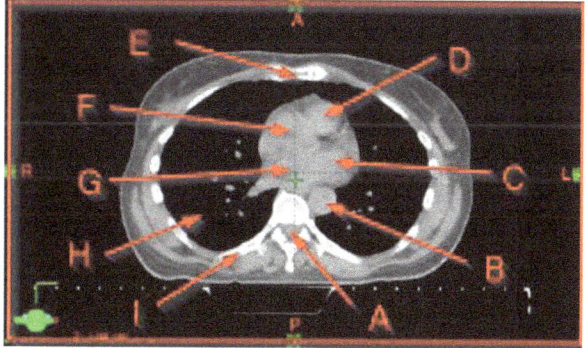

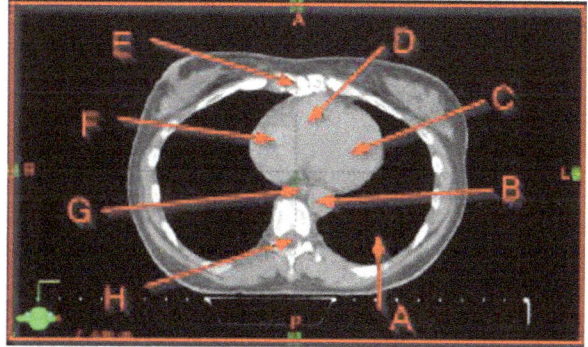

Fig. 12.3.9

Fig. 12.3.10

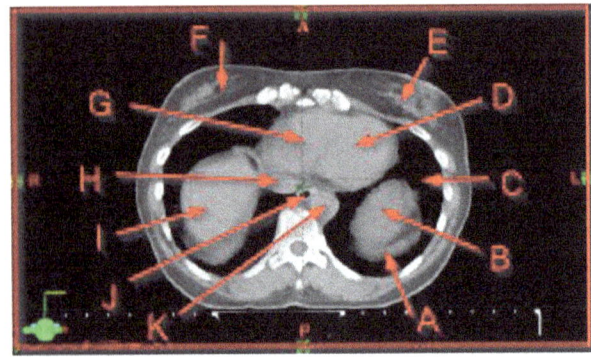

12.4 Abdomen (Questions)

Fig. 12.4.1

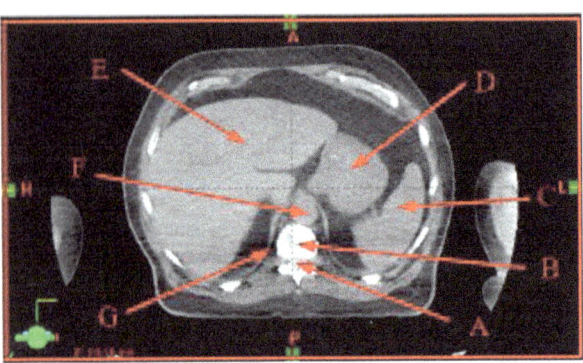

Fig. 12.4.2

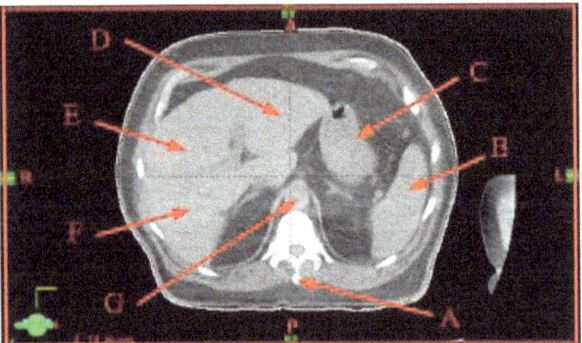

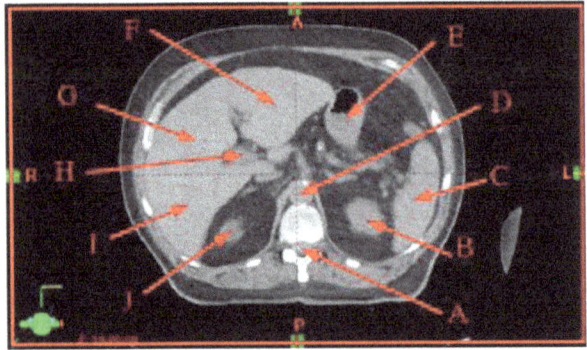

Fig. 12.4.3

12.4 Abdomen (Questions)

Fig. 12.4.4

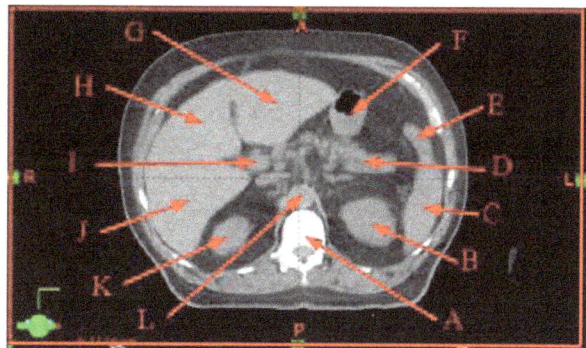

Fig. 12.4.5

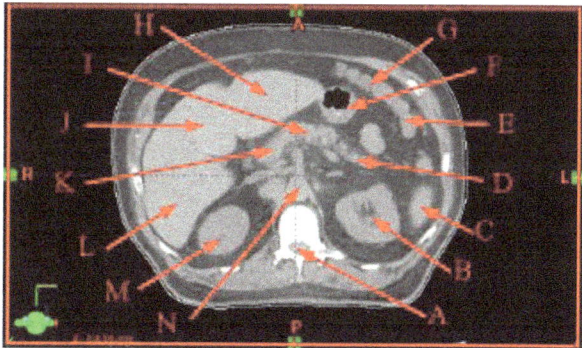

Fig. 12.4.6

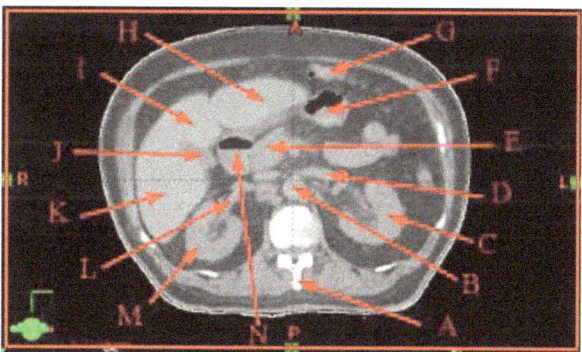

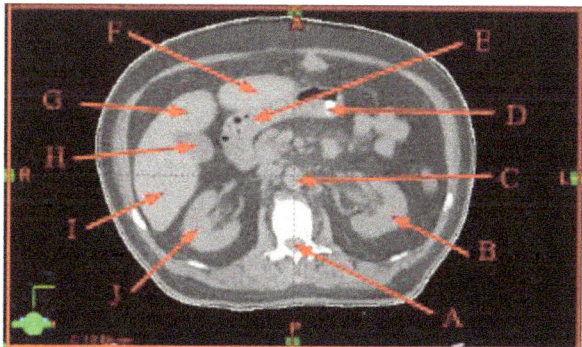

Fig. 12.4.7

Fig. 12.4.8

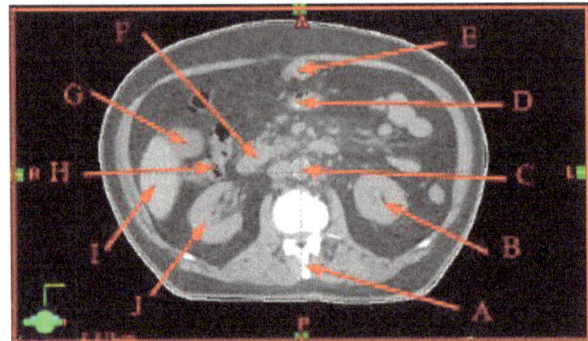

Fig. 12.4.9

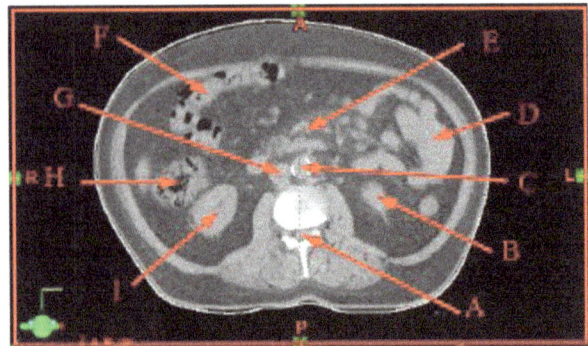

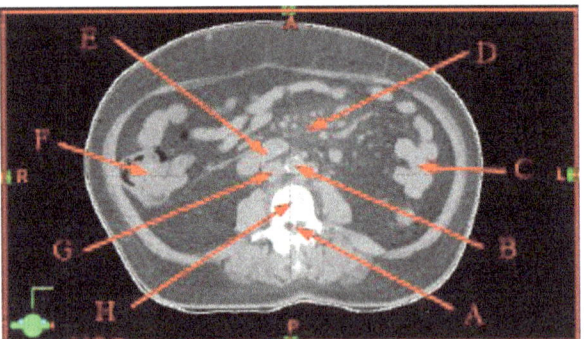

Fig. 12.4.10

12.5 Pelvis (Questions)

Fig. 12.5.1

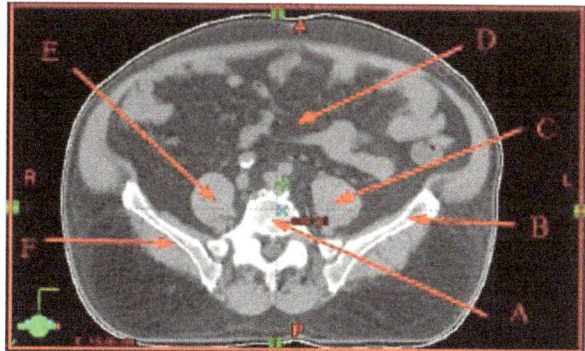

Fig. 12.5.2

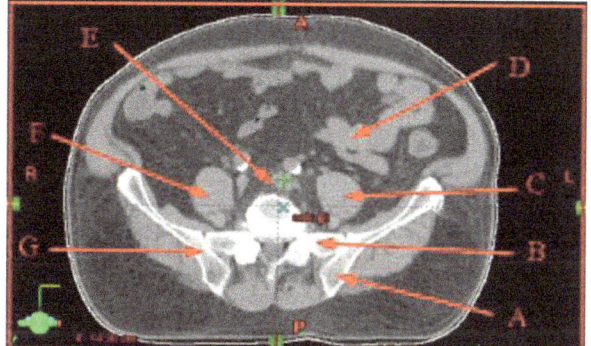

Fig. 12.5.3

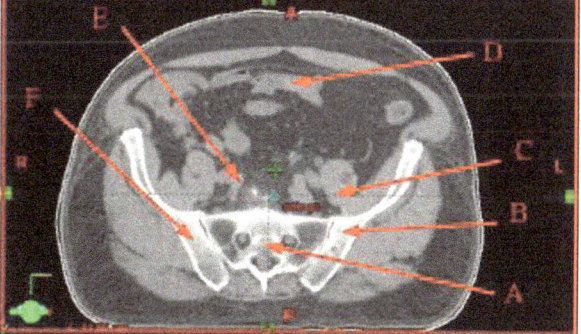

Fig. 12.5.4

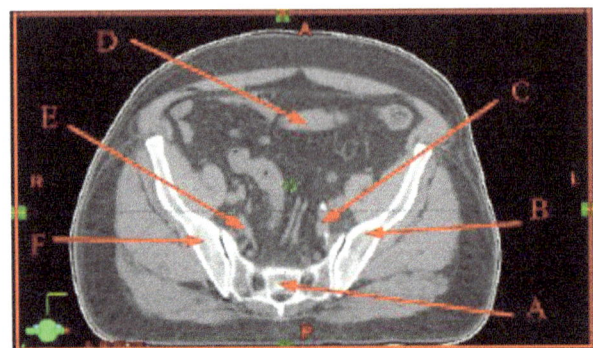

Fig. 12.5.5

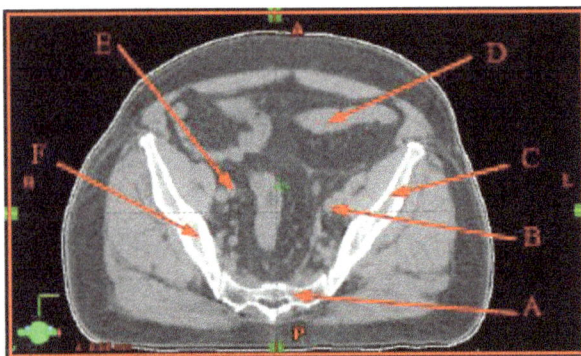

Fig. 12.5.6

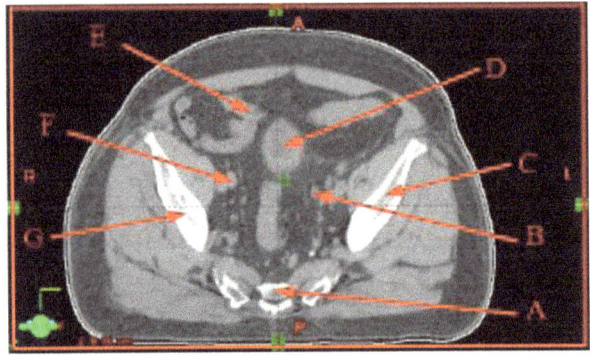

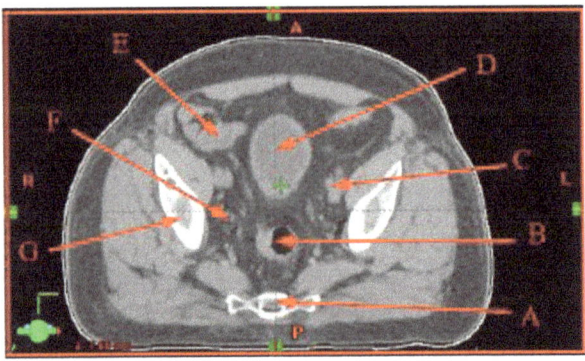

Fig. 12.5.7

12.5 Pelvis (Questions)

Fig. 12.5.8

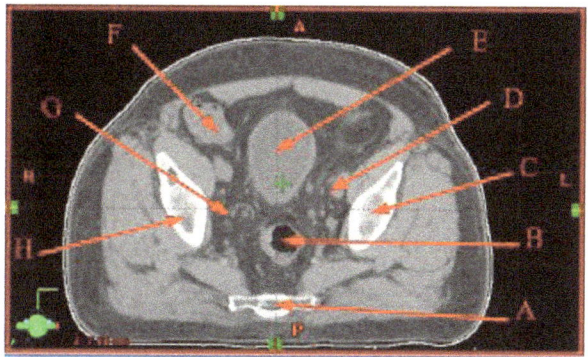

Fig. 12.5.9

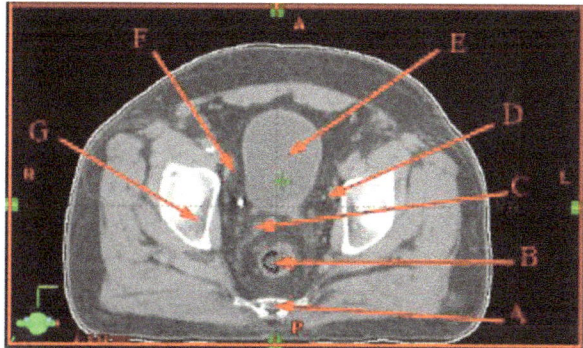

Fig. 12.5.10

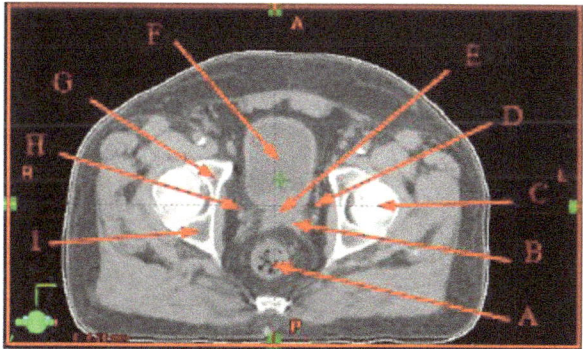

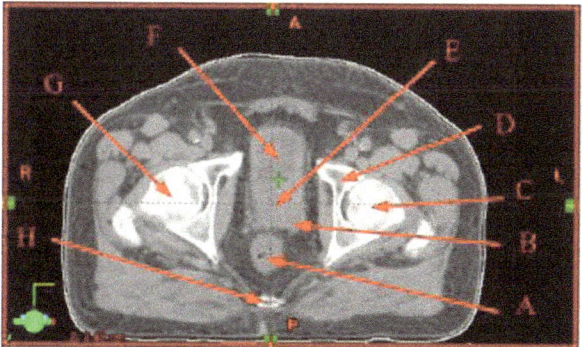

Fig. 12.5.11

Fig. 12.5.12

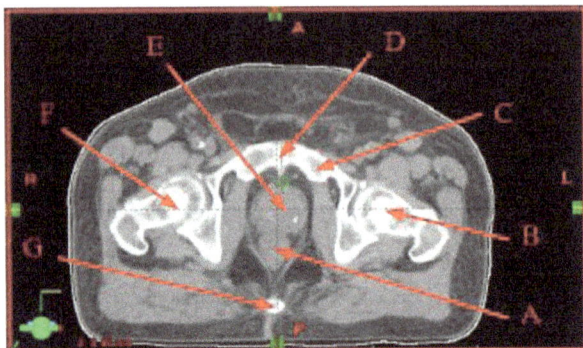

Fig. 12.5.13

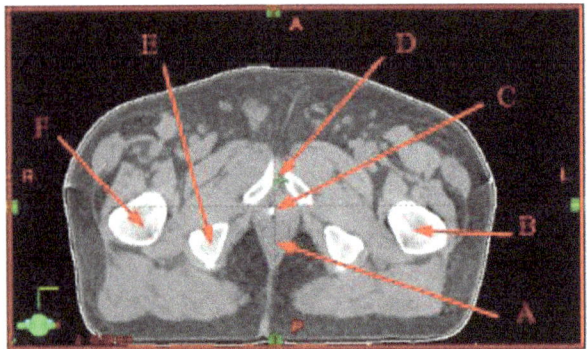

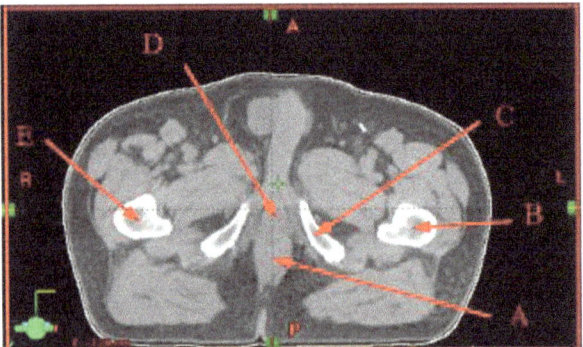

Fig. 12.5.14

12.6 Brain (Answers)

Fig. 12A.1.1

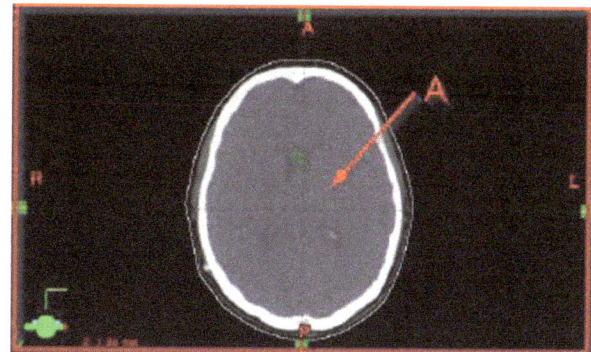

A. Brain

Fig. 12A.1.2

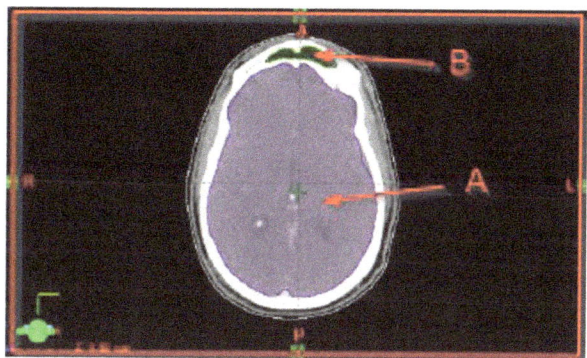

A. Brain
B. Frontal sinuses

Fig. 12A.1.3

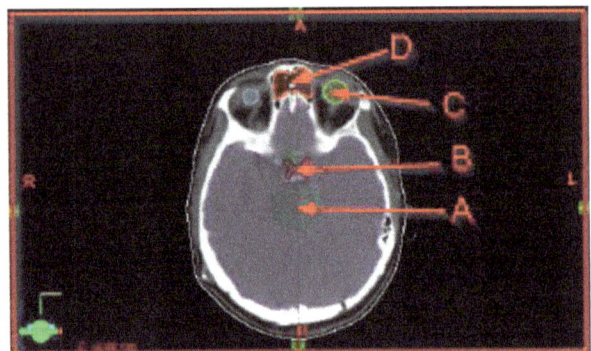

A. Brainstem
B. Optic chiasm
C. Left orbit
D. Ethmoid sinus

Fig. 12A.1.4

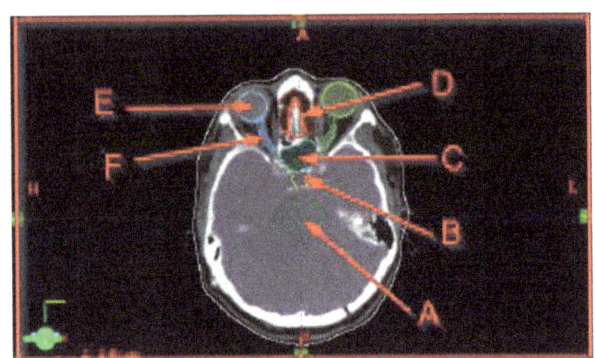

A. Brainstem
B. Pituitary gland
C. Sphenoid sinus
D. Ethmoid sinus
E. Right orbit
F. Right optic nerve

12.6 Brain (Answers)

Fig. 12A.1.5

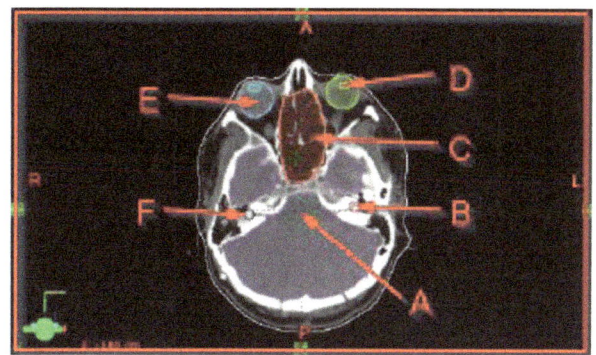

A. Brainstem
B. Left cochlea
C. Sphenoid sinus
D. Left lens
E. Right orbit
F. Right cochlea

Fig. 12A.1.6

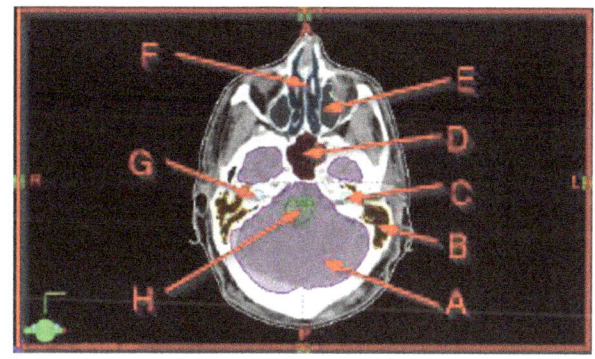

A. Brain
B. Mastoid air cells
C. Left cochlea
D. Sphenoid sinus
E. Maxillary sinus
F. Nasal cavity
G. Right cochlea
H. Brainstem

Fig. 12A.1.7

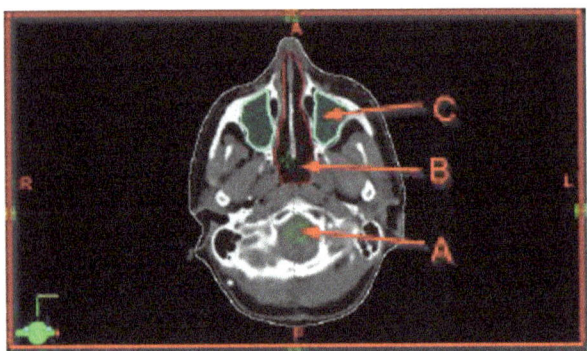

A. Brainstem
B. Nasal cavity
C. Maxillary sinus

12.7 Head and Neck (Answers)

Fig. 12A.2.1

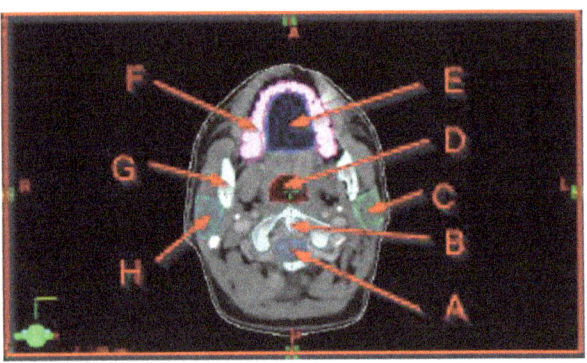

A. Spinal cord
B. C1
C. Left parotid
D. Trachea
E. Oral cavity
F. Tooth
G. Mandible
H. Right parotid

12.7 Head and Neck (Answers)

Fig. 12A.2.2

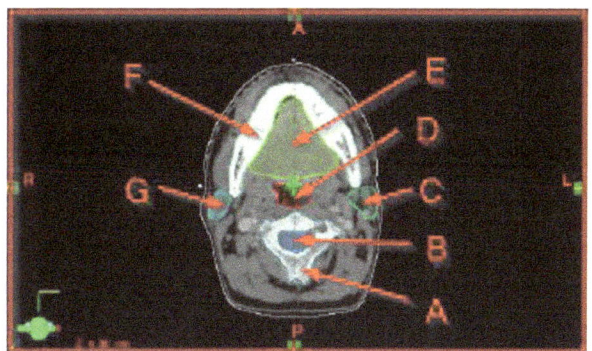

A. Vertebra
B. Spinal cord
C. Left parotid
D. Trachea
E. Oral cavity
F. Mandible
G. Right parotid

Fig. 12A.2.3

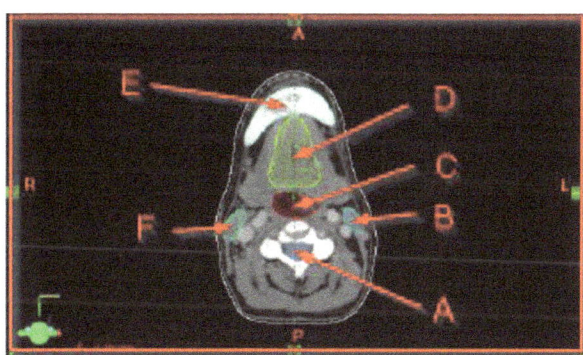

A. Spinal cord
B. Left parotid
C. Trachea
D. Tongue
E. Mandible
F. Right parotid

Fig. 12A.2.4

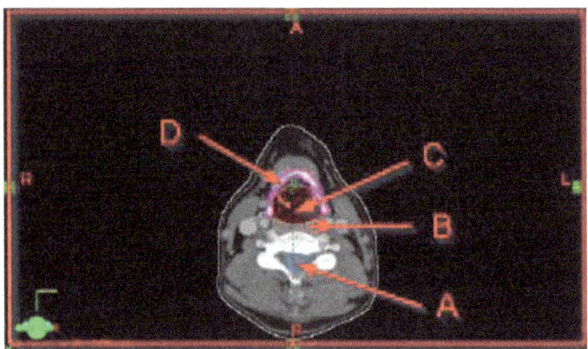

A. Spinal cord
B. Posterior pharyngeal wall
C. Epiglottis
D. Thyroid cartilage

Fig. 12A.2.5

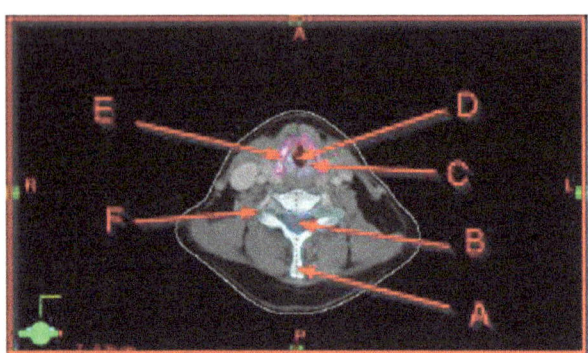

A. Spinous process of vertebra
B. Spinal cord
C. Cricoid cartilage
D. Epiglottis
E. Thyroid cartilage
F. Brachial plexus

12.7 Head and Neck (Answers)

Fig. 12A.2.6

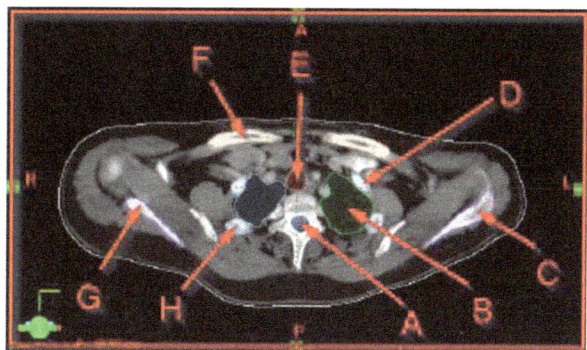

A. Spinal cord
B. Apex of the lung
C. Scapula
D. Rib
E. Trachea
F. Clavicle
G. Scapula
H. Rib

Fig. 12A.2.7

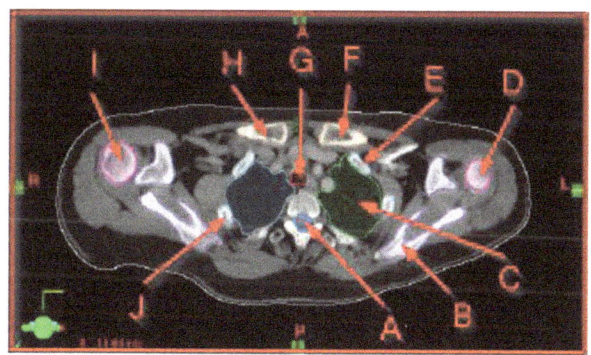

A. Spinal cord
B. Scapula
C. Apex of the lung
D. Left humeral head
E. Rib
F. Clavicle
G. Trachea
H. Clavicle
I. Right humeral head
J. Rib

12.8 Thorax (Answers)

Fig. 12A.3.1

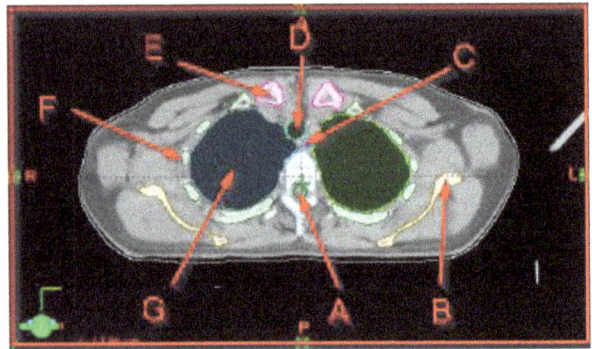

A. Spinal cord
B. Scapula
C. Esophagus
D. Trachea
E. Clavicle head
F. Rib
G. Apex of the lung

Fig. 12A.3.1

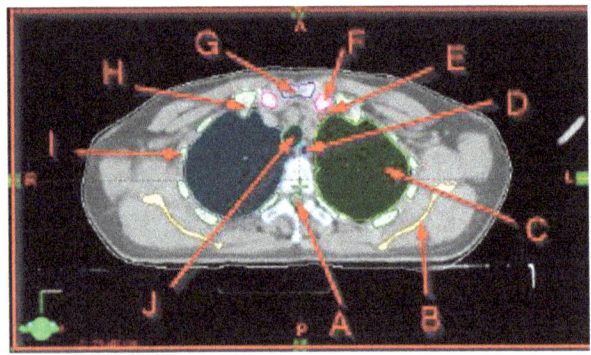

A. Spinal cord
B. Scapula
C. Apex of the lung
D. Esophagus
E. Internal mammary node
F. Clavicle head
G. Sternum
H. Rib
I. Rib
J. Trachea

12.8 Thorax (Answers)

Fig. 12A.3.2

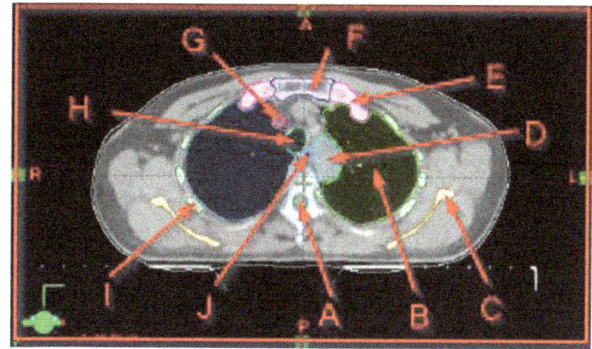

A. Spinal cord
B. Apex of the lung
C. Scapula
D. Aortic arch
E. First rib
F. Sternum
G. Superior vena cava
H. Trachea
I. Rib
J. Esophagus

Fig. 12A.3.3

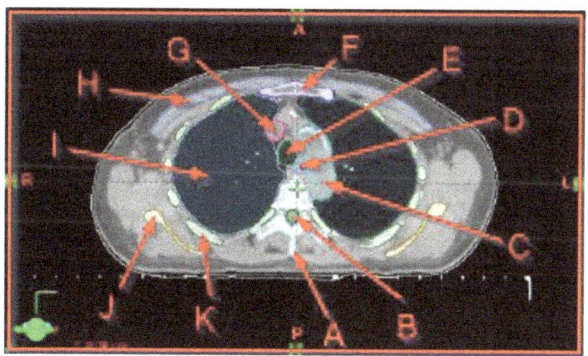

A. Spinal process
B. Spinal cord
C. Aortic arch
D. Esophagus
E. Trachea
F. Sternum
G. Superior vena cava
H. Pectoralis major
I. Lung
J. Scapula
K. Rib

Fig. 12A.3.4

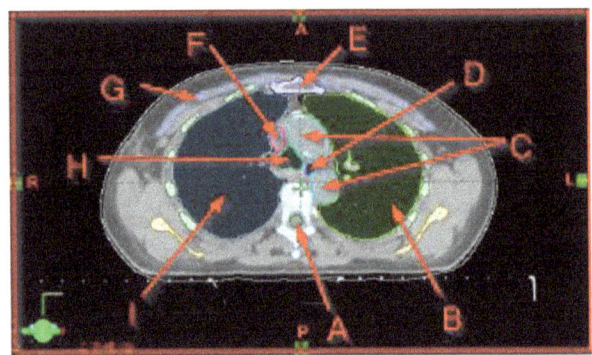

A. Spinal cord
B. Lung
C. Aortic arch
D. Esophagus
E. Sternum
F. Superior vena cava
G. Pectoralis major
H. Trachea
I. Lung

Fig. 12A.3.5

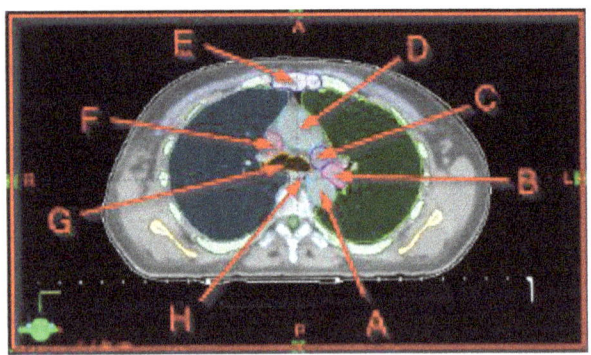

A. Aortic arch
B. Pulmonary artery
C. Pulmonary trunk
D. Aortic arch
E. Sternum
F. Superior vena cava
G. Bifurcation
H. Esophagus

Fig. 12A.3.6

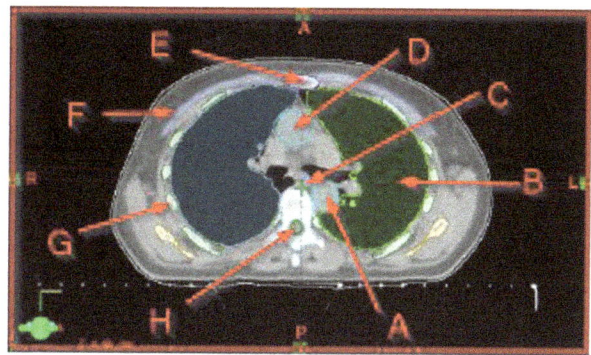

A. Aortic arch
B. Lung
C. Esophagus
D. Aortic arch
E. Sternum
F. Pectoralis major
G. Rib
H. Spinal cord

Fig. 12A.3.7

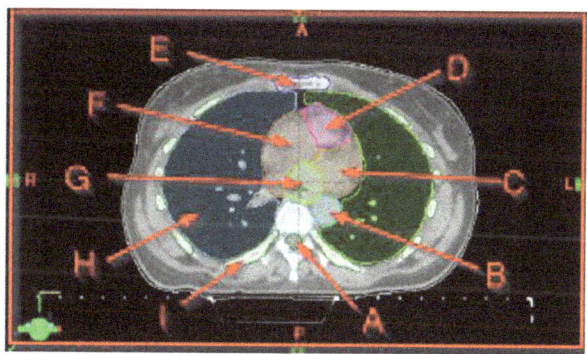

A. Spinal cord
B. Aortic arch
C. Left ventricle
D. Right ventricle
E. Sternum
F. Right atrium
G. Left atrium
H. Lung
I. Rib

Fig. 12A.3.8

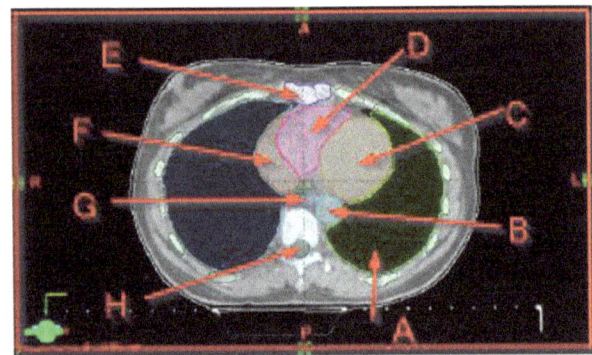

A. Lung
B. Aortic arch
C. Left ventricle
D. Right ventricle
E. Sternum
F. Right atrium
G. Esophagus
H. Spinal cord

Fig. 12A.3.9

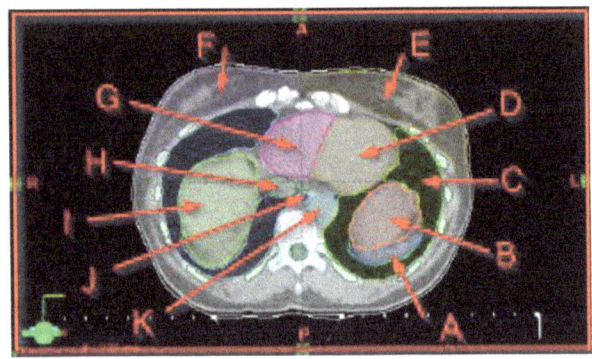

A. Spleen
B. Stomach
C. Lung
D. Left ventricle
E. Left breast
F. Right breast
G. Right ventricle
H. Inferior vena cava
I. Liver
J. Esophagus
K. Aortic arch

12.9 Abdomen (Answers)

Fig. 12A.4.1

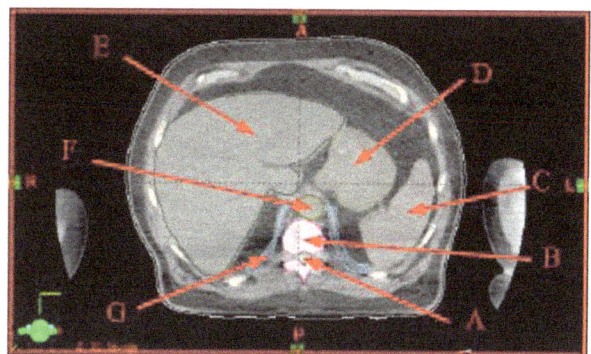

A. Spinal cord
B. Vertebra
C. Spleen
D. Stomach
E. Liver
F. Aorta
G. Diaphragmatic crus

Fig. 12A.4.1

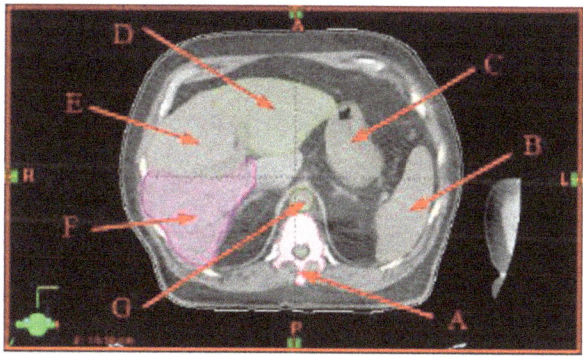

A. Spinal process
B. Spleen
C. Stomach
D. Left lobe of the liver
E. Caudate lobe of the liver
F. Right lobe of the liver
G. Aorta

Fig. 12A.4.2

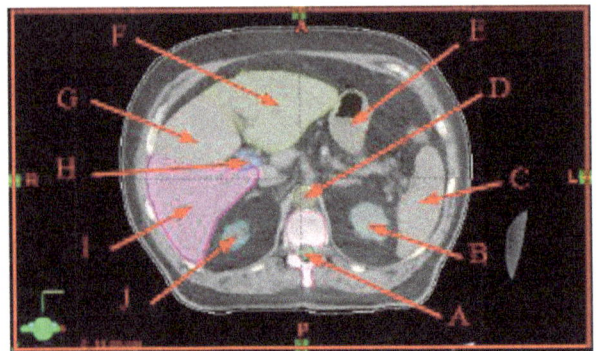

A. Spinal cord
B. Left kidney
C. Spleen
D. Aorta
E. Stomach
F. Left lobe of the liver
G. Caudate lobe of the liver
H. Hepatic vein
I. Right lobe of the liver
J. Right kidney

Fig. 12A.4.3

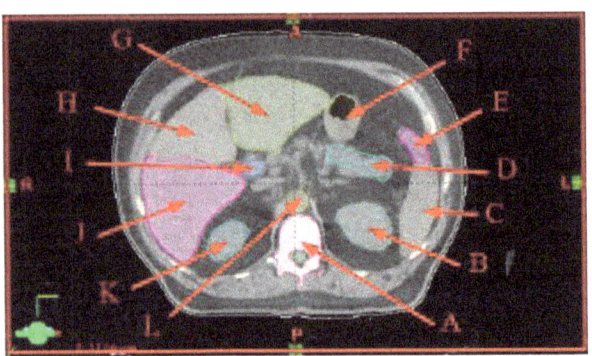

A. Body of the vertebra
B. Left kidney
C. Spleen
D. Tail of the pancreas
E. Descending colon
F. Stomach
G. Left lobe of the liver
H. Caudate lobe of the liver
I. Hepatic vein
J. Right lobe of the liver
K. Right kidney
L. Aorta

Fig. 12A.4.4

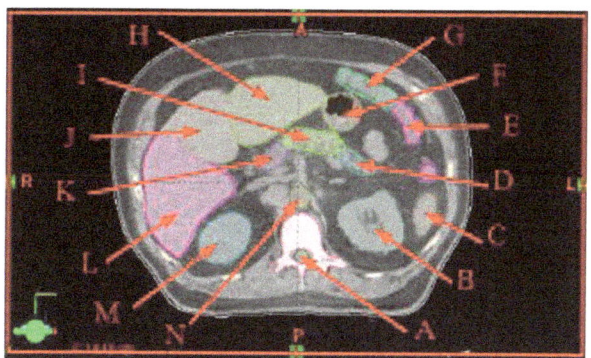

A. Spinal cord
B. Left kidney
C. Spleen
D. Tail of the pancreas
E. Descending colon
F. Stomach
G. Transverse colon
H. Left lobe of the liver
I. Body of the pancreas
J. Caudate lobe of the liver
K. Head of the pancreas
L. Right lobe of the liver
M. Right kidney
N. Aorta

Fig. 12A.4.5

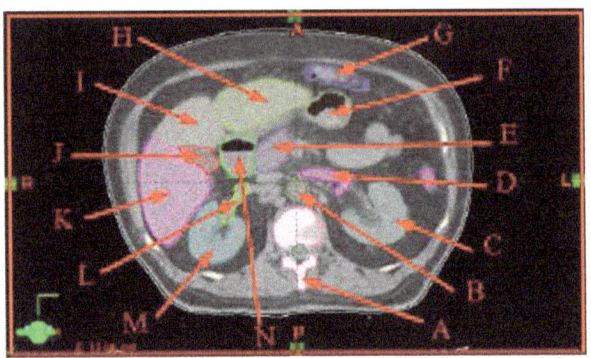

A. Spinal process
B. Aorta
C. Left kidney
D. Left renal artery
E. Head of the pancreas
F. Stomach
G. Transverse colon
H. Left lobe of the liver
I. Caudate lobe of the liver
J. Gallbladder
K. Right lobe of the liver
L. Right renal artery
M. Right kidney
N. Duodenum

Fig. 12A.4.6

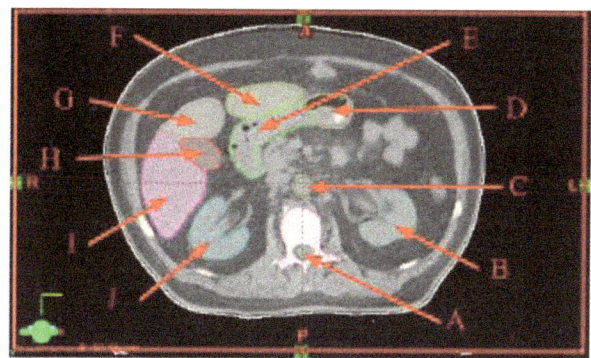

A. Spinal cord
B. Left kidney
C. Aorta
D. Stomach
E. Duodenum
F. Left lobe of the liver
G. Caudate lobe of the liver
H. Gallbladder
I. Right lobe of the liver
J. Right kidney

Fig. 12A.4.7

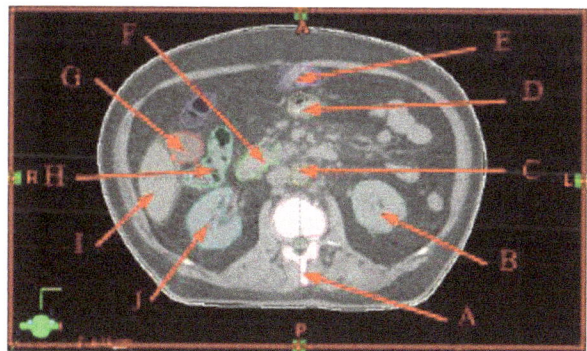

A. Spinal process
B. Left kidney
C. Aorta
D. Stomach
E. Transverse colon
F. Duodenum
G. Gallbladder
H. Bowel
I. Right lobe of the liver
J. Right kidney

Fig. 12A.4.8

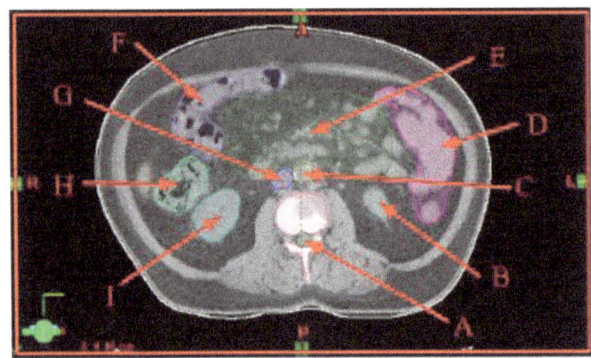

A. Spinal cord
B. Left kidney
C. Aorta
D. Descending colon
E. Small bowel
F. Transverse colon
G. Inferior vena cava
H. Colon
I. Right kidney

Fig. 12A.4.9

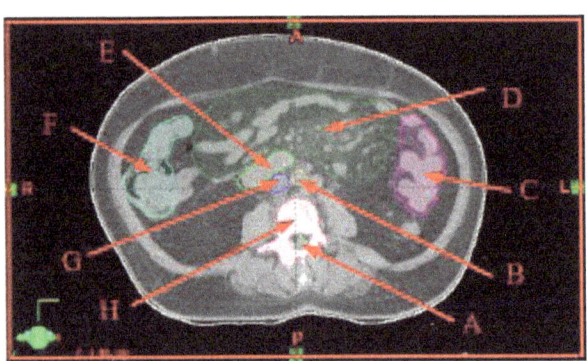

A. Spinal cord
B. Aorta
C. Descending colon
D. Small bowel
E. Duodenum
F. Colon
G. Inferior vena cava
H. Body of the vertebra

12.10 Pelvis (Answers)

Fig. 12A.5.1

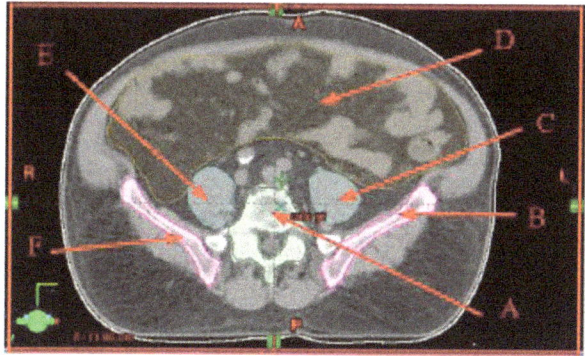

A. Body of the vertebra
B. Left iliac crest
C. Left kidney
D. Bowel
E. Right kidney
F. Right iliac crest

Fig. 12A.5.2

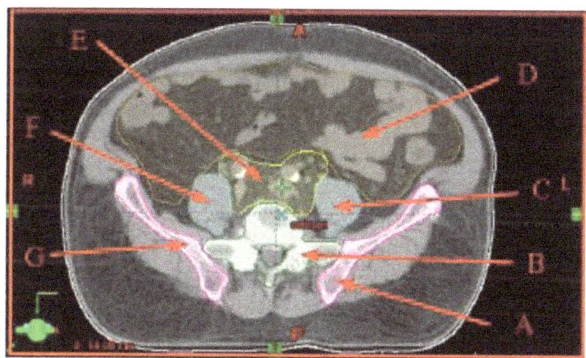

A. Left iliac crest
B. Transverse process of the vertebra
C. Left kidney
D. Bowel
E. Pelvic lymph nodes
F. Right kidney
G. Right iliac crest

Fig. 12A.5.3

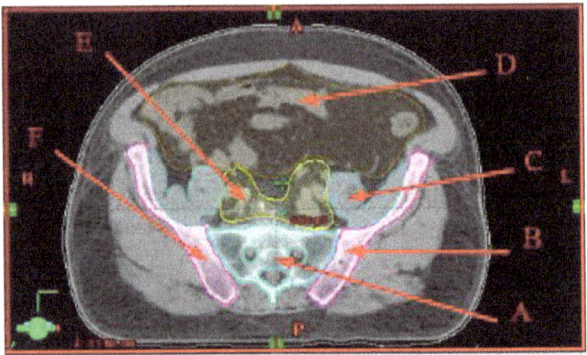

A. Sacrum
B. Left iliac crest
C. Iliopsoas muscle
D. Bowel
E. Pelvic lymph nodes
F. Right iliac crest

Fig. 12A.5.4

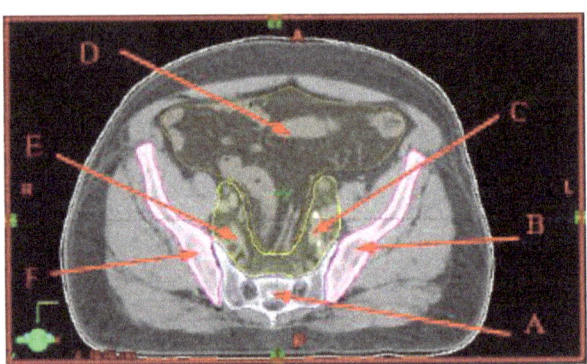

A. Sacrum
B. Left iliac crest
C. Right pelvic lymph nodes
D. Bowel
E. Left pelvic lymph nodes
F. Right iliac crest

Fig. 12A.5.5

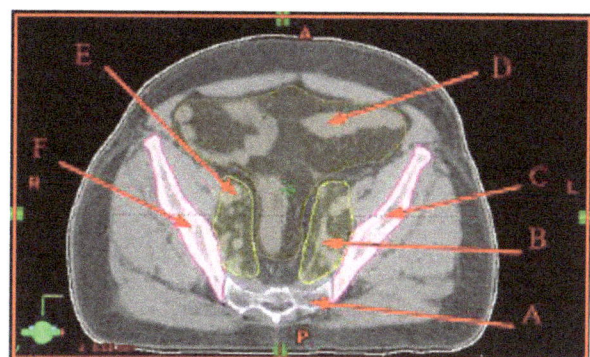

A. Coccyx
B. Pelvic lymph nodes
C. Left iliac crest
D. Bowel
E. Pelvic lymph nodes
F. Right iliac crest

Fig. 12A.5.6

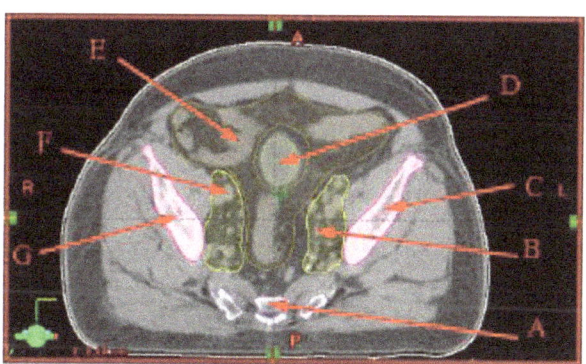

A. Coccyx
B. Pelvic lymph nodes
C. Left iliac crest
D. Urinary bladder
E. Bowel
F. Pelvic lymph nodes
G. Right iliac crest

Fig. 12A.5.7

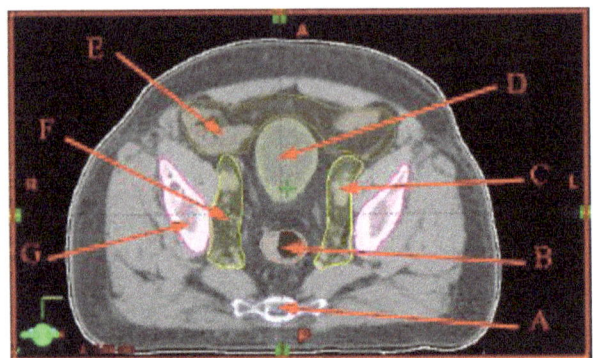

A. Coccyx
B. Rectum
C. Pelvic lymph nodes
D. Urinary bladder
E. Bowel
F. Pelvic lymph nodes
G. Ischium

Fig. 12A.5.8

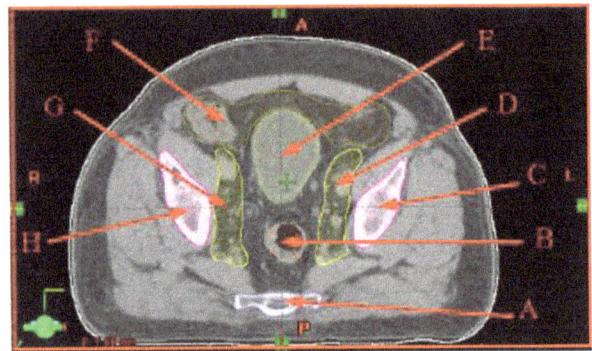

A. Coccyx
B. Rectum
C. Ischium
D. Pelvic lymph nodes
E. Urinary bladder
F. Bowel
G. Pelvic lymph nodes
H. Ischium

12.10 Pelvis (Answers)

Fig. 12A.5.9

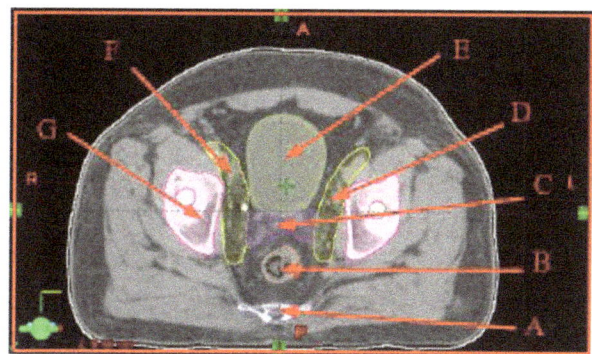

A. Coccyx
B. Rectum
C. Seminal vesicles
D. Pelvic lymph nodes
E. Urinary bladder
F. Pelvic lymph nodes
G. Ischium

Fig. 12A.5.10

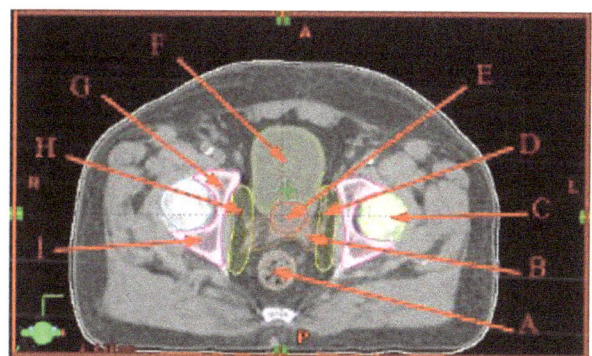

A. Rectum
B. Seminal vesicles
C. Left femoral head
D. Pelvic lymph nodes
E. Prostate
F. Urinary bladder
G. Ischium
H. Pelvic lymph nodes
I. Ischium

Fig. 12A.5.11

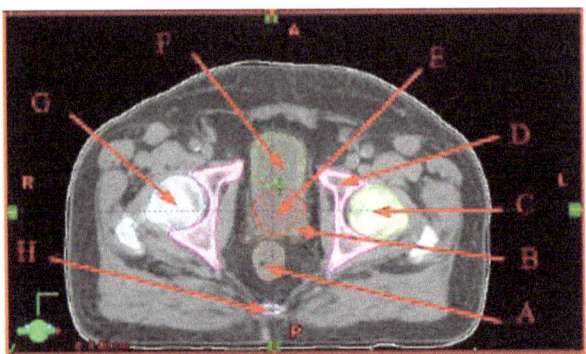

A. Rectum
B. Seminal vesicles
C. Left femoral head
D. Ischium
E. Prostate
F. Urinary bladder
G. Right femoral head
H. Coccyx

Fig. 12A.5.12

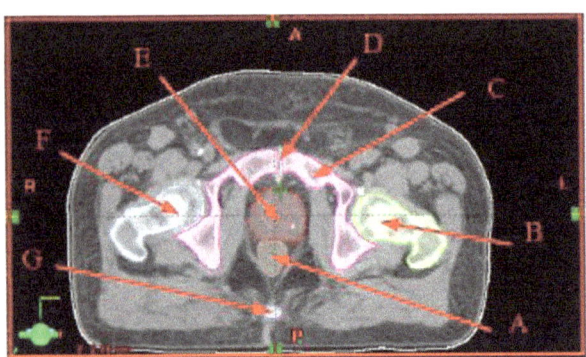

A. Rectum
B. Left femoral head
C. Ilium
D. Pubic symphysis
E. Prostate
F. Right femoral head
G. Coccyx

12.10 Pelvis (Answers)

Fig. 12A.5.13

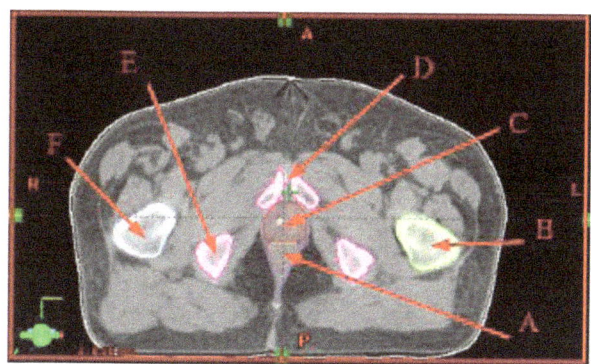

A. Rectum
B. Left femur
C. Prostate
D. Pubic symphysis
E. Ischium
F. Right femur

Fig. 12A.5.14

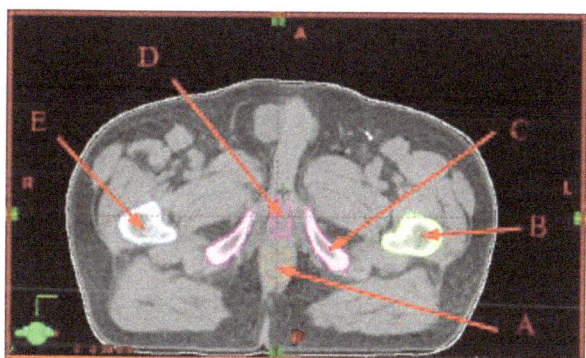

A. Anal canal
B. Left femur
C. Ischium
D. Penile bulb
E. Right femur

Imaging Modalities

Contents

13.1 Imaging Modalities (Questions) 723
13.2 Ultrasound (Questions) 733
13.3 Nuclear Medicine (Questions). 737
13.4 Positron Emission Tomography (PET) (Questions) 739
13.5 Imaging Modalities (Answers) 742
13.6 Ultrasound (Answers) 749
13.7 Nuclear Medicine (Answers). 752
13.8 Positron Emission Tomography (PET) (Answers) 754

13.1 Imaging Modalities (Questions)

Quiz 1 (Level 2)

1. A transverse tomography unit consists of:
A. A diagnostic x-ray tube and a film cassette that rotates simultaneously with the x-ray tube
B. A diagnostic x-ray tube and stationary circular array of detectors
C. A couch or table that moves in while the gantry rotates
D. A fixed diagnostic x-ray tube and movable circular array of detector

2. The difference between conventional tomography and transverse tomography is:
A. I, II, and III only
B. I and III only
C. II and IV only
D. IV only
E. All are correct
I. The orientation of the plane in focus.
II. A conventional tomography image is parallel to the long axis of the patient.
III. Transverse tomogram provides a cross-sectional image perpendicular to the body axis.
IV. Transverse tomogram provides a cross-sectional image lateral to the body axis.

3. The main disadvantage of conventional transverse tomography is:
A. Its cost
B. The speed at which it generates slices
C. The presence of blurred images resulting from structures outside the plane of interest
D. Inaccurate delineation of surface contour, internal structures, and target volume

4. Which of the following modalities can be used to accurately delineate target volumes and normal structures?
A. I, II, and III only
B. I and III only
C. II and IV only
D. IV only
E. All are correct
I. Magnetic resonance imaging (MRI)
II. Single-photon emission computed tomography (SPECT)
III. Positron emission tomography (PET)
IV. Ultrasound (US)

5. The most commonly used imaging modalities in radiation oncology are:
A. I, II, and III only
B. I, III, and IV only
C. II and IV only
D. IV only
E. All are correct
I. Magnetic resonance imaging (MRI)
II. Ultrasound (US)
III. Computed tomography (CT)
IV. Positron emission tomography (PET)

6. Which of the following is/are true about CT:
A. I, II, and III only
B. I and III only
C. II and IV only

D. IV only
E. All are correct
I. A CT image is reconstructed from a matrix of relative linear attenuation coefficients.
II. A single CT image typically consists of 512×512 pixels.
III. Each pixels measure the relative linear attenuation coefficient of the tissue.
IV. A CT image can be used to correct for tissue inhomogeneities.

7. Digital reconstructed radiographs (DRRs) are reconstructed images in planes other than:
A. I, II, and III only
B. I and III only
C. II and IV only
D. IV only
E. All are correct
I. Sagittal
II. Coronal
III. Oblique
IV. Transverse

8. Which of the following CT slice thickness is best to obtain high-quality DRRs?
A. 2–10 mm
B. 10 mm to 1 cm
C. 1–1.5 cm
D. >2 cm

9. Which of the following is *not* correct about spiral or helical CT?
A. Allows for continuous rotation of the x-ray tube as the patient is translated through the scanner aperture
B. Reduces the overall scanning time
C. Allows for the acquisition of a large number of thin slices required for high-quality CT images and the DRRs
D. Increases the overall scanning time due to numbers of reconstruction images

10. For radiation therapy treatment planning purposes:
A. I, II, and III only
B. I and III only
C. II and IV only
D. IV only
E. All are correct
I. The CT couch must be flat.
II. The CT couch could be of any type.
III. The patient must be setup in the CT in the same position as for actual treatment.
IV. A radiology CT scan setup can be used.

11. CT images can be processed to generate DRRs in which planes:
A. I, II, and III only
B. I and III only
C. II and IV only
D. IV only
E. All are correct
I. Sagittal.
II. Coronal.
III. Oblique.
IV. It cannot create oblique views.

12. A CT simulator is:
A. A CT scanner equipped with some additional hardware such as laser localizers, image registration devices, and a flat couch
B. A CT scanner used in a radiology department
C. A CT scanner that simulates the HDR room
D. A linac used to CT patients

13. In general, MRI is considered superior to CT for:
A. Contrast studies
B. Calcifications structures
C. Bony structures
D. Soft tissue discrimination

14. The most basic difference between CT and MRI is:
A. CT is related to electron density and atomic number, while MRI shows proton density distribution.
B. CT is related to proton density distribution, while MRI shows electron density and atomic number.
C. There is not any basic difference between CT and MRI.
D. CT spatial resolution is better than MRI.

15. MRI advantages include:
A. I, II, and III only
B. I and III only
C. II and IV only
D. IV only
E. All are correct
I. Soft tissue structures contrast.
II. Can be used to directly generate scans in axial, sagittal, coronal, or oblique planes.
III. No exposure to radiation.
IV. It is not susceptible to artifacts.

16. Which of the following modalities provides the best geometric accuracy?
A. Magnetic resonance imaging (MRI)
B. Ultrasound (US)
C. Positron emission tomography (PET)
D. Computed tomography (CT)

17. The major advantage of CT in radiation therapy treatment planning is:
A. 3D imaging.
B. Each voxel can be mapped to a specific electron density.
C. Histograms can be generated.
D. Contouring can be done easily.

18. A CT image is made of:
A. I, II, and III only
B. I and III only
C. II and IV only
D. IV only
E. All are correct
I. Pixels
II. Voxels
III. Field of view (FOV)
IV. DICOM

19. Image contrast can be achieved by:
A. Selecting the appropriate voxel, pixel, and matrix
B. Reconstruction of the CT image
C. Leveling and windowing the CT image
D. Selecting the Hounsfield number (H)

20. When windowing and leveling a CT image:
A. I, II, and III only
B. I and III only
C. II and IV only
D. IV only
E. All are correct
I. The operator selects a part of the gray scale to work with.
II. The operator selects the window width.
III. The operator selects the level of gray scale to visualize.
IV. The organ of interest must be taken in consideration.

21. When selecting a window on a CT image:
A. I, II, and III only
B. I and III only
C. II and IV only
D. IV only
E. All are correct
I. Anything above the window level would be white.
II. Anything below the window level would be black.
III. The contrast will be affected.
IV. Narrow window will have high contrast.

22. If the size of the detectors in the CT scanner are reduced and the number of pixels in the image is increased, what parameter is affected?
A. Contrast
B. Spatial resolution
C. Artifacts
D. Noise

23. Noise on a CT image or film is the:
A. Variation on the pixel readings
B. Incorrect leveling and windowing the CT image
C. Thickness of CT image
D. Incorrect field of view (FOV)

24. Field of view refers to:
A. The size of a pixel
B. A matrix
C. The diameter of the image reconstructed
D. The volume of a voxel

25. When converting attenuation readings from a detector to a digital image in a CT:
A. A reconstruction algorithm is employed.
B. The field of view is set.
C. A radiographic film is developed.
D. Window width is adjusted.

26. Hounsfield numbers range from:
A. 1 to 100
B. −100 to +500
C. −1,000 to +3,000
D. 0 to 1,000

27. The Hounsfield number (H):
A. I, II, and III only
B. I and III only
C. II and IV only
D. IV only
E. All are correct
I. Is related to a CT number
II. Is related to linear attenuation coefficients of different tissues
III. Represents a change of percentage in the attenuation coefficient of water
IV. Is related to homogeneity coefficient

28. The correct formula of Hounsfield number is:
A. $H = (\mu_{tissue} - \mu_{water})/\mu_{tissue} \times 1,000$
B. $H = 1,000 - \mu_{water}/\mu_{tissue}$
C. $H = (\mu_{tissue} - \mu_{water})/\mu_{water} \times 1,000$
D. $H = 1,000 - \mu_{water}/\mu_{tissue} \times 1,000$

13.1 Imaging Modalities (Questions) 729

29. Match the following Hounsfield number with its corresponding organ or tissue.

A.	Air	I.	−1,000
B.	Water	II.	+1,000
C.	Bone	III.	−100
D.	Fat	IV.	0
E.	Muscle	V.	+40

30. Some common considerations in obtaining treatment planning CT scans are:
A. I, II, and III only
B. I and III only
C. II and IV only
D. IV only
E. All are correct
I. A flat table top should be used.
II. A large diameter CT aperture (or bore) can be used to accommodate unusual arm positions or body parts.
III. Image artifacts should be avoided.
IV. Radiopaque markers should be used for external contour landmarks.

31. Which of the following organs has the lowest Hounsfield unit:
A. Fat
B. Lungs
C. Water
D. Muscle

32. A CT number assigned to a pixel represents:
A. The average linear attenuation coefficient of tissue in the voxel
B. The electron density in the voxel
C. The atomic number of tissue in the voxel
D. The atomic mass of tissue in the voxel

33. Disadvantages of MRI compared to CT include:
A. I, II, and III only
B. I and III only
C. II and IV only
D. IV only
E. All are correct
I. MRI provides lower spatial resolution.
II. Inability to image bone or calcifications.
III. Longer scan acquisition time.
IV. Technical difficulties due to small bore of the magnet and magnetic interference with metallic objects.

34. Which of the following is/are true about MRI:
A. I, II, and III only
B. I and III only
C. II and IV only
D. IV only
E. All are correct
I. It involves a phenomenon known as nuclear magnetic resonance.
II. It involves radiofrequency (RF) signal.
III. It involves nuclei that intrinsically possess spinning motion.
IV. It is most distinguished in nuclei with an odd number of protons.

Quiz 2 (Level 3)

1. Which of the following is the primary element used for MRI imaging that produces signals of sufficient strength?
A. 23Na
B. 13C
C. 31P
D. Hydrogen nuclei

2. Which of the following particles possess(es) properties of spin?
A. I, II, and III only
B. I and III only
C. II and IV only
D. IV only
E. All are correct
I. Photon
II. Electron
III. Positron
IV. Proton

3. Which of the following nuclei has an intrinsic magnetic moment and angular momentum?
A. Isotopes containing an even number of protons and/or even number of neutrons
B. Isotopes containing an odd number of protons and/or odd number of neutrons
C. Isotopes containing an even number of protons and/or odd number of neutrons
D. Isotopes of any classification

4. Magnetic fields:
A. I, II, and III only
B. I and III only
C. II and IV only
D. IV only
E. All are correct

13.1 Imaging Modalities (Questions)

I. Create a change in long axes spin direction of the nuclei (hydrogen)
II. Cause nuclei (hydrogen) to align their spin axes along the external magnetic field (H)
III. Cause nuclei (hydrogen) to orbit around the external magnetic field (H)
IV. Cause nuclei (hydrogen) to be deflected around the radiofrequency field in the transverse direction

5. The radiofrequency field is applied?
A. Horizontal to magnetic field
B. Perpendicular to magnetic field
C. Longitudinal to magnetic field
D. Same direction as magnetic field

6. A magnetic dipole moment takes place:
A. When charged particles relax
B. When spinning charged particles create a magnetic field from east to west poles
C. When spinning charged particles create a magnetic field from south to north poles
D. When a second radiofrequency field is applied to the magnetic field

7. T_2 relaxation is:
A. The time it takes the nuclei to return to the original longitudinal direction of the magnetic field
B. The time it takes the nuclei to change spin direction
C. The time it takes the nuclei to deflect from the longitudinal plane to transverse plane
D. The time it takes the nuclei to relax from transverse direction

8. Nuclear magnetic resonance signal is induced:
A. When the south and north poles are aligned
B. When proton spin is increased
C. When the radiofrequency field is turned on
D. When relaxation occurs

9. Localization of protons in MRI in a 3D space is achieved by?
A. RF gradient produced by magnetic field in two orthogonal planes
B. Applying magnetic field gradients produced by gradient RF coils in three orthogonal planes
C. T1 and T2 relaxation
D. Magnetic field gradients produced by gradient RF in two orthogonal planes

10. Which of the following MRI statements is/are true:
A. I, II, and III only
B. I and III only
C. II and IV only
D. IV only
E. All are correct

I. A body slice is imaged by applying field gradient along the axis of the slice and selecting a frequency range for readout.
II. The strength of the field gradient determines the thickness of the slice.
III. The greater the gradient, the thinner the slice.
IV. Most MR imaging uses a spin echo technique.

11. MRI image contrast can be affected by?
A. Adjusting T1 and T2 relaxation
B. Adjusting window and leveling
C. Adjusting echo time (TE) and repetition time (TR)
D. Adjusting kVp and mA

12. Which of the following combinations produces an MRI T1-weighted image?
A. A long TR and short TE
B. A long TR and a long TE
C. A short TR and a short TE
D. A short TR and a long TE

13. Which of the following units and ranges is used to measure the MRI magnetic field strength?
A. 0.5–3 T
B. 1–20 megahertz (MHz)
C. 0.2–3 megahertz (MHz)
D. 1–20 T

14. Which of the following contrast agents may be used in MRI to visualize the blood–brain barrier?
A. Gadolinium
B. Barium sulfate
C. Manganese
D. Perflubron

15. For safety precautions, which of the following items is/are not allowed in the MRI room?
A. I, II, and III only
B. I and III only
C. II and IV only
D. IV only
E. All are correct
I. Jewelry
II. Patient with pacemakers
III. Pregnant women
IV. Metal prosthesis

16. Hounsfield numbers DO NOT depend on:
A. Density of the material used
B. The mass attenuation coefficient
C. The linear attenuation coefficient
D. The energy of the photon in question

17. Which of the following variables is kept constant in a CT scan?
A. mA
B. kVp
C. mAs
D. Exposure time

18. A radiation oncology CT simulator must:
A. I, II, and III only
B. I and III only
C. II and IV only
D. IV only
E. All are correct
I. Contain a large gantry aperture so that all setups can be accomplished
II. Contain external lasers for setup reproducibility
III. Contain a flat table top similar to the linac couch
IV. Contain a contrast kit for patients who require a contrast study

19. Which of the following will happen when selecting thinner CT slices:
A. I, II, and III only
B. I and III only
C. II and IV only
D. IV only
E. All are correct
I. Lower noise
II. Better high-contrast (spatial) resolution
III. Poorer edge definition
IV. Less partial volume artifacts

13.2 Ultrasound (Questions)

Quiz 1 (Level 2)

1. Advantages of ultrasound over CT include:
A. I, II, and III only
B. I and III only
C. II and IV only
D. IV only
E. All are correct

I. Ultrasound does not involve ionizing radiation.
II. Ultrasound is less expensive than CT.
III. In some cases, ultrasound yields data of comparable value to CT.
IV. Ultrasound shows better detail of bony structure than CT.

2. Ultrasounds uses:
A. Radioactive material for imaging
B. X-rays for imaging
C. Magnetic field and radiofrequency pulses for imaging
D. High-frequency sound waves for imaging

3. Ultrasound produces images using:
A. I, II, and III only
B. I and III only
C. II and IV only
D. IV only
E. All are correct
I. Reflected ultrasound waves
II. Diffracted ultrasound waves
III. Transmitted ultrasound waves
IV. Using magnetic field, radio waves, and a computer

4. Which of the following units and ranges is used to measure diagnostic ultrasound frequencies?
A. 0.2–3 T
B. 1–20 megahertz (MHz)
C. 0.2–3 megahertz (MHz)
D. 1–20 T

5. Which of the following statements is/are true about ultrasound:
A. I, II, and III only
B. I and III only
C. II and IV only
D. IV only
E. All are correct
I. Acoustic impedance of a medium is defined as the product of the density of the medium and the velocity of ultrasound in the medium.
II. The larger the difference in acoustic impedance (Z) between two media, the greater the fraction of ultrasound energy reflected at the interface.
III. It is difficult to visualize structures lying beyond the bone (because the attenuation coefficient of ultrasound is very high for the bone).
IV. Water, blood, fat, and muscle are very good transmitters of ultrasound energy.

13.2 Ultrasound (Questions)

6. Where do strong reflections of ultrasound occur?
A. I, II, and III only
B. I and III only
C. II and IV only
D. IV only
E. All are correct
I. Air–tissue interfaces
II. Tissue–bone interfaces
III. Chest wall–lung interfaces
IV. Lung and air cavities interfaces

7. Ultrasonic waves are generated and detected by:
A. An ultrasound probe or transducer
B. An ultrasonic gantry
C. An ultrasound detector
D. A head coil

8. An ultrasonic probe or transducer is a device that:
A. Converts electrical energy into ultrasound energy, and vice versa
B. Converts wavelength into ultrasound energy, and vice versa
C. Converts radio frequency into electrical energy
D. Converts microwave into ultrasound

9. Which of the following is/are used in ultrasound imaging?
A. I, II, and III only
B. I and III only
C. II and IV only
D. IV only
E. None are correct
I. Laser effect
II. X-rays
III. Magnetic resonance
IV. Piezoelectric effect

10. The most common crystals used clinically in an ultrasound probe or transducer are:
A. I, II, and III only
B. I and III only
C. II and IV only
D. IV only
E. All are correct
I. Barium titanate
II. Lead zirconium titanate
III. Lead metaniobate
IV. Sodium iodine

11. The height of an ultrasound wave is called:
A. Frequency
B. Wavelength
C. Amplitude
D. Intensity

12. The ultrasound waves are:
A. I, II, and III only
B. I and III only
C. II and IV only
D. IV only
E. All are correct
I. Absorbed in the medium
II. Scattered in the medium
III. Reflected back toward the receptor
IV. Ionized the medium

13. In an ultrasound image, the pie-shaped scan can be accomplished by using?
A. A linear transducer or receiver
B. A convex transducer or receiver
C. A concave transducer or receiver
D. A combination of linear and convex transducer or receiver

14. Which of the following statements is/are true about ultrasound?
A. I, II, and III only
B. I and III only
C. II and IV only
D. IV only
E. All are correct
I. Lower frequency is used for deeper imaging.
II. Lower frequency produces worse detail.
III. The brightness depends on the strength of the echo and the time it takes to travel back to the receiver.
IV. Attenuation of sound pulses is lower in soft tissue than in the bone and air.

15. Which of the following mode is NOT used in ultrasound for image display?
A. A mode
B. L mode
C. B mode
D. M mode

16. The M mode in ultrasound image display:
A. Displays the signal amplitude of the wave
B. Displays the brightness of the cross-sectional image
C. Displays the motion of internal structures of the patient's anatomy
D. Displays the contrast of the image

17. When using ultrasound in radiotherapy, the cross-sectional information used for treatment planning is derived from:
A. A mode
B. B mode
C. M mode
D. L mode

18. The function of the gel applied to the patient's skin when ultrasound is used is:
A. To allow the probe to be moved smoothly across the skin area
B. To make the skin area sterile
C. To allow the probe to couple directly to the skin without any air gap
D. To minimize discomfort for patients

19. What is the approximate speed of an ultrasound wave in the soft tissue?
A. 330 m/s
B. 1,450 m/s
C. 1,540 m/s
D. 4,080 m/s

13.3 Nuclear Medicine (Questions)

Quiz 1 (Level 2)

1. Which of the following statements is/are true about nuclear medicine:
A. I, II, and III only
B. I and III only
C. II and IV only
D. IV only
E. All are correct
I. Nuclear medicine radioisotope images are dynamic and change with time.
II. Radioactive materials are absorbed in organs based on their physiological function.
III. Radioactive materials are used to create radiographic images.
IV. Most of radioactive materials used in nuclear medicine must be gamma emitters.

2. The half-life ($T_{1/2}$) of radioisotopes used in nuclear medicine must be?
A. Long so that it can be detected by the machine
B. Short to protect the patient and those around him
C. Long so that the radioisotope can penetrate the body and be absorbed by the organ of interest
D. Short so that it does not produce any pain when absorbed in the organ of interest

3. The effective half-life of radioisotopes used in nuclear medicine is:
A. Longer than actual half-life
B. The same as actual half-life
C. Shorter than actual half-life
D. Much longer than the actual half-life

4. Accelerator-produced radionuclides widely used in nuclear medicine for diagnostic procedures are:
A. I, II, and III only
B. I and III only
C. II and IV only
D. IV only
E. All are correct
I. Thallium-201 (^{201}TI)
II. Gallium-67 (^{67}Ga)
III. Iodine-123 (^{123}I)
IV. Xenon-133 (^{133}Xe)

5. What are some typical nuclear medicine modalities?
A. I, II, and III only
B. I and III only
C. II and IV only
D. IV only
E. All are correct
I. PET
II. SPECT
III. Planar gamma camera
IV. Cold spot

6. Which of the following organs will always appear to be "hot" in nuclear medicine study?
A. Brain
B. Liver
C. Bladder
D. Pancreas

7. Which of the following radionuclides is used to image the thyroid when performing a nuclear medicine study:
A. Thallium-201 (^{201}TI)
B. Gallium-67 (^{67}Ga)
C. Iodine-123 (^{123}I)
D. Xenon-133 (^{133}Xe)

8. Which of the following is used in nuclear medicine as a detector:
A. A circular array
B. A gamma camera
C. A magnetic field
D. A radiographic film

9. Nuclear medicine radionuclides usually enter the body via:
A. Oral cavity
B. Blood stream
C. Subcutaneous injection
D. Intracavity implant

10. Which of the following radioisotopes is the most widely used in nuclear medicine?
A. Technetium-99m
B. Gallium-67 (^{67}Ga)
C. Iodine-123 (^{123}I)
D. Xenon-133 (^{133}Xe)

11. What are some differences between nuclear medicine imaging and CT?
A. I, II, and III only
B. I and III only
C. II and IV only
D. IV only
E. All are correct
I. NM scans show functionality while CT shows anatomy.
II. CT has better spatial resolution than NM.
III. NM uses emission radiation while CT uses transmission radiation.
IV. NM uses collimation.

13.4 Positron Emission Tomography (PET) (Questions)

Quiz 1 (Level 2)

1. PET scan stands for:
A. Positron electron tomography
B. Positive emission tomography
C. Positron emission tomography
D. Proton electron tomography

2. Which of the following statement is/are true about PET scans:
A. I, II, and III only
B. I and III only
C. II and IV only
D. IV only
E. All are correct
I. The radioisotope undergoes positron emission decay.
II. The radioisotope emits gamma rays.
III. Metabolic sugars are linked to the radioisotope.
IV. Radioactive materials alone are absorbed in organs based on their physiological function.

3. Which of the following structures require(s) high sugar concentration:
A. I, II, and III only
B. I and III only
C. II and IV only
D. IV only
E. All are correct
I. Liver
II. Brain
III. Stomach
IV. Tumors

4. PET scan images are created because?
A. Circular gamma camera arrays around the patient detect photons created in an annihilation reaction produced by the positron when annihilating with an electron in the body.
B. Circular arrays opposed to the gantry detect x-rays when they pass through the patient's body.
C. A gamma camera with sodium iodine crystals detects gamma rays produced by a radioisotope.
D. Radiofrequency signals that are given off by protons are recorded.

5. The most commonly used drug for a PET scan is:
A. ^{18}FMISO
B. ^{18}FDG
C. ^{18}FAZA
D. ^{18}FLT

6. The lifetime for isotope ^{18}F is:
A. 8 days
B. 110 min
C. 74 days
D. 64 h

7. The isotope ^{18}F is generated from:
A. Fission remnant of nuclear plant
B. A cyclotron
C. A synchrotron
D. Different isotopes exposed to neutron beams

8. The energy for the γ-ray photons produced by positron annihilation is:
A. 0.511 MeV
B. 1.02 MeV
C. 256 keV
D. None of the above is correct

13.4 Positron Emission Tomography (PET) (Questions)

9. How long should a patient wait for the PET scan after being injected ^{18}FDG?
A. 10 min
B. Half a day
C. About 45 min to allow uptake
D. 110 min

10. A group of scientists want to do rat experiment with PET. Is this possible with clinical PET scanner?
A. They need to use microPET scanner.
B. As long as it is approved by the hospital.
C. Rats cannot tolerate the ^{18}FDG dose for human, which is necessary to do a scan.
D. They need larger animals.

Quiz 2 (Level 3)

1. Compared to CT scan, a PET scan has:
A. Better spatial resolution and better contrast resolution
B. Worse spatial resolution and worse contrast resolution
C. Better spatial resolution and worse contrast resolution
D. Worse spatial resolution and better contrast resolution

2. Can image quality of PET be improved with composite PET and CT scans with PET/CT scanner?
A. No. PET/CT is only for patient convenience as 2 scans are taken together.
B. Yes, because both PET and CT are internally fused.
C. Yes, because PET is reconstructed using the anatomical info in CT.
D. Yes, because more pathology info can be provided with the fused image.

3. The spatial resolution of PET is determined by:
A. I and II
B. I, II, III, and IV.
C. I, III, and IV.
D. All
I. Range of positron
II. The dose for 18FDG or whatever drug is used
III. Detector size of scanner
IV. Nonzero momentum of electron-positron pair to be annihilated
V. The effective thickness of anatomical tissue

4. The free path of positron in PET scan is:
A. Dependent on radionuclide and decay energy
B. Independent of radionuclide because it cannot be trapped until it reaches thermal level
C. Negligible because it is almost immediately trapped by an electron
D. Always 2 mm in the tissue

5. Suppose the size of detector can be extremely small. The natural limit for the spatial resolution of a typical clinical PET (80 cm in diameter) scanner is:
A. Around 2 mm, with consideration of different radionuclides
B. 4 mm
C. 1 mm
D. About 0.2 mm in this ideal case, because free path of positron becomes the major concern if detector size is zero

6. MicroPET (for animals) images have spatial resolution of approximately 1 mm, mainly because:
A. Better material (such as BGO) is used in detector.
B. Scanner is small in diameter; thus the non-colinearity effect is minimized.
C. Animal is much thinner than human.
D. Detector in scanner can be made quite smaller than a clinical PET scanner.

7. The difference between a dynamic PET scan and a static scan is:
A. They are the same in raw data but different in reconstruction binning.
B. They are different in both raw data and in reconstruction binning.
C. They are the same both in raw data and in reconstruction binning.
D. They used different reconstruct algorithms.

8. Three positron emitters are used: ^{18}F, ^{124}I, and ^{64}Cu. Which one will cause the largest non-colinearity in spatial resolution?
A. ^{18}F
B. ^{124}I
C. ^{64}Cu
D. Same, non-colinearity is independent of radioisotopes.

13.5 Imaging Modalities (Answers)

Quiz 1 (Level 2)

1. **A** A transverse tomography unit consists of a diagnostic x-ray tube and a film cassette that rotates simultaneously with the x-ray tube. The patient is positioned on the table so that the x-ray beam can pass through a desired transverse body cross-section only; the other cross-sectional slices are blurred. Modern CT scanners, such as spiral or helical CT, use an x-ray tube that rotates continuously as the patient is slowly translated through the CT aperture.

2. **A** The difference between conventional tomography and transverse tomography is the orientation of the plane in focus. A conventional tomography image is parallel to the long axis of the patient, while transverse tomogram provides a cross-sectional image perpendicular to the body axis.

13.5 Imaging Modalities (Answers)

3. C The main disadvantage of conventional transverse tomography is the presence of blurred images resulting from structures outside the plane of interest.

4. E All are correct. Each modality takes advantage of a different physical property to generate an image.

5. B The most commonly used imaging modalities in radiation oncology are magnetic resonance imaging (MRI), computed tomography (CT), and positron emission tomography (usually with CT, that is, PET/CT).

6. E All statements are correct. A CT image is reconstructed from a matrix of relative linear attenuation coefficients measured by the CT scanner. A typical CT image consists of 512×512 pixels, and each pixel contains information about the relative linear attenuation coefficient of the tissue. By proper calibration of the CT scanner, a relationship between pixel value and tissue density can be established allowing for pixel-by-pixel correction for tissue inhomogeneities in computing dose distributions.

7. D Digital reconstructed radiographs (DRRs) are reconstructed images in planes other than that of the original transverse image. A DRR is a simulated radiographic image that is generated from a CT scan. DRRs are used in radiation oncology to verify the positioning of the patient on the table since the DRR can be registered to the portal image acquired at the treatment machine.

8. A To obtain high-quality DRRs, not only images of high contrast and resolution are required, but the slice thickness must also be sufficiently small. A slice thickness of 2–10 mm is commonly used depending on the need. The DRR will be blurry if the transverse slice thickness is too large.

9. D Spiral or helical CT allows continuous rotation of the x-ray tube as the patient is translated through the scanner aperture, so it reduces the overall scanning time and allows acquisition of a large number of thin slices required for high-quality CT images and the DRRs.

10. B For radiation therapy treatment planning purposes, the CT couch must be flat to imitate the treatment room couch, and patients must be set up in the CT in the same position as for actual treatment. This allows for a reproducible daily setup at the linac. A radiology CT scan can be used to help the physician determine where the tumor or critical structures are, but it should not be used for treatment planning because the couch is typically curved to increase patient comfort and the radiology CT scan setup is different than the radiation therapy setup.

11. A CT images can be processed to generate DRRs in any plane. A DRR is generated by a ray tracing through the CT image to generate the DRR in the desired plane.

12. A   A CT simulator is a CT scanner equipped with some additional hardware such as laser localizers to set up the treatment isocenter, image registration devices, and a flat couch insert. A computer workstation with special software to process a CT data, plan beam directions, and generate DRRs allows CT simulation films with the same geometry as the treatment beams.

13. D   In general, MRI is considered superior to CT for soft tissue discrimination such us CNS tumors and abnormalities in the brain, also head and neck cancers, sarcomas, the prostate, and lymph nodes.

14. A   The most basic difference between CT and MRI is that CT is related to electron density and atomic number (actual representing x-ray linear attenuation coefficients), while MRI shows proton density distribution. MRI has an advantage over CT in that it does not use ionizing radiation to obtain an image; rather it uses a strong magnetic field and RF pulses to acquire an image. A downside to MRI is that an image acquisition takes longer than CT and, therefore, is susceptible to artifacts from patient movement. Both modalities have the same spatial resolution of around 1 mm.

15. A   The advantages of MRI are that soft tissue contrast is very good, images can directly generate (not reconstructed) in any plane, and there is no radiation exposure. MRI does suffer from artifacts that CT does not such as magnetic field inhomogeneities and distortions.

16. D   Computed tomography (CT) provides the best geometric accuracy which is one of the most important requirements in treatment planning.

17. B   All of these statements are true for CT imaging, but the major advantage for CT is that the voxels in the CT image can be directly mapped to an electron density. This means that heterogeneity corrections can be done during the treatment planning. MRI only has proton density information so to do heterogeneity corrections, the voxels have to be converted to electron density using an algorithm.

18. A   A CT image is made of pixels which are two dimensional representations of voxels. Voxels are composed of small discrete 3D volumes of imaged tissue.

19. C   Image contrast can be achieved by leveling and windowing the CT image which is an advantage of digital images. This does not change the resolution of the image or reduce the noise in the image as these depend on the physical design of the CT scanner and the scan and reconstruction parameters.

20. E   A CT image pixel typically contains 12 bits of information meaning that there are up to 4,096 different gray levels possible (2^{12}). The human eye can only visualize about 30–90 gray levels so windowing and leveling a CT image can help the operator visualize a particular organ or structure. To do

13.5 Imaging Modalities (Answers)

this the operator selects a particular level of the gray scale to work with and also the window width of gray scale to display.

21. E All statements are correct. When selecting a window on a CT image, anything above the window level is white, and everything below the window level is black. If high contrast is needed, a narrow window can be set, while a wide window will lower the contrast in the image.

22. B Spatial resolution CT image depends on many parameters including the size of the detector, the focal spot size, slice thickness, helical pitch, and the matrix size. The spatial resolution also depends on the reconstruction filters and algorithm the CT scanner uses. Windowing and leveling the image improves contrast as does increasing the mAs. Increasing the mAs increases the dose and also reduces the noise in the image since the signal-to-noise ratio (SNR) increases.

23. A Noise in a CT image or film is the variation in the pixel readings. The noise is affected by the number of photons traveling through each pixel where the noise is reduced as more photons travel through the pixel. The number of photons can be increased by increasing the mAs (more dose), increasing the slice thickness (reduced spatial resolution), or increasing the field of view with the same number of pixels (pixel size increases but spatial resolution decreases). There is always a trade-off in imaging. Remember that the ability to resolve contrast between objects is related to the noise in the image. The goal is to maximize the contrast-to-noise ratio (CNR).

24. C Field of view refers to the diameter of the CT image reconstructed. In CT imaging, there are almost always 512×512 pixels in an image so as the FOV increases, the pixel size increases, and the noise and spatial resolution both decrease.

25. A The reconstruction of an image by CT is a mathematical process of considerable complexity performed by a computer. The simplest method is called a filtered back projection. In simple terms, as the CT scanner rotates around the patient, many images, called projections, are acquired. Following the acquisition, the angle of each projection image in known and by drawing a ray from each detector with the intensity recorded by that detector back through a 3D matrix (positioned where the patient was), the intersection of these rays in the image matrix can be recorded. By summing all of the rays together from all of the projections, a 3D image can be reconstructed. The process involves other mathematical operations like filtering but that this is the basic principle of filtered back projection.

26. C Hounsfield numbers range from −1,000 for air to +3,000 for bone and contrast agents. Remember that a 12 bit pixel results in about 4,096 gray values.

27. **A** The Hounsfield number (H) is related to a CT number which is also related to linear attenuation coefficients of different tissues. The equation to calculate H is $H = 1,000 \times (\mu_{pixel} - \mu_{water})/\mu_{water}$. This equation shows that H also represents a change of percentage in the attenuation coefficient of water. The homogeneity coefficient is the ratio of the first to the second HVL in describing the quality x-ray beams.

28. **C** The correct formula of Hounsfield number is:
    $H = \mu_{tissue} - \mu_{water}/\mu_{water} \times 1,000$

29. A Hounsfield unit is an arbitrary unit of x-ray attenuation used for CT scan.
    - **A.** I. Air = −1,000
    - **B.** IV. Water = 0
    - **C.** II. Bone = +1,000
    - **D.** III. Fat = −100
    - **E.** V. Muscle = +40

30. **E** All are correct.

31. **B** Refer to question 29 above. Hounsfield unit or CT number.

Fat	(−100)
Lungs	(−700)
Water	(0)
Muscle	(35–50)

32. **A** A CT number assigned to a pixel represents the average linear attenuation coefficient of tissue in the voxel. By generating a CT to ED curve, the CT number can be related to an electron density.

33. **E** Disadvantages of MRI compared to CT are that the spatial resolution is slightly lower than CT, it is difficult to image the bone or calcifications, longer scan acquisition times increasing the possibility of motion artifacts, and technical difficulties with simulating patients (or claustrophobia) due to the small bore hole of the magnet and magnetic interference with metallic objects. Additionally, it can be difficult to obtain some of the special MRI contrast agents.

34. **E** MRI involves a phenomenon known as nuclear magnetic resonance, which is a resonance transition between nuclear spin states of certain atomic nuclei when subjected to a radiofrequency (RF) signal of a specific frequency in the presence of an external magnetic field. MRI involves only nuclei that intrinsically possess spinning motion or have angular momentum, and it is most distinguished in nuclei with an odd number of protons.

Quiz 2 (Level 3)

1. **D** Any nuclei with nonzero spin or angular momentum can be used for MRI imaging, but certain nuclei give larger signal than others. Because of its high intrinsic sensitivity and high concentration in tissues, hydrogen nuclei (protons) produce signals of sufficient strength for MRI imaging.

2. **E** Most particles have spinning properties. They can be either fermions or bosons depending on their constituents. Fermions have half-integer spin, and bosons have integer spin.

3. **B** All isotopes that contain an odd number of protons and/or odd number of neutrons have an intrinsic magnetic moment and angular momentum; in other words, they possess a nonzero spin. Isotopes with even number of protons and/or even number of neutrons do not spin.

4. **A** Magnetic fields create a change in long-axis spin direction of the nuclei (hydrogen) causing nuclei (hydrogen) to align their spin axes along the external magnetic field (H) as well as to orbit around the external magnetic field (H). A secondary radiofrequency wave is applied to cause the nuclei (hydrogen) to be deflected transverse direction. The return of the nuclei back to the stable position in the magnetic field results in a RF emission. This emission is detected and used to create the MR image.

5. **B** To cause the protons to flip, a RF field is generated by a radiofrequency coil. This field is applied perpendicular to magnetic field at the Larmor frequency.

6. **C** A magnetic dipole moment takes place when spinning charged particles create a magnetic field from south to north poles. When a RF field is applied to the protons in the magnetic field, they flip on along the longitudinal axis. Once the RF field is removed, the protons relax emitting a RF signal that can be detected. The length of the RF pulse determines how much the proton flips. This is called T1 relaxation.

7. **D** When the RF signal is turned off, the nuclei return to their original alignment around magnetic field. This is called relaxation. The turning off of the transverse radiofrequency field causes nuclei to relax in the transverse direction (T2 relaxation) as well as to return to the original longitudinal direction of the magnetic field (T1 relaxation). T2 relaxation is related to the surrounding magnetic fields created by other protons (spin–spin), while T1 is related to the time the RF pulse was applied and the properties of the material as a whole (spin–lattice). T1 is longer than T2.

8. **D** Nuclear magnetic resonance signal is induce when relaxation occurs. The relaxation times, T1 and T2, are actually time constants specific to each material.

9. **B** Localization of protons in MRI in a 3-D space is achieved by applying magnetic field gradients produced by gradient RF coils in three orthogonal planes. The three gradients are the slice select gradient, the frequency encode gradient, and the phase encode gradient. The slice select gradient works because the magnetic field is stronger at one end than the other meaning the protons at one end are spinning faster than at the other. The RF pulse will only cause the protons to flip that are rotating at the same frequency; therefore only one slice of tissue will be excited at a time. The frequency encodes gradient works in a similar fashion only in a direction perpendicular to the slice selection gradient. Now the redoubt pulses are localized in two dimensions. The third dimension is resolved with the phase encode gradient which is applied before the frequency encode but after the slice selection gradient to shift the phase of the signal in the last perpendicular direction.

10. **E** In MRI a body slice is imaged by applying field gradient along the axis of the slice and selecting a frequency range for readout, and the strength of the field gradient determines the thickness of the slice (the greater the gradient, the thinner the slice). Most MR imaging uses a spin echo technique in which a 180° RF pulse is applied after the initial 90° pulse, and the resulting signal is received at a time that is equal to twice the interval between the two pulses.

11. **C** MRI image contrast can be affected by adjusting echo time (TE) and repetition time (TR). TE is the echo time between when the RF pulse is applied and when the proton spins rephrase and emit a measurable RF signal. The TR is the repetition time between subsequent pulses. By adjusting TE and TR, one can take advantage of the different intrinsic T1 and T2 relaxation times of different tissues. Depending on what tissue one wants to see, TE and TR can be extended or reduced. Remember that T1 and T2 are intrinsic properties of each tissue and cannot be adjusted. Window and leveling are used to improve contrast in CT, and kVp and mA are used to improve contrast in diagnostic imaging.

12. **C** By adjusting TR and TE, image contrast can be affected. A long TR and short TE produce a proton (spin) density-weighted image. A short TR and a short TE produce a T1-weighted image, and a long TR and a long TE produce a T2-weighted image. Thus differences in proton density, T1, and T2 between different tissues can be enhanced by a manipulation of TE and TR.

13. **A** Tesla is the unit used to measure magnetic field strength. 0.5–3 T is the typical range of magnetic field strength used clinically. There are 7 T magnets that are used for research, but they are not common. Ultrasound waves of frequencies 1–20 megahertz (MHz) are used in diagnostic radiology.

14. **A** Gadolinium is the most commonly used MRI contrast agent for enhancement of vessels or for brain tumor associated with degradation of the blood–brain barrier. This agent works by changing the magnetic properties in the tissues near the agent. Barium sulfate can be used to lower T2 signal;

13.6 Ultrasound (Answers)

manganese can be used to enhance the T1 signal and has been used for the detection of liver lesions. Perflubron has been used as a gastrointestinal MRI contrast agent for pediatric imaging.

15. E For safety precautions, jewelry, patients with pacemakers, pregnant women, patients with a metal prosthesis, and any kind of metal objects should not be allowed in the MRI room.

16. D Hounsfield number depends on the density of the material used, the mass attenuation coefficient, and the linear attenuation coefficient.

17. B kVp is generally kept constant during a CT scan. Typical kVps range from 80 up to 140 kVp. 120 kVp is the most common. In the past mAs was held constant, but in order to reduce imaging dose, the current during the scan can be modulated so that it is lower in the AP direction and higher in the lateral direction to compensate for the change in thickness.

18. E A radiation oncology CT simulator must contain a large gantry aperture (bore) so that all setups can be accomplished such as large-breast patients, gynecological patients where the patient is required to be frog legged, and chest so that the arms can be flexed superiorly. The simulator must contain external lasers for setup reproducibility, a flat table top similar to linac couch, and a contrast kit for patients who require a contrast study.

19. C It is important to select an appropriate slice thickness due to a balance between edge definition (spatial resolution) and noise. Selecting thinner CT slices will create higher noise and poorer low-contrast resolution; on the other hand, it will create better edge definition, better high-contrast resolution (spatial resolution), and less partial volume artifacts.

13.6 Ultrasound (Answers)

Quiz 1 (Level 2)

1. A Ultrasound does not involve ionizing radiation, and it is also less expensive than CT study. A CT scan ranges from $1,200 to $3,200, while ultrasound depends on the area examined but usually ranges from $100 to $1,000. Ultrasound is usually not used for imaging bony structures; instead it is used for internal organs of the body. A disadvantage of ultrasound is that it cannot travel through air so it cannot be used for imaging in the lung.

2. D Ultrasound uses high-frequency sound waves for imaging. Nuclear medicine is a study where radioactive materials are used for imaging. CT scans as well as radiographic imaging use x-rays for imaging, and MRI uses a strong magnetic field and radiofrequency pulses for imaging.

3. B Ultrasound may be used to produce images by means of either transmission or reflection. However, in most clinical applications, use is made of ultrasound waves reflected from different tissue interfaces. Reflections or echoes are caused by variations in acoustic impedance of materials on opposite sides of the interfaces; in other words, ultrasonic waves are reflected at boundaries where there is a difference in acoustic impedance (Z) of the material on each side of the boundary. Ultrasound wave diffraction happens when a wave travels through a small hole in a barrier and bends around the edges.

4. B An ultrasound or ultrasonic wave is a sound wave having a frequency greater than 20,000 cycles per second or hertz (Hz). Ultrasound waves of frequencies 1–20 megahertz (MHz) are used in diagnostic radiology. Magnetic field strength in MRI is measured in units of tesla, and the strength ranges between 0.2 and 3 T.

5. E All the statements are correct about ultrasound.

6. A Strong reflections of ultrasound occur between air–tissue interfaces, tissue–bone interfaces, and chest wall–lung interfaces due to high impedance mismatch because the lung is composed of air. Lung and air cavity interfaces possess low-impedance mismatch so the reflection of ultrasound is weak.

7. A Ultrasonic waves are generated and detected by an ultrasound probe or transducer. The probe contains a piezoelectric material which converts electrical energy into sound energy and vice versa. When transmitting, an electrical current causes vibrations in the piezoelectric material which emits sound waves. During detection, the sound waves cause the piezoelectric material to vibrate which generates an electrical signal.

8. A An ultrasonic probe or transducer is a device that converts electrical energy into ultrasound energy and vice versa.

9. D The piezoelectric effect is a property in certain crystals in which a variation of an electric field across the crystal causes it to oscillate mechanically, thus generating acoustic waves. Conversely, pressure variations across a piezoelectric material result in a varying electrical potential across the opposite surface of the crystal.

10. A The most common crystals used clinically in an ultrasound probe or transducer are barium titanate, lead zirconium titanate, and lead metaniobate. Crystals of sodium iodine are found in nuclear medicine detectors to detect gamma rays and produce light (scintillating crystal).

11. C The amplitude is the height of an ultrasound wave. The frequency is the number of cycles per second, and the wavelength is the length of one cycle. The intensity is the rate at which energy passes through a material.

13.6 Ultrasound (Answers)

12. A The sound waves can be absorbed in the medium, scattered in the medium, or reflected back toward the receiver. When the sound waves collide against the receiver, oscillation occurs, causing electrical impulse to construct the image. Remember that ultrasound is not ionizing radiation, it is a sound wave.

13. B In an ultrasound image, the pie-shaped scan can be accomplished by using a convex transducer or receiver. A linear transducer or receiver provides a cross-sectional display from vertical parallel scan lines, and a combination of linear and convex transducers or receivers can be used, but a concave transducer or receiver does not exist.

14. E All are correct. Lower frequency is used for deeper imaging but produces worse detail. The higher the frequency, the better the spatial resolution in the direction of the wave. The penetration depth is greater with lower frequency because ultrasound waves lose their intensity at 0.5 dB per cm per MHz. That means for a 10 dB ultrasound wave, at 6 MHz the wave can travel about 3.3 cm (10 dB/(0.5 dB/cm×6 MHz)). At 12 MHz the same 10 dB wave can only travel 1.7 cm (10 dB/(0.5 dB/cm×12 MHz)). Remember that the wave has to travel to the interface and back so the actual penetration depth is half of the total distance the wave can travel. The brightness depends on the strength of the echo and the time it takes to travel back to the receiver, and attenuation of sound pulses is lower in the soft tissue than in the bone and air.

15. B As the ultrasound wave reflected from tissue interfaces is received by the transducer, voltage pulses are produced that are processed and displayed on the display in A, B, or M mode for image display.

16. C The M mode in ultrasound image displays the motion of internal structures of the patient's anatomy. The A mode displays the signal amplitude of the wave and the time on the abscissa which is related to distance or tissue depth, given the speed of sound in the medium. The B mode displays the brightness of the cross-sectional image and is the most commonly used mode.

17. B When using ultrasound in radiotherapy, the cross-sectional information used for treatment planning is derived from B-mode images.

18. C The function of the gel applied to the patient's skin when ultrasound is used is to allow the probe to couple directly to the skin without any air gap since air will cause the sound waves to reflect back to the transducer without any anatomic information.

19. C The approximate speed of an ultrasound wave in the tissue is 1,540 m/s. The speed of ultrasound waves in air is 330 and 4,080 m/s in the skull bone. 1,450 m/s is the speed of ultrasound waves in fat. In the liver it is approximately 1,555 and 1,600 m/s in the muscle.

13.7 Nuclear Medicine (Answers)

Quiz 1 (Level 2)

1. **E** All statements are true about nuclear medicine studies. Nuclear medicine radioisotope images are dynamic and change with time as the radiotracer is taken up by the tissue of interest and then washed out with biological and physical decay times. Nuclear medicine imaging also provides information about structure and function of the organ as opposed to structure only as in CT or most MRI imaging. The radiotracers (compound that is preferentially taken up by the tissue of interest but is also tagged with a radioactive isotope) are absorbed in organs based on their physiological function and are used to create radiographic images. Most of radioactive materials used in nuclear medicine must be gamma emitters so that it can penetrate the body and be detected by the nuclear medicine machine although positron emitters can be used because the annihilation photons, not the positron, are emitted and detected.

2. **B** The half-life ($T_{1/2}$) of radioisotopes used in nuclear medicine must be short to protect the patient and the general public since the patient is normally released once the study is completed. Nuclear medicine is safe, painless, and cost-effective.

3. **C** The half-life ($T_{1/2}$) of a radioactive substance is the time required for the activity or the number of radioactive atoms to decay to half their initial value. The formula is $T_{1/2} = \ln(2)/\lambda$ where λ is the decay constant for that particular isotope. The mean or average life is the average lifetime for the decay of radioactive atoms, and the formula is $T_a = 1.44 \times T_{1/2}$. The effective half-life is defined as the decay of a radioactive material via decay and biological excretion. Its formula is $1/T_e = 1/T_p + 1/T_b$. The effective half-life is always shorter than the physical half-life because the isotope is eliminated from the body in addition to the physical radioactive decay.

4. **E** All of these are used.

5. **A** Nuclear medicine imaging can be planar or 3 dimensional. 3D imaging like SPECT (single-photon emission computed tomography) and PET (positron emission tomography) generates images similar to CT in that a reconstruction algorithm uses projection images acquired at various angles around the patient to reconstruct a 3D image. The difference is how the rays are back projected into the 3D matrix. For CT, the photons are created from the x-ray generator and travel in a straight line to the detector. To back project, the ray from the detector is simply traced in a straight line back to the source (transmission-type reconstruction). In nuclear medicine, the source is inside the patient and

13.7 Nuclear Medicine (Answers) 753

emits radiation isotropically (in all directions), and the detectors are outside the patient (emission-type reconstruction). The big difference is how the lines or response is generated. In both planar gamma camera and SPECT imaging, physical collimators are used. Collimators are thick, high Z material devices that are placed in front of the gamma camera. The most common collimator is a parallel-hole collimator which consists of many long, straight holes through a high Z material plate. These holes only allow photons to enter in a straight line; any angle photons are attenuated and do not reach the scintillation crystal. Now, the rays can be back projected from the gamma camera because only photons from that direction could have made it to the crystal. Other collimators include pinhole, converging, and diverging. The difference between planar imaging and SPECT is that SPECT uses one or more gamma cameras, each with a collimator to acquire multiple projection images around the patient, while only one image is acquired for a planar image. PET does not use a physical collimator; rather, it uses electronic collimation. A PET system consists of a ring of gamma cameras around the patient. Since a positron emitter is used, the radiation emitted from the patient is a pair of 511 keV photons. By using special circuits, when a pair of photons is detected AT THE SAME TIME, a line of response can be created between the two detectors where the photons were detected since they are emitted 180° apart after annihilation.

6. C The radioisotope is filtered by the kidneys and sent to the bladder to be excreted from the body. Since the bladder will hold the radioisotope for a period of time before excretion, it will appear "hot" in the image.

7. C Iodine-123 (^{123}I) is used to image the thyroid when performing a nuclear medicine study due to the preferential uptake of iodine in the thyroid. Thallium-201 (^{201}Tl) is used to show myocardial ischemia; gallium-67 (^{67}Ga) is used to show inflammation and tumor activity, and xenon-133 (^{133}Xe) is used for lung ventilation studies. Remember, nuclear medicine used radiotracers that are compounds that preferentially accumulate in a particular tissue and are tagged with a radioactive isotope.

8. B A gamma camera is used in nuclear medicine as a detector. A scintillation crystal (sodium iodine, cesium iodine, bismuth germinate, etc.) or multiple crystals are positioned around the patient or rotated around the patient. The photons emitted from the patient interact in the crystal which produces visible light. This light is detected by a photomultiplier tube and converted into electrons that can be turned into an image. Remember that in SPECT and PET a 3D image is created from multiple projection images and for planar images a single gamma camera is used. In all cases, some type of collimator is needed to establish lines of response for the reconstruction algorithm. In CT, the detectors are always opposed to the source and rotate around the patient to acquire a transmission image. In MRI, magnetic fields and RF pulses are used to generate a 3D image.

9. B Nuclear medicine radionuclides are typically injected into the body via blood circulation although there are oral radiotracers and radiotracers that can be inhaled to image the lungs.

10. A 80 % of all nuclear medicine procedures are done using technetium-99 m due to its ideal characteristics. One of the most common uses is for myocardial perfusion studies to see how much blood is flowing to the cardiac muscle.

11. E All are correct. Nuclear medicine imaging is very useful because it shows how the particular organ is functioning rather than simple atomic structure. Nuclear medicine also has much poorer spatial resolution than CT. The spatial resolution is between 5 mm and 1 cm, whereas CT is around 1 mm. This is due to the resolution of the gamma camera and also, for PET, the positron as a range in the patient before it annihilates. NM does have much better contrast than CT. NM also uses some form of collimation, either physical or electronic. CT might have a small collimator to reduce the number of scatter photons, but it does not depend on this collimator to reconstruct the image.

13.8 Positron Emission Tomography (PET) (Answers)

Quiz 1 (Level 2)

1. C PET scan stands for positron emission tomography and is a nuclear medicine technique that produces a three-dimensional image of some body function.

2. B PET scans use radioisotope that emits positrons, which then interacts with an electron in an annihilation reaction creating two photons of 0.511 MeV traveling in opposite directions. A circular array of gamma cameras detects the photons. When using fluorodeoxyglucose (FDG), which is the most common radiotracer in PET, areas of high metabolic activity need sugar; therefore, this traces are uptaken into these areas preferentially which then are visible in the reconstructed image.

3. C Because of the high metabolic activity, the brain and tumors are structures that need high sugar concentration, and these are the two most common uses for FDG.

4. A PET scan images are created because a circular array of gamma cameras detects photons created in an annihilation reaction produced by the positron (emitted by radioisotope) captured by an electron in the body. Planar gamma camera or SPECT imaging uses gamma cameras with sodium

13.8 Positron Emission Tomography (PET) (Answers)

iodine crystals that detect gamma rays produced by a radioisotope. PET detectors do not use sodium iodine because they have lower Z, and the sensitivity to the high-energy 511 keV photons is very low. Instead, crystals like bismuth germinate (BGO) are used which have a higher Z and are more effective at stopping the 511 keV photons.

5. B Glucose labeled with positron emitting ^{18}F is normally used in PET as this is a metabolism tracer good for imaging tumors and brain activity.

6. B The half-life for F-18 is about 2 h. This means that it usually needs to be produced in a cyclotron relatively close to the hospital because of the short half-life.

7. B Positron emitters are typically generated in cyclotron.

8. A Two photons are generated; each has an energy of 0.511 MeV.

9. C Normally 40–60 min, the time is to allow the uptake of the drug. During this time the patient should be as inactive as possible to avoid uptake in muscle.

10. A MicroPET scanner has better spatial resolution and smaller size, which is good for animal studies. Remember that the clinical spatial resolution of PET is between 3 and 7 mm which are not sufficient for small-animal imaging.

Quiz 2 (Level 3)

1. D PET demonstrated excellent sensitivity; thus a tiny little amount of drug can make an image. However, the spatial resolution is poor due to the range of the positron and physical limitations in the gamma cameras.

2. C PET/CT has become the standard due to the additional anatomical information provided by the CT. The CT can also provide information to correct for attenuation in the patient. By using the CT numbers, the voxels deep in the patient can be increased, and the voxels near the edge of the patient can be reduced. The reduction in the number of counts is proportional to the total path length traveled by BOTH photons leaving the patient. Therefore, if attenuation is not correct, the edge of the patient appears very bright.
Answer B makes sense, but it has nothing to do with image quality. Similarly, D is right, but it will not help with image quality.

3. C There are three factors which limit the spatial resolution: free path of positron, non-colinearity of 2 annihilating photons, and detector size in the PET scanner.

Non-colinearity means the 2 photons are not exactly emitted 180° to each other since the momentum in the center-of-mass system is nonzero. Thus those 2 photons are almost back to back but within 2 small cones. The larger the scanner size, the larger the non-colinearity will be (because the cone becomes larger).

4. A Free path depends on the kinetic energy of positron, which is determined by the radioisotope. For ^{18}F (emission energy of 0.63 MeV), the free path is about 2 mm, which is quite small. Remember that electrons and positron lose about 2 MeV per cm in the tissue.

5. A 2 mm is the "natural limit" for spatial resolution, which is mainly contributed by the non-colinearity of the annihilation photons. For a typical PET scanner, the spatial resolution is around 4 mm because of the detector size and also the spread of light in the scintillator crystal.

6. B The contribution from non-colinearity is much smaller for microPET, simply because the scanner size is smaller. In this case, the detector size plays the major role, which can be controlled. Cost and computing power are issues with clinical PET scanners because they must be much larger and require many more crystals than a microPET system. It is possible to have a 1 mm or sub-mm spatial resolution for microPET scanner.

7. A The major difference is the binning in reconstruction. A dynamic scan in PET imaging is similar to a 4D CT scan where each slice is acquired multiple times and then binned according to some surrogate such as the breathing pattern or heartbeat. Each binned phase is reconstructed in the same manner as a static scan.

8. D When the positron is captured by an electron, its energy must be low enough, i.e., at thermal level; otherwise, it cannot be trapped. The typical process is that a positron collides with tissue and radiates Bremsstrahlung x-rays until it gradually slows down and is finally trapped by an electron.

When the electron and positron annihilate, the positron has "forgotten" its previous history because it has to be at thermal energy level. Thus non-colinearity has nothing to do with positron's initial energy, because it is an effect caused by annihilation. The energy of the positron will affect the spatial resolution of the image as the range increases with increasing energy.

Practice Test

14

Contents

14.1 Practice Test I: Questions 757
14.2 Practice Test II: Questions 785
14.3 Practice Test III: Questions 813
14.4 Practice Test IA: Answers 842
14.5 Practice Test IIA: Answers 850
14.6 Practice Test IIIA: Answers................................... 858

14.1 Practice Test I: Questions

1. Radiation protective barriers are designed:
A. To ensure that the dose equivalent received by any individual does not exceed the applicable maximum permissible value
B. To ensure that the dose equivalent received by radiation workers only does not exceed the applicable maximum permissible value
C. To ensure that no one is standing in a controlled or not controlled area
D. To protect against scatter radiation only

2. One atomic mass unit is equal to:
A. 1.66×10^{-27} kg
B. 1,862 MeV
C. 1.602×10^{-19} j
D. 0.511 MeV/c^2

3. The total body irradiation (TBI) with megavoltage photon beams is most commonly used in:
A. Mycosis fungoides
B. Bone marrow transplantation

C. The lung
D. Skin cancer

4. The energy needed to remove an electron from the shell is called:
A. The balance electrons
B. The binding energy
C. Transitions
D. Energy levels

5. What is the dose limit of leakage in locations surrounding the patient's room (hallway, adjacent patient room, etc.)?
A. 2 mrem/h.
B. 2 rem/h.
C. 10 mrem/h.
D. The dose rate surrounding the patient's room is never of concern.

6. The atoms are designated by atomic symbols; the A symbol represents:
A. I, II, and III only
B. I and III only
C. III and IV only
D. IV only
E. All are correct
I. Atomic number
II. Number of electrons
III. Mass number
IV. Number of protons and neutrons

7. What is the standard method for the patient to acquire iodine isotopes to treat thyroid cancer?
A. Injection of solutions with iodine ions.
B. Swallow iodine salt tabulates with juice.
C. Implant iodine seeds to thyroid.
D. Being exposed to radiation of iodine isotopes.

8. Which of the following is/are true?
A. I, II, and III only
B. II and IV only
C. I and II only
D. All are true
I. The activity per unit mass of a radionuclide is termed the half-life.
II. The number of atoms disintegrating per unit time is proportional to the number of radioactive atoms.
III. The time required for either the activity or the number of radioactive atoms to decay to half the initial value is termed specific activity.
IV. The average life or the mean life is the average lifetime for the decay of radioactive atoms.

9. The x-ray tube consists of:
I. A cathode
II. An anode
III. A glass envelope
IV. A tissue compensator
A. I, II, and III only
B. I and III only
C. II and IV only
D. IV only
E. All are correct

10. A nonsurgical, outpatient therapy that uses microscopic radioactive spheres to deliver high dose of radiation directly to the site of the liver tumors is named
A. Low-dose radiosurgery therapy (LDR)
B. High-dose radiosurgery therapy (HDR)
C. Selective internal radiation therapy (SIRT)
D. Stereotactic radiation therapy (SRT)

11. Which of the following statements is false?
A. The anode is made of a tungsten target.
B. The cathode is a tungsten filament.
C. Electrons are accelerated toward the cathode.
D. X-ray emerges through a thin glass beryllium window.

12. What is the difference between acceptance test and commissioning of equipment?
A. They are essentially the same.
B. They are totally irrelevant.
C. Acceptance test runs a small portion of dataset of commissioning.
D. Commissioning runs a small portion of dataset of acceptance test.

13. Which of the following statements about anode target is/are correct?
A. I, II, and III only
B. I and III only
C. II and IV only
D. IV only
E. All are correct
I. The anode target is made of tungsten.
II. The anode material atomic number (Z) is 74.
III. The target material must consist of high atomic number and high melting point.
IV. The target material must consist of high atomic number and low melting point.

14. The provability of Bremsstrahlung x-ray production fluctuates with:
A. The 1st power of the atomic number
B. Atomic mass^2 (A^2) of the target material
C. Atomic number^2 (Z^2) of the target material
D. Voltage applied to the tube

15. The thickness of an absorber required to attenuate the intensity of the beam to half its original value is a function of:
A. Energy absorption coefficient
B. Energy transfer coefficient
C. Attenuation coefficient
D. Half-value layer (HVL)

16. In coherent scattering:
A. The new photons have the same energy as the incoming photons but are scattered in different directions.
B. The new photons have the more energy than the incoming photons but are scattered in different directions.
C. The new photons have the same energy as the incoming photons and are scattered on the same directions.
D. The new photons have the less energy as the incoming photons but are scattered in different directions.

17. The probability of a photoelectric interaction depends on:
A. Atomic number (Z) and energy of the photon (E); the higher the Z of the material, the more likely the interaction, but the higher the energy of the photon, the less likely the interaction.
B. Atomic number (Z) and energy of the photon (E); the lower the Z of the material, the more likely the interaction, but the higher the energy of the photon, the less likely the interaction.
C. Atomic number (Z) and energy of the photon (E); the higher the Z of the material, the more likely the interaction, and the lower the energy of the photon, the less likely the interaction.
D. Atomic number (Z) and energy of the photon (E); the lower the Z of the material, the more likely the interaction, and the lower the energy of the photon, the less likely the interaction.

18. For pair production to take place, the threshold energy of the incident photon must be:
A. Equal to 0.51 MeV
B. Greater than 1.02 MeV
C. Greater than 2.04 MeV
D. Less than 1.02 MeV

19. The greatest limitation in using orthovoltage or deep therapy is:
A. Skin sparing
B. Skin surface dose
C. Cone size
D. Size and cost of the machine

20. Treatment parameters (gantry, collimator, field size, dose per fraction, total dose) to be used for a patient's treatment are controlled by
A. Ionization chamber (ion chamber is an instrument used in the measurement of the Roentgen according to its definition)
B. Calorimetry (calorimetry is a basic method of determining absorbed dose in a medium)

14.1 Practice Test I: Questions

C. Beam handling section (after electrons have been accelerated, they are redirected by the beam handling section which includes the bending magnet, target, scattering foil, or flattening filter)
D. Record and verify section (the record and verify section controls treatment parameters)

21. Which of the following parts is/are moved in front of the electron beam when the linear accelerator is in the electron mode?
    A. Scattering foil
    B. Flattening filter
    C. X-ray target
    D. Ion chamber

22. Ion chambers are made of
    A. High Z materials
    B. Low Z materials
    C. Tungsten
    D. Lead

23. Spine CyberKnife radiosurgery
    A. Uses external markers (tattoos) for preliminary alignment
    B. Uses implanting fiducials all the time
    C. Uses vest to track spine
    D. Uses mesh for spine tracking

24. Which of the following is the SI unit of mass?
    A. Second (s)
    B. Ampere (A)
    C. Kilogram (kg)
    D. Meter (m)

25. Which of the following formula is incorrect?
    A. Velocity (v) = length (l)/time (t)
    B. Acceleration (a) = Velocity (v)/time (t)
    C. Force (F) = mass (m) × acceleration (a)
    D. Power of work (P) = energy (E) × time (t)

26. The unit, SI unit, and special unit of kerma are
    A. j/kg, Gy, and RAD
    B. j/kg, Gy, and C kg
    C. Gy, Bq, and RAD
    D. j/kg, R, and C kg

27. Kerma is defined as
    A. I, II, and III only
    B. I and III only
    C. II and IV only
    D. IV only
    E. All are correct

I. The amount of kinetic energy transferred from photons to charge particles per unit mass
II. The sum of the initial kinetic energies of all the charged ionizing particles liberated by uncharged particles in a material of mass
III. The amount of kinetic energy transferred to the electrons
IV. The quantity of radiation for all types of ionizing radiation

28. PACS stands for
A. Picture active computer systems
B. Printer analog computer systems
C. Picture archiving and communication systems
D. Projection access communication systems

29. The percentage of the absorbed dose at any depth d to the absorbed dose at a fixed reference depth d0 along the central axis of the beam is the definition of:
A. Mayneord F factor
B. Percentage depth dose
C. Tissue-air ratio
D. Tissue-phantom ratio

30. The region between the surface and the point of maximum dose is called:
A. Skin-sparing effect
B. Dmax
C. Initial dose buildup region
D. Penumbra

31. The equivalent square formula can be used to calculate:
A. Circular-shaped fields
B. Irregular-shaped fields
C. Rectangular-shaped fields
D. Triangular-shaped fields

32. A PDD needs to be found for an equivalent square of a rectangular RT tangent breast of 20 cm by 14 cm. Which of the following answers is the equivalent square of the above RT breast tangent field?
A. 23.33
B. 41.11
C. 16.47
D. 4.11

33. A rectangular field is equivalent to a square field if:
A. Both have the same area/perimeter (A/P).
B. Both have different area/perimeter (A/P).
C. The rectangular is twice as bigger as the square.
D. Both have the same isocenter.

34. The increase in PDD with an increase on SSD can be found by:
A. Mayneord F factor formula
B. Equivalent square formula

C. Inverse square formula
D. Tissue-air ratio formula

35. $15^5 \times 10^3$ is equal to
A. 759,375,000
B. 8,000
C. 75,000
D. 22,781,250

36. Which the following metric system is equivalent to prefix deka?
A. 10^{-6}
B. 10^2
C. 10^{-12}
D. 10^1

37. What % of 60 Gy is 9?
A. 6.66 %
B. 5.40 %
C. 58 %
D. 15 %

38. 120 rad is equal to how many Gy?
A. 0.1 Gy
B. 1.2 Gy
C. 120 Gy
D. 30 Gy to rad

39. Radioactivity was first discovered by
A. Wilhelm Roentgen
B. Marie Curie
C. Henri Becquerel
D. Pierre Curie

40. Calculate the MU setting for an electron beam RT cheek treatment if the output cutout is 0.972 cGy/MU at Dmax and the physician wants to prescribe a dose of 250 cGy to the 85 % IDL.
A. 206 MU
B. 303 MU
C. 286 MU
D. 257 MU

41. Calculate the maximum practical range (Rp) of a 12 MeV electron if a tumor is to be treated with a dose of 250 cGy for 30 fractions.
A. 3 cm depth
B. 6 cm depth
C. 8 cm depth
D. 10 cm depth

42. Calculate the correction to an ionization chamber reading ($P_{t,p}$) if the treatment room temperature is 21 °C and the pressure is 772 mm mercury.
A. 1.980
B. 0.987
C. 0.980
D. 0.012

43. Which of the following IGRT systems enables visualization of the exact tumor location by integrating a CT imaging with a linac and involves acquiring multiple planar images?
A. BAT
B. Brainlab
C. Paired orthogonal planar imagers
D. CBCT

44. What will be the effect on the chamber reading for a given exposure if the temperature in the room decreases by 10 % and the pressure increase by 10 %?
A. Approximately 10 % decrease
B. Approximately 10 % increase
C. Approximately 5 % increase
D. Approximately 25 % decrease

45. Calculate the transmission factor if a lead block measuring 2.5 cm thickness and 10 mm HVL is used to block the esophagus on a patient at 100 SAD.
A. 4 %
B. 0.069 %
C. 2 %
D. 0.062 %

46. Calculate the wedge factor if the output of a beam is 0.700 without the wedge and 0.350 with the wedge.
A. 2.000
B. 0.500
C. 1.050
D. 0.350

47. Which of the following treatment devices is used to remove the small bower away from the treatment field?
A. Alpha cradle
B. Aquaplast mask
C. Belly board
D. Bite block

48. Calculate the hinge angle used in order to get the most homogeneous dose distribution in a wedged pair technique if 45° wedges are used.
A. 157.5°
B. 67.5°

C. 90°
D. 315°

49. Calculate the MU setting with a wedge in place if the wedge transmission factor is 0.640 and the MU setting for a field without wedge is 300.
A. 469 MU
B. 192 MU
C. 364 MU
D. 300.6 MU

50. Tongue and groove is used in MLC to
A. Reduce interleaf leakages
B. Correct for lack of divergence
C. Change the beam into a broad, clinically useful beam
D. Tilt the isodose lines through a specific angle

51. What is the dose rate (cGy/ min) a patient received in a cobalt 60 machine if the plan was done using 120 cGy/min at 80 SAD, but the patient was placed at 100 SAD?
A. 96 cGy/ min
B. 76.8 cGy/min
C. 150 cGy/min
D. 100 cGy/min

52. Calculate the output for a beam that delivers 300 cGy and the monitor unit set is 375.
A. 1.250
B. 0.800
C. 75
D. 80

53. Rotational therapy is best suited:
A. I, II, and III
B. I and III only
C. II and IV only
D. IV only
E. All are correct
I. For lateral tumors
II. For large tumor volumes
III. For external surface tumors
IV. For small, deep-seated tumors

54. Calculate the dose rate if a Co-60 machine delivers 400 cGy in 3 min.
A. 403 cGy/min
B. 0.007 cGy/min
C. 1,200 cGy/min
D. 133 cGy/min

55. Calculate the MU required to treat a patient whose dose is 180 cGy to the 84 % IDL and the output factor is 0.970 cGy/MU.
   A. 156 mu
   B. 186 mu
   C. 221 mu
   D. 147 mu

56. Calculate the prescribing dose if a dosimetrist evaluates a three-field rectum plan and concludes that the max dose in the plan is 277.5 cGy given to the 111 % IDL.
   A. 111 cGy
   B. 30.52 cGy
   C. 308 cGy
   D. 250 cGy

57. A plan was calculated for 200 cGy daily with an MU setting of 250 to a RT shoulder treatment at 100 SSD using a 20×20 field size at a depth of 9 cm, PDD of 78 %, 10 MV, Dmax at 2.5 cm. What would be the new PDD if the physician decided to treat at 115 cm SSD so that part of the ulna is included in the field?
   A. 103 %
   B. 78.0 %
   C. 79.1 %
   D. 89.7 %

58. Calculate the dose received by a patient if the output on a meditational treatment was 0.875 cGy/MU and the calculated MU was 195, but the machine broke and only delivered 105 MU.
   A. 91.8 cGy
   B. 171 cGy
   C. 79.2 cGy
   D. 120 cGy

59. Calculate the off-axis ratio or factor to be used if the tumor lies 10 cm deep and 6 cm lateral from the central axis. PDD at a depth of 10 cm along the central axis is 93.5 %, whereas PDD 6 cm lateral where the tumor lies is 87.3 %.
   A. 1.071
   B. 0.933
   C. 6.200
   D. 0.816

60. Calculate the penumbra width needed in a spine field where the source size is 1.5 cm, and the patient is treated at 100 cm SSD using a source to collimator distance of 75 cm.
   A. 3.50 cm
   B. 0.50 cm
   C. 2.00 cm
   D. 1.125 cm

14.1 Practice Test I: Questions

61. After completing TG-51 measurement, if the result is 3 % off, what should be done next?
A. Call the vendor to fix the machine.
B. Nothing, this is within the tolerance.
C. Adjust the corresponding potential meter to ensure the MU readout becomes correct.
D. Change the parameters in TPS since the machine output changes.

62. Calculate a craniospinal field gap if the thoracic spine field measures 38 cm×8 cm at 100 SSD and the lumbosacral field measures 20 cm×30 cm at 105 SSD using a depth of 7 cm.
A. 1.99 cm
B. 1.33 cm
C. 0.66 cm
D. 0.67 cm

63. Calculate the skin gap required if fields A/B are parallel opposed fields having a length of 25 cm and fields C/D are also parallel opposed fields having a length of 15 cm and all fields are treated at midplain, 100 SSD. Patient thickness is 20 cm.
A. 1.25 cm skin gap
B. 2 cm skin gap
C. 0.75 cm skin gap
D. 0.50 cm skin gap

64. The main interaction responsible for diagnostic imaging is
A. Coherent scattering
B. Compton effect
C. Photoelectric effect
D. Pair production

65. What would be the depth needed to calculate the exit dose if a patient is to be planned using a PA spine, max dose of 300 cGy at 2.5 cm depth? Patient thickness is 25 cm.
A. 15 cm depth
B. 12.5 cm depth
C. 22.5 cm depth
D. 25 cm depth

66. Deterministic effect is defined as:
A. The probability of occurrence of cancer is higher for higher doses, but the severity of any cancer is independent of dose.
B. The severity of a particular effect in an exposed individual increases with dose above the threshold for the occurrence of the effect.
C. The specified dose equivalent an individual is permitted to receive annually from working with radiation on the job.
D. The probability of occurrence of cancer is the same for any dose received, and late effect is always the case.

67. From the following table, calculate the total MU setting per fraction if a RT lower leg parallel opposed fields is planned using isocentric technique, patient separation of 12 cm, field size of 12 × 12, and dose to the isocenter of 180 cGy.

Table 14.1 Test 3

Depth	0	1	2	3	4	5	6
PDD	90	95	98	100	80	60	10

Output F	1.031 cGy/MU at 100 cm SSD, Dmax
Output F	1.075 cGy/MU at 100 cm SAD, Dmax

A. 182 MU
B. 190 MU
C. 231 MU
D. 152 MU

68. How many cm of lung is equivalent to 1 cm of water or tissue?
A. 5 cm
B. 3 cm
C. 2 cm
D. 10 cm

69. Calculate the effected path length used to plan a patient's treatment who has 5 cm of tissue from the skin to the center of the leg where a titanium metal replaces the bone measuring 3 cm, and then from the bone to the back of the femur, there is a separation of 7 cm tissue. Total thickness is 15 cm.
A. 9 cm tissue
B. 15 cm tissue
C. 16.5 cm tissue
D. 20 cm tissue

70. Radioactivity is defined as
A. An emission of radiation from unstable nuclei of element in the form of particles, electromagnetic radiation, or both
B. Radiation in which a particle carries energy capable of removing electrons from an atom producing free radicals
C. The rate of energy loss per unit path length
D. The rate of decay of a radioactive material

71. A plot of the volume of a given structure receiving a certain dose or higher as a function of dose is the definition of
A. Differential DVH
B. Cumulative integral DVH
C. Dose volume histogram (DVH)
D. Beam's eye view

72. A tumor at a depth of 3–4 cm is best treated with
A. 6 MeV
B. 9 MeV
C. 12 MeV
D. 18 MeV

73. Which of the following is/are correct according to the following DVH graph?
A. I, II, and III
B. I and III only
C. II and IV only
D. IV only
E. All are correct

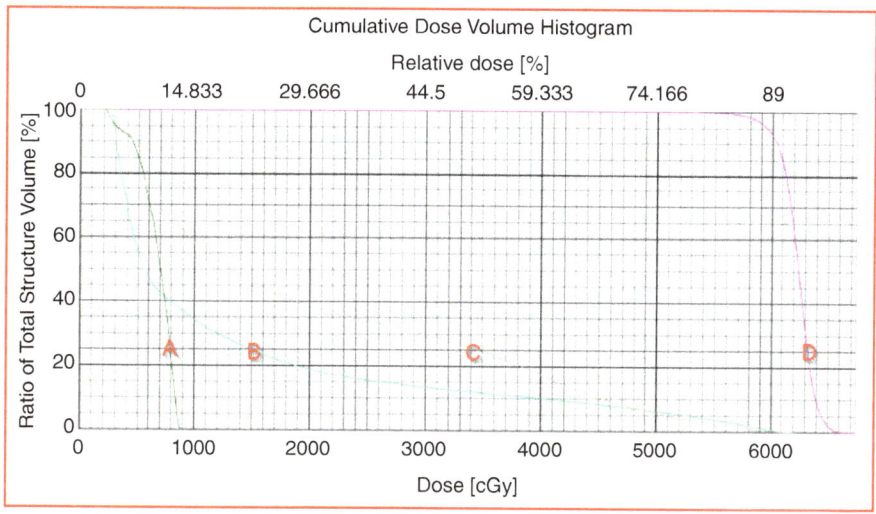

Fig. 14.1 Test 1 (Courtesy of University of Miami, Sylvester Cancer Center)

I.   Line A, max dose is approximately 9 Gy.
II. Line B, V20 was achieved.
III. Line C, 30 % of the volume receives at least 30 Gy.
IV. Linac D, RX dose of 60 Gy was not achieved.

74. Which of the following scenarios will not include a DVH?
A. 3-D conformal planning
B. IMRT planning
C. IMRT ARC planning
D. Electron clinical setup

75. Which of the following statements is/are true?
A. The dose at any depth is greatest on the central axis of the beam and gradually decreases toward the edges of the beam.
B. The dose at any depth is lower on the central axis of the beam and gradually increases toward the edges of the beam.
C. Near the field edges, the dose rate increases rapidly as a function of lateral distance from the beam axis.
D. Isodose curves at specified depth are not of concern when defining physical penumbra.

76. If the exposure rate at 3 cm from a source of ^{137}Cs is said to be 3.62 R·cm^2/h·mg, what would be the exposure rate at 7 cm from the source?
A. 0.66 R·cm^2/h·mg
B. 19.71 R·cm^2/h·mg
C. 1.55 R·cm^2/h·mg
D. 0.051 R·cm^2/h·mg

77. Horns are
A. I, II, and III
B. I and III only
C. II and IV only
D. IV only
E. All are correct
I. High-dose areas near the surface in the periphery of the field
II. Low-dose areas near the surface in the periphery of the field
III. Are created by the flattening filter
IV. Are created by the scatter in the body

78. Which of the following parameters affect(s) the isodose distribution?
A. I, II, and III
B. I and III only
C. II and IV only
D. IV only
E. All are correct
I. Beam energy
II. Source size, SSD, and SDD
III. Collimation
IV. Field size

79. Which of the following has the greatest influence in determining the shape of the isodose curves?
A. Field size
B. Flattening filter
C. Source-to-skin distance (SSD)
D. Beam energy

80. Which of the following should a medical dosimetrist do?
A. I, II, and III only
B. I and III only
C. II and IV only
D. IV only
E. All are correct
I. Perform radiation treatment planning
II. Recognize and resolve equipment problems and treatment discrepancies
III. Recommend when treatment should be withheld until a physician and physicist can be consulted
IV. Sign radiation prescriptions if the physician and/or physicists are not available

81. The most commonly used isodose beam-modifying device is
A. Block
B. Wedge filter
C. Cutout
D. Bolus

82. A professor asks one of his graduate students to ship a source from one lab to another lab. The student puts the source into the trunk of his car. Is this OK?
A. Nope. The professor should always ship the source himself.
B. Yes. It is always fine to use private transportation vehicles.
C. Only if the student has the proper training on radioactive material handling.
D. The package should never be handled by a student.

83. Which of the following is/are correct about wedges?
A. I, II, and III
B. I and III only
C. II and IV only
D. IV only
E. All are correct
I. Tilt the isodose curves toward the thin end.
II. Tilt the isodose curves toward the thicker end.
III. The degree of tilt depends on the slope of the wedge filter.
IV. The degree of tilt depends on the position of the wedge (RT, LT, in or out)

84. This DVH graph represents

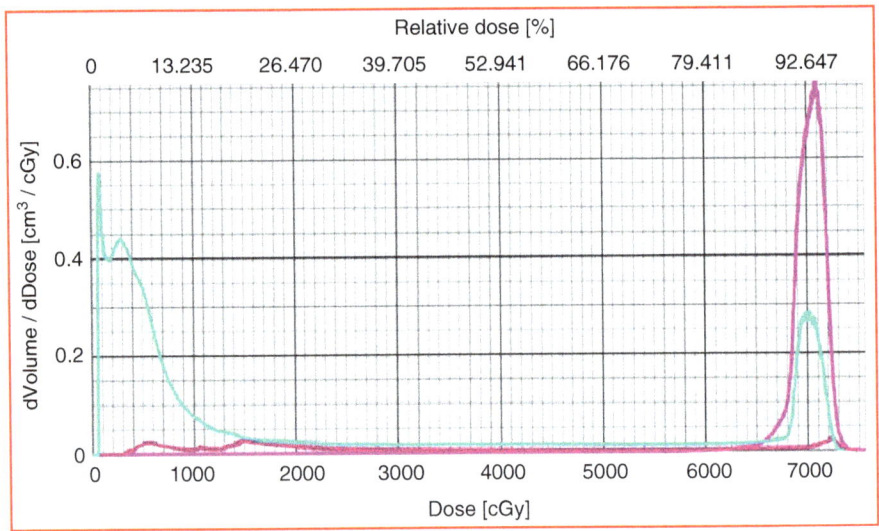

Fig. 14.2 Test 1

A. Differential DVH graph absolute dose
B. Cumulative DVH graph absolute dose
C. Differential DVH graph % dose
D. Cumulative DVH graph absolute volume

85. The isodose uniformity distribution depends on
A. I, II, and III
B. I and III only
C. II and IV only
D. IV only
E. All are correct
I. Patient thickness
II. Beam energy
III. Beam flatness
IV. Correct weighting

86. What electron energy in MeV should be selected if a tumor is located at 4 cm depth?
A. 6 MeV electron energy
B. 9 MeV electron energy
C. 12 MeV electron energy
D. 16 MeV electron energy

87. The most clinical useful energy range for electrons is
A. 12–24 MeV
B. 6–12 MeV
C. 6–20 MeV
D. 16–20 MeV

14.1 Practice Test I: Questions   773

88. Source-to-skin distance is
A. SSD = SAD − d
B. SSD = SAD + d
C. SSD = SAD/d
D. SSD = SAD × d

89. cos30° equals
A. 84.3
B. 0.34
C. 0.87
D. 36

90. The rate of electron energy loss depends primarily on
A. Electron density of the medium
B. Type of cutout used
C. Electron energy
D. Type of collision

91. On Bremsstrahlung interaction, the rate of energy loss on an electron beam per cm is proportional to
A. I, II, and III
B. I and III only
C. II and IV only
D. IV only
E. All are correct
I. Electron energy
II. Electron mass
III. Square of the atomic number (Z^2)
IV. Rest mass of an electron 0.511

92. As electron beam energy increases,
A. I, II, and III
B. I and III only
C. II and IV only
D. IV only
E. All are correct
I. Dose increases.
II. Surface penumbra decreases.
III. Penumbra at depth increases.
IV. Surface penumbra increases.

93. Which of the following energies generates the highest surface dose or less skin-sparing effect?
A. 6 MeV
B. 9 MeV
C. 12 MeV
D. 16 MeV

94. Which of the following is/are the result of removing an orbital electron in the K, L, or M shell by a direct hit of an incoming electron?
A. Photoelectric effect
B. Characteristic x-rays
C. Bremsstrahlung x-rays
D. Compton effect

95. If the treatment depth on an electron is in doubt, the dosimetrist should:
A. Use a bigger cutout
B. Use a bigger cone size
C. Use higher electron energy
D. Treatment depth is not important

96. Uniformity or flatness of the electron beam is usually specified:
A. I, II, and III
B. I and III only
C. II and IV only
D. IV only
E. All are correct
I. In a plane perpendicular to the beam axis
II. Horizontal to the beam axis
III. At the depth of the 95 % isodose beyond the depth of dose maximum
IV. At Dmax

97. Advantages of inverse treatment planning IMRT (ITP) over standard forward panning IMRT include:
A. I, II, and III
B. I and III only
C. II and IV only
D. IV only
E. All are correct
I. Improved dose homogeneity inside the target volume
II. Increased speed and lesser complexity of the proposed solution
III. A quantitative introduction of cost functions, often incorporating dose volume constraints and biological functions
IV. Adjustment of the optimal treatment planning to the actual dose delivery technique

98. Which of the following IMRT treatment modes is referred as the sliding window mode?
A. Segmented MLC mode (SMLC)
B. Dynamic MLC mode (DMLC)
C. Intensity-modulated arc therapy (IMAT)
D. Synchronize MLC mode (SYMLC)

99. IMRT stands for:
A. Intensity-multiple radiation therapy
B. Intensity-modulated rotational therapy
C. Intensity-modulated radiation therapy
D. Irregular-modulated radiation therapy

14.1 Practice Test I: Questions 775

100. Which of the following statements about magnetron and klystron is/are true?
A. Both devices produce microwaves.
B. Both devices can be used in high-energy (>10 MV) linacs.
C. The magnetron produces microwaves, and the klystron is a microwave amplifier.
D. Magnetron is more expensive and has a long life span.

101. IMRT refers to:
A. Radiation therapy technique in which nonuniform fluence is delivered to the patient from any given position of the treatment beam to optimize the composite dose distribution
B. Radiation therapy technique in which uniform fluence is delivered to the patient from one to maximum of ten field positions of the treatment beam to optimize the composite dose distribution
C. Radiation therapy technique in which beams of radiation used in treatment are shaped to match the tumor
D. Radiation therapy technique in which treatment planning is limited to generating dose distributions in a single or a few planes of the patient's target volume

102. What is the purpose of IMRT optimization?
A. I, II, and III
B. I and II
C. I and III
D. I only
E. All are correct
I. To minimize the dose in normal tissue
II. To maximize the dose in target volume
III. To generate a dose fluence
IV. To reduce the treatment time

103. The prescription for mediastinum lymphoma is 36 Gy, treated in 20 fractionations. The physician decided to treat the patient with AP/PA instead of IMRT. The reason could be:
A. AP/PA gives fewer doses to normal tissue than IMRT.
B. To save time, because it might take too long to plan and treat with IMRT.
C. There is no need to use IMRT because the prescription dose is low.
D. AP/PA has better outcome for mediastinum lymphoma.

104. The physician needs an SBRT plan with the target in the abdomen. The patient has been treated before. In this case, is VMAT the better choice over standard IMRT?
A. Not necessarily, because the main advantage for VMAT is fast delivery of dose.
B. No. Standard IMRT is better because normal tissue can be avoided by choosing appropriate beam angles by beam's eye view (BEV).
C. Yes. VMAT is generally better over standard IMRT in SBRT, because the factional dose of SBRT is huge and VMAT may distribute dose to surrounding normal tissues and reduce the probability normal tissue complication.
D. Either is a really bad option because the patient was treated before.

105. Does an IMRT plan use wedges or EDWs?
- A. Yes, to achieve a homogeneous dose, compensators are always needed.
- B. No, an IMRT plan does not care dose homogeneity.
- C. Yes, IMRT has its limitations so wedges are still needed.
- D. No, IMRT can achieve homogeneity with DMLCs.

106. Which of the following is the mean-life formula?
- A. $\tau = 1.44\, T_{1/2}$
- B. $N = N_0 e^{-\lambda \tau}$
- C. $A = -\lambda N$
- D. $T_{1/2} = 0.693/\lambda$

107. What is the normal request for PTV in terms of prescription in an IMRT plan?
- A. 100 % of PTV is covered with 100 % of prescription dose.
- B. 100 % of PTV is covered with 95 % of prescription dose.
- C. 95 % of PTV is covered with 100 % of prescription dose.
- D. 95 % of PTV is covered with 95 % of prescription dose.

108. Which of the following statements is/are true about parallel-opposed beams on TBI treatments?
- A. I, II, and III
- B. I and III only
- C. II and IV only
- D. IV only
- E. All are correct
- I. The higher the beam energy, the greater the dose uniformity for any thickness patient.
- II. The higher the beam energy, the lower the dose uniformity for any thickness patient.
- III. For patients of thickness greater than 35 cm, energies higher than 6 MV should be used to minimize the tissue lateral effect.
- IV. For patients of thickness less than 35 cm, energies higher than 6 MV should be used to minimize the tissue lateral effect.

109. Which of the following techniques can be used to treat TBI?
- A. I, II, and III
- B. I and III only
- C. II and IV only
- D. IV only
- E. All are correct
- I. Bilateral total body irradiation
- II. AP/PA total body irradiation
- III. Recline AP/PA total body irradiation
- IV. Oblique total body irradiation

110. Compensator design for TBI is complex because of:
- A. I, II, and III
- B. I and III only

14.1 Practice Test I: Questions

C. II and IV only
D. IV only
E. All are correct
I. Large variation in body thickness
II. Lack of complete body immobilization
III. Internal tissue heterogeneities
IV. Thickness of compensator

111. Unlawful physical contact or touching of a person without permission is the definition of:
A. Assault
B. False imprisonment
C. Battery
D. Invasion of privacy

112. $\sqrt[3]{27}$ is equal to
A. 2
B. 5
C. 10
D. 3

113. Stereotactic radiosurgery (SRS) is:
A. A single radiation therapy procedure for treating intracranial lesions
B. Multiple-dose-fraction procedure for treating intracranial lesions (stereotactic radiotherapy (SRT))
C. A single radiation therapy procedure for treating lung lesions
D. Multiple radiation therapy procedure for treating spine lesions

114. Which of the following devices is used in a stereotactic radiosurgery linac treatment for immobilization?
A. Stereotactic Aquaplast mask
B. Stereotactic alpha-credo
C. Stereotactic frame
D. Stereotactic bolus

115. 15 cm-long circular cones are used on SRS linac treatments to
A. Minimize geometric penumbra
B. Increase the distance (SSD)
C. Maximize the noncoplanar arcs
D. Shape the beam's eye aperture

116. The maximum channel diameter or field size on a Gamma Knife helmet is
A. 4 mm
B. 8 mm
C. 14 mm
D. 18 mm

117. When using film for stereotactic radiosurgery (SRS) dosimetry, care must be taken because
A. I, II, and III
B. I and III only
C. II and IV only
D. IV only
I. Films have a size limitation.
II. Films show energy dependence.
III. Films show possible directional dependence.
IV. Films have great statistical uncertainty.

118. Some of the major components of treatment QA for stereotactic radiosurgery (SRS) include:
A. I, II, and III
B. I and III only
C. II and IV only
D. IV only
E. All are correct
I. Stereotactic frame accuracy
II. Pedestal or couch mount
III. Frame alignment with gantry and couch eccentricity
IV. Congruence of target point with radiation isocenter

119. Hepatic metastases and primary neoplasms are often
A. Focal and regular in shape
B. Focal and irregular in shape
C. Multifocal and regular in shape
D. Multifocal and irregular in shape

120. Which of the following radioisotopes is used on selective internal radiation therapy (SIRT)?
A. Iridium-192 (Ir-192)
B. Yttrium-90 (Y-90)
C. Iodine-125 (I-125)
D. Phosphrus-32 (P-32)

121. Which organ would be the major concern for normal tissue complication if the patient is treated with Y-90?
A. Gallbladder
B. Lung
C. Stomach
D. Pancreas

122. Which of the following isotope of iodine is used to treat thyroid cancer?
A. I-123
B. I-124
C. I-125
D. I-131

123. Which of the following treatments requires an alpha cradle mold for patient immobilization?
A. Head and neck nasopharynx
B. Rt Lower leg sarcoma
C. RT chest wall
D. Whole brain

124. Patient's positioning and device used depend on:
A. I, II, and III
B. I and III only
C. II and IV only
D. IV only
E. All are correct
I. Patient's medical condition
II. CT scanning aperture dimension
III. Location of the disease
IV. Patient's preference

125. Image-guided radiotherapy (IGRT) refers to:
A. A patient anatomy image technique just before or during delivery of a fraction of radiotherapy to improve accuracy of radiotherapy delivery to the target and avoidance of organs at risk
B. View of patient from the target, through the beam portal showing patient anatomy within treatment beam
C. A combined radiation therapy in which a single portal is irradiated both with an electron and a photon beam
D. An x-ray film taken on the treatment machine with the patient in treatment position and with the beam settings as used for treatment

126. The nucleus of an atom is composed of
A. I, II, and III only
B. I and III only
C. II and III only
D. IV only
E. All are correct
I. Electrons
II. Protons
III. Neutrons
IV. Positron

127. The advantage of megavoltage beams for CBCT is:
A. The beams come from the linac beam line and thus no additional equipment is required to produce the cone beam.
B. It does produce better soft tissue contrast.
C. It can rotate a full 360°.
D. It can produce radiographic and fluoroscopic images.

128. Name the structure label C

Fig. 14.3 Test 1

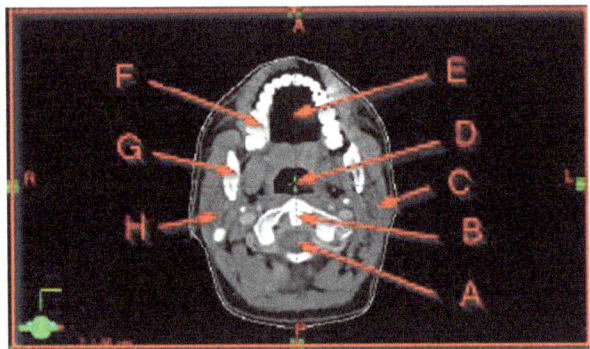

129. IMRT QA involves
A. I, II, and III only
B. I and III only
C. II and IV only
D. IV only
E. All are correct
I. The irradiation of a phantom to verify dose distribution versus dose plan
II. Verification of hand MU calculations
III. Verification of treatment safe parameters
IV. Verification of calculation point not to be close to MLC or in high-dose gradient

130. Name the structure label D

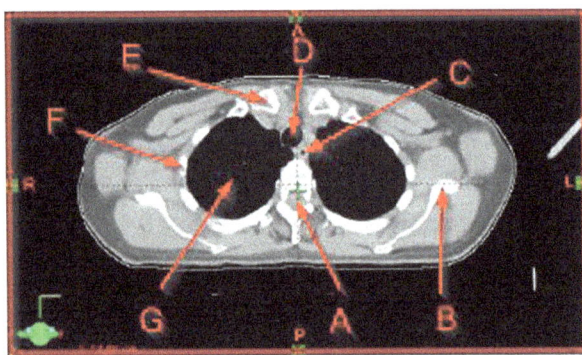

Fig. 14.4 Test 1

131. A patient threw away his immobilization mask before being treated to the neck with a boost plan, what would the therapists do? Assume the linear machine is capable of KeV imaging.
A. Make the patient another mask at linear accelerator couch, and treat with the boost plan.
B. Redo a CT with a new mask, and ask the dosimetrist to redo the boost plan with the new CT.
C. Forget about the mask since it was already lost. Ask the dosimetrist to do a simple plan like bilateral or AP/PA for the same dose.
D. Treat the patient without the mask.

132. Transient equilibrium is achieved when
A. The half-life of the daughter is much longer than the half-life of the parent
B. The half-life of the parent is much longer than the half-life of the daughter
C. The parent and daughter decay at their own respective half-lives
D. The half-life of the parent is not much longer than the half-life of the daughter

133. Adaptive radiotherapy was proposed in recently, which requested a replanning once every 1–3 fractions in hyperfractionation. Will this method help in minimizing the setup uncertainty?
A. Not really, since it focuses on replanning due to targets changing with time.
B. Sure, replanning reduces the setup uncertainty because the new plan follows the change of target.
C. Actually, it depends on whether the target changes with time or not.
D. It is too early to judge this since it is too new.

134. Name the structure label F.

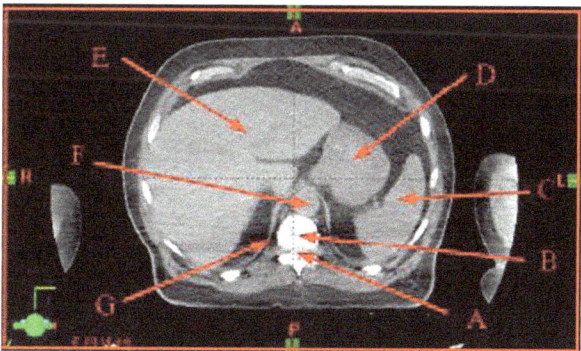

Fig. 14.5 Test 1

135. Which of the following statements is/are true about brachytherapy?
A. I, II, and III
B. I and III only
C. II and IV only
D. IV only
E. All are correct
I. Sources may be left in place for a limited period of time to irradiate the tissues.
II. Brachytherapy delivers fractionated doses of 120–400 cGy multiple times separated by many hours or days (teletherapy).
III. Brachytherapy uses sealed sources of ionizing radiation placed within the patient.
IV. Brachytherapy is an external beam radiation therapy (teletherapy).

136. The definition of absorbed dose is
A. Energy loss by electrons per unit path length of a material
B. Energy absorbed from all ionizing radiations per unit mass of materials
C. Charge liberated by ionization radiation per unit mass air
D. Rate at decay of radioactive material per unit time (second)

137. Exposure rate constant Γ ($R cm^2/mCi-h$) of ^{226}Ra is
A. 8.25
B. 3.28
C. 10.15
D. 2.38

138. An opposed AP/PA isocenter abdomen plan is done using 20×20 cm field size, 6 MV, patient separation of 40 cm, daily dose of 180 cGy and MU 195, and total number of fractions of 35. The patient is treated to 30 fractions and loses 4 cm due to weight loss. Approximately what will be the new MU correction for the last 5 fractions if separation changed from 40 to 36 cm?
A. 23 MU
B. 171 MU
C. 189 MU
D. 218 MU

139. The basal dose is defined as
A. The average of the maximum dose between sources
B. The average of the minimum dose between sources
C. The maximum dose in the plane of treatment (state dose)
D. The total dose contribution from each point

140. The source used for COMS eye plaque is/are:
A. I, II, and III
B. I and III only
C. II and IV only
D. IV only
E. All are correct
I. Radium-226 (^{226}Ra)

II. Iodine-125 (^{125}I)
III. Gold-198 (^{198}Au)
IV. Palladium-103 (^{103}Pd)

141. Which of the following radionuclide(s) is/are actually used for permanent radioactive seed implants?
A. I, II, and III
B. I and III only
C. II and IV only
D. IV only
E. All are correct
I. Palladium-103 (^{103}Pd)
II. Iridium (^{192}Ir)
III. Iodine-125 (^{125}I)
IV. Radium (^{226}Ra)

142. Which of the following dose volume histograms (DVH) has been found to be more useful and more commonly used?
A. Differential
B. Cumulative integral
C. Isodose curve
D. Beam's eye view

143. Which of the following procedures is/are recommended for intracavitary sources and manual afterloading source identification?
A. I, II, and III only
B. I and III only
C. II and IV only
D. IV only
E. All are correct
I. Source physical length
II. Source diameter
III. Source serial number
IV. Source color coding

144. Which of the following is the comprehensive AAPM TG Report for permanent prostate seed implant brachytherapy?
A. TG-43
B. TG-40
C. TG-64
D. TG-128

145. ALARA stands for:
A. As low as radiation association
B. At lower absolute radiation achievable
C. As low as reasonably achievable
D. As longer as radiation acquired

146. HDR pretreatment safety checks must be performed:
A. Once a week
B. On any day that the HDR procedure is scheduled
C. Once a month
D. Before each patient's treatment

147. Calculate the MU required to deliver 250 cGy to the 90 % IDL if the RT breast electron cutout has an output of 1.07 cGy/MU.
A. 260 MU
B. 234 MU
C. 241 MU
D. 268 MU

148. Which of the following radiation monitoring instruments is best suitable to search for lost clinical radioactive implant sources?
A. Ionization chambers (Cutie Pie)
B. Thermoluminescent dosimeters (TLD)
C. Photographic film
D. Geiger-Müller counters

149. Which of the following methods is used to check jaw symmetry?
A. Graph paper
B. Pack film
C. Machinist's dial indicator
D. Wiggler point

150. A Cutie Pie survey meter
A. I, II, and III only
B. I and III only
C. II and IV only
D. IV only
E. All are correct
I. Measures dose rate around an implanted patient and patient room
II. Surveys in and around the storage area in which radioactive materials are kept
III. Surveys areas around radiation-producing machines such as ^{60}Co units
IV. Calibrates linear accelerators or ^{60}Co units

151. Which of the following is the discipline dealing with what is good or bad, right or wrong, and moral principles that apply values and judgments to the practice of medicine?
A. Legal concepts
B. Ethics
C. Moral ethics
D. Fidelity

152. The F factor is:
A. I, II, and III only
B. I and III only

C. II and IV only
D. IV only
E. All are correct
I. The Roentgen-to-rad conversion factor
II. Relate dose in air to dose in tissue
III. Conversion of exposure to absorbed dose
IV. The rad-to-Roentgen conversion factor

153. One bit is equal to
A. A binary digit (0 or 2)
B. A single digit (1)
C. A binary digit (0 or 1)
D. A decimal digit (0–9)

154. Which of the following technologies is the most rapid in data transportation?
A. Modem
B. ISDN
C. DSL
D. SS7

155. The maximum number of electrons that can occupy a specific energy level is determined using the formula:
A. $E^{kl}photon = E_k - E_l$
B. $E = mc^2$
C. $2n^2$
D. $T_{1/2} = Ln2/\lambda$

14.2 Practice Test II: Questions

1. The advantage(s) of parallel opposed fields is
A. I, II, and III
B. I and III only
C. II and IV only
D. IV only
E. All are correct.
I. Simplicity and reproducibility of setup
II. Homogeneous dose to the tumor
III. Less chances of geometrical miss
IV. Excessive dose to normal tissues and critical organs above and below the tumor

2. If the temperature is 22 °C and the pressure is 750 mm of mercury, the correction needed to an ionization chamber would be
A. 0.8622
B. 119.79
C. 1.0133
D. 0.0133

3. Which of the following elements have the same # of neutrons but different # of protons?
   A. Isotopes
   B. Isotones
   C. Isobars
   D. Isomers

4. What is the difference between acceptance test and commissioning of equipment?
   A. They are essentially the same.
   B. They are totally irrelevant.
   C. Acceptance test runs a small portion of dataset of commissioning.
   D. Commissioning runs a small portion of dataset of acceptance test.

5. The most stable atoms are
   A. Atoms with even # of protons and odd # of protons
   B. Atoms with odd # of protons and even # of neutrons
   C. Atoms with even # of protons and even # of neutrons
   D. Atoms with odd # of protons and odd # of neutrons

6. Which of the following is a corresponding characteristic of electron capture?
   A. Z ≥82, same nuclear structure of an $_2^4He$, atomic number (Z) decreases by 2, atomic mass (A) decreases by 4, and particle composed of two protons and two neutrons.
   B. Excessive number of neutrons, high neutron-to-proton (n/p) ratio; reduce n/p ratio by converting a neutron into a proton, negatron, and antineutrino; atomic number (Z) increases by 1, but atomic mass (A) remains the same.
   C. Deficit of neutrons, low neutron-to-proton (n/p) ratio, increase n/p ratio by converting a proton into a neutron and a positron or by capturing an orbital electron; atomic number (Z) decreases by 1, but atomic mass (A) remains the same; consists of a continuous energy distribution.
   D. Deficit of neutrons, low neutron-to-proton (n/p) ratio, increase n/p ratio by capturing one of the orbital electrons by the nucleus transforming a proton into a neutron; often called K capture; gives rise to characteristic x-ray with emission of Auger electrons.

7. Calculate the projection of field size on a film if on the patient skin measures 20×15 and the magnification factor is 1.45.
   A. 21.7×29
   B. 29×21.75
   C. 21.45×16.45
   D. 13.8×10.34

8. Intracavitary applicators internal positioning may be examined by
   A. Orthogonal radiographs
   B. Visual inspection
   C. No internal structure exam is required
   D. CT scan

14.2 Practice Test II: Questions

9. CyberKnife image tracking system
A. I, II, and III
B. I and III only
C. II and IV only
D. IV only
E. All are correct
I. Images patient at 45° orthogonal angle
II. Uses two diagnostic x-ray sources plus two ASI image detectors (cameras)
III. Uses real-time, live images compared against DRRs generated from CT
IV. The robot adjusts position based on the image/DRR comparison

10. If an HVL of 2.5 mm tin (Sn) is assigned to a specific machine, what will be approximately the percentage of the radiation beam transmitted through a 15 cm tin (Sn)?
A. 1.56 %
B. 0.89 %
C. 98.44 %
D. 0.015 %

11. The physicist on your department needs to use I-125 with an activity of 17.8095 mCi on November 10th, but they need to place the order 10 days before (November 1st). What is the activity of I-125 at the time of shipping (November 1st)?
A. 20 mCi
B. 0.0116 mCi
C. 59.6 mCi
D. 25 mCi

12. If penetration power of the beam is needed:
A. Added filtration and/or decreased voltage across the tube can be used.
B. Added filtration and/or increase voltage across the tube can be used.
C. Inherent filtration and/or decreased KV_P across the tube can be used.
D. Inherent filtration and/or increase MAS can be used.

13. If a Compton photon interacts with an orbital electron by direct hit,
A. No energy is transferred.
B. Electron will receive maximum energy, and scatter photon will leave with minimum energy.
C. Photon with energy of 0.511 MeV.
D. Incoming photon with energy up to 50 KeV.

14. The basal dose is defined as
A. The average of the maximum dose between sources
B. The average of the minimum dose between sources
C. The maximum dose in the plane of treatment (state dose)
D. The total dose contribution from each point

15. Which of the following is/are indirect ionization?
A. X-rays
B. γ-rays
C. Neutrons
D. All are correct.

16. The lateral distance between two specified isodose curves at specified depth is used to estimate
A. Tissue lateral effect
B. Transmission penumbra
C. Physical penumbra
D. Beam profiled

17. Closed-circuit television and audio monitoring systems
A. I, II, and III only
B. I and III only
C. II and IV only
D. IV only
E. All are correct
I. Are required in treatment rooms
II. Should be checked daily for proper operation
III. Should be turned on for all treatments
IV. Are not necessary if any tracking system (calypso, respiratory gating, etc.) is used

18. CyberKnife path is defined as
A. Preassigned points in space where the linac can deliver radiation from multiple beam angels
B. Preassigned points in space where the manipulator is allowed to stop in order to deliver radiation dose
C. A fixed and predetermined workspace where the robotic arm can move
D. The geometric isocenter where the beam is aimed

19. 1 mg-Ra eq is equal to
A. 8.25×10^{-4} mR/h at 1 m
B. 8.25×10^{-4} R/h at 1 m
C. 8.25×10^{-2} R/h at 1 m
D. 8.25×10 R/h at 1 m

20. The point of intersection of the collimator axis and the axis of rotation of the gantry is known as:
A. Secondary collimator
B. SSD
C. Wiggler point
D. Isocenter

21. A source is considered to be leaking if a presence of
A. 0.5 μCi or more of removable contamination is measured
B. 0.05 μCi or more of removable contamination is measured
C. 0.005 μCi or more of removable contamination is measured
D. 0.0005 μCi or more of removable contamination is measured

14.2 Practice Test II: Questions

22. The most frequently used TLD material for clinical dosimetry is
    A. Lithium borate ($Li_2B_4O_7$)
    B. Calcium fluoride ($CaF_2:M_n$ and nat)
    C. Calcium sulfate ($C_aS_{o4}:M_n$)
    D. Lithium fluoride (LIF)

23. The 90 % depth dose of a 16 MeV occurs at
    A. 2 cm
    B. 4 cm
    C. 5 cm
    D. 8 cm

24. Radiochromic films' response depends on
    A. Humidity
    B. Pressure
    C. Temperature
    D. Chemical processing

25. Outside the geometric limits of the beam and the penumbra, the dose variation is the result of
    A. I, II, and III
    B. I and III only
    C. II and IV only
    D. IV only
    E. All are correct
    I. Side scatter from the field
    II. Lateral scatter from the medium
    III. Leakage and scatter from the collimator
    IV. Leakage from the head of the machine

26. What is the difference between 3D-CRT hyperfractionation strategy and IMRT hyperfractionation strategy?
    A. Both are efforts to minimize normal tissue complications, and IMRT does a better job.
    B. Both are efforts to enhance better treatment outcomes, and IMRT does a better job.
    C. IMRT does a better job in both minimizing normal tissue complications and treatment outcomes.
    D. Both are efforts to enhance treatment outcomes and to minimize normal tissue complications and IMRT does a better job in both of them.

27. Determine the treatment time to deliver 150 cGy (rad) at the center of rotation of an arc treatment where the dose rate in free space at SAD is 80.5 cGy/min and the average TAR is 0.550.
    A. 3 min
    B. 3.39 cGy/min
    C. 3.39 min
    D. 5 min

28. Field shaping can be accomplished in electron beam therapy by using
A. MLC
B. Cones
C. Cutout
D. Wedges

29. SAR depends on:
A. I, II, and III only
B. I and III only
C. II and IV only
D. IV only
E. All are correct
I. Beam energy
II. Depth
III. Field size
IV. SSD

30. Which of the following diseases is/are primarily treated with radiosurgery CyberKnife treatment?
A. I, II, and III
B. I and III only
C. II and IV only
D. IV only
E. All are correct
I. Meningiomas
II. Acoustic neuroma
III. Gliomas
IV. Trigeminal nerve

31. The rate of kinetic energy loss per unit path length of charged particle is
A. Mass stopping power
B. Stopping power
C. LET
D. Activity

32. For Gamma Knife, CyberKnife, standard IMRT, and VMAT, if all normalized to body maximum, which one of following is correct for reasonable isodose lines to be chosen?
A. 60 %, 70 %, 95 %, 90 %
B. 50 %, 70 %, 95 %, 90 %
C. 60 %, 70 %, 98 %, 90 %
D. 50 %, 60 %, 95 %, 90 %
E. 50 %, 70 %, 95 %, 90 %

33. Which of the following corresponds to the diagram?
A. TMR
B. PDD
C. SAR
D. BSF

Fig. 14.6 Test 2

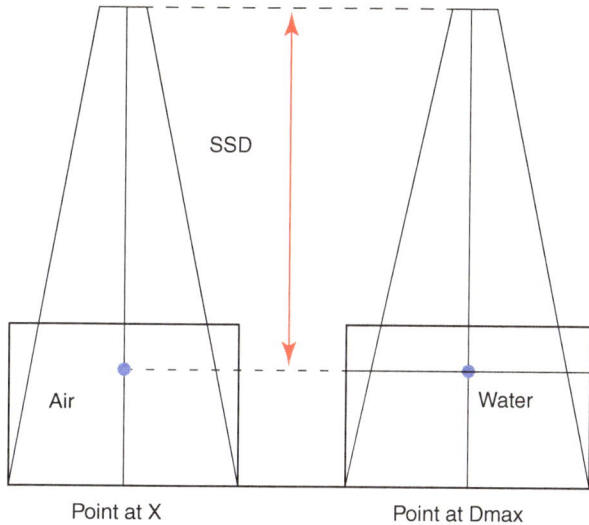

34. How could therapy with Y-90 selectively treat hepatocellular carcinoma (hcc) alone in the liver without putting a lot of dose to the most healthy part of the liver?
A. Hepatocellular carcinoma selectively absorbs Y-90 solution.
B. There uptakes of Y-90 in other parts of the liver are negligible although blood flowing through carries Y-90.
C. Blood which flows carrying Y-90 mainly passes through the part of the organ which has a disease.
D. Tumor is more sensitive to radiation than healthy normal tissues in the organ.

35. What is the range of a TI in mR/h at 1 m from the surface?
A. 1–100
B. 1–20
C. 1–10
D. 1–5

36. Scatter-maximum ratio (SMR):
A. I, II, and III only
B. I and III only
C. II and IV only
D. IV only
E. All are correct
I. Is the quantity designated specifically for the calculation of scattered dose in a medium
II. Is the ratio of the scattered dose at a given point in the phantom to the effective primary dose at the same point at Dmax.
III. Is a variable of SAR
IV. Is the ratio of the scattered dose at a given point in the phantom to the effective primary dose at any point

37. The relationship between wavelength, frequency, and velocity for photons is given by the formula
A. $E = h\nu$
B. $E = hc/\lambda$
C. $C = \nu \cdot \lambda$
D. $A = -\lambda N$

38. A PA field is clinically set up at 70 SSD using 20×25 cm, but the whole area is not included, and the SSD needs to be moved to 95. What is the new field size at 95 SSD?
A. 34×27
B. 27×34
C. 332.5×266
D. 45×50

39. Nowadays, hypofractionation has been gradually picked up again, although this strategy had been vanished for decades (if we do not consider SRS was hypofractionated since it was indeed a different modality), the reason for this situation is:
A. Actually, it is still controversial since hypofractionations caused a lot of normal tissue complications (NTC) in the early time of radiotherapy.
B. Technologies for on-site imaging, e.g., IGRT, have been greatly improved; thus, a much smaller margin can be used, in which the chance for NTC has been significantly minimized.
C. After treating patients with radiotherapy for a century, people have a much better understanding on NTCs; thus, hypofractionation is no longer dangerous.
D. Gamma Knife has proved that high fractional dose is fine with patients as long as the target is precisely located; thus, hypofractionation can be picked up again.

40. Calculate the magnification factor to use in the construction of a block if the field size at SAD was 13×15 cm and the image projection on the film is 15.6×18 cm.
A. 0.833 cm
B. 28.6 cm
C. 2.6 cm
D. 1.2 cm

14.2 Practice Test II: Questions

41. Calculate the therapeutic range of a 16 MeV electron if a tumor is to be treated with a dose of 250 cGy for 30 fractions.
A. 1.5 cm depth
B. 3 cm depth
C. 4 cm depth
D. 5 cm depth

42. The energy range of Compton effect photon interaction is
A. 150 KeV to over 50 MeV
B. Greater than 1.02 MeV
C. 1–50 KeV
D. Few electron volts to over 1 MeV in high atomic number elements

43. Calculate the 50 % IDL of a 12 MeV electron if a tumor is to be treated with a dose of 180 cGy for 35 fractions.
A. 2.57 cm depth
B. 3.86 cm depth
C. 5.15 cm depth
D. 6.86 cm depth

44. One kilobyte equals
A. 1,048,576 bytes
B. 1,024 bytes
C. 1,073,741,824 bytes
D. 32 bytes

45. Calculate the correction to an ionization chamber reading ($P_{t,p}$) if the treatment room temperature is 21°C and the pressure is 772 mm mercury.
A. 1.980
B. 0.987
C. 0.980
D. 0.012

46. Calculate the MU required to deliver 250 cGy to the 90 % IDL if the RT breast electron cutout has an output of 1.07 cGy/MU.
A. 260 MU
B. 234 MU
C. 241 MU
D. 268 MU

47. Inherent filtration refers to:
A. Absorption of the photons through a filter placed externally to the tube
B. Absorption of the photons through the target, glass walls of the tube, or thin beryllium window
C. The placement of a flattening filter in the beam path.
D. Shielding against leakage radiation

48. Calculate the linear attenuation coefficient of an aluminum material placed in the beam path if the thickness of the material is 1.5 mm.
A. 1.03
B. 0.46
C. 2.16
D. 2.19

49. The average life of a radionuclide is
A. The sum of the lifetimes of all the individual atoms divided by the total number of atoms present originally
B. Number of disintegrations per second of a radioactive source (activity)
C. The thickness of a given material needed to reduce the intensity of a photon beam to 50 % of its initial value (HVL)
D. The time necessary for a radioactive material to decay to 50 % of its original activity (half-life)

50. TAR at Dmax is equal to:
A. PDD
B. BSF
C. TPR
D. SAR

51. Calculate the hinge angle used in order to get the most homogeneous dose distribution in a wedged pair technique if 45° wedges are used.
A. 157.5°
B. 67.5°
C. 90°
D. 315°

52. One method for correcting tissue inhomogeneities and used to remove the SSD dependence is:
A. SAR
B. Clarkson's method
C. TAR
D. TMR

53. Use the following table to calculate the dose (cGy) received at 7 cm if a plan was done using 180 cGy at a depth of 5 cm, 100 SSD, 20×20 field size, and 10 MV to a PA spine.

Table 14.2. Test 2

Depth/PDD	6×6	15×15	20×20
5	91.8	92.3	92.5
7	83.2	84.5	84.9
10	71.8	74	74.7
Output Dmax			
100 SSD	0.972	1.034	1.053
100 SAD	1.025	1.072	1.094

A. 197 cGy
B. 165 cGy
C. 152 cGy
D. 213 cGy

54. What will be the percentage change in PDD if a patient is planned with 10 MV using 110 SSD at a depth of 15 cm but the physician changes the treatment area to be extended 4 cm more and the SSD changes to 120 cm?
A. 1.6 % increase
B. 0.9 % increase
C. 1.6 % decrease
D. No change in PPD%

55. Calculate the dose received by each field if a patient is treated using opposed fields AP/PA RT hip weighted 2:1 at the isocenter for a daily dose of 250 cGy.
A. AP: 125 cGy, PA: 125 cGy
B. AP: 200 cGy, PA: 50 cGy
C. AP: 170 cGy, PA: 80 cGy
D. AP: 167 cGy, PA: 83 cGy

56. The appropriate device to check a spill area is:
A. Geiger-Müller counters
B. Ionization chambers
C. Cutie Pie
D. Proportional counters

57. Which of the following statements is/are true?
A. Coherent scattering probability decreases with high atomic number (Z) materials and with photons of low energy.
B. Photoelectric effect probability increases with low atomic number (Z^3) materials and with higher energy photons (E^{-3}).
C. Compton scattering probability also increases with decreasing energy (E^{-1}); it depends on the number of electrons per gram of material and is independent of Z.
D. Pair production probability decreases with increasing atomic number (Z) and at lower energy photons greater or equal to 1.02 MeV.

58. Planning with 5-field fixed-gantry-angle IMRT for prostate cancer, normalized to body maximum, what is the typical isodose line to be chosen?
A. It depends on cases, but normally 95 % or better.
B. Normally around 90 %.
C. Above 99 %.
D. A perfect IMRT plan should use 70 % isodose line.

59. Calculate the dose received by each field if a patient is planned using three-field rectum technique, PA/ RT/LT lateral weighted 3:2:1 at the isocenter for a daily dose of 200 cGy.
A. PA, 78 cGy; RT, 68 cGy; LT, 54 cGy
B. PA, 33 cGy; RT, 67 cGy; LT, 100 cGy
C. PA, 100 cGy; RT, 67 cGy; LT, 33 cGy
D. PA, 200 cGy; RT, 1 cGy; LT, 1 cGy

60. The personal badge holder open window will determine:
A. Alpha particles
B. Beta particles
C. Photon beam energies
D. Gamma particles

61. The decay constant of Co-60 is higher than the decay constant of Cs-137.
A. True
B. False

62. Calculate the new TMR if a patient is treated to the LT hip using 6 MV, 12 × 12 field size for 250 cGy to midplain, SSD of 92.5, 98 % IDL, separation of 15 cm, and TMR of 0.685, but the SSD is changed to 110 cm.
A. 0.685
B. 0.814
C. 0.484
D. 0.772

63. CyberKnife IGRT uses:
A. I, II, and III
B. I and III only
C. II and IV only
D. IV only
E. All are correct
I. A set of paired orthogonal x-ray imagers to determine the location of the lesion in the room coordinate system
II. Axial CT images that serve as a base for the determination of a set of digitally reconstructed radiograph (DRR) images
III. A coordinate system that communicates to the robotic arm, which adjusts the pointing of the linac beam to maintain alignment with the target
IV. Online tracking of target motion

64. An LT breast plan is done using 200 cGy daily for 25 TX to 100 % to the isocenter. The plan reveals a hot spot of 108 %. How hot does the plan will become if the physician decides to renormalize it to 90 % IDL to the isocenter?
A. 108 %
B. 120 %
C. 83 %
D. 140 %

65. A Microtron generator is
A. A device that accelerates electrons in a circular orbit using a magnetic field with an accelerating tube shaped like a hallow doughnut
B. An electron accelerator that combines the principles of both the linear accelerator and the cyclotron
C. A charged particle accelerator, mainly used for nuclear physics research
D. A device that uses radioisotope sources to treat at extended distances

14.2 Practice Test II: Questions

66. On a brachytherapy treatment of the cervix, Point A is defined as
A. 2 cm superior to the lateral vaginal fornix and 2 cm lateral to the cervical canal
B. 2 cm superior to the external cervical os and 2 cm lateral to the cervical canal
C. 2 cm superior to the internal cervical os and 2 cm lateral to the cervical canal
D. 2 cm inferior to the lateral vaginal fornix and 2 cm lateral to the cervical canal

67. Calculate the total dose at Dmax if a dose of 200 cGy at midline is delivered using parallel-opposed brain fields, field size of 20×20, output factor of 1.089, TMR of 0.858, and RT/LT lat SSD 90 cm with a block covering the face (tray factor of 0.980).
A. 136.9 cGy
B. 69.9 cGy
C. 206.8 cGy
D. 230.2 cGy

68. Calculate the wedge factor if the output of a beam is 0.700 without the wedge and 0.350 with the wedge.
A. 2.000
B. 0.500
C. 1.050
D. 0.350

69. How many cm of lung is equivalent to 1 cm of water or tissue?
A. 5 cm
B. 3 cm
C. 2 cm
D. 10 cm

70. Which of the following Cerrobend cutout thickness will be optimal to adequately stop an electron beam using 12 MeV energy?
A. 6 mm Cerrobend thickness cutout
B. 7.2 mm Cerrobend thickness cutout
C. 8 mm Cerrobend thickness cutout
D. 4.5 mm Cerrobend thickness cutout

71. Which of the following is a general reaction for α particle decay process?
A. $^{A}_{Z}X \rightarrow {^{A}_{Z-1}}Y + {^{0}_{-1}}b + n + Q$
B. $^{A}_{Z}X \rightarrow {^{A}_{Z-1}}Y + {^{0}_{1}}\beta + v + Q$
C. $^{A}_{Z}X \rightarrow {^{A-4}_{Z-2}}Y + {^{4}_{2}}He + Q$
D. $^{A}_{Z}X + {^{0}_{-1}}e \rightarrow {^{A}_{Z-1}}Y + v + Q$

72. Some strategies used to maximize dose to the tumor while minimizing dose to surrounding tissue are
A. I, II, and III
B. I and III only
C. II and IV only
D. IV only
E. All are correct

I. Increasing the number of fields
II. Selecting appropriate beam direction
III. Adjusting beam weights
IV. Using appropriate beam energy

73. The ionization chamber used for isodose measurements should
A. I, II, and III
B. I and III only
C. II and IV only
D. IV only
E. All are correct
I. Be small (sensitive volume less than 15 mm long and inside diameter of 5 mm or less)
II. Be energy dependent
III. Be energy independent
IV. Be as big as possible to cover the beam

74. The treatment planning process is based on
A. I, II, and III
B. I and III only
C. II and IV only
D. IV only
E. All are correct
I. Pathology
II. Staging
III. Diagnostic exams
IV. Karnofsky score

75. What would be approximately the wedge angle (in degree) used to get the most homogeneous dose distribution for the following diagram?

Fig. 14.7 Test 2

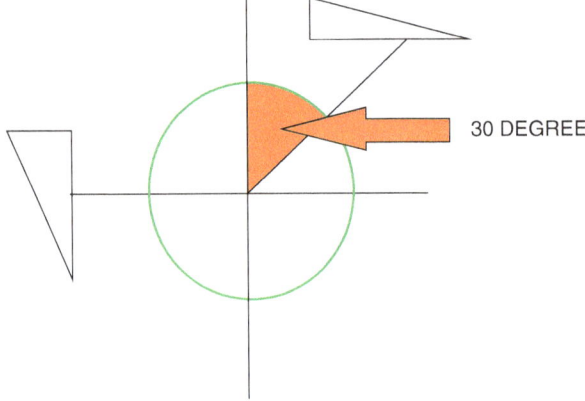

A. 60
B. 45
C. 30
D. 15

76. The gross tumor volume (GTV)
A. Demonstrates the tumor(s) if present and any other tissue with presumed tumor or microscopic disease
B. Demonstrates the extent and location of the visible tumor only
C. Compensates for internal physiological movements and variation in size, shape, and position of the CTV
D. Includes CTV with ITV and setup margin for patient movement and setup uncertainties

77. Which of the AAPM TG report refers to brachytherapy source dose calculation?
A. TG-51
B. TG-43
C. TG-21
D. TG-40

78. The highest dose in the target area that covers a minimum of 2 cm² is called:
A. Hot spots
B. Mean target dose
C. Maximum target dose
D. Modal target dose

79. What is the energy of a photon emitted from a characteristic process where a transition involved an electron descending from the L shell with a binding energy of 1.100 KeV to the K shell with a binding energy of 8.980 KeV?
A. 8.163 KeV
B. 7.880 KeV
C. 10.08 KeV
D. 9.878 KeV

80. An electron beam emanates from:
A. The physical source
B. The virtual point
C. The target
D. The cutout

81. Electron beam obliquity tends to:
A. I, II, and III
B. I and III only
C. II and IV only
D. IV only
E. All are correct
I. Increase side scatter at Dmax
II. Decrease the depth of penetration
III. Shift Dmax toward the surface
IV. Shift Dmax away from the surface

82. The correct fractional weighted contribution for two fields (RT_LT laterals) is
A. RT Lat=RT/RT−LT; LT Lat=LT/LT−RT
B. RT Lat=RT−RT/LT; LT Lat=LT−RT/LT
C. RT Lat=RT/RT+LT; LT Lat=LT/LT+RT
D. RT Lat=RT×RT−LT; LT Lat=LT×LT−RT

83. Bolus is often used in electron beam therapy to:
A. I, II, and III
B. I and III only
C. II and IV only
D. IV only
E. All are correct
I. Flatten out an irregular surface
II. Reduce the penetration of the electrons in parts of the field
III. Increase the surface dose
IV. Increase the depth dose

84. The required thickness of Cerrobend is approximately
A. 50 % greater than that of pure lead
B. 30 % greater than that of pure lead
C. 20 % greater than that of pure lead
D. Equal to that of pure lead

85. As a rule of thumb, the minimum thickness of lead required for blocking of electrons in mm is given by
A. Electron energy in MeV/4
B. Electron energy in MeV/2
C. Electron energy in MeV×2
D. Electron energy in MeV +4

86. The penumbra of a Cobalt-60 teletherapy beam is
A. Smaller than that of a linear accelerator
B. Bigger than that of a linear accelerator
C. Same as that of a linear accelerator
D. Smaller on the on position and bigger on the off position than that of the linear accelerator

87. Which of the following is the key device to form a LAN of a series of computers, iPhones, and printers?
A. Phone lines
B. Router
C. Operating system for multiple users
D. Outlets

88. Which of the following cases has the most substantial change of dose due to electron backscatter?
A. Lung–tissue interface
B. Shielding shape
C. Tissue-lead interface
D. Bone–tissue interface

89. A linear accelerator vault is designed to be within ALARA level 1, as a rule of thumb, what is normal shielding on walls?
A. 1TVL or 3.2HVLs
B. 2TVLs
C. 3TVLs
D. 4TVLs

90. The physician wants to treat the lower lip which measures 2 cm thick using a 9 MeV electron beam. What is the thickness of lead required in order to protect the structures beyond the lips?
A. 2 mm
B. 2.5 cm
C. 2.5 mm
D. 4.5 cm

91. A superficial tumor along curve surfaces such as chest wall or ribs is better treated with
A. Multiple abutting electron fields
B. Electron arc therapy
C. Rapid arc photon therapy
D. Pseudo-arc technique

92. The benchmark test indicates
A. Creating a patient model based on the standard CT data
B. That all beam technique functions work, using a standard beam description provided by the vendor (beam description)
C. The dose calculations for single- and multiple-source implant (brachytherapy dose calculations)
D. The accuracy of the dose calculation algorithm under very specific circumstances with specific beam data

93. Gamma Knife and CyberKnife are all for radiosurgery; however, the difference between those two modalities is:
A. Gamma Knife is equivalent to 3D-CRT, whereas CyberKnife is equivalent to IMRT in linear accelerator.
B. Gamma Knife can treat larger lesions.
C. CyberKnife plans are more conformal because there are more beams.
D. Gamma Knife has better homogeneity in dose.

94. What is the goal of IMRT optimization?
A. Find the local minimum of the cost function.
B. Find the global minimum of the cost function.
C. Find the local maximum of the cost function.
D. Find the global maximum of the cost function.

95. Consider the margin from CTV to PTV, which statement below is right?
A. IMRT has smaller margin than 3D-CRT, because IMRT uses optimization.
B. The margin is irrelevant to modality either IMRT or 3D-CRT.
C. IMRT can use IGRT, whereas 3D-CRT cannot; thus, IMRT has smaller PTV than 3D-CRT.
D. Those two modalities of treatment are not comparable.

96. A tumor 10 cm deep needs to be treated using 100 SSD, 25×20 cm field size on the tumor. If a 1 cm bolus is placed on the skin, what will be the new field size on the tumor?
A. 25×20
B. 20.45×16.36
C. 22.5×18
D. 30.5×24.4

97. Penumbra is independent of:
A. Source-to-diaphragm distance
B. Source diameter
C. Field size
D. Source-to-surface distance

98. Planning with VMAT for prostate cancer, normalized to body maximum, what is the typical isodose line to be chosen?
A. It depends on cases, but normally 95 % or better.
B. Normally around 90%.
C. Above 99 %.
D. A perfect IMRT plan should use 70 % isodose line.

99. What is the name of the optimization object of IMRT?
A. IMRT fluence
B. Cost function
C. MLC optimization algorithm
D. Iteration function

100. The main component(s) of the Gamma Knife unit is/are
A. I, II, and III
B. I and III only
C. II and IV only
D. IV only
E. All are correct
I. Radiation unit with an upper hemispherical shield and a central body
II. An operating table and sliding cradle
III. A set of four collimator helmets providing circular beams
IV. A robotic arm that holds the gantry

101. Which of the following parts of the x-ray tube contains the filament and focusing cup?
A. The anode
B. The cathode
C. The transformer
D. The rectified

102. Which of the following dose is categorized as low-dose TBI?
A. Single fraction or up to six fractions of total dose 1,200 cGy
B. Ten to fifteen fractions of 10–15 cGy each
C. Single fraction of 8 Gy delivered to the upper or lower half body
D. Twenty fractions with total dose of 40 Gy

103. Phantom scatter factor (Sp)
A. I, II, and III only
B. I and III only
C. II and IV only
D. IV only
E. All are correct
I. Takes into account the change in scatter radiation originating in the phantom at a reference depth as the field size is changed
II. Is the ratio of the dose rate for a given field at a reference depth to the dose rate at the same depth for the reference field size, with the same collimator opening
III. Is related to changes in the volume of the phantom irradiated for a fixed collimator opening
IV. If backscatter factors can be measured, Sp at Dmax may be defined as the ratio of BSF for the given field to that for the reference field.

104. Which of the following are total body irradiation techniques?
A. I, II, and III
B. I and III only
C. II and IV only
D. IV only
E. All are correct
I. Two short SSD parallel opposed beams
II. A dedicated TBI Cobalt-60
III. Extended SSD with patient standing
IV. Extended SSD with patient on a stretcher

105. Calculate the MU setting for each beam if a total of 250 cGy is to be delivered at a depth of 15 cm using a 12 × 12 cm field size, 10 MV from parallel opposed brain fields. The patient has been setup at 100 cm SAD.

TMR = (12 × 12 at depth 15) = 0.731

Output factor at 100 SAD = 1.023 cGy/MU

Backscatter factor (BSF) 12 × 12 = 1.035

PDD (12 × 12, depth 15 cm, 100 SSD) = 58.5
A. 97 MU
B. 33 MU
C. 323 MU
D. 162 MU

106. The formula to approximate the mean or average energy of the photon is:

A. $E = h\nu$
B. $E_{avg} = 1/5\, E_{max}$
C. $E_{avg} = 0.33/E_{max}$
D. $E_{avg} = 1/3\, E_{max}$

107. Which of the following dosimetric parameters is/are considered on large total skin electron irradiation (TSEI)?
A. I, II, and III
B. I and III only
C. II and IV only
D. IV only
E. All are correct
I. Field flatness at Dmax
II. Electron beam output at dose calibration point
III. PDDs measured at a depth of 15 cm
IV. TMR measured at a depth of 15 cm

108. Which of the following statements is/are true about intraoperative radiotherapy (IORT)?
A. I, II, and III
B. I and III only
C. II and IV only
D. IV only
E. All are correct
I. IORT is a single-fraction special radiotherapeutic technique.
II. IORT delivers radiation dose of the order of 10–20 Gy.
III. IORT combines surgery and radiotherapy conventional modalities of cancer treatment.
IV. Once the IORT is performed, external beam radiotherapy cannot be done in the same area.

109. Endorectal treatments technique includes
A. I, II, and III
B. I and III only
C. II and IV only
D. IV only
E. All are correct
I. Short SSD technique of the order of 4 cm
II. Tumor dose 80 Gy delivered in two or three fractions of 20–30 Gy given 2 weeks apart
III. Long SSD technique of the order of 20 cm
IV. Short SSD technique of the order of 10 cm

110. Stereotactic radiosurgery CyberKnife treatments require
A. I, II, and III
B. I and III only
C. II and IV only

D. IV only
E. All are correct
I. High precision
II. Steep gradient
III. Reliability
IV. Reproducibility

111. The F factor is:
A. The Roentgen-to-rad conversion factor
B. Relate dose in air to dose in tissue
C. Conversion of exposure to absorbed dose
D. The rad-to-Roentgen conversion factor

112. Which of the following planning system is used in CyberKnife?
A. AAA calculation
B. Pencil beam calculation
C. Monte Carlo calculation
D. Acuros

113. In the film badge or OSL badge, there are three small pieces of metals inside (copper, tin, and aluminum). What are the functions of those metal pieces?
A. To attenuate the radiation
B. To monitor the energy of the radiation
C. To frame the badge
D. To generate secondary particles for imaging

114. The source-to-axis distance (SAD) on a CyberKnife machine is
A. 150 cm SAD
B. 100 cm SAD
C. 80 cm SAD
D. 50 cm SAD

115. Which of the following isotopes of iodine is used to treat thyroid cancer?
A. I-123
B. I-124
C. I-125
D. I-131

116. What is Calypso® 4D localization systems used for?
A. Intra-fractional prostate motion tracking
B. Inter-fractional prostate motion tracking
C. Intra-fractional prostate motion monitoring
D. Inter-fractional prostate motion monitoring

117. What technique is used to find the solution in IMRT optimization?
A. Least square
B. Stimulated annealing
C. Standard deviation

D. Analytic methods

118. Which of the following are components of Calypso® 4D systems?
A. I, II, III, and IV
B. II, III, and IV
C. I, III, and IV
D. All of them
I. 4D electromagnetic array
II. Implanted electromagnetic transponders
III. 4D console inside treatment room
IV. 4D tracking system
V. Infrared cameras and optic targets

119. TAR depends on:
A. I, II, and III only
B. I and III only
C. II and IV only
D. IV only
E. All are correct
I. Field size
II. Depth
III. SAD
IV. Distance

120. IGRT adaptive radiotherapy:
A. Modifies dose delivery for subsequent treatment fractions of a course of radiotherapy
B. Modifies patient position for subsequent treatment fractions of a course of radiotherapy
C. Alternates CBCT and orthogonal x-ray images for subsequent treatment fractions of a course of radiotherapy
D. Alternates CBCT and ultrasound images for subsequent treatment fractions of a course of radiotherapy

121. A treatment setup is done at 100 SSD using a 110×150 mm on the skin; what is the field size 25 in. below the surface where the tumor lies?
A. 125×187.5 mm
B. 179.3×245.25 mm
C. 179.3×245.25 cm
D. 125×187.5 cm

122. IGRT adaptive radiotherapy is useful on
A. I, II, and III
B. I and III only
C. II and IV only
D. IV only
E. All are correct
I. Tumor shrinkage
II. Patient loss of weight
III. Increased hypoxia due to fractionated treatment

IV. Patient movement

123. A patient is planning using 250 cGy/fx at 100 SSD to the spine at a depth of 5 cm; what will be the dose received at 5 cm depth if the optical distance indicator (ODI) is misled and the therapist read 100 SSD when in reality it is 115 SSD?
A. 189 cGy
B. 217 cGy
C. 330 cGy
D. 200 cGy

124. CyberKnife treatment robot couch
A. Contains six degrees of freedom.
B. Contains three degrees of freedom.
C. It is not able to pitch.
D. Can rotate but no translation is allowed.

125. Which of the following electron fields has the highest PDD?
A. I only
B. II only
C. III only
D. IV only
E. All have the same PDD
I. 10×10
II. 10×15
III. 10×20
IV. 20×20

126. Which of the following equations is/are correct?
A. I, II, and III
B. I and III only
C. II and IV only
D. IV only
E. All are correct
I. $SinX° = OPP/HYP$
II. $TangX° = OPP/ADJ$
III. $CosX° = ADJ/HYP$
IV. $CosX° = HYP/ADJ$

127. CyberKnife robot motion is based on
A. Isocenter rotation only
B. Gantry angles designed by the planner
C. Spiral rotation
D. Path and nodes

128. Adaptive radiotherapy was proposed in recently, which requested a replanning once every 1–3 fractions in hyperfractionation. Will this method help in minimizing the setup uncertainty?
A. Not really, since it focuses on replanning due to target's changing with time.
B. Sure, replanning reduces the setup uncertainty because the new plan follows the change of target.
C. Actually, it depends on whether the target changes with time or not.
D. It is too early to judge this since it is too new.

129. Source-to-skin distance is
A. SSD=SAD−d
B. SSD=SAD+d
C. SSD=SAD/d
D. SSD=SAD×d

130. An abdomen AP/PA field technique was calculated using 30° wedges (transmission factor of 0.82), hinge angle of 120° for a total of 244 MU to deliver 200 cGy to the isocenter. What is the dose received by the patient if the therapist forgot to insert the AP wedge and the patient was treated?
A. 364
B. 182
C. 100
D. 222

131. Compare standard IMRT to 3D conformal radiotherapy.
A. Standard IMRT is superior in both curing the disease and sparing normal tissue doses than 3D CRT.
B. Standard IMRT is superior in sparing normal tissue dose but unnecessarily better in curing the disease than 3D CRT.
C. 3D CRT is superior in curing the disease but worse in sparing normal tissue dose than standard IMRT.

132. The exposure rate of a radionuclide at any particular point is
A. Proportional to the product of its mass and its exposure rate constant
B. Proportional to the product of its activity and its exposure rate constant
C. Proportional to its milligram of radium equivalent
D. Proportional to the air-kerma strength

133. An ^{125}I source implant was performed on a patient on June 15, 2012, with the intention to deliver 70 Gy to the tumor. Due to an emergency, the sources were removed on September 1, 2012. Calculate what dose was delivered to the tumor.
A. 89 cGy
B. 5,987 cGy
C. 4,187 cGy
D. 7,210 cGy

14.2 Practice Test II: Questions

134. Stochastic effect is defined as:
A. The probability of occurrence increases with increasing absorbed dose, but the severity in affected individuals does not depend on the magnitude of the absorbed dose.
B. The probability increases in severity with increasing absorbed dose in affected individuals.
C. The probability of occurrence decreases with increasing absorbed dose, but the severity in affected individuals does not depend on the magnitude of the absorbed dose.
D. The probability of occurrence increases with decreasing absorbed dose as well as severity in affected individuals.

135. Which of the following organizations established or proposed a general dose-specification system to be adopted universally?
A. International Commission on Radiation Units and Measurements (ICRU).
B. Nuclear Regulatory Commission (NRC).
C. National Council on Radiation Protection and Measurements (NCRP).
D. Atomic Energy Commission (AEC).
E. 3D CRT is superior in both curing the disease and in sparing normal tissue dose than standard IMRT.

136. The optical density, OD, is defined as:
A. $\log (I_0 \times I_t)$
B. $\log (I_0/I_t)$
C. $\log (I_0 - I_t)$
D. $\log (I_0 + I_t)$

137. The optical density of the film is measured by
A. Densitometer
B. Extrapolation chamber
C. Electrometer
D. TLD

138. ALARA stands for:
A. As low as radiation association
B. At lower absolute radiation achievable
C. As low as reasonably achievable
D. As longer as radiation acquired

139. CyberKnife offers the following improvements over standard radiosurgical techniques:
A. I, II, and III
B. I and III only
C. II and IV only
D. IV only
E. All are correct
I. It allows frameless radiosurgery.

II. It monitors and tracks the patient's position continuously.
III. It allows for frameless radiosurgical dose delivery to extracranial targets such as spine, lung, and prostate.
IV. It allows the patient to move during treatment without affecting the treatment.

140. The best method to reduce the neutron influence incident at the door is:
A. By building a maze of any dimension
B. By building a maze longer than 5 m
C. By adding lead shielding to the door
D. By adding steel shielding to the door

141. Some of the benign lesions treated by stereotactic radiosurgery (SRS) are
A. I, II, and III
B. I and III only
C. II and IV only
D. IV only
E. All are correct
I. Meningiomas
II. Acoustic neuromas
III. Arteriovenous malformations (AVM)
IV. Gliomas

142. Calculate the MU per field setting to deliver a total of 200 cGy at midline if parallel-opposed brain fields are used, field size is 20×20, output factor is 1.089, TMR at 10 cm depth is 0.863, and RT/LT lat SSD is 90 cm with a block covering the face (tray factor of 0.980).
A. 215 MU
B. 218 MU
C. 94 MU
D. 109 MU

143. The initial activity of Au-198 is 15 mCi; what is the activity in 20 days if its half-value layer is 2.5?
A. 0.2556 mCi
B. 0.09036 mCi
C. 2.8931 mCi
D. 2,490 mCi

144. What is the standard method for the patient to acquire iodine isotopes to treat thyroid cancer?
A. Injection of solutions with iodine ions
B. Swallow iodine salt tabulates with juice
C. Implant iodine seeds to thyroid
D. Being exposed to radiation of iodine isotopes

145. How is the QA for whether collimator rotation influences light field centricity done?
A. Use crosshair aligned with graph paper; rotate couch 90°.
B. Use crosshair aligned with graph paper; rotate collimator 90°.
C. Use crosshair aligned with graph paper; rotate collimator 180°.
D. Use crosshair aligned with graph paper; rotate gantry 90°.

146. The major advantage of proton therapy is:
A. Good distribution of depth (Bragg peak)
B. Very sharp penumbra region
C. Range modulation
D. High-energy radiation therapy

147. The mass defect is defined as
A. A defect in the number of protons in the nucleus.
B. Every gram atomic weight of a substance contains the same number of atoms.
C. The difference in mass between an atom and the sum of the masses of its constituent particles.
D. The propagation of energy through space or a material medium.

148. A binary digit used by computer operating system is referred to as
A. Byte
B. Bit
C. Bin
D. Megabyte

149. Belly boards' main advantage(s) is/are
A. I, II, and III
B. I and III only
C. II and IV only
D. IV only
E. All are correct
I. Minimize lung dose
II. Reduce pelvic tilt
III. Reproducibility
IV. Minimize small bowel dose

150. What comes out right after IMRT optimization?
A. IMRT fluence for each field
B. IMRT dose-volume histogram
C. IMRT MLC motion file
D. MU numbers

151. What is the maximum number of electrons can 2p subshell hold?
A. 2
B. 6
C. 8
D. 18

152. Intracranial radiosurgery is better treated with:
A. Gamma Knife machine
B. Cobalt-60 radiosurgery machine
C. HDR brachytherapy
D. CyberKnife

153. Calculate the MU needed to deliver a prostate treatment using a 354° arc technique if the average TMR is known to be 0.570 and the prescription dose to the isocenter is 180 cGy.
A. 621 MU
B. 354 MU
C. 103 MU
D. 316 MU

154. Name structure C.
A. Esophagus
B. Scapula
C. Bifurcation
D. Trachea

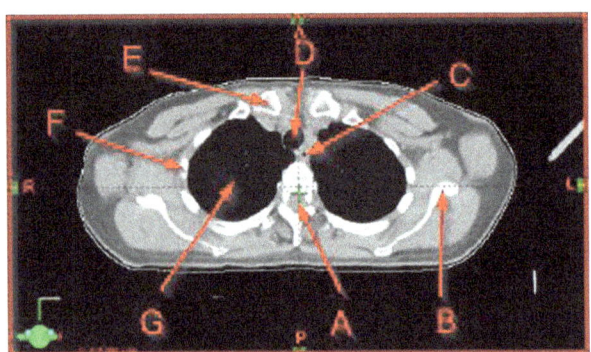

Fig. 14.8 Test 2

155. Name structure E.
A. Rectum
B. Prostate
C. Urinary bladder
D. Seminal vesicles

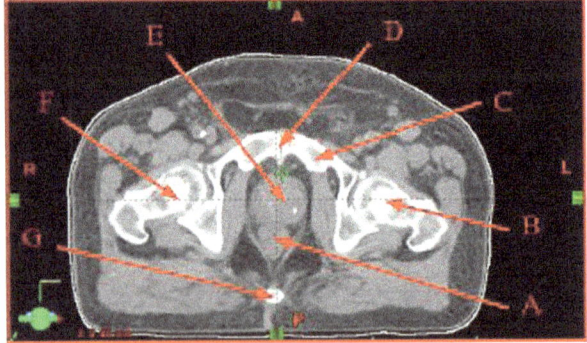

Fig. 14.9 Test 2

14.3 Practice Test III: Questions

1. Which of the following wedge types should be avoided in the medial tangent of a breast treatment?
A. I, II, and III
B. I and III only
C. II and IV only
D. IV only
E. All are correct
I. Dynamic wedge
II. Asymmetric wedge
III. Universal wedge
IV. Physical wedge

2. CyberKnife geometric isocenter
A. Is a reference point in the room which serves as the origin for several coordinate systems used within the CyberKnife application
B. Refers to an isocentric treatment to a target
C. Refers to the isocenter selected on the planning system
D. Refers to the robot cough isocenter

3. Calculate the number of atoms/g of cobalt if its atomic weight (Aw) is 58.93.
A. 3.549×10^{25}
B. 1.0220×10^{22}
C. 1.220×10^{23}
D. 9.7845×10^{23}

4. The main advantage of selective internal radiation therapy (SIRT) over a traditional method is
A. Low toxicity
B. No adverse effects
C. Curative treatment
D. Fewer treatments

5. For a polyenergetic beam,
A. $HVL_1 > HVL_2$.
B. $HVL_1 < HVL_2$.
C. $HVL_1 = HVL_2$.
D. $HVL_1 \leq HVL_2$.

6. Which of the following devices is/are used for immobilization in CNS patients?
A. Sandbags
B. Belly board
C. Wing board
D. Duncan face mask

7. According to TG-51 protocol, which of the following is calibrated with an ionization chamber in water at a depth of 10 cm?
A. Electron

B. Photon
C. Proton
D. Neutron

8. The smallest component of an element having the chemical properties of the element is
A. Element
B. Atom
C. Nucleus
D. Quarks

9. Gamma Knife and CyberKnife are all for radiosurgery; however, the difference between those 2 modalities is:
A. Gamma Knife is equivalent to 3D-CRT, whereas CyberKnife is equivalent to IMRT in linear accelerator.
B. Gamma Knife can treat larger lesions.
C. CyberKnife plans are more conformal because there are more beams.
D. Gamma Knife has better homogeneity in dose.

10. Which of the following is/are advantages of CyberKnife treatment?
A. I, II, and III
B. I and III only
C. II and IV only
D. IV only
E. All are correct
I. Frameless treatment
II. Non-isocentric
III. Fractionated treatment
IV. More complex and conformal treatment

11. Permanent prostate pre-implant treatment plan worksheet includes
A. I, II, and III
B. I and III only
C. II and IV only
D. IV only
E. All are correct
I. Number of needles to be used
II. Number of seeds in each needle
III. Template coordinates
IV. Size of the needles to be used

12. As per TG-135, which of the following QAs must be done daily on a CyberKnife machine?
A. I, II, and III
B. I and III only
C. II and IV only
D. IV only
E. All are correct

14.3 Practice Test III: Questions

I. Safety interlocks
II. Accelerator output
III. Accelerator warm-up
IV. Imager alignment

13. Suppose the rest mass of electron is m_0, and the speed is $v=0.6c$; its kinetic energy is
A. $m_0v^2/2$
B. Smaller than $m_0v^2/2$
C. Larger than $m_0v^2/2$
D. 0.511 MeV/c^2

14. Which of the following decay process is due to deficit of neutrons?
A. Internal conversion
B. Electron capture
C. Alpha particles
D. Beta minus

15. Hounsfield numbers range from
A. 1 to 100
B. −100 to +500
C. −1,000 to +1,000
D. 0 to 1,000

16. As filtration increases,
A. Higher average energy and lower penetrating power
B. Lower average energy and greater penetrating power
C. Higher average energy and greater penetrating power
D. Lower average energy and lower penetrating power

17. Which of the following methods is/are used in calculating the dose in an SAD technique?
A. I, II, and III only
B. I and III only
C. II and IV only
D. IV only
E. All are correct
I. TAR and dose rate in air
II. PDD
III. TPR and TMR
IV. Clarkson's method

18. Which of the following is the definition of ablative treatment radiosurgery?
A. Single large doses
B. Multiple small doses
C. Several large doses
D. Single small doses

19. During CyberKnife treatments, after the orthogonal x-ray images are compared to DRRs generated from CT,
A. The couch automatically adjusts its position based on the results of the comparison.
B. The patient adjusts his/her position based on the results of the comparison.
C. The robot automatically adjusts the beam's position based on the results of the comparison.
D. The therapist moves the couch based on the results of the comparison.

20. Which of the following statements are/is true about pair production?
A. I, II, and III only
B. I and III only
C. II and IV only
D. IV only
E. All are correct
I. Incident photon energy must be greater than 1.02 MeV.
II. Photon interacts with atom.
III. Photon gives up all its energy in the process.
IV. A negative electron (e−) and a positive electron (e+) are created.

21. For standard ^{60}Co source change, all 201 sources of 6600Ci in total need to be replaced. What type of shipping package is needed?
A. NRC has to handle this since the activity is too strong.
B. Type C package.
C. Type B package.
D. Type A package.
E. Strong tight container.

22. The BAT system is most commonly used for:
A. Prostate localization
B. Liver mets localization
C. Brain boost localization
D. Pancreas localization

23. From the following table, calculate the MU setting to deliver 200 cGy using 10 MV at a depth of 7.5–25×25 cm field size at 100 SSD.
A. 215 MU
B. 195 MU
C. 221 MU
D. 200 MU

Table 14.3. Test 3

	F.S	6×6	10×10	15×15	20×20	30×30
PDD	2	98.0	98.0	99.0	99.0	99.5
	5	91.8	92.1	92.3	92.5	92.7
	10	71.8	73.0	74.0	74.7	75.7
	15	56.2	57.9	59.3	60.4	61.8
	18	48.5	50.4	52.0	53.1	54.8

14.3 Practice Test III: Questions

Table 14.3. (continued)

TMR	2	0.970	0.970	0.980	0.980	0.985
	5	0.963	0.966	0.968	0.970	0.972
	10	0.824	0.838	0.850	0.858	0.869
	15	0.701	0.723	0.741	0.753	0.772
	18	0.634	0.659	0.680	0.695	0.717
Output at 2 cm, SSD 100		1.030	1.045	1.063	1.070	1.085
Output at 2 cm, SAD 100		1.042	1.051	1.072	1.089	1.120

24. According to the atomic mass unit, the mass of a neutron is
A. No mass
B. 1.00727 amu
C. 0.000548 amu
D. 1.00866 amu

25. What is the purpose of using klystron?
A. I and II
B. III and IV
C. I, III, and IV
D. All
I. To increase the amplitude of accelerating voltage
II. To increase the total number of electrons in waveguide
III. To make electrons in waveguide into bunches thus to pulse the x-ray
IV. To increase the energy of electrons in waveguide

26. A group of bytes is
A. A bit
B. A field
C. A file
D. A record

27. The reference point used to record target dose recommended by the ICRU for parallel opposed, unequally weighted beams
A. Should be specified at the center of rotation in the principal plane
B. Should be on the central axis midway between the beam entrances
C. Should be specified on the central axis placed within the PTV
D. Should be at the intersection of the central axes of the beams placed within the PTV

28. Hydrogen gas is filled into thyratron; what is the correct pressure and what is the gas for?
A. 0.5 psi, used as conductor
B. 0.5 Torr, used as conductor
C. 0.5 psi, used as insulator
D. 0.5 Torr, used as insulator

29. Which of the following parameters is/are considered during the radiation survey performed by the physicist after installation on new equipment?
A. I, II, and III only
B. I and III only
C. II and IV only
D. IV only
E. All are correct
I. Dose rate output
II. Machine on time
III. Use factor
IV. Occupational factors

30. Inherent filtration refers to:
A. Absorption of the photons through a filter placed externally to the tube
B. Absorption of the photons through the target, glass walls of the tube, or thin beryllium window
C. The placement of a flattening filter in the beam path
D. Shielding against leakage radiation

31. What are the differences between LDR and HDR system?
A. LDR devices use multiple sources, together with inactive spacers, to achieve typical treatment dose rates of about 0.4–2 Gy/h; HDR systems use a single source, with a typical activity of 10–20 Ci.
B. LDR systems use a single source, with a typical activity of 0.4–2 Gy/h; HDR devices use multiple sources, together with inactive spacers, to achieve typical treatment dose rates of about 10–20 Ci.
C. LDR devices use multiple sources, together with inactive spacers, to achieve typical treatment dose rates of about 0.4–12 Gy/h; HDR systems use a single source, with a typical activity of 0.4–2 Gy/h.
D. LDR systems use a single source, with a typical activity of 0.4–12 cGy/h; HDR devices use multiple sources, together with inactive spacers, to achieve typical treatment dose rates of about 0.4–2 cGy/h.

32. Which of the following is/are true about the five Rs of radiotherapy?
A. I, II, and III
B. I and III only
C. II and IV only
D. IV only
E. All are correct
I. Cells repopulate while receiving fractionated doses of radiation.
II. Redistribution in proliferating cell populations throughout the cell cycle phases increases the cell kill from a fractionated treatment relative to a single session treatment.
III. Reoxygenation of hypoxic cells occurs during a fractionated course of treatment, making them more radiosensitive to subsequent doses of radiation.
IV. Cells can repair from radiation damage.

33. The basal dose is defined as
A. The average of the maximum dose between sources

14.3 Practice Test III: Questions   819

B. The average of the minimum dose between sources
C. The maximum dose in the plane of treatment (state dose)
D. The total dose contribution from each point

34. Ring dosimeters:
A. I, II, and III only
B. I and III only
C. II and IV only
D. IV only
E. All are correct
I. Should be worn when there is a possibility of significant exposure to the hand
II. Should be worn on the hand that is favored
III. Should be usually worn on the index finger, which receives the greatest exposure
IV. Should be worn under gloves to protect it from contamination

35. TMR is a special case of:
A. TPR
B. SAR
C. SMR
D. Backscatter factor

36. CyberKnife safety zone is
A. The distance between the robot position and virtual obstacle
B. The distance between the robot point of radiation and the personnel
C. Where radiation is bellow tolerance
D. The distance between the robot and the couch

37. CyberKnife IGRT is based on:
A. A pair of orthogonal x-ray images to determine the location of the lesion in the target relative to the room's coordinate system
B. A cart-based ultrasound unit positioned next to a linac treatment table to image the target volume prior to each fraction of a patient's radiotherapy
C. A reflective marker array attached to an ultrasound probe using an infrared tracking system relative to reflective markers attached to patient
D. A conventional x-ray tube mounted on a retractable arm at 90° to the high-energy treatment beam and a flat panel x-ray detector mounted on a retractable arm opposite the x-ray tube

38. Clarkson's method is used to calculate:
A. Circular fields
B. Irregular fields
C. Rectangular fields
D. Square fields

39. SAD is equal to
A. SSD−depth
B. SSD+depth

C. SSD/depth
D. SSD×depth

40. For pair production to take place, the threshold energy of the incident photon must be:
A. Equal to 0.51 MeV
B. Greater than 1.02 MeV
C. Greater than 2.04 MeV
D. Less than 1.02 MeV

41. Which of the following materials is used for the measurement of HVL?
A. Aluminum (AL), Cerrobend, or tin (Sn)
B. Aluminum (AL), copper (Cu), or tungsten
C. Lipowitz copper (Cu) or tin (Sn)
D. Aluminum (AL), copper (Cu), or tin (Sn)

42. The International Commission on Radiation Units and Measurements (ICRU) recommends that dose delivered to a tumor to be
A. Within 5.0 % of the prescribed dose
B. Within 8.0 % of the prescribed dose
C. Within 10.0 % of the prescribed dose
D. Within 15.0 % of the prescribed dose

43. From the following Helman brain field, calculate the effective equivalent square.
A. 14.9 cm2
B. 14.3 cm2
C. 2.5 cm2
D. 16 cm²

Fig. 14.10 Test 3

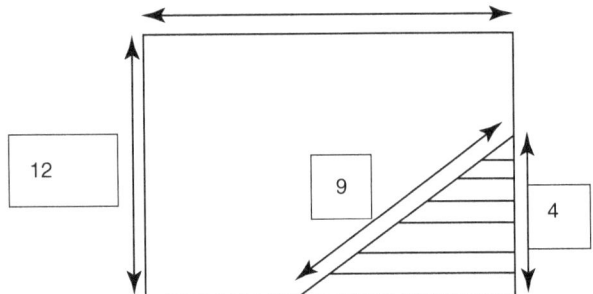

44. Which of the following is/are correct about planning organ at risk (OR)?
A. I, II, and III
B. I and III only
C. II and IV only
D. IV only
E. All are correct

I. It needs adequate protection.
II. All organs at risk need the same margins.
III. It needs margins to compensate for its movements, internal as well as setup.
IV. It is not of importance if abutting with the plan tumor volume (PTV).

45. CyberKnife skull tracking has an accuracy of:
A. 5 mm translation error; 5° rotation error
B. 0.5 mm translation error; 0.5° rotation error
C. 0.5 mm translation error; 10° rotation error
D. 10 mm translation error; 0.5° rotation error

46. Tomotherapy system includes:
A. I, II, and III
B. I and III only
C. II and IV only
D. IV only
E. All are correct
I. IMRT treatment using 6MV linear accelerator
II. A CT type gantry ring that rotates around the patient
III. A couch that advances the patient through the gantry bore
IV. IMRT treatment using dual energy (6 and 18 MV)

47. What is the annual occupational maximum permissible dose (MPD) for the lens of eye?
A. 50 mSv or 5 rem/year.
B. 15 mSv or 150 rem/year.
C. 5 mSv or 0.5 rem/year.
D. 150 mSv or 15 rem/year.

48. On Bremsstrahlung interaction, the rate of energy loss on an electron beam per cm is proportional to
A. I, II, and III
B. I and III only
C. II and IV only
D. IV only
E. All are correct
I. Electron energy
II. Electron mass
III. Square of the atomic number (Z^2)
IV. Rest mass of an electron 0.511

49. A patient threw away his immobilization mask before being treated to the neck with a boost plan, what should the therapists do? Assume the linear accelerator has KV imaging capabilities.

A. Make a new mask for the patient at linear accelerator couch, and treat with the original boost plan.
B. Redo a CT with a new mask, and ask the dosimetrist to replan the boost using the new CT.
C. Forget about the mask since it was already lost. Ask the dosimetrist to do a simple plan like bilateral or AP/PA fields for the same dose.
D. Treat the patient without the mask.

50. Calculate the collimator rotation required to align a 20×20 cm craniospinal field isocentric at 100 SAD with an adjacent PA spine field which is 40 cm in length at 100 SSD.
A. 21.8°
B. 11.3°
C. 78.7°
D. 15.2°

51. Which of the following particles is emitted on a beta plus (β^+) decay process?
A. Internal conversion
B. An electron
C. A positron
D. An alpha particle
E. A negatron

52. A temporary implant of ^{192}Ir has been scheduled for Monday, 1st at 8:00 a.m. in your department; the physician wants to deliver 15 Gy and the initial dose rate of ^{192}Ir source is 0.6 Gy/h. When must the source be removed so that the patient receives the correct dose?
A. Wednesday, 3rd at 8:00 a.m.
B. Monday, 1st at 10:00 p.m.
C. Tuesday, 2nd at 9:00 a.m.
D. Thursday, 4th at 10:00 a.m.

53. A meson is composed of
A. A quark and an antiquark of the same flavor
B. A quark and an antiquark of different flavors
C. 2 quarks or 2 antiquarks of different flavors
D. 2 quarks or 2 antiquarks of the same flavor

54. The appropriate device to check a spill area is:
A. Geiger-Müller counters
B. Ionization chambers
C. Cutie Pie
D. Proportional counters

14.3 Practice Test III: Questions   823

55. Calculate the correction to an ionization chamber reading ($P_{t,p}$) if the treatment room temperature is 21 °C and the pressure is 772 mm mercury.
A. 1.980
B. 0.987
C. 0.980
D. 0.012

56. Calculate the MU setting with a wedge in place if the wedge transmission factor is 0.640 and the MU setting for a field without wedge is 300.
A. 469 MU
B. 192 MU
C. 364 MU
D. 300.6 MU

57. Which of the following particle is composed of two protons and two neutrons?
A. Hydrogen's nuclear
B. ^3He nuclear
C. Alpha particle
D. Beta minus

58. In regard to the CyberKnife's image tracking system,
A. I, II, and III
B. I and III only
C. II and IV only
D. IV only
E. All are correct
I. The patient is imaged at 45° orthogonal angles.
II. Uses two diagnostic x-ray sources and two ASI image detectors
III. Uses live x-ray images compared against DRRs generated from a CT
IV. The robot adjusts its position based on the image/DRR comparison.

59. Calculate the dose received by each field if a patient is planned using three-field rectum technique, PA/RT/LT lateral weighted 3:2:1 at the isocenter for a daily dose of 200 cGy.
A. PA, 78 cGy; RT, 68 cGy; LT, 54 cGy
B. PA, 33 cGy; RT, 67 cGy; LT, 100 cGy
C. PA, 100 cGy; RT, 67 cGy; LT, 33 cGy
D. PA, 200 cGy; RT, 1 cGy; LT, 1 cGy

60. As per NCRP recommendations, what is the maximum accumulated dose a 50-year-old occupational worker can have?
A. I, II, and III
B. I and III only

C. II and IV only
D. IV only
E. All are correct
I. 500 mSv
II. 10 mSv
III. 50 rem
IV. 1 mSv

61. Calculate the total dose at Dmax if a dose of 200 cGy at midline is delivered using parallel-opposed brain fields, field size of 20×20, output factor of 1.089, TMR of 0.858, and RT/LT lateral SSD 90 cm with a block covering the face (tray factor of 0.980).
A. 136.9 cGy
B. 69.9 cGy
C. 206.8 cGy
D. 230.2 cGy

62. The benchmark test indicates
A. Creating a patient model based on the standard CT data.
B. That all beam technique functions work, using a standard beam description provided by the vendor (beam description)
C. The dose calculations for single- and multiple-source implant (brachytherapy dose calculations)
D. The accuracy of the dose calculation algorithm under very specific circumstances with specific beam data

63. Calculate the skin dose using the following 12 MeV PDD table if a dose of 250 cGy is delivered to a tumor at a depth of 4 cm from the skin and 1 cm bolus is used.
A. 417 cGy
B. 376 cGy
C. 277 cGy
D. 225 cGy

Table 14.4 Test 3

Depth	0	1	2	3	4	5	6
PDD	90	95	98	100	80	60	10

64. What is the standard method for the patient to acquire iodine isotopes to treat thyroid cancer?
A. Injection of solutions with iodine ions.
B. Swallow iodine salt tabulates with juice.
C. Implant iodine seeds to thyroid.
D. Being exposed to radiation of iodine isotopes.

14.3   Practice Test III: Questions   825

65. Which of the following isodose lines (IDLs) in a penumbra represents the field edge or border?
A. 100 % isodose line of calculation point
B. 75 % isodose line of the prescription dose
C. 50 % isodose line of the prescription dose
D. Cannot be identified

66. On a brachytherapy treatment of the cervix:
A. The longest tandem length as well as the largest set of ovoids that fit the patient's anatomy should always be used.
B. The longest tandem length but the smallest set of ovoids should always be used.
C. The smallest tandem length as well as the smallest set of ovoids should always be used.
D. The tandem length and the size of the ovoids are not important on a brachytherapy treatment of the cervix.

67. Which of the following about isodose cures is/are correct?
A. I, II, and III
B. I and III only
C. II and IV only
D. IV only
E. All are correct
I. Are lines passing through points of equal dose
II. Are expressed as a percentage of the dose at a reference point
III. Represent levels of absorbed dose
IV. Represent the hot spot location

68. If a disagreement between the vendor and the user source calibration is within ±5 %,
A. The user calibration should be used.
B. The vendor calibration should be used.
C. The source would require recalibration by the vendor.
D. The source would require recalibration by the user.

69. When using wedge pair technique,
A. I, II, and III
B. I and III only
C. II and IV only
D. IV only
E. All are correct
I. The high-dose region (hot spot) is moved to the thick end of the wedges (hill).
II. The high-dose region (hot spot) is moved to the thin end of the wedges (toe).
III. The high-dose region (hot spot) decreases with field size and wedge angle.
IV. The high-dose region (hot spot) increases with field size and wedge angle.

70. Which of the following organizations established or proposed a general dose-specification system to be adopted universally?
A. International Commission on Radiation Units and Measurements (ICRU)
B. Nuclear Regulatory Commission (NRC)
C. National Council on Radiation Protection and Measurements (NCRP)
D. Atomic Energy Commission (AEC)

71. The dynamic collimator on CyberKnife is called
A. IRIS
B. MLC
C. Jaw
D. EDW

72. The gross tumor volume (GTV)
A. Demonstrates the tumor(s) if present and any other tissue with presumed tumor or microscopic disease
B. Demonstrates the extent and location of the visible tumor only
C. Compensates for internal physiological movements and variation in size, shape, and position of the CTV
D. Includes CTV with ITV and setup margin for patient movement and setup uncertainties

73. Which of the following is/are correct about treatment volume?
A. I, II, and III
B. I and III only
C. II and IV only
D. IV only
E. All are correct
I. It is larger than the planning target volume.
II. It is a margin added to the target volume to allow for limitations of treatment technique.
III. It depends on a particular treatment technique.
IV. It is larger than the irradiated volume.

74. Electrons interact with atoms through
A. I, II, and III
B. I and III only
C. II and IV only
D. IV only
E. All are correct
I. Inelastic collisions with atomic electrons
II. Inelastic collisions with nuclei
III. Elastic collisions with atomic electrons
IV. Elastic collisions with nuclei

14.3 Practice Test III: Questions

75. Methods of inhomogeneity corrections for photon beams are:
A. I, II, and III only
B. I and III only
C. II and IV only
D. IV only
E. All are correct
I. TAR
II. Effective SSD method
III. Isodose shift method
IV. Coefficient equivalent thickness

76. How is the QA for whether collimator rotation influences light field centricity done?
A. Use crosshair aligned with graph paper; rotate couch 90°.
B. Use crosshair aligned with graph paper; rotate collimator 90°.
C. Use crosshair aligned with graph paper; rotate collimator 180°.
D. Use crosshair aligned with graph paper; rotate gantry 90°.

77. The rate of electron energy loss depends primarily on
A. Electron density of the medium
B. Type of cutout used
C. Electron energy
D. Type of collision

78. One kilobyte equals
A. 1,048,576 bytes
B. 1,024 bytes
C. 1,073,741,824 bytes
D. 32 bytes

79. As electron beam energy increases,
A. I, II, and III
B. I and III only
C. II and IV only
D. IV only
E. All are correct
I. Dose increases
II. Surface penumbra decreases
III. Penumbra at depth increases
IV. Surface penumbra increases

80. If the linear attenuation coefficient for 23× is 0.046 mm^{-1} lead, what is the HVL thickness?
A. 0.03 mm lead
B. 15 mm lead

C. 0.066 mm lead
D. 10 mm lead

81. The tail of the electron depth dose curve at the point where it becomes straight is due to:
A. Photoelectric effect interactions of electrons with the collimator system
B. Bremsstrahlung interactions of electrons with the collimator system
C. Bremsstrahlung interactions of electrons with the target
D. Bremsstrahlung interactions of electrons with the flattening filter

82. In an electron treatment, energy should be selected based on:
A. I, II, and III
B. I and III only
C. II and IV only
D. IV only
E. All are correct
I. Depth of target volume
II. Minimum target dose required
III. Clinically acceptable dose to critical organs
IV. Field size used

83. Which of the following radiation monitors can give instantaneous reading as needed?
A. I, II, and III only
B. I and III only
C. II and IV only
D. IV only
E. All are correct
I. Pocket dosimeter
II. Thermoluminescence dosimetry (TLD)
III. Silicon diodes
IV. Film badge (radiographic film)

84. The physician wants to treat the lower lip which measures 2 cm thick using a 9 MeV electron beam. What is the thickness of lead required in order to protect the structures beyond the lips?
A. 2 mm
B. 2.5 cm
C. 2.5 mm
D. 4.5 cm

85. IMRT stands for:
A. Intensity-multiple radiation therapy
B. Intensity-modulated rotational therapy

C. Intensity-modulated radiation therapy
D. Irregular-modulated radiation therapy

86. Which of the following is/are the best method to use on radiation protection?
A. I, II, and III
B. I and III only
C. II and IV only
D. IV only
E. All are correct
I. Using the appropriate radiation monitor
II. Using the personal monitoring device at all time on the collar
III. Using a lead apron around radioactive patients
IV. Maximizing the distance

87. In standard model, a quark may have the following interactions:
A. Strong, electromagnetic, and weak
B. Strong and electromagnetic
C. Strong and weak
D. Strong only

88. What technique is used to find the solution in IMRT optimization?
A. Least square
B. Stimulated annealing
C. Standard deviation
D. Analytic methods

89. What is the name of optimization object of IMRT?
A. IMRT fluence
B. Cost function
C. MLC optimization algorithm
D. Iteration function

90. Calculate the brain field collimator angle needed to match a PA spine divergence on a craniospinal treatment where the upper spine field length is 36 cm × 8 cm at 100 SSD and the brain field is 14 cm in length by 21 cm width at midplain (100 SAD).
A. 0.18°
B. 79.7°
C. 10.2°
D. 15°

91. How many fix collimators does the CyberKnife have?
A. 5 fix collimators
B. 10 fix collimators
C. 12 fix collimators
D. 15 fix collimators

92. A plot of the volume of a given structure receiving a certain dose or higher as a function of dose is the definition of
A. Differential DVH
B. Cumulative integral DVH
C. Dose volume histogram (DVH)
D. Beam's eye view

93. What is the output factor?
A. The transmission of radiation through the edges of the collimator blocks
B. Used to bent the electron beam 90° or 270° from its original direction
C. Measure of ionization produced per unit mass on air
D. The energy absorbed in a material per unit mass

94. The source-to-axis distance (SAD) on a CyberKnife machine is
A. 150 cm SAD
B. 100 cm SAD
C. 80 cm SAD
D. 50 cm SAD

95. Calculate the dose received by each field if a patient is treated using opposed lateral fields RT/LT larynx weighted 3:1 at the isocenter for a daily dose of 180 cGy.
A. RT, 45 cGy; LT, 135 cGy
B. RT, 135 cGy; LT, 135 cGy
C. RT, 179 cGy; LT, 45 cGy
D. RT, 150 cGy; LT, 30 cGy

96. In compliance with the NRC regulations, the leakage radiation levels outside the HDR unit
A. Should not exceed 1 R/h at a distance of 10 mm with the source in the shielded position
B. Should not exceed 10 mR/h at a distance of 5 cm with the source in the shielded position
C. Should not exceed 1 mR/h at a distance of 10 cm with the source in the shielded position
D. Should not exceed 10 mR/h at a distance of 10 mm with the source in the shielded position

97. What is the function of the circulator in the microwave transmission waveguide?
A. To block the microwave reflected from klystron to accelerating waveguide
B. To allow one-way passing from klystron to accelerating waveguide
C. To isolate the N_2 (or Freon) in the transmission waveguide to the vacuum of accelerating waveguide
D. To avoid sparkles inside the transmission waveguide

98. The purpose of the MDCB Scope of Practice is to define the scope of practice of medical dosimetrists in order to:
A. I, II, and III only
B. I and III only
C. II and IV only
D. IV only

E. All are correct
I. Delineate areas of technical service.
II. Educate professionals in the fields of health care, education, and other communities of interest regarding the expectations of medical dosimetrists.
III. Assist medical dosimetrists in their efforts to provide appropriate and high-quality services to those in need of radiation therapy.
IV. Establish a reference for curriculum review of educational programs in medical dosimetry.

99. To treat hepatocellular carcinoma (hcc), to which part of the body is the Y-90 microsphere solution injected with the image guidance of angiography?
A. Femoral artery
B. Hepatic artery
C. Splenic artery
D. Pulmonary vein

100. Patient's positioning and device used depend on:
A. I, II, and III
B. I and III only
C. II and IV only
D. IV only
E. All are correct
I. Patient's medical condition
II. CT scanner bore dimension
III. Location of the disease
IV. Patient's preference

101. Calculate the effected path length used to plan a patient's treatment who has 5 cm of tissue from the skin to the center of the leg where a titanium metal replaces the bone measuring 3 cm, and then from the bone to the back of the femur, there is a separation of 7 cm tissue. Total thickness is 15 cm.
A. 9 cm tissue
B. 15 cm tissue
C. 16.5 cm tissue
D. 20 cm tissue

102. The dose on a fixed SSD technique is usually normalized at:
A. The surface of the patient
B. The isocenter
C. At Dmax
D. The tissue surrounding the target

103. Which of the following devices is/are used for immobilization of head and neck radiation treatment?
A. I, II, and III
B. I and III only
C. II and IV only

D. IV only
E. All are correct
I. Aquaplast mask
II. Shoulder straps
III. Head rest
IV. Bite block

104. Which of the following is the unit of absorbed radiation dose?
A. Becquerel (Bq)
B. Curie (Ci)
C. Gray (Gy)
D. Roentgen (R)

105. Calculate the brain couch angle needed to match a PA spine divergence on a craniospinal treatment where the upper spine field is 30×5 cm, the lower spine field is 18×15 cm at 100 SSD, and the RT/LT lateral brain fields are 18×20 cm at 93 SSD and the separation of the patient head is 14 cm.
A. 5.14°
B. 4.57°
C. 5.48°
D. 0.15°

106. Which of the following are components of Calypso® 4D systems?
A. I, II, III, and IV
B. II, III, and IV
C. I, III, and IV
D. All of them
I. 4D electromagnetic array
II. Implanted electromagnetic transponders
III. 4D console inside treatment room
IV. 4D tracking system
V. Infrared cameras and optic targets

107. The electron scattering power varies
A. I, II, and III
B. I and III only
C. II and IV only
D. IV only
E. All are correct
I. Inversely as the electron mass
II. Approximately as the square of the atomic number (Z^2)
III. Approximately as the square of the kinetic energy
IV. Inversely as the square of the kinetic energy

108. The angle of the sloping isodose curve on a dynamic wedge is determined by:
A. The speed with which the gantry moves
B. The dose rate

14.3 Practice Test III: Questions 833

C. The speed with which the collimator leaf moves
D. The amount of monitor units delivered

109. Stationed wave (SW) accelerator has a shorter accelerating waveguide than traveling wave (TW) accelerator. This is because:
A. In SW accelerator, coupling cavities are put aside the waveguide.
B. SW is more energetic in accelerating electrons.
C. TW accelerator has higher energy; thus, it takes longer to accelerate electrons.
D. SW has higher amplitude in accelerating voltage.

110. Which of the following factors should be considered when irradiating a pregnant woman?
A. I, II, and III
B. I and III only
C. II and IV only
D. IV only
E. All are correct
I. Fetal doses below 100 mGy should not be considered a reason for terminating a pregnancy.
II. Any therapeutic procedure for pregnant women be planned to deliver the minimum dose to any embryo or fetus.
III. Radiotherapeutic procedures causing exposure of the abdomen or pelvis of women who are pregnant or likely to be pregnant be avoided unless there are strong clinical indications.
IV. The magnitude and type of fetal damage is a function of dose and stage of pregnancy.

111. BAT stands for:
A. Brain acquisition and targeting system
B. B-mode acquisition and targeting system
Z Best algorithm treatment system
D. B-section alteration tolerance

112. The Xsight Spine algorithm used in CyberKnife:
A. Uses external markers (tattoos) for preliminary alignment
B. Uses implanted fiducials
C. Uses LED markers attached to a vest on the patient to track the spine
D. Uses features of the patient's vertebrae to track the target

113. Tongue and groove is used in MLC to
A. Reduce interleaf leakages
B. Correct for lack of divergence
C. Change the beam into a broad, clinically useful beam
D. Tilt the isodose lines through a specific angle

114. Horns are
A. I, II, and III

B. I and III only
C. II and IV only
D. IV only
E. All are correct
I. High-dose areas near the surface in the periphery of the field
II. Low-dose areas near the surface in the periphery of the field
III. Created by the flattening filter
IV. Created by the scatter in the body

115. Depending on the type of tumor being treated, which of the following targeting and tracking methods system can be used on CyberKnife treatment?
A. I, II, and III
B. I and III only
C. II and IV only
D. IV only
E. All are correct
I. 6D Skull Tracking System
II. Xsight Spine and lung Tracking System
III. Fiducial Tracking System
IV. In Tempo Adaptive Imaging System

116. The process by which an atomic nucleus of unstable atom become more stable by emitting particles and/or electromagnetic radiation is called
A. Half-life
B. Transmutation
C. Radioactive decay
D. Electron equilibrium

117. Electron beam obliquity tends to:
A. I, II, and III
B. I and III only
C. II and IV only
D. IV only
E. All are correct
I. Increase side scatter at Dmax
II. Decrease the depth of penetration
III. Shift Dmax toward the surface
IV. Shift Dmax away from the surface

118. For safety precautions, which of the following items is/are not allowed in the MRI room?
A. I, II, and III only
B. I and III only
C. II and IV only
D. IV only
E. All are correct

14.3 Practice Test III: Questions

I. Jewelry
II Patient with pacemakers
III Pregnant women
IV Metal prosthesis

119. The SI unit of the reference air-kerma rate is
A. Gy/s
B. cGy/h.
C. Curie (Ci)
D. Becquerel (Bq)

120. The anterior rectal wall and the sigmoid colon dose can be minimized by
A. I, II, and III only
B. I and III only
C. II and IV only
D. IV only
I. Using a rectal retractor
II. Using packing
III. Using a tandem with appropriate degree of angulation
IV. Minimizing the treatment time

121. Use the following table to calculate the total dose received at midplain on the RT femur, ignoring off-axis ratio, if the separation is 8 cm and the treatment involves also RT hip with a central axis separation of 16 cm and the dose delivered is 300 cGy for 10 treatments.
A. 2,695 cGy
B. 333.9 cGy
C. 3,340 cGy
D. 3,433 cGy

Table. 14.5. Test 3

Depth	1.5 cm	4 cm	6 cm	8 cm	16 cm
PDD	100 %	91 %	83.9 %	75.7 %	61.5 %
TMR	1.000	0.963	0.919	0.865	0.756

122. Increasing the kVp will:
A. I, II, and III only
B. I and III only
C. II and IV only
D. IV only
E. All are correct
I. Increase the intensity of an x-ray beam.
II. Decrease image noise.
III. Increase Compton effect interaction.
IV. Contrast will remain the same.

123. Delivery of IMRT treatments can be accomplished via:
A. I, II, and III
B. I and III only
C. II and IV only
D. IV only
E. All are correct
I. Segmented MLC mode (SMLC)
II. Dynamic MLC mode (DMLC)
III. Intensity-modulated arc therapy (IMAT)
IV. Synchronized MLC mode (SYMLC)

124. Which of the following planning system is used in CyberKnife?
A. AAA calculation
B. Pencil beam calculation
C. Monte Carlo calculation
D. Acuros

125. LET stands for
A. Linear energy transfer
B. Lateral equivalent tumor
C. Linear electron therapy
D. Linear excitation tissue

126. A physician wants a treatment done using 30 mCi-min of ^{125}I, but the documents must be filled out in mg-Ra eq-hr. How many mg-Ra eq-hr. should be documented?
A. 318.54 mg-Ra eq-min
B. 10,171 mg-Ra eq-hr.
C. 5.309 mg-Ra eq-hr.
D. 318.54 mg-Ra eq-hr.

127. What is the difference between 3D-CRT hyperfractionation strategy and IMRT hyperfractionation strategy?
A. Both are efforts to minimize normal tissue complications, and IMRT does a better job.
B. Both are efforts to enhance better treatment outcomes, and IMRT does a better job.
C. IMRT does a better job in both minimizing normal tissue complications and treatment outcomes.
D. Both are efforts to enhance treatment outcomes and to minimize normal tissue complications, and IMRT does a better job in both of them.

128. Calculate the MU required to deliver 250 cGy to the 90 % IDL if the RT breast electron cutout has an output of 1.07 cGy/MU.
A. 260 MU
B. 234 MU
C. 241 MU
D. 268 MU

14.3 Practice Test III: Questions 837

129. Calculate the dose to point P from sources A, B, and C using the following table and description.
A. 7.83 cGy/h.
B. 60.30 cGy/h.
C. 18.75 cGy/h.
D. 17.30 cGy/h.

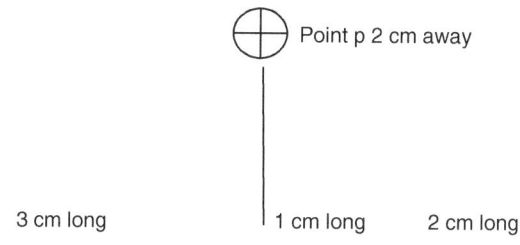

3 cm long   1 cm long   2 cm long

| Source A: 15 mg | Source B: 10 mg | SourceC: 5 mg |

Table 14.6. Test 3

Away	Distance along source, cm					
Cm	0	1.0	1.5	2.0	2.5	3
1.0	6.69	4.11	2.48	1.54	0.99	0.68
2.0	1.89	1.56	1.25	0.97	0.74	0.57
3.0	0.86	0.77	0.70	0.60	0.51	0.42
4.0	0.49	0.46	0.43	0.39	0.35	0.31
5.0	0.31	0.30	0.29	0.27	0.25	0.22

130. Which of the following parameters affect(s) the isodose distribution?
A. I, II, and III
B. I and III only
C. II and IV only
D. IV only
E. All are correct
I. Beam energy
II. Source size, SSD, and SDD
III. Collimation
IV. Field size

131. What are somatic effects?
A. Harm that exposed individuals suffer during their lifetime.
B. Radiation-induced mutations to an individual's genes and DNA that can contribute to the birth of defective descendants.
C. The probability of occurrence increases with increasing dose, but the severity in affected individuals does not depend on the dose.

D. Increases in severity with increasing dose, usually above a threshold dose, in affected individuals.

132. The 90 % depth dose of a 16 MeV occurs at
A. 2 cm
B. 4 cm
C. 5 cm
D. 8 cm

133. What comes out right after IMRT optimization?
A. IMRT fluence for each field
B. IMRT dose-volume histogram
C. IMRT MLC motion file
D. MU numbers

134. What will be the total dose required to kill 90 % of tumor population if the dose (D_o) given to the tumor is 5 Gy?
A. 11.5 Gy
B. 3.46 Gy
C. 115 Gy
D. 34.65 Gy

135. Calculate the percentage change in dose rate if the distance is increased from 100 to 120 cm.
A. 0.8333
B. 1.4444
C. 0.6944
D. 1.2222

136. If OSL dosimeter is used to monitor individual exposure, how frequent should it be replaced normally?
A. 2 weeks
B. 1 month
C. 2 months
D. 3 months

137. A wedge angle refers to:
A. The angle between the central axes of the two beams (hinge angle)
B. The angle of the isodose tilt at Dmax
C. The angle through which an isodose curve is tilted at the central axis of the beam at a specified depth
D. The physical degree angle of the wedge (15, 30, 45, or 60)

138. Which of the following radioisotopes is used on selective internal radiation therapy (SIRT)?
A. Iridium-192 (Ir-192)
B. Yttrium-90 (Y-90)

C. Iodine-125 (I-125)
D. Phosphorus-32 (P-32)

139. Which of the following is/are true about ^{137}Cs and ^{137m}Ba?
A. I, II, and III only
B. I and III only
C. III and IV only
D. IV only
E. All are correct
I. They belong to the same element.
II. They possess the same mass number.
III. They are considered isotopes.
IV. They possess the same atomic number.

140. Secondary barrier is said to be:
A. I, II, and III
B. I and III only
C. II and IV only
D. IV only
E. All are correct
I. A barrier sufficient to attenuate the useful beam to the required degree
II. A barrier sufficient to attenuate leakage and scatter radiation
III. A barrier capable to attenuate neutron radiation
IV. A barrier sufficient to attenuate stray radiation

141. After how long will Ir-192 decay to 99.5 % of its original activity?
A. 5.37 days
B. 0.537 days
C. 53.7 h
D. 1 day

142. Which of the following is/are considered liver-directed treatments?
A. I, II, and III
B. I and III only
C. II and IV only
D. IV only
E. All are correct
I. Conformal radiation therapy
II. Hepatic arterial infusion chemotherapy (HAC)
III. Transarterial chemoembolization (TACE)
IV. Radioembolization (RE) using yttrium-90

143. Geometric field size is defined as:
A. The intersection of the 50 % isodose line and the surface
B. The intersection of the collimator axis and the axis of rotation
C. The region between the surface and maximum dose or Dmax
D. Region near the edge of the field margin, where the dose falls rapidly

144. Calculate the new TMR if a patient is treated to the LT hip using 6 MV, 12 × 12 field size for 250 cGy to midplain, SSD of 92.5, 98 % IDL, separation of 15 cm, and TMR of 0.685, but the SSD is changed to 110 cm.
A. 0.685
B. 0.814
C. 0.484
D. 0.772

145. Calibration of survey meters must be done at intervals not exceeding
A. Every 6 months
B. One year
C. Two years
D. Five years

146. Which of the following is/are considered portable radiation survey instruments?
A. I, II, and III only
B. I and III only
C. II and IV only
D. IV only
E. All are correct
I. Pocket dosimeter
II. Cutie Pie
III. Film badge
IV. Geiger-Muller counter

147. What is the goal of IMRT optimization?
A. Find the local minimum of the cost function.
B. Find the global minimum of the cost function.
C. Find the local maximum of the cost function.
D. Find the global maximum of the cost function.

148. How many kinds of neutrino exist in nature?
A. 6
B. 3
C. 1
D. 2

149. Beneficence means:
A. The ethical principle of doing no harm to a patient by a medical professional.
B. Patients who has a condition of being independent, freedom, or self-government.
C. Health-care professionals must act in the best interest of a patient, even at some inconvenience and sacrifice to themselves. The state of quality of being kind, charitable, or beneficial.
D. The principle of fairness and equity is maintained for all individuals.

14.3 Practice Test III: Questions

150. Which of the following is true about IMRT treatment planning?
A. I, II, and III
B. I and III only
C. II and IV only
D. IV only
E. All are correct
I. Each beam is divided into large number of beamlets.
II. The treatment planning determines the fields' fluencies.
III. The treatment planning determines the fields' weight.
IV. The treatment planning is based on inverse planning.

151. After 10 HVL, the intensity of the beam is reduced by
A. $I = I_0(0.1)^n$
B. $I = I_0(0.5)^n$
C. $I^n = I_0(0.5)^n$
D. $I = I_0(10)^n$

152. Calculate the effective half-life of a radionuclide if the physical half-life is 7 h. and the biological half-life is 14 h..
A. 15 h.
B. 3.26 h.
C. 16 h.
D. 4.66 h.

153. Which of the following IGRT systems enables visualization of the exact tumor location by integrating a CT imaging system with a linac and involves acquiring multiple planar images?
A. BAT
B. Brainlab
C. Paired orthogonal planar imagers
D. CBCT

154. What is the Hounsfield number of water?
A. −1,000
B. 60
C. 40
D. 0

155. The mass defect is defined as
A. A defect in the number of protons in the nucleus
B. Every gram atomic weight of a substance that contains the same number of atoms
C. The difference in mass between an atom and the sum of the masses of its constituent particles
D. The propagation of energy through space or a material medium

14.4 Practice Test IA: Answers

1. A

2. A

3. B

4. B

5. A

6. C The symbol A represents the mass number, which is equal to the # of protons plus neutrons.

7. B

8. B

9. A

10. C

11. C

12. C Acceptance test is done when new device is delivered or installed, which contains only a portion of commissioning procedures.

13. A The target must have high atomic number and high melting point (3,3700 °C).

14. C

15. D Half-value layer (HVL) evaluates the thickness of an absorber required to attenuate the intensity of the beam to half its original value.

16. A

17. A

18. B

19. B

20. D

21. A Scattering foil is moved by a carrousel in front of the electron beam when the linear accelerator is in the electron mode. The flattening filter and x-ray target are moved away. The ion chamber always stays in the beam path.

14.4 Practice Test IA: Answers

22. B

23. D

24. C

25. D

26. A   The unit for kerma is the same as for dose, j/kg, SI unit is Gy, and its special unit is rad.

27. A

28. C   Picture archiving and communication systems

29. B

30. C

31. C

32. C $ESF = 2\,(L \times W)/L + W$ or $ESF = 4 \times A/P$

33. A

34. A

35. A

36. D $10^1 = \text{deka} = 10 = \text{ten}$

37. D   15 %

38. B   120 rad = 1.2 Gy

39. C

40. B

41. B   Maximum practical range of an electron is energy (MeV)/2 or around 2 MeV/cm.

42. C

43. D

44. B

45. D

46. B

47. C

48. C Hinge angle is the angle between the central rays of the two beams.

Fig. 14.11 Test 3

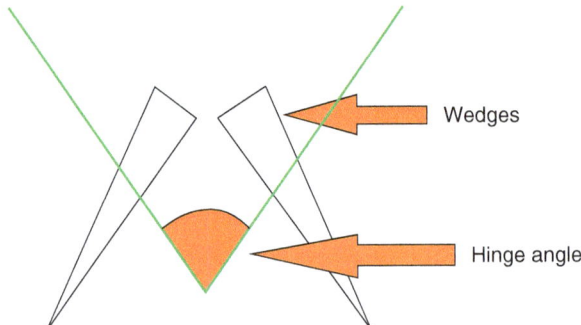

49. A

50. A

51. B

52. B

53. D

54. D

55. C

56. D

57. C

58. A

59. B

60. B

61. C

62. A

14.4 Practice Test IA: Answers

Fig. 14.12 Test 1A

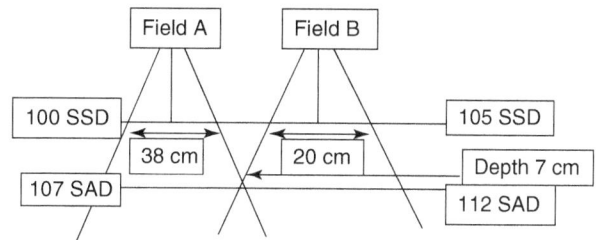

63. B

64. C

65. C

66. B

67. A   MU = (Dose/FX)/(output factor (SAD) × TMR at iso)

68. B

69. C

Fig. 14.13 Test 1A

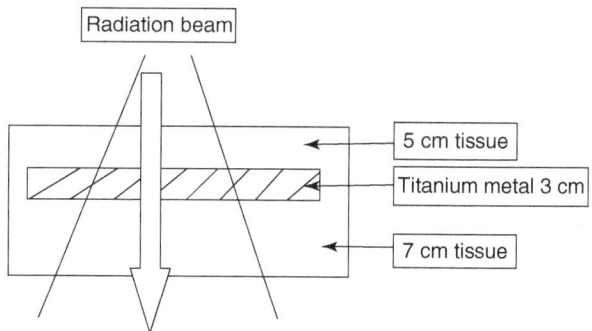

70. A

71. B

72. C   The rule of thumb states that electrons treat to a depth in cm of energy (MeV)/3 to energy (MeV)/4 approximately.

73. E

74. D

75. A

76. A

77. B

78. E

79. B

80. A

81. B

82. C

83. B

84. A

85. D

86. C   As a rule of thumb, the electron energy in MeV should be three times the maximum depth of a given tumor; that is, for a 4 cm treatment depth, a 12 MeV electron beam should be used.

87. C

88. E

89. C

90. A

91. B

92. A

93. D

94. B

95. C

96. B

97. E

98. B

99. C

100. C   The magnetron is a device that produces microwaves, and the klystron is not a generator of microwave but rather a microwave amplifier.

101. A

102. A

103. C

104. C

105. D

106. A

107. C

108. B

109. A

110. A

111. C

112. D

113. A

114. C

115. A

116. D

117. C

118. E

119. D

120. B

121. B   Lung dose is the major concern, due to the blood flow.

122. D

123. **B**

124. **A**

125. **A**

126. **C**   The nucleus of an atom is composed of protons and neutrons; these protons and neutrons are termed nucleons.

127. **A**

128. **C**   Parotid

Fig. 14.14   Test 1A

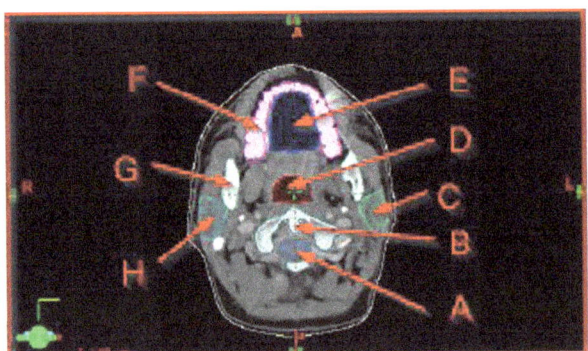

129. **B**

130. **D**   Trachea

Fig. 14.15   Test 1A

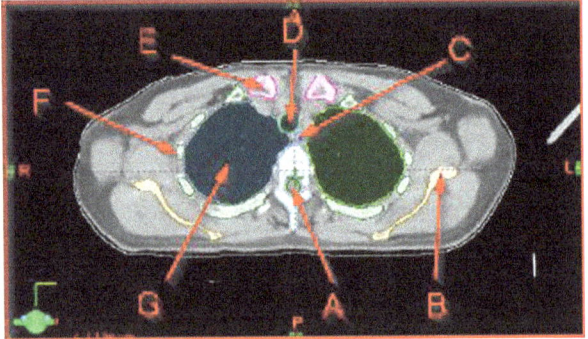

131. **B**

132. **D**

14.4 Practice Test IA: Answers

133. A

134. F   Aorta

Fig. 14.16 Test 1A

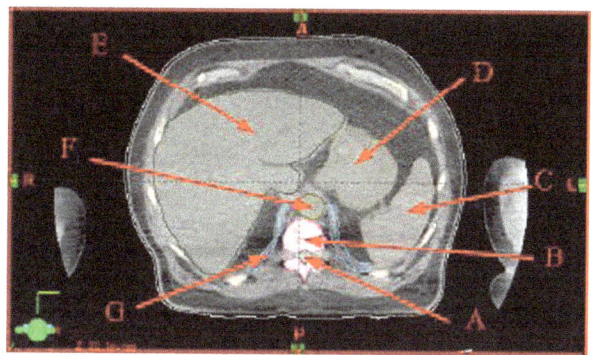

135. B

136. B

137. A   Exposure rate constant Γ (Rcm2/mCi-h) of 226Ra is 8.25.

138. B

139. B

140. C

141. B

142. B   Of the two forms of DVH, the cumulative DVH has been found to be more useful and more commonly used than the differential one.

143. E

144. B   AAPM TG-43 is the essential report for brachytherapy dose calculations.

Radiation Protection

145. C   ALARA is a philosophy of maintaining personnel radiation exposure as low as reasonably achievable.

146. B

147. A

148. D

149. C

150. A

151. B

152. A

153. C   One bit is equal to a binary digit of two possible values, 0 or 1, which all computer data is stored.

154. C

155. C

14.5 Practice Test IIA: Answers

1. A

2. C $C_{tp} = (760/p)(273 + t/295)$

3. B

4. C

5. C   The most stable atoms are the ones that have even # of protons and even # of neutrons with 165 isotopes.

6. D

7. B

8. A

9. E

10. A

14.5 Practice Test IIA: Answers

11. A

12. B

13. B If Compton photon makes a direct hit with the electron, the electron will travel forward 0° receiving maximum energy, and the scattered photon will travel backward 180° left with minimum energy.

14. B

15. D

16. C

17. A

18. C

19. B

20. D

21. C

22. D

23. C The 90 % depth dose takes place at about 1/3 of the electron energy (MeV).

24. C

25. B

26. A

27. C

28. C

29. A

30. E

31. B

32. B

33. **D**

34. **C**

35. **C**

36. **A**

37. **C** $c = \nu\lambda$ is the formula that establishes the relationship between wavelength (λ), frequency (ν), and velocity (c).

38. **B**

39. **B**

40. **D**

41. **C**   The rule of thumb states that the therapeutic range or 90 % IDL of an electron is energy (MeV)/4.

42. **A**

43. **C**   The rule of thumb states that the 50 % IDL of an electron is energy (MeV)/2.33.

44. **B**   One kilobyte equals 1,024 bytes.

45. **C** $C_{T,P} = (760/P)(273.2 + T/273.2 + 22)$

46. **A**

47. **B**

48. **B**   Linear attenuation coefficient $\mu = 0.693/\text{HVL}$

49. **A**

50. **B**

51. **C**   Hinge angle = $180° - (2 \times \text{wedge angle})$

52. **C**

53. **B**

54. **A**   Mayneord factor formula must be used to find PDD.

$$F = \left[(SSD_2 + D\max/SSD_1 + D\max) \times (SSD_1 + d/SSD_2 + d)\right]^2$$

New PDD = Old PDD × 0.986

14.5 Practice Test IIA: Answers

55. D Fractional contribution from AP field:

$$AP = AP / AP + PA$$

Fractional contribution from PA field:

$$PA = PA / AP + PA$$

56. A The appropriate device to check a spill area is the Geiger-Müller counters (G-M)

57. C

58. A

59. C Fractional contribution from PA field:

$$PA = PA / PA + RT + LT$$

Fractional contribution from RT field:

$$RT = RT / PA + RT + LT$$

Fractional contribution from LT field:

$$LT = LT / PA + RT + LT$$

60. B

61. A

62. A

63. E

64. B

65. B

66. B

67. C Total dose at Dmax = entrance dose at Dmax + exit dose at Dmax
Entrance dose at Dmax = dose from one field × (TMR at Dmax/TMR at 10 cm) × (distance 2/distance 1)2
Exit dose = dose from one field × (TMR at 18 cm/TMR at 10 cm) × (distance 2/distance 1)2

68. B WF = measurement with wedge/measurement without wedge

69. B

70. B As a rule of thumb, MeV/2 or half of the energy should be the lead cutout thickness in mm to stop the energy in question.

71. **C**

72. **E**

73. **B**

74. **E**

75. **C** Wedge angle = 900−(0.5×hinge angle)

76. **B**

77. **B** AAPM TG-43 is the essential report for brachytherapy dose calculations.

78. **C**

79. **B** Formula $h\nu = E_k - E_L$, where E_k and E_L are the electron-binding energies of the K and L shell.

80. **B**

81. **A**

82. **C**

83. **A**

84. **C**

85. **B**

86. **B**

87. **B**

88. **C**

89. **C** 3TVLs is the rule of thumb for vault shielding.

90. **C** The practical range (Rp) must be found first = 9 MeV/2 = 4.5 cm.

The most probable energy at the lead-lower lip interface (2 cm depth) is found by using the following formula:

$$E_z = E_0\left(1 - z/R_p\right)$$

14.5 Practice Test IIA: Answers

91. B
92. D
93. A
94. B
95. B
96. A
97. C
98. B
99. B
100. A
101. B
102. B
103. E
104. E
105. D   MU = dose per beam/output × BSF × TMR
106. D
107. A
108. A
109. A
110. E
111. A   The F factor is the Roentgen-to-rad conversion factor.
112. C
113. B
114. C

115. D I-131 with a lifetime of 8 days is ideal to treat thyroid cancer.

116. C

117. B

118. D

119. A

120. A

121. B

122. A

123. A $I_1/I_2=(SSD_2/SSD_1)^2$

124. A CyberKnife treatment robotic couch has six degrees of freedom (anterior/posterior, superior/inferior, left/right, roll, pitch, and yaw).

125. E

126. A

127. D

128. A

129. A $SSD=SAD-d$

130. D

131. B There is no evidence that IMRT is better in local control of disease than 3D-CRT.

132. B

133. C Cumulative implant dose formula: $D_c=D_{total}(1-e^{-t/tavg})$

134. A

135. A In 1978, the International Commission on Radiation Units and Measurements (ICRU) Report No.50 and 62 (24, 25)

136. B $OD=\log(I_0/I_t)$, where I_0 is the amount of light collected without film and it is the amount of light transmitted through the film.

14.5 Practice Test IIA: Answers

137. A

138. C

139. A

140. B

141. A

142. D MU = (dose/FX)/(output cGy/MU at SAD) × TMR × TF

143. B

144. B

145. B

146. A

147. C

148. B

149. D

150. A

151. B

152. D

153. D MU = dose/TMR

154. A Esophagus

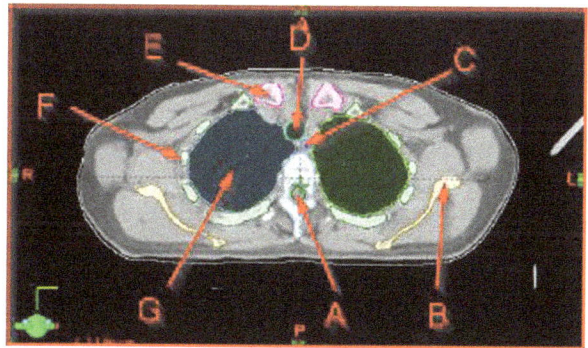

Fig. 14.17 Test 2A

155. B Prostate

Fig. 14.18 Test 2A

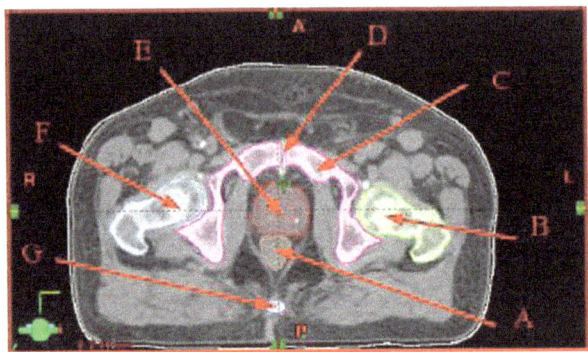

14.6 Practice Test IIIA: Answers

1. **D** Physical wedge is usually made of lead, which produces scatter on the contralateral breast.

2. **A**

3. **B** Number of atoms/g = N_A/A_w

4. **A**

5. **B**

6. **D**

7. **B**

8. **B** An atom is defined as the smallest component of an element having the chemical properties of the element.

9. **A**

10. **E**

11. **A**

12. **A**

13. **C**

14.6 Practice Test IIIA: Answers

14. B Electron capture decay is produced due to a radionuclide deficit of neutrons, low neutron-to-proton (n/p) ratio.

15. C Hounsfield numbers range from −1,000 for air to +1,000 for bone.

16. C

17. B

18. A

19. C

20. E

21. C Type B package is for ^{60}Co shipment. There is no Type C package.

22. A

23. C

24. D

25. C Klystron is a microwave amplifier. It bunches the electrons and hence generates high-amplitude voltage pulses.

26. B

27. C

28. D Thyratron is a fast on/off HV switch; thus, it is filled with gas working as insulator. 1 atm = 760 mmHg = 760 Torr.

29. E

30. B

31. A

32. E

33. B

34. E

35. A TMR is a special case of TPR where the reference depth is chosen to be at Dmax.

36. **A**

37. **A**

38. **B** Clarkson's method is used to calculate irregular fields. Circular, rectangular, and square fields are not considered irregular fields.

39. **B** SAD = SSD + depth

40. **B**

41. **D**

42. **A**

43. **A**

44. **B**

45. **B**

46. **A**

47. **D**

48. **B**

49. **B**

50. **B**

51. **C**

52. **C**

53. **B**

54. **A**

55. **C** $C_{T,P} = (760/P)(273.2 + T/273.2 + 22)$

56. **A** MU = field without wedge MU/wedge factor

57. **C**

14.6 Practice Test IIIA: Answers

58. E

59. C

60. B

61. C

62. D The benchmark test indicates the accuracy of the dose calculation algorithm under very specific circumstances with specific beam data.

63. B

64. B

65. C

66. A

67. A

68. B

69. C

70. A

71. A

72. B

73. A

74. E

75. B

76. B

77. B Rule of thumb: the energy loss rate of electrons per cm in water is roughly about 2 MeV/cm of water.

78. B One kilobyte equals 1,024 bytes.

79. A

80. B Half-value layer is related to the linear attenuation coefficient (μ) by the equation HVL = .693/μ.

81. B The tail of the electron depth dose curve at the point where it becomes straight is due to Bremsstrahlung interactions of electrons with the collimator system.

82. A

83. B

84. C

85. C

86. D

87. A

88. B

89. B

90. C

91. C The 12 collimator diameters are 0.5, 7.5, 10, 12.5, 15, 20, 25, 30, 35, 40, 50, and 60 mm.

92. B

93. C

94. C CyberKnife SAD is 800 mm or 80 cm; linac accelerator used to be 80 cm and most of them are now 100 cm SAD.

95. B

96. C

97. B

98. E

99. A

14.6 Practice Test IIIA: Answers   863

100. A

101. C

102. C

103. E

104. C Absorbed dose is energy absorbed from all ionizing radiations per unit mass of materials; its SI unit is gray (Gy), and the old unit is rad.

105. A

106. D

107. C

108. C

109. A

110. E

111. B BAT stands for B-mode acquisition and targeting system.

112. D

113. A

114. B

115. A

116. C

117. A

118. E

119. A The SI unit of the reference air kerma rate is the Gy/s; curie (Ci) is the unit of activity; and becquerel (Bq) is the SI units of apparent activity.

120. A

121. **C**

122. **B**

123. **A**

124. **C**

125. **A**

126. **D** # mg-Ra eq. radionuclide = Γ radionuclide/Γ ^{226}Ra × activity.

127. **A**

128. **A** MU = dose/fx/output (PDD/100).

129. **B** Dose to point $P = 60.30$ cGy/h.

130. **E**

131. **A**

132. **C** The 90 % depth dose takes place at about 1/3 of the electron energy (MeV).

133. **A**

134. **C** $D_{10} = \log_{10} \times D_0$. The total dose for 10 decades is $11.5 \times 10 = 115$ Gy.

135. **C**

136. **C** As usual, an OSL dosimeter should be replaced every 2 months; whereas a film badge dosimeter should be replaced monthly.

137. **C**

138. **B**

139. **A**

140. **C**

141. **B**

142. **E**

14.6 Practice Test IIIA: Answers

143. A

144. A

145. B

146. C

147. B

148. A

149. C

150. E

151. B

152. D

153. D

154. D — Hounsfield unit is an arbitrary unit of x-ray attenuation used for CT scan. Each voxel is assigned a value on a scale in which air has a value of −100; water, 0; and compact bone, +100.

155. C

References

1. Bentel GC (1996) Radiation therapy planning, 2nd edn. McGraw-Hill Professional, New York, 0-07-005115-1
2. Bushberg JT, Anthony Siebert J, Leidholdt EM, Boone JM (2002) The essential physics of medical imaging, 2nd edn. Lippincott Williams & Wilkins, Philadelphia, 0-683-30118-7
3. Clifford Chao KS, Perez CA, Brady LW (1999, 2002) Radiation oncology: management decisions, 2nd edn. Lippincott Williams & Wilkins, Philadelphia, 0-78173222-0
4. Hall EJ, Giaccia AJ (2006) Radiobiology for the radiologist, 6th edn. Lippincott Williams & Wilkins, Philadelphia, 0-7817-4151-3
5. Khan FM (2003) The physics of radiation therapy, 3rd edn. Lippincott Williams & Wilkins, Philadelphia, 0-7817-3065-1
6. Stanton R, Stinson D (1996) Applied physics for radiation oncology. Medical Physics Publishing, Madison, WI, 0-944838-60-X (softcover), 0-944838-61-8 (hardcover)

CPSIA information can be obtained
at www.ICGtesting.com
Printed in the USA
LVHW080812100520
655298LV00001B/1